MANAGEMENT OF TRAUMA:
Pitfalls and Practice

MANAGEMENT OF TRAUMA:
Pitfalls and Practice

ALEXANDER J. WALT

ROBERT F. WILSON
Wayne State University
Detroit, Michigan

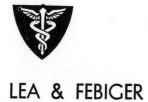

LEA & FEBIGER · *Philadelphia 1975*

Library of Congress Cataloging in Publication Data

Walt, Alexander J.
    The management of trauma.

    1. Medical emergencies. 2. Wounds—Treatment. I. Wilson, Robert Francis, 1934—
joint author. II. Title. [DNLM: 1. Wounds and injuries—Therapy. W0700 W23lm]
RC87.W25   1975   617.1   74-22475
ISBN 0-8121-0318-1

Published in Great Britain by Henry Kimpton Publishers, London

PRINTED IN THE UNITED STATES OF AMERICA

To *all the generations of Wayne State University interns and residents who have served in "the pits" at Detroit General (Receiving) Hospital with so much private commitment and so little public recognition.*

PREFACE

TRAUMA is a ubiquitous problem which recognizes no boundaries drawn by custom or specialty boards. Experience in a busy emergency room is therefore vital to the education of every physician even if only to develop the ability to make important decisions rapidly and rationally. These initial decisions often dramatically determine the ultimate outcome. Death, deformity and medicolegal entanglements may flow from vacillation or error. When decisions are approached with confidence, logic and technical skill, the associated mortality rate, preventable complications, permanent disability and economic loss may be strikingly reduced.

The need to improve our management of trauma has gained national acceptance in recent years. Many hospitals in the United States treat as many victims each week as does a busy military hospital in a combat zone. Basic principles exist which are vital to optimal recovery. Uncertainty, inactivity, and inappropriate investigation by the physician are all detrimental to the patient. Recurrent pitfalls tend to be ignored or forgotten and need to have mental "flags" placed around them. Certain hallowed traditional concepts need to be abandoned and new approaches learned. These are our justifications for adding yet another new

book to the burgeoning literature on trauma.

At Detroit General (Receiving) Hospital, our residents and staff have treated approximately 100,000 to 120,000 patients in the emergency room annually for many years. Many of these patients are victims of injuries. During the past decade, with improved ambulance service and resuscitation measures, patients have been brought to emergency departments with severe injuries which would previously have caused early death. The number of destructive lesions caused by firearms has increased alarmingly, demanding that we learn to translate the appropriate observations made by military surgeons.

The emergency department is the living laboratory where the sophisticated physiologic concepts of the research laboratories are applied. It is essential that physicians working in emergency departments are thoroughly conversant both with the application of basic clinical principles and with the new technical equipment which provides support of the various organ systems during the initial critical period. Despite deep interest and extensive experience in this broad field of patient care, we are constantly faced with decisions to which we have only tentative and often disputed approaches. Even more disturbing, when we analyze these decisions later, it is apparent that frequently there is a need to amend our thinking. The premise that each patient who dies represents something of a defeat or failure is chastening, but it also constantly forces a redefinition of clinical approach.

No detailed review of all traumatic conditions is possible in a single volume. It has been our purpose to present a broad approach to the management of patients who have suffered major trauma, to draw attention to some prevailing errors and, above all, to define for ourselves where we stand today on common problems, especially those which are incompletely solved. We have deliberately omitted extensive historical references in the interest of brevity. As compensation, however, selected references for additional reading have been appended to most chapters.

All of our contributors are members of the faculty of Wayne State University, and all would agree that we have learned as much from our residents as we have taught them. At the same time, both groups, together with countless nursing, administrative and other personnel, have had the personal and professional satisfaction of providing service to almost 1,500,000 patients in the emergency department over the past decade. In an era when universities are frequently chastised for inadequate involvement with their communities, this book bears testimony to the long association between Wayne State University and the citizens of Detroit.

While there are a great many people who merit special thanks for their patience, encouragement and plain hard work in the preparation of this manuscript, we would particularly like to express our appreciation to Mrs. Karen Lloyd, Mr. Dennis Gibson and Miss Grace Marks.

ALEXANDER J. WALT, M.D.

ROBERT F. WILSON, M.D.

Detroit, Michigan

CONTRIBUTORS

Agustin Arbulu, M.D.

Professor of Surgery
Wayne State University
School of Medicine

Graeme C. Baker, M.D.

Resident in Plastic Surgery
Yale University School of Medicine
Formerly Assistant Professor of Surgery
Wayne State University
School of Medicine

G. Jan Beekhuis, M.D.

Professor of Otolaryngology
Wayne State University
School of Medicine

Phillip M. Binns, M.D.

Associate Professor and Acting Chairman
Department of Otolaryngology
Wayne State University
School of Medicine

Lucy M. Brand, R.N., M.S.

Associate Professor
Wayne State University
School of Nursing

Oscar Brown, M.D.

Clinical Professor of Ophthalmology
Wayne State University
School of Medicine

Ralph Cushing, M.D.

Assistant Professor of Internal Medicine
Wayne State University
School of Medicine

Tommy N. Evans, M.D.

Professor and Chairman
Department of Obstetrics and Gynecology
Wayne State University
School of Medicine

Stefan H. Fromm, M.D.

Clinical Assistant Professor of Surgery
University of Puerto Rico
Formerly Assistant Professor of Surgery
Wayne State University
School of Medicine

Elisha S. Gurdjian, M.D.

Professor Emeritus of Neurosurgery
Wayne State University
School of Medicine

David M. Hirsch, Jr., M.D. (deceased)

Surgeon, Springfield, Massachusetts
Formerly Assistant Professor of Surgery
Wayne State University
School of Medicine

Kamil Imamoglu, M.D., Ph.D.

Associate Professor of Surgery
Wayne State University
School of Medicine

H. John Jacob, M.D.

Resident in Otolaryngology
Wayne State University
School of Medicine

John R. Kirkpatrick, M.D.

Assistant Professor of Surgery
Wayne State University
School of Medicine

Ronald L. Krome, M.D.

Associate Professor of Surgery
Wayne State University
School of Medicine

Raymond S. Kurtzman, M.D.

Professor of Radiology
Wayne State University
School of Medicine

Robert D. Larsen, M.D.

Clinical Associate Professor of Surgery
Wayne State University
School of Medicine

L. Phillip LeBlanc, M.D.

Surgeon, Guelph, Ontario
Formerly Associate Professor of Surgery
Wayne State University
School of Medicine

James R. Lloyd, M.D.

Clinical Assistant Professor of Surgery
Wayne State University
School of Medicine

Charles E. Lucas, M.D.

Associate Professor of Surgery
Wayne State University
School of Medicine

Eberhard F. Mammen, M.D.

Professor of Physiology and Professor of Pathology
Wayne State University
School of Medicine

James McKenna, M.D.

Clinical Assistant Professor of Surgery
Wayne State University
School of Medicine

Frank Monaco, D.D.S.

Clinical Professor of Oral Surgery
University of Detroit
School of Dentistry

Martin L. Norton, M.D.

Associate Professor of Anesthesiology
Boston University School of Medicine
Formerly Associate Professor of Anesthesiology
and Associate Professor of Law
Wayne State University

James M. Pierce, M.D.

Professor and Chairman
Department of Urology
Wayne State University
School of Medicine

John C. D. Plant, M.D.

Assistant Professor of Surgery
Wayne State University
School of Medicine

Irwin K. Rosenberg, M.D.

Professor of Surgery
Wayne State University
School of Medicine

Jerry C. Rosenberg, M.D.

Professor of Surgery
Wayne State University
School of Medicine

James R. Ryan, M.D.

Assistant Professor of Orthopedic Surgery
Wayne State University
School of Medicine

Suryanarayanan Sankaran, M.D.

Assistant Professor of Surgery
Wayne State University
School of Medicine

Vishwanath M. Sardesai, Ph.D.

Associate Professor of Surgery and Associate
    Professor of Biochemistry
Wayne State University
School of Medicine

Irwin J. Schatz, M.D.

Professor of Internal Medicine
University of Michigan School of Medicine
Formerly Professor of Internal Medicine
Wayne State University
School of Medicine

Yvan J. Silva, M.D.

Associate Professor of Surgery
Wayne State University
School of Medicine

Zwi Steiger, M.D.

Associate Professor of Surgery
Wayne State University
School of Medicine

John Y. Teshima, M.D.

Associate Professor of Obstetrics and Gynecology
Wayne State University
School of Medicine

L. Murray Thomas, M.D.

Professor and Chairman
Department of Neurosurgery
Wayne State University
School of Medicine

Norman W. Thoms, M.D.

Associate Professor of Surgery
Wayne State University
School of Medicine

Alexander J. Walt, M.D.

Grover Penberthy Professor and Chairman
Department of Surgery
Wayne State University
School of Medicine

Arthur W. Weaver, M.D.

Associate Professor of Surgery
Wayne State University
School of Medicine

Jacqueline A. Wilson, R.N., M.S.

Formerly Nursing Director
Critical Care Units
Harper Hospital
Detroit, Michigan

Robert F. Wilson, M.D.

Professor of Surgery
Wayne State University
School of Medicine

Paul Zamick, M.D.

Assistant Professor of Surgery
Wayne State University
School of Medicine

James Yao, M.D., Ph.D.

Associate Professor of Surgery
Northwestern University
School of Medicine
Formerly Assistant Professor of Surgery
Wayne State University
School of Medicine

CONTENTS

Part 5   COMPLICATIONS OF TRAUMA

Part 6   MEDICOLEGAL IMPLICATIONS OF TRAUMA

Part 1

PREPARATION AND PLANNING FOR EMERGENCIES AND TRAUMA

1 THE ORGANIZATION OF THE MODERN EMERGENCY DEPARTMENT

R. L. KROME
R. F. WILSON
A. J. WALT

"Once upon a time when emergency rooms first 'happened,' it was accepted that they should be poorly lit and overcrowded, serving primarily as catchment areas for patients who are poor."

A. J. WALT AND R. L. KROME[6]

Physicians have a vested interest in ensuring that emergency services are efficiently organized, and are being increasingly drawn into the field of planning for emergency health care. The deplorable quality of emergency services has attracted governmental scrutiny and public clamor in recent years. While much of this criticism has been directed at the poor state of department facilities, organization and staffing, there has recently been increased recognition of the need to improve ambulance services[1] and to define the type and level of training to be given to those who first see and transport the injured.[2] At the same time, critical surveys of the functioning of emergency departments (E.D.)[3] are being undertaken with a view to the establishment of minimal standards of care and subsequent quality control.

One of the first of these surveys was taken in 1970 under the auspices of the Greater Detroit Area Hospital Council. The 35 hospitals with emergency facilities in the Detroit metropolitan area were evaluated by means of questionnaires and on-site inspection teams. Although the care provided was generally quite good, many deficiencies came to light. Only 74% of the emergency departments were fully equipped with resuscitation equipment; 6% did not have endotracheal tubes, 17% did not have a defibrillator, and 23% did not have an electrocardiograph. Medical and nurse staffing patterns in the E.D. varied widely; however, 14% did not have 24-hour physician coverage and 31% did not have 24-hour coverage by registered nurses. The availability of "back-up" medical staff in the hospital is one measure of the hospital's ability rapidly to expand its medical services. It was found that 24-hour in-house physician coverage was available for internal medicine in 51% of hospitals, for general surgery in 43%, for obstetrics in 43%, and for orthopedics in 11%. Operating-room teams were present around the clock in only 31%, and anesthetists were present at all times in only 40%.

Many communities are at last adopting a broader, more ecumenical view of their emergency needs and are pooling their resources and applying a systems approach to these problems.[4] Recently, much of this concern has crystallized in the formation of the University Association for Emergency Medical Services and the American College of Emergency Physicians.

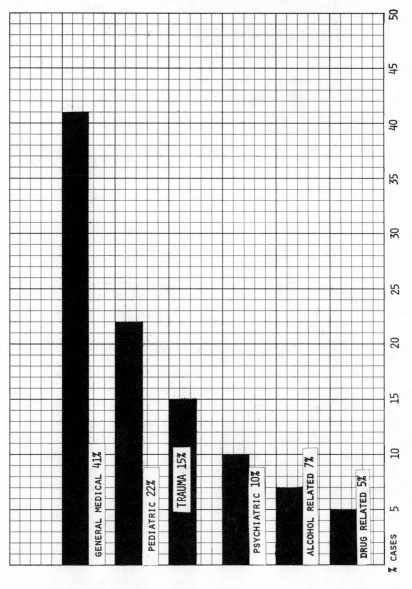

FIG. 1. 15% of our cases are trauma related. The greatest percentage are nontrauma, general medical (41%) and pediatric (22%).

While trauma has certain unique aspects, it can be managed with consistent efficiency only when the emergency department is organized to take care of all varieties of illness expeditiously, using an orderly pre-determined system. For such a system to operate smoothly, appropriate physical facilities and a department director are necessary. These essentials have often been neglected in the past. This chapter directs itself to these requirements and is based on experience at the Detroit General (Receiving) Hospital where over 120,000 emergencies, of which approximately 15% are traumatic in origin, are treated annually (Fig. 1).

THE ORGANIZATION OF
THE EMERGENCY DEPARTMENT

The modern E.D. is the nerve center of today's hospital and has become its most socially and politically sensitive area. The obsolete concept of the "emergency room," where limited and often dilatory care was given by junior members of the house staff, is rapidly being replaced because of intense public and governmental pressure. Accreditation inspections to ensure quality control and regionalization of emergency facilities have begun in some parts of the United States[3,5] and will undoubtedly spread rapidly. The change in public attitude makes it mandatory that E.D.s be given the same attention and degree of organization as the ambulatory clinics and inpatient sections of the hospital complex.

The main operating suite, blood bank, and x-ray department should all be within easy reach of the emergency department. When elevators must be used to reach any of these, special keys should be available so that the elevators can be rapidly

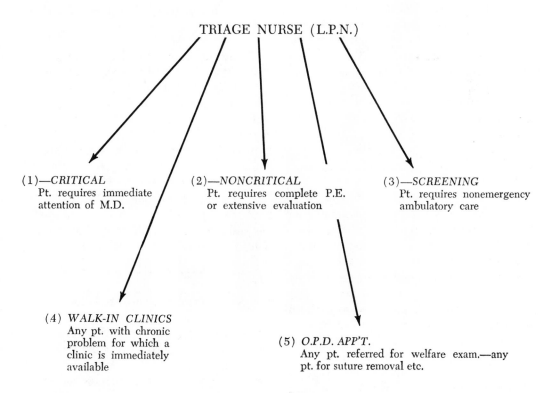

FIG. 2. DGH Triage System.

obtained and controlled during an emergency. The intensive-care unit, coronary-care unit, and burn unit should also be readily accessible to the E.D.

The E.D. should be planned and set up to provide for: good medical care, orderly flow patterns, security for patients and personnel, immediate availability of charts, and an environment in which high staff morale can be maintained. It should have a well-lighted, clearly marked, secure ambulance entrance separated from the general hospital entrance and easily accessible from major roads in the area.

Triage

All patients, whether ambulatory or on stretchers, should enter the emergency department past one central checkpoint for both administrative and medical reasons. At Detroit General Hospital, the triage station is the hub from which all patient care emanates (Fig. 2). Patients in critical condition are directed immediately to the appropriate treatment areas; the less seriously ill or injured are first seen by the triage physician. This initial triage, by either an experienced physician or a nurse, can greatly increase the efficiency of the E.D. and help to establish priorities of treatment.

PITFALL
IF TRIAGE IS NOT PERFORMED ON VIRTUALLY ALL PATIENTS SOON AFTER ARRIVAL IN THE E.D., THE CRITICALLY ILL MAY HAVE TO WAIT WHILE OTHERS WHO ARRIVED EARLIER WITH LESS SERIOUS PROBLEMS ARE TREATED.

If a physician is always used to perform the initial triage, the operation can become increasingly costly financially and from the standpoint of physician utilization. In times of disaster, however, the function of triage officer is so important that it may be wise to use the best and most experienced personnel while these special conditions exist.

Treatment Areas

The requirements of individual E.D.s will vary with the demands placed on them, but may be divided into the following broad areas for patient care and related facilities:

1. a major trauma section, situated close to the ambulance entrance, for injured patients requiring immediate resuscitation;
2. a minor trauma section for injuries not requiring resuscitation, such as lacerations, closed fractures, etc.;
3. a nontrauma section for medical, neurologic, gynecologic, etc. problems;
4. a pediatric section;
5. a psychiatric section;
6. an observation ward for patients requiring short-term care or observation;
7. clinical laboratories;
8. x-ray facilities;
9. a cast room;
10. an operating room which has major capabilities but is usually used only for minor surgery such as insertion of chest tubes.

Treatment rooms should be flexible. This means that fixed partitions and fixed wall units of any sort should be kept to a minimum. The more "fixed" the equipment and walls, the less possible it is for the emergency department to adjust its operations to meet the varied demands of a disaster.

Psychiatric-care Units and Quiet Areas

The needs of emotionally disturbed patients are very often ignored. Special facilities and personnel should be available at all times to deal with them. With drug prob-

---

PITFALL
IF NO SPECIAL PROVISION IS MADE TO SEQUESTER PSYCHIATRICALLY DISTURBED PATIENTS, THE NOISE AND COMMOTION UNAVOIDABLY ASSOCIATED WITH THEM GREATLY DISTURBS THE E.D. PERSONNEL AND THE OTHER PATIENTS AND THEIR FAMILIES, INTERFERING WITH MEDICAL CARE, LOWERING MORALE, AND BRINGING CRITICISM ON THE HOSPITAL.

---

lems increasing and numerous psychiatric problems being brought to emergency departments, a quiet psychiatric-care unit should be available.

Separating excessively loud patients allows other patients who are acutely ill to be treated effectively in a peaceful, organized environment by a less stressed staff.

Observation Ward

The availability of a separate observation ward within the emergency department may greatly expedite the handling of patients. Such a ward, where patients with conditions such as acute alcoholism or mild head injury may be kept for up to 12 hours, will avoid many unnecessary admissions to the hospital.

PITFALL

IF THE OBSERVATION WARD IS ABUSED, IT RAPIDLY BECOMES A NO-MAN's-LAND WHERE PATIENTS LINGER AND WHERE INDECISION AMONG PHYSICIANS IS ENCOURAGED WHILE THE NURSING STAFF BECOMES INCREASINGLY EXASPERATED.

Office Space

Traditionally the E.D. has been grossly understaffed and cramped for space with little or no provision for physicians' offices in the areas where they work. Ample space should also be available for teaching of house staff, students, nurses and paramedical personnel, and for the privacy of those being interviewed.

Visitors' Room

A comfortable, large, cheerful visitors' room should be constructed adjacent to the E.D. but isolated and far enough away to discourage excessive and unapproved visiting. Not uncommonly there are more problems, and time spent, with friends and relatives than with the patient himself. Social workers, volunteers, and security officers can help relay information to visitors and relieve their anxieties.

Medical Records

PITFALL

IF THERE IS NO READY ACCESS TO THE PATIENT's HOSPITAL RECORD, ESPECIALLY IF NO HISTORY IS AVAILABLE FROM THE PATIENT, FAMILY, OR FRIENDS, TREATMENT MAY BE INAPPROPRIATE OR DANGEROUSLY DELAYED.

A system whereby the patient's chart is immediately available and follows him wherever he goes in the hospital is essential. Computerization of records is highly desirable, and systems to achieve this are being devised. The quality of the entries in the chart often reflect the quality of the medical care delivered. Regular audit of randomly selected charts from the E.D. helps to maintain quality control and to reduce medicolegal liabilities. In addition to the immediate improvement in patient care which good records provide, an efficient record system assists greatly with the implementation of accurate billing.

Security

Security personnel must be available in sufficient numbers to control visitors and safeguard the privacy of the patients. Under certain conditions, they may also have the responsibility of ensuring the safety of the personnel in the E.D.

Relationship to the Outpatient Department

PITFALL

IF, BY DEFAULT, AN INSTITUTION FORCES THE E.D. TO DOUBLE AS AN AMBULATORY CLINIC, BOTH THE E.D. AND AMBULATORY CLINIC SUFFER BADLY.

Paradoxically, the magnet of an improved E.D. draws increased numbers of patients from the surrounding community and, without the safety valve of an efficient triage system and ambulatory clinic, the deserving E.D. undeservedly ensures its own failure. The national experience shows that 65% of patients entering the emergency department between the hours of 8:00 a.m. and 6:00 p.m. could be evaluated and treated in an outpatient facility.[6] The relationship between the outpatient department and the emergency department must, therefore, be a close one. Modification of the treatment or administrative policies of either the E.D. or the ambulatory clinic often influences the function of the other. Nonemergency patients should have a "walk-in" clinic available to them separate from the E.D., so that the E.D. is not forced to function as a substitute ambulatory clinic. Where this dual role for the E.D. is thought to be unavoidable at night or on weekends, clear arrangements with the ambulatory clinic for the subsequent receipt of patients and their records are important.

THE PERSONNEL OF THE EMERGENCY DEPARTMENT

Director of the Emergency Department

PITFALL

IF INSTITUTIONS DO NOT APPOINT AND SUPPORT AN E.D. DIRECTOR WHO HAS BOTH PROFESSIONAL AND MANAGERIAL INTERESTS, THEY WILL BE UNLIKELY TO PROVIDE THE ENVIRONMENT NECESSARY FOR IMPLEMENTING MODERN CONCEPTS OF BROAD-BASED EDUCATION AND PATIENT CARE.

Ideally, the director must be a physician "for all seasons." Charged with the responsibility for the entire department, he must also be given commensurate authority. This authority includes (1) a seat on the executive committee of the hospital, (2) the right to discipline anyone employed in the E.D. who fails to meet predetermined standards, (3) the invitation to build his own annual budget for presentation to the hospital administration, (4) the opportunity to determine priorities when fiscal support is not completely adequate, (5) participation in the recruitment and the control of those assigned to the E.D. from various services of the hospital, such as the clinical departments, social service, housekeeping, nursing, and administration, (6) disposition of patients to the ambulatory clinic, into the hospital or back to their homes, (7) the chance to recruit his own medical staff for consideration for appointment to the hospital by the executive committee. At Detroit General Hospital, the E.D. director is department chief and is responsible to the executive committee and the administration of the hospital. He works through existing supervisory staff but is responsible for developing and implementing departmental policy (Fig. 3).

As the E.D. is the most sensitive interface between the hospital and the community, the director should identify and interpret the needs of each to the other. These needs will vary with the location of the institution. In the urban environment, problems of acute alcoholism, psychiatric breakdown, and chronic geriatric care may predominate; in both cities and suburbs, problems of drug abuse, trauma, and mass casualties are always relevant. In any community planning to ameliorate these and to devise practical systems whereby such patients enter the health-care system, the E.D. director is probably best placed to be the hospital representative and is in a sense a public-relations officer.

In a delineation of his role in more detail, the E.D. director has been examined as physician, manager, leader, educator, and synthesizer. In view of the delicate relationships of the E.D. to the clinical departments, the ambulatory clinics, the hospital administration and the departments of nursing, social work, and pharmacy, the director must have a broad understanding of the entire operation of the hospital and the personal sensitivities of its patients and personnel.

The discipline in which the director has received his professional training is less important than his ability to gain the profes-

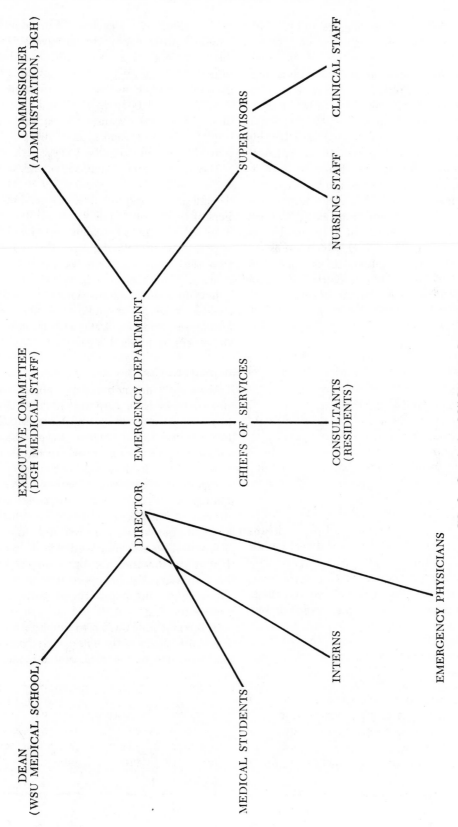

FIG. 3. Organization, DGH Emergency Department

sional respect of his colleagues and his willingness to adopt an ecumenical view of the many services working in the E.D. In some institutions, a surgeon may be best suited to this task, in others an internist, and, in still others, an individual interested in community or family medicine. In academic institutions, the director will receive his academic appointment from the department of his discipline, and he should be encouraged to continue to see and to treat patients in his professional field in order to preserve his own skills.[6] At the same time, he must give appropriate attention to the vital managerial aspects of the E.D. which are essential to the rejuvenation, reformation and solvency of this often embattled and usually neglected sector of the hospital.

Medical Staff

The medical staff should consist of mature well-trained physicians whose sole responsibility while on duty is to care for patients in the E.D.

These physicians must be capable of determining quickly the extent of a patient's injury or illness with a minimum of laboratory and radiographic study. Staffing of the emergency department with incompletely trained, uninterested or unenthusiastic physicians is now recognized to be totally inconsistent with good medical care. The physician's ability to detect subtle changes in the patient's general appearance and vital signs and to institute appropriate treatment rapidly may well be the major determinant of the patient's eventual outcome.

PITFALL

IF THE MEDICAL AND NURSING STAFF IN THE E.D. IS NOT ADJUSTED ACCORDING TO THE PEAK LOADS IN THE E.D., INEFFICIENT UTILIZATION OF PERSONNEL WILL OCCUR WITH THE STAFF BEING RELATIVELY INACTIVE PART OF THE TIME AND OVERWORKED AT OTHER TIMES.

Staffing patterns developed from data on patient load at various hours have allowed more efficient utilization of physicians and nurses. For example, in many hospitals the greatest number of patients are seen on the 3:00 to 11:00 p.m. shift and yet, out of tradition and because it is easier to recruit for daytime hours, the 7:00 to 3:00 p.m. shift usually has the largest staff.

Day-to-day supervision and chart auditing must be closely overseen by the E.D. director and well-trained, experienced members of the hospital staff. It is vital, furthermore, that E.D. physicians be given the opportunity to follow-up on the patients they see, especially those admitted to the hospital. The special training which emergency physicians should be given so they can recognize acute medical problems and initiate appropriate treatment is now in the process of being defined.

Nursing Personnel

Vigorous and enthusiastic nurses who specialize in E.D. care should be trained to function as a part of the team. Modern E.D. nurses should not only be capable of performing all the usual nursing duties but should also be trained to insert intravenous catheters and endotracheal tubes and to begin cardiac massage and other resuscitative measures. If a physician is not immediately available, nurses may be required to exercise initiative and independence of action. If they are to perform in this manner, however, they need the support of their supervisory staff and relevant and current in-service training.

A nursing staff unable to function at this level in treating acute emergencies reduces the efficiency of the E.D. and the quality

---

PITFALL

IF THESE SPECIALLY TRAINED E.D. NURSES ARE NOT ASSIGNED FULL TIME TO THE E.D., THEIR MORALE MAY DETERIORATE AND THEIR SKILLS MAY DIMINISH RAPIDLY BECAUSE OF LACK OF PRACTICE.

---

of care available to its patients. Current nursing policies and training need to be redefined in the light of these expanding concepts for the health-care team.

Not uncommonly nurses choose to work full time in the E.D. because they enjoy the rapid pace and challenge. If they are pulled out to cover nursing shortages in other parts of the hospital, they may become depressed and less effective.

Paramedical Personnel

PITFALL

IF ATTENDANTS ARE NOT AVAILABLE TO MOVE PATIENTS RAPIDLY, THE DELAYS IN OBTAINING TESTS AND ADMITTING PATIENTS RESULT IN OVERCROWDING AND REDUCED EFFICIENCY OF ALL PERSONNEL.

The ability of physicians to function in an efficient manner has become increasingly dependent on the enthusiasm, industry, and ability of the paramedical staff. This is especially true in the E.D. where a number of procedures are ideally done concurrently for severely injured and desperately ill patients.

The role of the emergency medical technician is expanding rapidly. Many technical functions—taking electrocardiograms, drawing blood, splinting fractures, starting I.V.s, passing nasogastric tubes, and inserting urinary catheters—can all be done by specially-trained technicians. Even though the nurses may not be required to do these tasks, they should be capable of performing and supervising them.

Other paramedical personnel who wish to specialize in E.D. care should be encouraged to develop their capabilities to the fullest and should be provided adequate compensation and a realistic and inviting career structure.

Social Workers

Frequently overlooked but vitally necessary to any large E.D. are the social work-

ers. Their functions are to aid in: (1) locating family and friends, (2) obtaining medical history from family and friends, and (3) making arrangements for post-hospital care and follow-up, including placement in nursing homes for continued convalescent care. The expeditious movement of patients who have been treated out of the E.D. by the social workers improves its overall function dramatically; the acutely ill and injured may be seen more rapidly in a less crowded environment. This in turn will help diminish the accusations of excessive delay in giving care to individual patients. Finally, and often most important of all, appropriate attention can be directed to the nonmedical needs of the patient. In the case of the poor and the aged, the social worker may be the patient's only friend.

SUMMARY

A detailed examination of the place and requirements of a modern E.D. and its director and other personnel has been attempted. Rhetoric alone, however, is not

TABLE 1. MOST FREQUENT ERRORS

Failure to provide an adequate department organizational structure with responsibility and authority vested in a director.

Failure to provide an adequate system of triage to ensure the treatment of the critically injured first.

Failure to provide an adequate area for sequestration of the psychiatrically ill.

Failure to adequately control the use of an observation ward so that patients do not linger in the emergency department for prolonged periods.

Failure to ensure access to the patient's previous medical records.

Failure to segregate the nonemergency patient from the critically ill and injured.

Failure to adjust the staffing schedule to the patient load.

Failure to provide a corps of specially trained physicians, nurses, and emergency medical technicians.

Failure to provide adequate numbers of paramedical staff to do technical tasks.

---

enough. If the injured patient is to obtain rapid and intelligent treatment, a fundamental reorientation of current conceptual thinking and organizational structure in the emergency department is vital. Table 1 lists the most frequent causes of failure to achieve this goal.

REFERENCES

1. *Accidental Death and Disability: The Neglected Disease of Modern Society.* Washington, National Academy of Sciences–National Research Council, 1966.
2. Farington, S. D., and Hampton, O. P.: A curriculum for training emergency medical technicians. Bull. Amer. Coll. Surg., 5:273, 1969.
3. Youmans, R. S., and Brose, R. A.: A basis for classifying hospital emergency services. JAMA, 213:147, 1970.
4. Gibson, G.: *Emergency Medical Services in the Chicago Area.* Chicago, Center for Health Administration Studies, Univ. of Chicago, 1970.
5. Skudder, P., McCorroll, J., and Wade, P. A.: Hospital emergency facilities and services, A survey. Bull. Amer. Coll. Surg., 46:40, 1961.
6. Walt, A. J., and Krome, R. L.: Of wicked stepmothers, ugly sisters and academic Cinderellas. J. Trauma, 11:554, 1971.
7. Krome, R. L., Schron, S. R., and Wilson, R. F.: Survey preludes regional planning. Hospitals, 47:135, 1973.
8. Krome, R. L., Schron, S. R., and Wilson, R. F.: A study of emergency medical services in the Detroit metropolitan area. J. Amer. Coll. Emer. Physicians, 2:177, 1973.

Suggested Reading

1. *Emergency Department: A Handbook for the Medical Staff.* Chicago, American Medical Association, 1966.
2. *Recommendations of the Conference on the Guide Lines for the Categorization of Hospital Emergency Capabilities.* Chicago, American Medical Association, 1971.
3. *Emergency Department Management Guide.* East Lansing, American College of Emergency Physicians, 1971.
4. *Guidelines for Organization of a University Emergency Department.* East Lansing, University Association for Emergency Medical Services, in press.
5. Poticha, S. M.: The role of the emergency room in the education of medical students (editorial). J. Trauma, 11:1091, 1971.
6. Wiegenstein, J. G.: The need for training physicians in emergency medicine. J. Trauma, 13:375, 1972.
7. Boyd, D. R., et al.: The Illinois plan for a statewide system of trauma centers. J. Trauma, 13:24, 1973.
8. Hampton, O.: Unresolved questions about fulltime physicians in hospital emergency departments (editorial). J. Trauma, 13:1027, 1973.

2 DISASTER PLANNING: A MODERN REALITY

A. J. WALT
R. F. WILSON

Every hospital must have a disaster plan which has been developed and tested long before any calamity strikes. Since disasters may have different origins and vary in degree, all plans must be versatile, flexible, and, above all, easily understood. The system adopted must be realistic in terms of the hospital's capabilities, with careful consideration of its location, personnel, and equipment. The place of the hospital within the regional plan for the community must be clearly defined; competition with other institutions for patients is to be discouraged.

Conventional disaster plans have traditionally been geared to meet the emergency of a sudden explosion, storm or transportation accident with a sudden influx of a large number of patients. These plans assume the presence of a uniformly cooperative and sympathetic citizenry, the immediate mobilization of all community resources, and relatively free-flowing transportation. More recently, additional plans for nuclear disasters have been made in close cooperation with civil-defense authorities; these plans assume widespread destruction of large areas with drastically limited communications, forcing surviving hospitals to be virtually self-supporting.

Although these plans were given much thought and seemed adequate for handling most disasters, the major civil disturbances in many of our large cities during the past few years have caused a number of unexpected problems. Casualties may arrive over a period of many days and nights in staccato manner (Table 1). Hazardous roads and an uncooperative or even hostile citizenry may force casualties to await police or military authorities for safe escort. Essential hospital personnel may find it impossible to get to work, and others already at the hospital may have similar difficulty in returning home for a number of days. Patients with minor injuries must be rapidly treated and discharged, but this may not be easy to accomplish if the hospital is situated close to the area of violence. The hospital may be forced to admit large numbers of prisoners and innocent victims simultaneously and must provide for the security of both groups. Although there is a strong tendency to focus attention only on the disaster and its victims, provisions must also be made for continued care of in-hospital patients and new patients not involved in the disaster (Table 2).

To provide optimal care for patients during a disaster, a number of steps should be taken: (1) long before the disaster, (2) immediately on being notified of an impending or actual disaster, and (3) during the influx of patients into the hospital.

TABLE 1.   TIME DISTRIBUTION OF PATIENTS
(12:01 a.m. July 23, through 11:59 p.m. July 28, 1967)*

	Gunshot wounds	Lacerations or stab wounds	Other	Total trauma	Total non-trauma	Total patients
Sunday						
a.m.	2	14	34	50	65	115
p.m.	3	46	23	72	104	176
Monday						
a.m.	21	58	34	113	28	141
p.m.	32	64	30	126	40	166
Tuesday						
a.m.	35	21	18	74	40	114
p.m.	4	33	17	54	57	111
Wednesday						
a.m.	3	10	13	26	50	76
p.m.	8	21	23	52	107	159
Thursday						
a.m.	5	7	19	31	46	77
p.m.	3	17	27	47	64	111
Friday						
a.m.	0	7	6	13	65	78
p.m.	5	34	31	70	81	151
TOTALS	121	332	275	728	747	1,475

* From Walt, A. J., et al.[1] Used with permission.

TABLE 2.   EMERGENCY ROOM (E.R.) PATIENTS
(12:01 a.m. July 23, through 11:59 p.m. July 28, 1967)*

	Admitted to hospital bed	Discharged from E.R. after treatment	Dead on or soon after arrival in E.R.	Total
Gunshot wounds	58	38	25	121
Lacerations or stab wounds	25	305	2	332
Other trauma	32	240	3	275
TOTAL TRAUMA	115	583	30	728
Nontrauma	129	602	16	727
TOTAL PATIENTS	244	1,185	46	1,475

* From Walt, A. J., et al.[1] Used with permission.

PREPARATIONS BEFORE THE DISASTER

Preparations which should be made by all hospitals long before a disaster occurs include: (1) development and testing of a disaster plan, (2) development of clear communication arrangements, and (3) storage of special supplies.

Development and Testing of a Disaster Plan

All hospitals must have a disaster committee, composed of the heads of all hospital departments, which shall develop a "written plan for the proper and timely care of casualties arising from external disasters, and shall periodically rehearse this plan."[2] Its plan for emergency casualty care should reflect the hospital's capabilities to: (1) provide simple first aid, (2) prepare casualties for transfer elsewhere, or (3) administer definitive care.

This plan must be developed in conjunction with other emergency medical facilities in the community and with local civil authorities to establish an effective chain of command, make appropriate jurisdictional provisions, obtain efficient disaster-site triage and distribution of patients, and identify the hospital's resources to the community, local police, rescue squads and ambulance teams.

The vital need for police and other civil and military authorities in the hospital has been neglected in the past. Future planning committees, charged with the task of designing comprehensive disaster plans, should have high-level representation from the police and fire departments of their cities.[1]

PITFALL

IF A DISASTER PLAN IS NOT CHECKED PERIODICALLY TO BE SURE THAT DESIGNATED SUPPLIES HAVE NOT BEEN USED FOR OTHER PURPOSES AND THAT PERSONNEL ASSIGNED TO SPECIFIC RESPONSIBILITIES HAVE NOT LEFT OR BEEN TRANSFERRED TO OTHER DEPARTMENTS, CONFUSION MAY SUPERVENE WHEN THE HOSPITAL IS PUT TO A GENUINE TEST.

Realistic disaster-plan drills should be conducted at least twice a year, preferably as part of a coordinated drill with other community emergency service agencies. The drills must involve the medical staff and administrative, nursing and other hospital employees. All personnel should be provided with identification cards which also indicate, as a reminder, the assigned station for the individual during a disaster. A checklist for the disaster plans and drills is invaluable, but only if it is actually periodically checked (Table 3).

TABLE 3. CHECKLIST FOR A HOSPITAL CIVIL DISTURBANCE PREPAREDNESS PROGRAM*

GENERAL CONSIDERATIONS

1. Have you updated your disaster plan to include civil disturbances?
2. Have you made arrangements for additional emergency power to use in the event of power failure at the hospital?
3. Are you prepared for the possibility that persons in the riot area may seek refuge in the hospital? Experience of hospitals during riots has been that, particularly if there are widespread fires, persons living in the area are likely to look upon a hospital as a refuge even though they are uninjured. If a hospital believes it is able to accommodate only a limited number of such persons, contact should be made with other nearby institutions the facilities of which may also be put to such use.
4. Have you alerted your employees to the fact that some patients may be militant?

OPERATING PLANS

5. Have you established an emergency operation center from which you will be in command of the situation?
6. Have you notified department heads and supervisory personnel that they should be geared for a five-day emergency?
   Inasmuch as such emergencies can last for a long time, it is important that personnel understand this possibility and be prepared for it.
7. Have you made arrangements to contact your key personnel during the emergency—by telephone if the system is operable, by alternate methods if the system is not—to report for duty?
8. Have you notified the staff that everyone may be working 12-hour shifts during the emergency period?
9. Have you made specific arrangements for patterns of responsibility and for the individuals assigned these responsibilities?

*From *Accreditation Manual for Hospitals.*[3] Reprinted with permission of the American Hospital Association.

TABLE 3. CHECKLIST FOR A HOSPITAL CIVIL DISTURBANCE PREPAREDNESS
PROGRAM *(Continued)*

10. Have you alerted your department heads and supervisory personnel to prepare for a high absentee rate during the first days of the emergency?
11. Have you informed receiving-area personnel that the number of patients coming in is likely to increase as darkness approaches?
12. Have you alerted staff to the fact that routine visits to the emergency room will all but stop?
13. Have you made arrangements to house, feed, and care for the families of employees, within the hospital or its environs, if this becomes necessary in order to maintain adequate staffing by key personnel?
14. Have you made arrangements to feed the police and the military as well as any special security forces on duty in the institution?

Patient Care and Hospital Services

15. Do personnel in the receiving area understand that policemen, firemen, and military patients must be kept separate from patients who participate in the riots?
16. Have you made arrangements for the continuity of regular hospital services?
17. Have you made arrangements to increase your bed capacity?
18. Have you established a plan to discharge patients who can be sent home and to evacuate the hospital should it become necessary?
19. Have you made arrangements to cancel all elective surgery until further notice?

Supplies

20. Have you contacted your local blood source in order to arrange adequate deliveries?
21. Have you contacted the American National Red Cross regarding the availability of cots and blankets?
22. Have you contacted the military establishments in your area concerning the availability of supplies and personnel?
23. Has the purchasing department stockpiled supplies that are used in the treatment of gunshot wounds, lacerations, fractures, and burns?
24. Have you made arrangements to increase the supply of linen available?
25. Have you made arrangements to use disposable products—dishes and utensils—in the dietary department?

Transportation

26. Have you established, in conjunction with the police department, emergency routes that will be used to transport employees, patients, physicians, and supplies to the hospital?
27. Have pick-up points been established for employees so that employees will have protection and transportation to the hospital?
28. Have you made arrangements with the police department for police personnel to drive the transportation vehicles? If police cannot provide this service, have you arranged for alternate methods?

Visiting Regulations

29. Have you met with the local ministerial association to establish an identification system for their memberships and to set up a priority system for visitations in order to reduce the number of clergy in the hospital during the emergency?
30. Have you curtailed visiting privileges except in cases in which the condition of the patient necessitates a visit by the family?

Medical Records

31. Have you made specific plans for handling riot emergency medical records and informed personnel that such records should be as complete as possible? The record should include such information as the type of wound (the bullet should be retained in case of a gunshot wound), cause of injury, location of patient when picked up, means of transportation to the hospital, whether the patient appeared to be intoxicated or under the influence of drugs, and the medical care provided.

COMMUNICATIONS

Communication Systems

32. Do you have adequate telephone communications with, and among, the receiving area, the operating suite, and the intensive-care unit?

TABLE 3. CHECKLIST FOR A HOSPITAL CIVIL DISTURBANCE PREPAREDNESS
PROGRAM (Continued)

33. Does your paging system operate independently of the switchboard? Independent operation is essential, inasmuch as a switchboard may become jammed or inoperable during a civil disturbance.
34. Have you established supplemental means of communication between your office and critical departments, e.g. engineering, x-ray?
35. Have you made arrangements with the telephone company to install additional lines or to restrict the use of certain lines for hospital business or for employees wishing to ascertain the safety of their families?
36. Have you established two-way radio communications with the local police department, civil-defense authorities, other hospitals, and hospital associations?
37. Have you purchased walkie-talkies for key personnel and instructed them in their use in order to facilitate internal communications?

Internal Communications

38. Do you have individuals within the hospital who can keep you informed of the "mood" of employees and of persons outside the hospital?
39. Have you arranged for frequent meetings with key personnel for the purpose of quelling or confirming rumors during an emergency?

External Communications

40. Have you requested the cooperation of local radio and television stations in contacting employees during an emergency?
41. Have you named one person responsible for releasing news and given this person's name to the news media?
42. Have you determined the type of news and photographs that can be released? Have you arranged for the delayed release of information that might be detrimental to the situation?

SECURITY

43. Have you impressed on the local police the necessity of protecting your building and grounds? Some community hospitals are located in areas more vulnerable to riots and vandalism than other hospitals. If the hospital is damaged or if patient care is hindered or disrupted in any way, the hospital will be unable to carry out its responsibility to the community even if it has a most effective disaster-riot plan.
44. Have you initiated an employee identification program, which includes photo identification, to make it possible for employees to cross police lines or to be allowed through protective barriers?
45. Have you made efforts to establish a strong security force and, where possible, to have this force deputized?
46. Have you established with the local police the fact that the hospital has no responsibility for restraining prisoners who are patients?
47. Have you made arrangements to prohibit the use of pay telephones in order to eliminate outside calls by patients or by other unauthorized persons? Militant patients or publicity seekers have been known to call for help or to contact the news media from within the hospital. It may be necessary to have the telephone company disconnect telephones or for the hospital to make these telephones inoperable through "out-of-order" signs, etc.
48. Have you assigned security guards to protect supplies kept in outdoor areas—particularly the oxygen supply?
49. Have you instructed your employees to lock all doors and windows in the hospital, leaving only the receiving area as the entrance to and exit from the building? Experience has shown that militants often attempt to gain entrance to a hospital for the purposes of vandalism or revenge.
50. Have you instructed your employees to draw the blinds and drapes at dusk and to use the minimum amount of light throughout the hospital?
51. Have you instructed your staff that patients must be confined to their beds and that if a patient must get up he must be in the company of a hospital employee? Militant patients have been known to throw things from windows at persons below waiting for treatment.
52. Have you advised your staff that only *known* volunteers should be accepted for service during a riot emergency?

While every town and every disaster is slightly different, it is important to think and plan in terms of general principles. These should be based on what is in fact at hand—not what might be wished or planned for the future. Disaster plans must be constantly reviewed in light of personnel changes and the availability of back-up personnel. Any plan should take into account the total facilities in terms of physical plant, physicians, trained nurses, supporting personnel, administrative organization, supplies, foodstuffs, communications, transport, auxiliary lighting, and security. No hospital should view itself in isolation, and yet it should be able to function on its own if absolutely necessary.

It must be recognized that the disaster may occur suddenly or unfold gradually. Explosions fall into the former group, civilian disorders in the latter. Furthermore, it may not be possible to forecast how long—hours or days—the disaster, especially a civil disturbance, may last. There must, consequently, be a series of plans for each phase of the emergency and for varying degrees of severity to avoid premature and unnecessary alarm while at the same time ensuring maximal preparedness.

Communication Systems

PITFALL

IF COMMUNICATIONS AMONG ALL AREAS OF THE HOSPITAL AND AUTHORITIES OUTSIDE ARE NOT WELL ESTABLISHED AND CONTINUOUS, EFFORTS CANNOT BE COORDINATED, CONTROL IS LOST AND CHAOS ENSUES.

Proper communication systems to all areas within the hospital and to important areas outside the hospital are vital to smooth operation during any emergency. Communications with local civil authorities, police, ambulances and other hospitals must be well established. Within the hospital there must be clear communication arrangements between the emergency department and the wards and operating rooms.

The communication channels through which notification of a potential or continuing emergency will be provided must be clearly understood. Certain key personnel should have private telephones separated from the hospital switchboard so that they can make and receive calls without delay. Within the hospital, the utilization of walkie-talkies for selected individuals with predetermined areas of responsibility is invaluable.

There should be one central communications center or command post where ambulances and individual hospitals can report, where rerouting can be done, and where rumors can be confirmed or denied. From and to this command post, there must be uninterrupted radio communication. Experts in the field of communication, whether police, civilian, or civil-defense personnel, should be consulted and the appropriate equipment installed.

Supplies

PITFALL

IF THE DISASTER SUPPLIES ARE NOT CHECKED PERIODICALLY, THEY MAY BE OUTDATED, INEFFECTIVE, OR GONE WHEN A DISASTER ACTUALLY OCCURS.

A special cache of supplies for disasters should always be kept on hand, specifically marked and periodically inspected to be sure it has not been depleted for everyday use within the hospital. Special attention should be given to the adequacy of those items most likely to be inadequately stocked—chest tubes, suction apparatus, I.V. fluids, and dressings.

Basic to the efficient functioning of the hospital is the knowledge that, although 85% of those treated will be discharged home, the hospital population of personnel, patients, relatives, police, and sometimes troops may increase tremendously in times of emergency. These groups will need to be fed and sometimes accommodated, espe-

discharged immediately, while
o are not acutely ill but who still
ospitalization may be transferred
oring institutions which have not
gnated to receive casualties. The
he remaining patients should be
tely marked by a code denoting
ity of illness so that, if the need
beds becomes critical later during
gency, there is no disagreement
tion about the order of priority of
This obviates the need for harassed
s, unacquainted with the patients,
hurried decisions if the eventual
beds exceeds the anticipated de-
he cleared wards should be in a
nt area of the hospital close to the
cy room and the operating rooms
ld be designated as preoperative,
ion, and postoperative wards.[1]

on of Treatment Areas

lished hospitals must of necessity
disaster plans to the architectural
f their individual emergency rooms
rds. These plans influence the effi-
of the operation and provisions
be made accordingly. Although large
may be aesthetically displeasing,
invaluable for the rapid suturing of
umbers of patients on litters, for
l utilization of nurses and for the
n of a police guard when violent
rs are present. Many small rooms
the efforts of the professional per-
and cause delay. On the other hand,
ly injured patients are best treated
uscitation teams in single rooms
are large enough to accommodate
or stretcher and at the same time
e unrestricted mobility for medical
rsing personnel.[1]

vision should be made for defined and
ted areas where patients with spe-
najor injuries such as burns, severe
res, or chest wounds requiring ventil-
care may be concentrated. Prisoners,
isoners, and law-enforcement officials
her police, national guard, or federal

troops) should be assigned to
areas. This helps to relieve the
the nursing service and permits
tration of effort. The mixing of
assault and their alleged assailts
for many social and administrive
culties.

Security

During a civil disturbance, inter
and external security of the hital m
be maintained. The immedienviron
at least, must be well guarded the hos
pital is a focal point to which ny prisoners may be brought. In the stages
of the civil disturbance in D in 1967,
a number of people wandnto the
hospital freely with no obvpurpose.
These could have included plly dangerous individuals with the city
inflict further injury on helpsualties
and on unsuspecting hospitalnel. All
entrances should be sealed prevent
the entry of unauthorized inals and
to ensure an orderly flow of nt traffic
to and within the hospital, implies
that inpatients should be con to their
wards during the period of gency to
keep the hospital corridors and to
prevent any violence or disrup.

Special provision must be me for visitors, often angry and distraugh who cannot be allowed into the area activity.
The hospital has the responsibih of supplying immediate information to anxious
relatives of injured patients on the nature
of the injury, current status, and rognosis.
If visitors need to be taken to se a specific
patient, they should be escorted y a member of the hospital staff. Identication of
employees of the hospital should be unequivocal so that there is no infiltration
from without of individuals or groups who
may be ill motivated. (As mentioned earlier,
all hospital personnel, as part of the preplanning, should have been given identification cards with their pictures and initial
assignments.)

Prisoners present a special problem.

...ally at night, if there is a curfew or no
...ublic transport. In addition, there will be
...n extra demand for the services of the
...hospital by day if other medical care in
...the area has been disrupted.

ACTION TAKEN UPON NOTIFICATION OF A DISASTER

Some of the actions which must be taken
as soon the hospital has been notified of
a disaster include:

1. ...ification of key personnel;
2. ...egorization of the in-hospital and ... patients;
3. ...paration of treatment areas;
4. ...vision for security;
5. ...vision for decontamination;
6. ...vision for a temporary morgue;
7. ...cking of local supplies of blood, ...ma, and other fluids;
8. ...cking of food supply;
9. ...vision for visitors;
10. ...vision for the press.

Notification of Key Personnel

The ...idity with which a disaster can
occur... its size may vary tremendously.
It may difficult but it is obviously important attempt to gauge the seriousness
of the circumstances early. It is helpful to
have ... phases of alert, with the hospital
disaster chief determining the level of
emergency after consultation with the central communications officer of the area. A
phase-I alert is called if an incident has
occurred which might become a disaster
or lead civil strife; phase II constitutes
an established milieu in which many casualties may suddenly develop and where
a serious disruption of order is threatened;
in phase III the disaster or civil disturbance
has occurred and an influx of patients is
imminent.

PITFALL

ALTHOUGH IT IS IMPORTANT NOT TO DELAY
A PHASE-III ALERT, IF IT IS PREMATURELY DE-
CLARED CLINICS ARE UNNECESSARILY CLOSED,
PATIENTS ARE EVACUATED, FURTHER TENSION
IS GENERATED AND MORALE IS UNDERMINED.

Hospital ...
cerned abo...
own famili...
get home a...
of phase-I ...
compromise ...
partments a...
tential disas...
necessary p...
alarm should ...

The hospit...
cial list of ke...
mediately of ...
aster; this sh...
hospital depa...
turn can then...
the alert, not...
staff to come ...
propriate pre...
in consultatio...
ing plans and ...
the basis of f...
cerning the ex...

If the street...
escorts are sca...
ment elsewhere...
shift may have ...
hours so that ...
leave the hospi...
who live at a ...
may of necessi...
hospital for the ...
The need to pr...
sleeping accomm...
pated while con...
tively free and ...
addition, since m...
occurs at night, ...
hospital personn...
10:00 p.m. and ...
the increased nu...
can be anticipated

Categorization of In-... and E.D. Patients

Beds must be ...
injured from the s...
actual disaster, th...
pital who are we...

should be ...
others wh...
require h...
to neighb...
been des...
beds of ...
appropria...
the sever...
for more ...
the eme...
or vacilla...
transfer. ...
physician...
to make ...
need for ...
mand. T...
convenie...
emergen...
and sho...
observat...

Preparat...

Estab...
fit their ...
design ...
and wa...
ciency ...
should ...
rooms ...
they ar...
large ...
maxima...
provisi...
prisone...
diffuse...
sonnel ...
serious...
by re...
which ...
a bed...
provid...
and n...

Pro...
separa...
cific ...
fractu...
atory ...
nonpr...
(whe...

Those who are admitted into the hospital should be placed in specially designated wards for purposes of security. Others, having been treated, will be taken into custody by law-enforcement officers. In a busy emergency, however, there may be a substantial time interval between completion of the prisoner's treatment and his transfer. Again, a special area should be designated and the responsibility for the security of this group placed squarely on the police. It is important to have this segment of the patient population sequestered from the rest of the hospital to avoid disruption of normal facilities and to separate the prisoner from the nonprisoner population.

Where radioactive materials, tear gas or similar noxious chemicals have been used on patients brought to the hospital, it is important to have an area where they may be washed down before entering the emergency department. Otherwise, the patients may represent a health hazard to those around them, and the concentration of these agents may rapidly rise to the point where hospital personnel become unable to take care of their patients. The availability of a showering or douching area must be ensured before an emergency arises; sudden improvisation may be extremely difficult. (No attempt will be made to discuss the peculiar needs for decontamination in case of a nuclear disaster.)

Provision for a Temporary Morgue

A temporary morgue may be needed for patients who are either dead on arrival or die within the emergency department or the hospital. This should be situated in a cool area, properly marked and under guard. The proper and rapid disposition of the bodies requires the cooperation and preplanning of the medical examiner's office, the police, and the hospital.

Supplies of Blood, Plasma, and Other Fluids

At first word of impending disaster, the local supplies of blood, plasma and other fluids, both within the hospital and in the city, should be checked. Provision must be made for access to whatever is available and, in the case of civil disturbances, this must be done as soon as possible, before communications become difficult. Special arrangements for emergency donors should also be made.

Food

The usual sources of food supply may be closed as the emergency extends. Since the hospital may have to feed a greatly increased population of patients, their families, hospital personnel, and law-enforcement officers, and since the length of the emergency cannot be predicted, a form of rationing may well be instituted from the start.

Visitors

Provision must be made for a predictable and large influx of anxious relatives and friends of the injured. For reasons of efficiency and security, these individuals cannot be allowed to wander through the hospital in search of patients, and yet they deserve rapid replies to their inquiries. An area of the hospital should be designated for this purpose and staff, particularly chaplains and social workers, should be assigned to it. Many citizens who appear at the hospital are not certain whether the person whom they seek is in fact in the hospital; consequently it is of vital importance that meticulous records be kept so that information may be obtained accurately and without delay. Many with next of kin who are severely injured will insist on staying in the hospital for long periods of time, and arrangements may have to be made to provide them with food and toilet facilities.

News Media

At times of disaster, the news media are active and there may be considerable invasion of privacy. Television cameras may suddenly appear within the hospital, focusing on individual patients and on the general activity. Apart from the social implications, the cables and bulky apparatus will often hamper rapid medical care. It is appropriate that reporters be given full details of the general situation within the hospital, including numbers and types of injury, but it is essential that the rights of privacy of the patient be preserved. A press room should be provided and a press secretary from among the hospital staff may be assigned to the collection and distribution of information. Newsmen and television cameramen should be prohibited from roaming freely through the hospital.

ACTIONS TAKEN DURING THE INFLUX OF PATIENTS

When disaster patients begin to enter the hospital: (1) the triage site must become operational, (2) treatment teams and staff schedules must be set up, (3) treatment must be continued for nondisaster victims, and (4) communication and consultation among key personnel must continue.

Triage

The triage officer is universally recognized as filling an essential role in any disaster. In addition to broad medical knowledge, he should possess an equable temperament, sound judgment, a large commanding voice, and physical stamina.[1] While his main function is the rapid assessment of the degree of injury suffered by each casualty, he must also be responsible ultimately for traffic regulation in the triage area. A rapid flow of traffic is essential so that maximal use of strained resources is ensured; consequently only authorized vehicles and personnel can be permitted in the hospital area. Entering ambulances must be controlled so that the casualties may be unloaded at the triage point in an orderly manner. Where possible, this is best done in a well demarcated area outside the emergency room. This should be well lit, as many patients will arrive at night. If the area is exposed to potential sniper fire,

alternative positions for transporting patients directly into the emergency room must be available. In addition to teams of physicians, the triage officer requires assistance in the form of clerks and orderlies whose duty it is to attach the vital information to each entering patient and to ensure that each is taken to the appropriate area of the emergency room.

At times the work of the triage officer may be hampered by large groups of interested individuals—medical, paramedical, press, radio, and television personnel—who collect around each vehicle bringing new casualties. The curiosity and excessive enthusiasm of persons legitimately in the hospital but not assigned to the triage area must be curbed. It is probably wise, early in the disaster, to define lines beyond which only specially designated persons can proceed.

Formation of Treatment Teams

PHYSICIANS. As part of the hospital disaster plan, all physicians should have been given initial assignments to specific wards, operating rooms, clinics, and emergency areas. Constant reappraisal of the needs for patient care is ultimately under the control of the disaster chief during the period of the emergency. Temporary reassignment of personnel and alterations in departmental anatomy may be essential to the smooth functioning of the hospital team under these strenuous conditions.

At first glance, it often appears that surgical demands will be the dominant factor during an emergency, but in fact other services play at least an equal part. For one thing, commonplace illnesses such as diabetic coma, myocardial infarction, gastrointestinal and vaginal hemorrhage, seizures and strokes continue to occur; since physicians' offices will often be closed and communications disrupted, these may all be channeled to a few emergency departments in the community.

It is important, therefore, that a series of teams be arranged, each with its own function and area of responsibility. For example, in a long emergency physicians should work in shifts for maximal efficiency. If numbers permit, schedules which allow for regular hours of rest should be arranged and should be enforced as far as possible over the protests of those who, temporarily stimulated by the situation, overestimate their own physical endurance. We greatly underestimated the duration of the emergency in Detroit in 1967. This led to avoidable fatigue among key personnel and to an excessive number of relatively unoccupied assistants impeding patient traffic during the many hours of intermittent calm. Fortunately, an abundance of skilled help permitted this relatively inefficient utilization of our human resources. In other circumstances, however, this well might have been detrimental to the overall performance.

Under strain and in times of fatigue, personal prejudice may sometimes be aroused. Further, some physicians may be unable to withstand with equanimity the insults they may be forced to absorb from patients whom they are treating. In these cases, the physician should be moved to another area. He will also need to remind himself that, in times of civil disturbance, individuals cannot be prejudged. Some who are in police custody are in fact innocent, while others who appear as free citizens may in fact have been guilty of gross violence.

Another problem which may militate against optimal performance is the physician's private concern for his own family.

In the course of handling many casualties it is very easy to neglect to record accurate medical findings, especially the details of wounds, and to instruct and record the after-care to be followed, such as drugs prescribed or return visits to the clinic. Medicolegal embarrassment may follow later in these cases.

NURSES. A change to 12-hour shifts should be instituted immediately for increased efficiency. During civil disturbances, this will also allow movement in and

out of the hospital to occur in daylight. Staging areas outside the trouble spots should be designated where personnel can be met and safely delivered in the morning and evening by hospital transport, traveling in convoy if necessary. A redistribution of nurses on duty at any time may have to be undertaken, because of the likelihood that the influx of casualties will be greater at night. Provision must be made for the possibility that many nurses may be absent from work if they live in areas of disturbance or are unable to leave their homes or children. Conversely, personnel may be unable to leave the hospital at the end of their shift, in which case sleeping and washing facilities should be available. Periodic dissemination of information on the current situation to heads of nursing sections is invaluable so that they may pass information on to their personnel, thereby dispelling rumors which might otherwise rapidly erode morale.

While the principles outlined above may need modification depending on the individual's type of work, similar problems pertain to all hospital personnel including laboratory and x-ray technicians, social workers, and clerks.

Nondisaster Victims

Preoccupation with plans for surgical emergencies should not distract attention from the need to provide treatment for emergencies not connected with the riot. An adequate number of beds should be kept for gynecologic and medical admissions, as a number of such patients will require urgent treatment. Whereas virtually no cases of the more common surgical emergencies, such as appendicitis, cholecystitis, and gastroduodenal perforation, were seen during the six days of the 1967 Detroit riots, a significant number of medical patients required admission.[1] In particular, a rapid and fairly sudden influx of patients with diabetic acidosis and epilepsy was noted after the first 48 hours, presumably attributable to the inaccessibility of various drugs and to personal neglect in a time of disturbed routine.

Teamwork

It is axiomatic that intelligent teamwork at all levels is essential to the successful management of a disaster. The administrator of the hospital and the medical director of the disaster service must be in close communication throughout the period. The former is faced with the need to act as liaison officer with the news media, the police, and the military authorities, and must deploy the nursing, administrative, and paramedical staff. Fresh calls for special supplies, supplementary nurses, and ancillary personnel develop constantly, and improvisation is often required to meet the situation.

CONCLUSION

Disaster plans and disaster drills are essential features of the modern hospital. While an influx of massive numbers of casualties may occur only once in a generation, the need for clear planning remains vital. In an era of large aircraft, huge factories and restless populations, the realities of unpredicted disaster may be unpleasant to contemplate but should not obscure the recognition that many of our traditional concepts may require urgent revision.

REFERENCES

1. Walt, A. J., et al.: Anatomy of a civil disturbance. JAMA, 202:394, 1967.
2. *Accreditation Manual for Hospitals.* Hospital Accreditation Program. Chicago, Joint Commission on Accreditation of Hospitals, 1970.

Suggested Reading

1. Mustell, P.: Packaged disaster hospitals. New Eng. J. Med., 285:125, 1971.

2. Dressler, D. P., Hozid, J. L., and Giddon, D. B.: The physician and mass casualty care: A survey of Massachusetts physicians. J. Trauma, 11:260, 1971.
3. Brown, B. L., Jr.: Hospital disaster plan meets 40 hour test during racial rioting. Mod. Hosp., 115:85, 1970.
4. Rumage, W. T., Jr.: The disaster medical care committee of the council on national security of the American Medical Association. J. Trauma, 10:515, 1970.
5. Rairley, J.: Mass disaster schemes. Brit. Med. J., 4:571, 1969.
6. Bouzarth, W. F., and Mariano, J. P.: Philadelphia regional emergency medical disaster operations plan (PREMDOP). Arch. Environ. Health, 18:203, 1969.
7. Phillips, A. W.: Burn therapy: V Disaster management—To treat or not to treat? Who should receive intravenous fluids? Ann. Surg., 168:986, 1968.
8. Editorial: Disaster planning: An unexercised responsibility. New Eng. J. Med., 278:847, 1968.
9. *Model Plan Metropolitan Area Emergency Health Service.* Bulletin 1071-A-7, U.S. Dept. of Health, Education and Welfare. Washington, Public Health Service, 1968.
10. *Manual on Hospital Emergency Preparedness.* Boston, National Fire Protection Association (NFPA), No. 3M, 1970.
11. *Central Station Protective Signaling Systems.* Boston, National Fire Protection Association (NFPA), No. 71, 1972.
12. *Principles of Disaster Planning for Hospitals.* Chicago, American Hospital Association, 1967.
13. *Hospital Planning for National Disaster.* Washington, U.S. Public Health Service Publication Number 1071-G-1, 1968.
14. Nissan, S., and Eldar, R.: Organization of surgical care of mass casualties in a civilian hospital. J. Trauma, 11:974, 1971.
15. Saha, A. L.: Epidemiological first aid and follow-up in natural calamities. Indian J. Public Health, 16:156 1972.
16. Rock, J. L.: A disaster drill for a psychiatric hospital. Hosp. Community Psychiat., 24:314, 1973.
17. Collidge, T. T.: Rapid city flood medical response. Arch. Surg., 106:770, 1973.
18. Rutherford, W. H.: Experience in the accident and emergency department of the Royal Victoria Hospital with patients from civil disturbances in Belfast 1969-72 with a review of disaster in the United Kingdom. Injury, 4:189, 1973.

3 INTENSIVE-CARE UNITS: PLANNING AND PRACTICE

R. F. WILSON
J. A. WILSON
L. BRAND
A. J. WALT

The intensive-care unit is a specific area of the hospital designed to provide maximum surveillance and treatment of patients with acute, but reversible, life-threatening impairments of single or multiple vital systems.[1] In a sense, the intensive-care unit (I.C.U.) is an extension of the emergency department (E.D.). The results of special or heroic treatment in the E.D. and operating room may ultimately be vindicated or vitiated by the quality of care provided in the I.C.U.

Of the 700,000 persons who die each year in the United States from medical and surgical emergencies, many might be saved if they could be transported to treatment centers with adequate facilities for critical care.[1] The treatment of critically ill and injured patients in specialized units should not only help to reduce mortality and morbidity but should also enhance teaching and research and promote efficient utilization of highly trained personnel and sophisticated monitoring and resuscitation equipment.

It can be argued with some justification that all I.C.U.s have the common denominator of intense illness—whether peritonitis or pulmonary disease, cardiac or cerebral—and no special features are required to care for the victims of trauma. Such a view, however, fails to take into account the multiplicity of injury, the spectrum of concomitant physiologic derangements, and the variety of specialists who may be involved with a single case of trauma.

The planning and administration of the intensive-care unit should be done by a special intensive- or critical-care committee. This committee should include at least an anesthesiologist, surgeon, internist and/or pediatrician, one of the nursing directors for the hospital, the head nurse of the unit, a member of the hospital administration, and a senior house physician. The physicians on the committee should have extensive experience with the management of life-threatening injuries and illnesses. When a physician has been selected to be medical director for the unit, he should also be on this committee, preferably as its chairman.

In planning for an intensive-care unit a number of factors have to be considered:

1. What is the need for the unit?
2. How big should it be?
3. How much will it cost?
4. How much space is needed?
5. What personnel are needed?
6. What equipment is needed?
7. What policies and procedures should it have?

WHAT IS THE NEED FOR AN I.C.U. IN THE HOSPITAL?

Intensive-care facilities should probably be developed in most hospitals with busy emergency rooms and which perform major abdominal, thoracic and neurologic operations. Attempts to provide sophisticated care in understaffed and underutilized facilities, merely to enhance reputation or status, may be hazardous for the patient; however, all hospitals should make some provision for the treatment of severely ill or injured patients, even if a sophisticated I.C.U. is not feasible.

Gann and Zuidema point out that "the morbidity of trauma can be ascribed in part to the specific injury sustained and in part to major complications . . . Some of these factors may be treated specifically and others may be prevented by early recognition . . . The implication is that satisfactory intensive care of the trauma patient depends upon basing therapeutic decisions on an integrated overall view of the behavior, physiologic compensation, and pathologic decompensation of the many organ systems within the body."[2]

HOW BIG SHOULD THE I.C.U. BE?

The number of special-care beds needed at a given hospital depends on the number of critically ill or injured patients likely to be present at any one time. A rather detailed survey should be made over a period of several months to determine the number of patients with acute reversible organ failure who would have benefited from the maximal surveillance and care an I.C.U. can provide. These include patients requiring respiratory assistance or frequent (every ½ to 2 hours) monitoring of blood pressure, pulse, central venous pressure (CVP), and urine output. Patients with recent multiple severe injuries, shock, severe hypotension, massive gastrointestinal bleeding, and those in the immediate postoperative period after cardiac surgery also require constant observation.

In addition to the I.C.U., critical or special care is often also provided simultaneously in several hospital areas, including the emergency department, the postoperative recovery room, cardiac-care unit, and special areas such as the renal dialysis unit. The relationships among these areas must be defined in advance in order to maintain flexibility and provide optimal patient care in the face of varying patient problems and patient loads. Certainly if critical-care facilities and personnel are already available in the E.D. and recovery rooms there is less need for a large I.C.U. However, many experts in the field of criti-

TABLE 1.   HOSPITAL AND I.C.U. CENSUS, HARPER HOSPITAL, DETROIT, MICHIGAN

| | Yearly census | | Average I.C.U. monthly census | Average I.C.U. daily census | Average patient stay (days) |
Year	Entire hospital	I.C.U.			
1964	24,531°		33		
1965	24,936°	528	44		
1966	24,227°	576	48		
1967	22,650°	621	51		
1968	20,009°	566	47	6.0	
1969	17,584	650	54	6.6	
1970	17,629	693	58	6.2	3.5
1971	17,240	771	64	7.5	3.6

° Includes obstetric patients.

cal care believe that there are definite advantages in efficiency and economy in having all these facilities combined into one large critical-care area utilizing common personnel, supplies, and laboratory facilities.

The number of patients requiring intensive care after the I.C.U. has been in operation will almost always be greater than initial estimates. When the benefits derived from the unit become apparent, the demand for its services tend to increase progressively. At Harper Hospital, a 700-bed private hospital in Detroit, for example, only 528 patients were treated in the I.C.U. during its first full year; since then its yearly census has increased about 8% per year (Table 1). The requests for admissions have increased so much that an intermediate-care area is now being started to help handle the increased patient load.

Furthermore, critically ill or injured patients who in the past might have died soon after admission now, because of better observation and care, either survive or are kept alive for much longer periods of time. The need for prolonged maximal care is particularly evident in critically injured patients. At Detroit General Hospital, the total number of trauma patients treated in the I.C.U. has remained relatively constant, but their length of stay has progressively increased, thereby reducing the total number of admissions possible (Table 2). The patients most apt to be treated in the I.C.U. for prolonged periods are those with gunshot wounds of the abdomen (Table 3). These patients tend to develop septic and respiratory complications requiring meticulous care which cannot usually be provided in general ward beds.

Since an intensive-care unit supplying maximal care and surveillance functions optimally with about six to ten beds, need for more special care is probably best provided by an intermediate-care area adjacent to the I.C.U. These two units can work synergistically and help prevent the sudden reduction in care and observation which often occurs when a patient is transferred from the I.C.U.

If the decision to establish an intermediate-care facility is made, it is important

TABLE 2. TOTAL ADMISSIONS TO THE I.C.U. OF DETROIT GENERAL HOSPITAL

Year	Total admissions	Total trauma admissions	Total trauma deaths
1968	363	82	25
1969	267	73	21
1970	189	62	11
1971	192	80	26

TABLE 3. TYPES OF TRAUMA AND TIME OF DEATH FOR INJURED PATIENTS TREATED IN THE I.C.U. DETROIT GENERAL HOSPITAL (1968-1971)

Type of trauma	No. of patients	No. of deaths in the I.C.U.	Number of patients dying in the I.C.U. at various time intervals		
			1-4 days	5-10 days	11 or more days
Stab of the chest	21	0	—	—	—
Stab of the abdomen	8	2	1	—	1
Gunshot wound of the chest	50	5	3	2	—
Gunshot wound of the abdomen	103	36	17	9	10
Auto accidents and other blunt trauma	97	25	13	7	5
Burns	24	11	9	0	2
TOTAL	303	79	43	18	18

that this unit be under the direction and supervision of the same physician and nursing personnel as the I.C.U. Without such an arrangement, effective coordination of efforts will not be possible.

HOW MUCH WILL THE I.C.U. COST?

Once it has been determined that the hospital needs an I.C.U. for improved patient care and an estimate of its probable patient load has been made, a number of difficult decisions will have to be made regarding space, personnel, and equipment. In making these decisions, the individuals involved should keep a number of basic principles in mind. We refer to these as our "ten platitudes":

1. "You get what you pay for."
2. "A Cadillac requires more gas than a Volkswagen."
3. "The unit is only as good as the people who work in it."
4. "Nurses are made, not born."
5. "People have more potential and ability than we ordinarily give them credit for."
6. "The nurse-liberation movement is on."
7. "Nurses belong with their patients."
8. "If the patient is to get adequate care, the nurse must be given enough time to take care of him."
9. "Monitoring is not new."
10. "Policies and procedures must be clearly spelled out."

"YOU GET WHAT YOU PAY FOR." In this time of skyrocketing hospital costs, it is important that the very purpose for which the I.C.U. was established not be subverted. It must be recognized that the initial cost for space, personnel, and equipment to give proper care to the critically ill and injured is usually much more than that required to deliver other patient services. Commitment by all concerned to this philosophy is a prerequisite to quality care. If for economic reasons high standards are sacrificed, the I.C.U. is likely to be only a convenient place to congregate the more seriously ill.

"A CADILLAC REQUIRES MORE GAS THAN A VOLKSWAGEN." Once the original investment is made, it must be realized that the continued operation of an I.C.U. is also extremely costly. If the I.C.U. is to provide optimal surveillance and care, it requires many well-trained and highly motivated personnel, especially nurses. Furthermore, these nurses should be properly compensated for their advanced training and the increased demands of their work. Other expenses, especially for laboratory tests, will also be much higher for I.C.U. patients.

At Detroit General Hospital, many of the patients need far more care than is usually required or available at other hospitals. During 1969-70, the average calculated cost per patient day in the I.C.U. was $424.02 and in the C.C.U. was $336.15 compared with $107.12 for the remainder of the hospital patients (Table 4). The costs for subsequent years appear to be rising about 10% per year. The nurse-patient ratio in the I.C.U. was about six times greater and the number of laboratory tests performed was about eight times greater than for patients on the general wards (Table 5).

Although these costs seem prohibitive, there is no question that this I.C.U. and its personnel have saved many critically injured patients who almost surely would have died elsewhere. Attempts to economize on I.C.U. expenses unfortunately are reflected very quickly in the quality of care rendered, rapidly reducing the morale and confidence of all individuals concerned. Using L.P.N.s and technicians to replace some of the R.N.s may economize, but only a few of these individuals will ever develop the expertise and attitude of the well-trained and well-motivated R.N.s.

HOW MUCH SPACE IS NEEDED?

Maximum surveillance and easy access to the patient are of utmost importance. The design should provide a minimum of 200 net square feet per bed in open multiple-bed areas, and 250 square feet for isolation beds.[1] Individual isolation rooms or small

TABLE 4. COSTS IN 1969-70 (ADD 10% FOR 1970-71)

	Cost per patient day			Cost per patient day			Total
	I.C.U.	C.C.U.	General beds	I.C.U.	C.C.U.	General beds	
Nursing	199.44	214.44	32.01	359,000.00	193,000.00	4,875,000.00	5,427,000
Laboratory	76.10	19.02	8.68	136,972.00	17,121.60	1,321,905.60	1,476,000
Dietary	8.81	8.81	8.81	15,845.60	7,922.80	1,342,231.60	1,366,000
Operating room	8.63	8.63	8.63	15,520.80	7,760.40	1,314,718.20	1,338,000
Admitting	7.53	7.53	7.53	13,537.20	6,768.60	1,146,694.20	1,167,000
Interns and resident	28.51	28.51	6.76	51,318.40	25,659.20	1,029,022.40	1,106,000
Radiology	5.06	5.06	5.06	9,106.00	4,553.00	771,341.00	785,000
Anesthesiology	4.03	4.03	4.03	7,238.40	3,619.20	613,142.40	624,000
Administration	4.00	4.00	4.00	7,192.00	3,596.00	609,212.00	620,000
Housekeeping	7.26	3.63	3.59	13,061.60	3,265.40	546,673.00	563,000
Pharmacy	26.81	6.70	3.06	48,256.00	6,032.00	465,712.00	520,000
Repair and maint.	5.74	5.74	2.82	10,324.00	5,162.00	429,514.00	445,000
Central supply	16.67	5.56	2.60	29,997.60	4,999.60	396,002.80	431,000
Medical records	7.48	4.99	2.42	13,467.60	4,489.20	369,043.20	387,000
Linen	2.59	2.59	1.27	4,663.20	2,331.60	194,005.20	201,000
Cafeteria	1.06	1.06	1.06	1,902.40	951.20	161,146.40	164,000
Depreciation	0.97	0.97	0.97	1,740.00	870.00	147,390.00	150,000
Social service	0.89	0.89	0.89	1,600.80	800.40	135,598.80	138,000
Blood and plasma	6.91	0.86	0.79	12,435.20	777.20	120,787.60	134,000
Special salaries	1.44	1.44	0.71	2,598.40	1,299.20	108,102.40	112,000
Misc. supplies	0.48	0.48	0.48	870.00	435.00	73,695.00	75,000
Physical med.	0.35	0.35	0.35	638.00	319.00	54,043.00	55,000
Blood bank	2.78	0.35	0.32	5,011.20	313.20	48,675.60	54,000
EKG	0.16	0.32	0.16	290.00	290.00	24,420.00	25,000
EEG	0.26	0.13	0.06	464.00	116.00	9,420.00	10,000
Clothes room	0.06	0.06	0.06	116.00	58.00	9,826.00	10,000
TOTAL	424.02	336.15	107.12	763,236.00	302,535.00	16,317,229.00	17,383,000

AVG = $112.15

TABLE 5. RELATIVE USE OF SERVICES

	I.C.U.	C.C.U.	General beds
Nursing	6×	7×	1×
Laboratory	8×	2×	1×
Dietary	1×	1×	1×
Operating room	1×	1×	1×
Admitting	1×	1×	1×
Interns and residents	4×	4×	1×
Radiology	1×	1×	1×
Anesthesiology	1×	1×	1×
Administration	1×	1×	1×
Housekeeping	2×	1×	1×
Pharmacy	8×	2×	1×
Repair and maintenance	2×	2×	1×
Central supply	6×	2×	1×
Medical records	3×	2×	1×
Linen	2×	2×	1×
Cafeteria	1×	1×	1×
Depreciation	1×	1×	1×
Social service	1×	1×	1×
Blood and plasma	8×	1×	1×
Nurse specialist salaries	2×	2×	1×
Misc. supplies	1×	1×	1×
Physical med.	1×	1×	1×
Blood bank	8×	1×	1×
EKG	1×	2×	1×
EEG	4×	2×	1×
Clothes room	1×	1×	1×

wards must be provided in or adjacent to the main unit for patients with communicable diseases as well as for those in reverse isolation.

A minimum support space of 100 square feet per bed for storage and equipment and utility rooms should also be provided. We have yet to see an I.C.U. provided enough convenient storage space to handle needed supplies and equipment properly. The man-hours lost requesting and obtaining these materials are wasteful and can be exasperating.

A number of other facilities important to the I.C.U. also require space. These include:

1. sleeping rooms in or immediately adjacent to the unit for physicians on call,
2. offices for the unit director, his secretary, and the head nurse,
3. a conference room for discussion of patients by the unit staff and for in-service training programs,
4. a nurses' lounge within the unit, and
5. a waiting room for relatives and visitors adjacent to the unit.

WHAT PERSONNEL ARE NEEDED?

Director of the Intensive-care Unit

The J.C.A.H. recommendations on special-care units call for appointment of a physician director. The success or failure of the unit to a large extent will depend on his ability and enthusiasm. If the hospital has a large number of critically ill or injured patients, such a physician should direct the critical-care units on a full-time basis. He should be chosen on the basis of experience, competence, interest and availability rather than specialty affiliation. He should have completed residency training in one of the major clinical specialties (anesthesiology, medicine, surgery, pediatrics) and should have acquired advanced skills and knowledge in life-support techniques and patient monitoring.[1] If a large number of trauma patients are seen in the hospital, a general surgeon with extensive trauma experience is generally a good choice as head of the I.C.U. He should be responsible directly to the I.C.U. committee, the executive committee of the medical staff and the administration of the hospital. Associate or co-directors, whose primary specialty may be different from that of the director, may share full-time supervision and responsibility for training and patient care.

The I.C.U. director or his designate should approve, in consultation with the head nurse, all admissions and discharges; he should be responsible for surveillance, resuscitation and basic life support of all patients; and he should ensure that patient care involving multiple services is coordinated for efficient use of time and space.

The director should have the right to request consultation from other physicians or services, and to determine which patients require isolation facilities.

Training and continuing education of personnel assigned to the unit should be the responsibility of the director. He should supervise the recording of important statistical information for evaluation of the unit's effectiveness, and in some instances he may also propose an annual budget to the I.C.U. committee and hospital administration.

PITFALL

IF THE I.C.U. RECORDS AND THE EFFECTIVENESS OF CARE ARE NOT PERIODICALLY REVIEWED, DETERIORATION OF CARE AND SUBOPTIMAL UTILIZATION OF PERSONNEL AND FACILITIES MAY GO UNNOTICED.

Medical Staff of the Intensive-care Unit

Optimal surveillance and management of patients in the I.C.U., especially those with multiple injuries, can often be best provided by a team of physicians, nurses, and allied health personnel. The team of physicians should include the patient's personal physician, the director of the unit or his designate, the house physicians assigned to the I.C.U. and any specialists required by the patient's condition. The importance of teamwork in the I.C.U. cannot be stressed enough. Only rarely can the physician spend the hours at the bedside that the nurses and other personnel must spend there treating and observing the patient.

The house staff providing the 24-hour coverage in the I.C.U. should be in at least their second year of specialty training and should be competent in: airway care; artificial ventilation; resuscitation; arrhythmia control; fluid, acid-base, and electrolyte therapy and the treatment of shock. These physicians should be responsible to the director of the unit and, if possible, should be assigned full time to the I.C.U. without other responsibilities. All orders

should be channeled through a member of the unit's full-time physican staff, or a resident physician assigned full time to the unit. Management of critically ill patients by inexperienced junior house staff or by physicans who do not remain with the patient should be strongly discouraged. The patient's personal physician can either retain responsibility for his patient's general care (provided he is available at all times for guidance of the team) or delegate his role to a specialist who is available at all times and familiar with critical care.

To provide optimal service to the patient and the operation of the unit, it is advisable to have a list of consulting specialists in neurology, bronchoesophagology, neurosurgery, orthopedic surgery, infectious diseases, renal and metabolic diseases, physical medicine, psychiatry, and radiology. Such specialists should have an interest in applying their specific skills to patients with life-threatening illnesses and injuries, and be known to work cooperatively with members of the unit staff.[1] It should be kept in mind that the care of the patient with multiple injuries should not be partitioned among the various specialists involved. One individual, preferably a general surgeon, should coordinate all these activities.

Nursing Staff

In most hospitals, the I.C.U. is primarily a special nursing unit.

"THE UNIT IS ONLY AS GOOD AS THE PEOPLE WHO WORK IN IT." Working in an I.C.U. is an extremely demanding job, mentally, physically, and emotionally. The nurses working in this unit should possess a number of important characteristics including:

1. a good general nursing training and experience,
2. intelligence and an inquiring mind,
3. physical strength and endurance,
4. ability and courage to exercise initiative,
5. an emotionally stable nature.

Unfortunately, the emotional trauma inflicted on I.C.U. nurses is not generally appreciated. Because of the close and constant individual patient contact, the nurse often becomes strongly attached psychologically and emotionally to her patients. Since the death rate in these critically ill patients is high, the nurse is apt to feel a strong and repeated sense of grief and failure. Strong support from her supervisors and the physicians is essential for optimal care and morale. However, it must be remembered that, although the emotional trauma may be stressful, it is this same closeness of feeling that frequently stimulates ideas to improve care.

"NURSES ARE MADE, NOT BORN." Once a nurse with the desired characteristics and experience has been carefully selected to work in the I.C.U., she must be trained properly and must be provided continuing education by a strong program of in-service training. Ideally, the new I.C.U. nurse should be given three to six weeks of training under a unit teacher; about 75% of her time should be spent on practical problems and 25% on theory. She can then be gradually worked into the usual staffing patterns.

The contents of the initial course and continuing in-service training should include:

1. cardiovascular system, including monitoring (BP, P, CVP, EKG), catheter care, drug actions, defibrillators, and pacemakers;
2. respiratory system, including blood gas patterns, airway management (endotracheal tubes, tracheostomy), and control of respirators;
3. renal system, including urine output, drug effects, and dialysis;
4. metabolism and fluid and electrolytes, including intravenous hyperalimentation;
5. sepsis, antibiotics, and isolation techniques;
6. management of the patient with multiple injuries, especially those with head, spinal-cord, and orthopedic injuries;
7. psychologic needs of patients, family, and nurses;
8. basic instrumentation; nurses must understand the basic construction and operation of the instruments used in the I.C.U. Otherwise they are apt to develop a sense of insecurity, and will tend to view the machines as monsters.

The I.C.U. nurses should be available to provide consultation, act as resource people, and help with the in-service training of nurses in other parts of the hospital. This helps to defuse tension and allay jealousies among the "out group." It must be remembered at all times, however, that the nurse's main responsibility is direct patient care and the carrying out of the physician's orders.

It quickly became apparent that I.C.U. nurses are "a special breed of cat." As their training, experience, and knowledge have improved, their role has also expanded considerably.

"PEOPLE HAVE MORE POTENTIAL AND ABILITY THAN WE ORDINARILY GIVE THEM CREDIT FOR." The physician who has patients in an I.C.U. must learn to listen carefully to the observations and ideas of nurses and other personnel. Given encouragement and support, they can often make important suggestions for improving care. All individuals working with the patient should be motivated to improve their skills and assume increasing responsibility and initiative. Furthermore, if the plan and theory of the treatment to be used are explained to the members of the team, implementation can proceed in a more intelligent and effective manner. The highest quality care can be achieved when all personnel working in the I.C.U. feel the right and responsibility to contribute. This interchange of ideas not only fosters an esprit de corps but encourages a striving for excellence on the part of all concerned.

"THE NURSE-LIBERATION MOVEMENT IS ON." The role of nurses in many areas of patient care, especially the I.C.U., is expanding rapidly. The morale and pride of the nurses in the I.C.U. will usually reflect the energy and perceptiveness of the head nurse or nursing supervisor. This is the key figure who is called to account by such disparate individuals as the administrator, the nursing office, the directors of training programs, and a constellation of physicians, some of whom are less well informed on intensive medical care than she is.

Her responsibilities, training and level of decision making place her in a category far removed from that of the traditional nurse, and she should be paid accordingly. While she may be physically present 40 to 48 hours per week, she assumes constant responsibility for the unit seven days a week, just as a surgeon does for his patient, and is in a sense permanently on call. She is not only quarterback but is also required to run interference for her team of nurses. For this to be accomplished, she needs the strong support of physicians available, both day and night, for all emergencies, few of which follow any circadian rhythm.

"NURSES BELONG WITH THEIR PATIENTS." We should do our utmost to keep the nurse with her patients. Her observations and care, especially of the trauma patient, are often the most important benefits to be derived from a critical-care unit. Ancillary personnel should be trained to perform as many of the nurse's other duties as possible.

PITFALL

IF THE NURSES ARE NOT INFORMED AS TO THE LESIONS OR COMPLICATIONS WHICH MAY DEVELOP LATER IN THE ACUTELY INJURED PATIENT, OR IF THEY ARE TOO BUSY TO OBSERVE THE PATIENT CLOSELY, ADDITIONAL INJURIES WHICH WERE NOT APPARENT DURING THE INITIAL RESUSCITATION EFFORTS MAY BE MISSED UNTIL THEIR TREATMENT BECOMES DIFFICULT OR IMPOSSIBLE.

"IF THE PATIENT IS TO GET ADEQUATE CARE, THE NURSE MUST BE GIVEN ENOUGH TIME TO TAKE CARE OF HIM." If a nurse is required to care for more than one or two critically ill or injured patients at a time, her effectiveness is greatly reduced. Certainly two such patients should be all that one nurse should be required to care for during the day and afternoon shifts when the routine is constantly being broken for tests and examination and treatment by physicians. Furthermore, there are many duties to perform in an I.C.U. besides direct care of the patient. These include scheduling personnel, secretarial tasks, ordering supplies and diets, arranging for x-rays, filing the lab slips and other reports, and talking with the physicians and relatives. All these activities, plus inhalation therapy, equipment maintenance, electrical safety, and checking for drug incompatibilities, take a great deal of time. Sufficient support personnel in the form of ward clerks, unit managers, administrative assistants, and nursing supervisors must be supplied if patient care is to be adequate.

Ancillary Staff

Inhalation therapists, chest physiotherapists, biomedical electronic technicians and engineers, and various technicians and technologists should be part of the critical-care team. With proper supervision, they can bring a variety of valuable skills to the patient, upgrade nursing and medical care, and provide increased time for the bedside nurse to perform her specific functions.

Unfortunately, there is often some conflict of roles between the nurses and the ancillary staff, especially the respiratory technicians and inhalation therapists. As the inhalation therapists have gained advanced knowledge and experience in their field, they have become increasingly independent and possessive of their position. Because patient care of the critically ill cannot be segmented or divided among "interested groups" without sacrificing quality, the roles and responsibilities of all personnel must be clearly outlined in the unit's policy-and-procedure manual. Should conflicts arise, they should be dealt with immediately, with assistance from the I.C.U. committee as needed.

Currently much of our intensive care in trauma patients is directed toward management of pulmonary problems, sepsis or stress bleeding. Our ability to control or treat shock and cardiovascular abnormalities has progressively improved over the past five to six years.[2,4] Many patients who previously would have died soon after injury or in the operating room now survive after successful management of a long series of serious complications or die at a much later time. Many of these patients develop a severe progressive respiratory failure which may not become apparent until 12 to 96 hours after the injury.[5-7] If sepsis supervenes, the problem is magnified.

Treatment of these individuals requires early recognition of the problem and intensive respiratory care. Many physicians treating patients with respiratory failure have little training or experience with pulmonary physiology, blood gases, or respirators. Under these circumstances the inhalation therapist may be required to make all or many of the decisions concerning the operation of the respirator. Although the therapist certainly should be encouraged to participate in the patient's care and offer suggestions, the treatment itself should be determined and ordered by a physician with special skill in this field.

Administrative Staff

A clerk-typist and unit manager should assist the head nurse during the daytime shifts to facilitate handling of patient and administrative records, purchase orders, phone calls and physician page calls. A clerk or aide should also be available on all shifts, including nights and weekends, to handle phone communications and records. One member of the hospital administration staff should serve as coordinator of administrative functions and budgets for the unit and should be a member of the I.C.U. committee.

WHAT EQUIPMENT IS NEEDED?

Laboratory Facilities

A 24-hour laboratory service must be readily available for rapid measurement of pH, blood gas tensions, electrolytes, blood glucose, and for routine hematologic, urine, and microbiologic studies. Total protein, serum enzyme levels, serum and urine osmolality, blood oxygen content or saturation, cardiac output, pulmonary function tests (minute volume, vital capacity, and analysis of mixed expired gas) and pulmonary artery catheterization should also be available in the larger trauma hospitals on a 24-hour basis. This is most readily achieved by the location of a core laboratory within the unit or immediately adjacent to it. Such a laboratory should be supervised by the director or his designate.

Monitoring Equipment

The monitoring equipment used in any unit will vary considerably. Certainly cardioscopes and central venous pressures are now used extensively. Intra-arterial and pulmonary wedge pressures are being measured more frequently, and in some centers more sophisticated tests, including cardiac output and oxygen consumption, may also be performed.

Before deciding on the purchase of monitoring equipment, several things must be considered:

1. How badly is it needed?
2. How much will the physicians, nurses and other personnel use the additional data provided?
3. How much does it cost?
4. How simple is it to use?
5. How durable is the machine and how well will it be serviced?

For example, many physicians have asked us if their hospital should buy the instruments needed to measure cardiac output. In general, the cardiac output is seldom needed to decide the type of therapy to be used; it is primarily a research tool. Simpler observations usually suffice. Furthermore, there are several technical points in performing the measurement that must be carefully observed. Unless a full-time physician is interested in this field, cardiac output determinations may be unreliable and of little use.

"MONITORING IS NOT NEW." We have always monitored our patients in terms of blood pressure, pulse, temperature, urine output, and weight. The main danger of the newer instruments, including those that can record physiologic data at a distance, is that we may be seduced into believing that equipment can replace rather than supplement or enhance the direct observations of trained personnel.

WHAT POLICIES AND PROCEDURES ARE NEEDED?

"POLICIES AND PROCEDURES MUST BE CLEARLY SPELLED OUT." Written policies and procedures are essential. Some of the most significant areas to be covered are: admission and discharge policies, authority to write orders, lines of authority, and activities that personnel can do independently, both routinely and in emergencies. The following example of the I.C.U. policy and procedure proposed for Harper Hospital in the Detroit Medical Center may apply to many large hospitals with medical and surgical residents but no full-time intensivists.

I. *Criteria for Admission to the I.C.U.*

Physicians tend to use the I.C.U. as a convenient place to send all their extremely sick patients, regardless of the surveillance and treatment required. Not uncommonly it is used to show the family that the doctor is doing everything he can, even if the patient has irreversible disease. These problems often develop because our sophisticated medical care is capable of keeping terminal patients alive for extended but often unwarranted periods of time. The difficulties of readjusting traditional interpersonal medical relationships should not be sidestepped. This is a sensitive issue, but if optimal care of the individual patient is the ultimate objective, specific agreements should be reached.

A. Patients eligible for admission to the I.C.U. include those with acute reversible life-threatening problems requiring constant monitoring of the following vital systems:

cardiovascular (BP or CVP every ½ hour or oftener; cardioscope)
respiratory (respirator, blood gases)
neurologic
renal (urinary output).

Examples of trauma patients requiring intensive care include those who have had:

multiple severe injuries
shock or severe hypotension
moderate to severe hemorrhage
cardiac surgery
medical problems making them extremely poor risks, especially severe fluid and electrolyte problems
severe acute respiratory failure.

B. The necessity for transfer to or from the I.C.U. should be based on the quality of nursing care needed by the patient and also on his prognosis.

C. Patients who should *not* be admitted to the restricted clean I.C.U. include those with:

1. terminal conditions such as:
   a. brain death (unless an effort is to be made to use the kidneys of the patient for transplantation, especially if he is a young trauma victim)
   b. terminal malignancies.
2. infectious problems such as
   a. those from Staphylococcus aureus
   b. purulent drainage of any kind (these patients are often the sickest in the hospital and should be treated in a separate room or ward)
   c. tuberculosis.
3. myocardial infarctions or severe arrhythmias without other intensive-care problems. If no bed is available in the coronary-care unit, they should probably be treated in a private room with special nurses and monitoring equipment.

II. *Procedure for Admission and Transfer to the I.C.U.*

In hospitals treating large numbers of trauma victims and other emergencies, it is wise to leave at least one to two I.C.U. beds available each night for new admissions and to categorize the other I.C.U. patients in order of priority of transfer.

1. The physician who wishes to transfer a patient to the I.C.U. will dis-

cuss the problem with the physician director or his designate and the nurse in charge of the I.C.U. for that shift. They will determine if the patient meets the criteria for admission to the I.C.U., if a bed is or can be made available, and outline the monitoring and care needed.

2. If the patient is accepted, the physician or his resident and a nurse should accompany the patient to the I.C.U.. The physician(s) must rewrite the orders and review the patient's condition and orders with the nurse who will take care of the patient.

3. Patients transferred to the I.C.U. from other units should be transported to the I.C.U. on an I.C.U. bed.

4. Should the need for a bed in the I.C.U. arise at a time when no bed is available, and the patient is eligible for admission, the attending physician requesting admission should contact the physician director, his alternate, or the senior resident assigned to the I.C.U. to explore the possibility of releasing a bed in the unit by transfer of another patient from the unit. If the senior resident and the nurse in charge agree that the new patient should be admitted to the I.C.U., it should be the responsibility of the senior resident to discuss the problem with the attending physician who is treating the patient presently in the I.C.U.

5. Controversial decisions regarding I.C.U. admissions and transfers should be referred immediately to the physician director, the chairman of the I.C.U. committee or his designated representative, who should discuss the problem with the attending physicians involved as soon as possible.

6. When a patient is transferred to the I.C.U., a bed should not be reserved for him in another part of the hospital.

7. There should be no direct admission to the I.C.U. from outside the hospital unless the patient is first examined by his attending physician. In the absence of examination by the attending physician, the patient should be examined in the emergency room by the I.C.U. physician or senior medical or surgical resident on call. The decision of whether to transfer the patient to the I.C.U. should be made at that time in consultation with the patient's physician.

III. *Procedure for Transfer from the I.C.U.*

1. Requests for beds for patients to be transferred from the I.C.U. should be given top priority by the admitting office.

2. Upon transfer from the I.C.U., all orders must be rewritten by the attending physician or house officer.

IV. *Professional Supervision*

In addition to the guidelines mentioned earlier, certain details of the professional supervision of the patient's care should be stressed. A designated physician member of the I.C.U. committee should be expected to make rounds in the unit daily with the nursing supervisor or her designated representative to evaluate care and functioning of the unit. Recommendations or suggestions for improving care on individual patients should be made as needed by the I.C.U. physician on the progress notes or on special I.C.U. forms.

One medical and one surgical resident in at least their second year of training should be assigned to the I.C.U. as the sole or major portion of their clinical duties. They will be expected to be familiar with the condition of all patients in the I.C.U. on their respective services. These residents will communicate relevant information to their senior medical and surgical residents on call prior to leaving the hospital each day. During the night and on weekends, the senior medical and surgical residents on call will be responsible for the house-staff coverage in the I.C.U.

Progress notes must be made daily by the attending physician or his resident on each patient's chart.

V. *Functions of the I.C.U. Nurse*

A. The I.C.U. nurse should not only provide optimal nursing care but should also, with proper training, assist the physician in evaluating the patient and guiding therapy.

B. Standing orders from individual staff physicians for medications and treatment may be followed after these orders are written and approved by the I.C.U. committee.

C. If the attending physician or house officer is not available, I.C.U. nurses should have the training and experience, especially in emergencies, to:
1. order, begin, or increase the administration of oxygen;
2. use equipment (e.g. manual breathing bag) to assist ventilation;
3. order or make adjustments in the ventilation of patients on respirators, in consultation with the inhalation therapist if available, if blood gas analyses indicate inadequate or excess ventilation or oxygenation;
4. diagnose cardiac arrest or ventricular fibrillation and begin closed-chest cardiac massage and artificial ventilation;
5. use the defibrillator if the patient has ventricular fibrillation;
6. obtain EKG tracings as needed; order EKGs if necessary;
7. order chest x-rays as needed;
8. request routine laboratory tests such as blood gases, electrolytes, or CBC when needed;
9. administer and adjust I.V. lidocaine and other medications to control cardiac arrhythmias;
10. adjust cardiac pacing equipment to maintain the pacing requested by the physician;
11. administer I.V. drugs or infusions requested by the physician;
12. start I.V.s as needed if I.V. technicians are not available;
13. draw venous blood (even if no I.V. catheter is in place);
14. draw blood from established arterial or intravenous lines;
15. apply tourniquets in acute pulmonary edema or use automatic rotating tourniquet apparatus;
16. regulate I.V. fluids to maintain requested levels of blood pressure, CVP, or urinary output;
17. take smears, cultures, and sensitivities as needed;
18. enforce isolation procedures on infected cases.

VI. *Private-duty Nurses*

Patients will not be permitted to have private-duty nurses except for those approved by the nursing office and I.C.U. committee.

INTERMEDIATE-CARE UNITS
I. *Objective*

The objective of the intermediate-care unit is to provide a specific area for continued concentrated nursing care for patients with acute reversible conditions which do not require admission to the I.C.U. but still require more surveillance and therapy than would generally be available on the general wards.

II. *Criteria for Admission to the Intermediate-care Unit*
   A. Patients requiring *frequent* monitoring of the following vital systems:
   cardiovascular (BP or CVP every one to two hours, cardioscope)
   respiratory (respirator, blood gases)
   neurologic
   renal (hourly urinary output).
   Typical examples of conditions requiring intermediate care include:
   postoperative thoracotomy
   postoperative brain surgery
   postoperative vascular surgery
   moderately poor-risk patients after surgery
   those on respirators
   peritoneal dialysis
   metabolic problems, such as diabetic acidosis without coma.
   Patients with infections requiring frequent or constant monitoring may be admitted to the special intermediate-care beds provided for this.
   B. Patients who should not be admitted to the intermediate-care unit include:
   terminal conditions such as brain death or terminal liver failure, or malignancies.
All other policies and procedures for the intermediate-care unit should be identical with those in the intensive-care unit.

REFERENCES

1. Downes, J. J.: Guidelines for organization of critical care units. The Committee on Guidelines of the Society for Critical Care Medicine, May, 1971.
2. Gann, D. S., and Zuidema, C. D.: Intensive care of the trauma patient. Med. Clin. N. Amer., 55:1171, 1971.
3. Thal, A. P., and Wilson, R. F.: Shock. Curr. Probl. Surg., September:1, 1965.
4. Wilson, R. F., and Fisher, R. R.: The hemodynamic effects of massive steroids in clinical shock. Surg. Gynec. Obstet., 127:769, 1968.

5. Wilson, R. F., et al.: Clinical respiratory fail-
    ure after shock or trauma: Prognosis and meth-
    ods of diagnosis. Arch. Surg., 98:539, 1969.
6. Wilson, R. F., et al.: Physiologic shunting in
    the lung in critically ill or injured patients.
    J. Surg. Res., 10:571, 1970.
7. McCarthy, G., et al.: Sub-clinical fat embo-
    lism: A prospective study of fifty patients with
    extremity fractures. J. Trauma, in press.

Suggested Reading

1. Lee, B.: Shock room: Equivalent of military
    field hospital. Mod. Hosp., 118:92, 1972.
2. Maddox, D.: Community hospital gears up to
    provide intensive care. Mod. Hosp., 118:100,
    1972.
3. Michaels, D. R.: Too much in need of sup-
    port to give any? Amer. J. Nurs., 71:1932,
    1971.
4. Todd, J. S.: Symposium on intensive care
    units. Med. Clin. N. Amer., 55:5, 1971.
5. Clark, L.: Can the nursing workload be
    measured? Supervisor Nurse, 1:7, 1970.
6. Kinney, J. M.: Intensive care of the critically
    ill: A foundation for research. J. Trauma, 10:
    949, 1970.
7. Erickson, S.: Infant I.C.U.'s save lives—but
    too many units may add cost and hamper
    growth. Mod. Hosp., 115:80, 1970.

8. Rakkaner, P.: Intensive care unit of an acci-
    dent hospital. Acta Chir. Scand., 135:197,
    1969.
9. Sheppard, L. C., et al.: Automated treatment
    of critically ill patients. Ann. Surg., 168:596,
    1968.
10. Maloney, J. V.: The trouble with patient
    monitoring. Ann. Surg., 168:605, 1968.
11. Lambertsen, E. C., and Strauss, A.: Sympo-
    sium on intensive care nursing. Nurs. Clin. N.
    Amer., 3:1, 1968.
12. *The Planning and Operation of an I.C.U.*
    Battle Creek, W. K. Kellogg Foundation, 1961.
13. Blowers, R.: General aspects of infection con-
    trol in the operating room and intensive care
    unit. Int. Anesth. Clin., 10:23, 1972.
14. Walker, W. F.: Surgical intensive care. Ann.
    Roy. Coll. Surg. Eng., 53:50, 1973.
15. Fleming, W. H., et al.: Evolution of an in-
    tensive care unit in Viet Nam. Ann. Surg.,
    39:422, 1973.
16. Weinsaft, P.: Maximum and acute care units
    where aged doesn't mean expendable. Geri-
    atrics, 28:162, 1973.
17. Morgan, A., et al.: Dollar and human costs of
    intensive care. J. Surg. Res., 14:441, 1973.
18. Korbelak, R., et al.: An improved critical care
    record. J. Trauma, 13:65, 1973.

Part 2
PHYSIOLOGIC CONSIDERATIONS

4 METABOLIC AND NUTRITIONAL CONSIDERATIONS IN TRAUMA

R. F. WILSON

G. BAKER

V. SARDESAI

A. J. WALT

J. C. ROSENBERG

"Fat serves as man's caloric buffer, protein as his machinery, and carbohydrate reserves as an emergency energy supply."

G. F. CAHILL, JR.[1]

The modern physician treating injured patients must be as sensitive to the basic metabolic changes following trauma as doctors of past generations have been to the more obvious anatomic damage. The physiologic activities through which the organism derives energy essential to the repair of injured tissues are affected by many reflexes and neurohumoral substances. The stimuli for these changes arise both directly from the damaged tissues and indirectly from hemodynamic alterations. The purpose of this chapter is to explore some practical aspects of these metabolic changes in terms of the clinical picture and management of the patient.

NEUROHUMORAL RESPONSES AFTER TRAUMA

The main neurohumoral responses after trauma include: (1) the sympatho-adrenal response, (2) the renin-angiotensin-aldosterone response, (3) the antidiuretic-hormone response, (4) the adrenocorticotropic hormone (ACTH) response, and (5) the responses caused by the injured tissue.

The Sympatho-adrenal Response to Trauma

The sympathetic nervous system and the adrenal medulla are stimulated to release catecholamines by reduction of the blood pressure or the oxygen content of blood. Afferent impulses from the heart, lungs, and aorta are carried by the vagus nerves while stimuli from the carotid sinus and carotid body travel along Hering's nerve to the vasomotor center located in the reticular substance of the medulla and pons. When blood pressure falls or hypoxia occurs, the vasomotor center is released from its normal inhibition; it then sends impulses down all the sympathetic nerves, including those to the adrenal medulla, resulting in release of increased amounts of epinephrine and norepinephrine.[2] Other pathways of inhibition and excitation of the vasomotor center exist in other areas of the brain, e.g. the cerebral cortex and hypothalamus. These areas are, in turn, influenced by stimuli arising from injured, painful areas, adding to the effects of hypotension and hypoxia.[3]

The sympatho-adrenal response has profound hemodynamic and metabolic effects. The hemodynamic changes have been divided into "alpha" and "beta" receptor responses.[4] The alpha effects consist of arteriolar vasoconstriction maximal in those tissues most resistant to hypoxia and a relatively generalized venous constriction, especially in the capacitance veins. The beta effects consist of a mild arteriolar vasodilation in striated muscle, constriction of capacitance veins and an increase in the rate and force of myocardial contraction. Of the various drugs used to alter cardiovascular function, norepinephrine has about 90% alpha and 10% beta effect; epinephrine has about 50% alpha and 50% beta effect; and isoproterenol has an almost pure beta effect.

The Renin-angiotensin-aldosterone Response to Trauma

Renin is a proteolytic enzyme synthesized in the macula densa or juxtaglomerular apparatus located adjacent to the afferent arteriole of the glomerulus. A decrease in the "effective blood volume" as manifested by a decreased perfusion of the kidney increases renin secretion.[5] The decapeptide angiotensin I, which is biologically inactive, is produced by the action of renin on an alpha globulin in the plasma. Angiotensin I is then converted to angiotensin II, an octapeptide, which is a potent vasopressor agent and the major stimulus for aldosterone release from the adrenal cortex.[6] Although aldosterone secretion is virtually always greatly increased following trauma, it can be partially reduced by adequate administration of fluids and electrolytes.[7]

Antidiuretic-hormone Secretion Following Trauma

Antidiuretic-hormone (ADH) secretion is strikingly affected by neurogenic stimuli and the osmolality of the blood. A decrease in tone of the left atrial wall removes the inhibiting effect of its stretch receptors on ADH release, thereby increasing ADH secretion.[8] Other neurogenic stimuli releasing ADH include painful stimuli from any part of the body. ADH is also released if the blood coming into contact with osmoreceptors in the hypothalamus and along the internal carotid artery has increased osmolarity.[9]

ADH promotes the resorption of water from the distal tubules and collecting ducts into the hypertonic renal medullary interstitial spaces. This reabsorbed water increases plasma volume and thereby reduces plasma osmolality. At high concentrations, ADH also has a vasopressor effect.

Trauma can increase ADH secretion for several days,[10] resulting in a smaller volume of more concentrated urine, expansion of the extracellular fluid compartment and a dilutional hyponatremia. After trauma the usual controlling mechanisms are somewhat depressed. Overhydration does not suppress ADH secretion, probably because the neurogenic stimuli, especially from pain, are still active.

Adrenocorticotropin (ACTH) Activity Following Trauma

Soon after surgery or trauma there is an increase in the blood and urine concentration of hydrocortisone-like compounds.[10] Adrenocorticotropin (ACTH), a polypeptide substance elaborated by the basophilic cells of the anterior pituitary gland, is the major stimulus for the secretion of adrenocortical hormones. ACTH is released by corticotropic-releasing factor (CRF) which is elaborated by the axons of large neurons in the hypothalamus when a stressful stimulus reaching the cerebral cortex interferes with the sustained inhibition of the reticular formation upon hypothalamic centers. CRF then passes into the hypophyseal-portal circulation and promotes ACTH secretion from the anterior pituitary. When ACTH reaches the adrenal cortex, enzymatic systems responsible for the biosynthesis of steroid hormones are activated, and the secretory activity and size of the adrenal cortex increase.

Glucocorticoids promote gluconeogenesis (particularly carbohydrates from proteins) and depress glucose utilization, resulting in a mild to moderate diabetic-like state. Cortisol (hydrocortisone), the major glucocorticoid secreted by the adrenal cortex, also increases plasma amino acids by stimulating protein catabolism in muscles. The amino acids are then utilized by the liver to synthesize glucose or new protein.

The Wound as a Source of Stimuli

PITFALL

IF THE EXCISION OF LOCALIZED AREAS OF EXTENSIVE TISSUE DAMAGE, NECROSIS, OR INFECTION IS UNDULY DELAYED BECAUSE OF "THE POOR CONDITION OF THE PATIENT," FURTHER DETERIORATION OF THE PATIENT MAY OCCUR BECAUSE OF CONTINUED ABSORPTION OF TOXINS AND VASOACTIVE SUBSTANCES INTO THE GENERAL CIRCULATION.

There is increasing awareness that the wound may act as an important source of neurogenic and hormonal stimuli. Pain causes direct stimulation of the hypothalamus and other neurogenic centers, and the local inflammatory response in the injured tissue releases proteolytic enzymes and polypeptides which have profound hemodynamic effects and can act as blood-borne stimuli to all parts of the body.

SOURCES OF ENERGY DURING STARVATION AND FOLLOWING TRAUMA

Carbohydrate

Of the three main potential fuels (carbohydrate, fat, and protein) carbohydrate is essential for survival in emergencies. The glycogen stored in liver and muscle can be rapidly mobilized to supply energy for sudden bursts of activity or stress. These glycogen stores provide high-energy phosphates rapidly, primarily by anaerobic glycolysis. This anaerobic glycolysis occurs with hypoxia, ischemia, or sudden need for increased energy, but is very inefficient. Under anaerobic conditions, the glucose is incompletely oxidized to lactate, producing only four moles of high-energy phosphate (ATP) in contrast to the 36 moles released when the glucose is completely oxidized. The 50 to 75 gm of liver glycogen and 200 gm of muscle glycogen present in the average adult male could provide only twelve hours of basal caloric need. Consequently prolonged glucose requirements cannot be met by glycogen breakdown alone and the patient must rely also on fat and gluconeogenesis from protein.

Protein

Although protein is an important source of energy in traumatized patients, a "labile protein pool" serving as an expendable nitrogen depot probably does not exist.[1] Protein exists in the body chiefly in muscle (the ratio of tissue protein to serum protein is approximately 30 : 1), and during the response to injury the protein in the muscle is broken down to amino acids which are subsequently changed by the liver and kidneys to urea. Although it might be felt that some of this accelerated protein catabolism is related to increased energy and oxygen demands, Kinney has shown only a slight rise in oxygen consumption following trauma.[11]

Fat

Fat is the most important potential fuel in the body as it is almost all labile as far as physiologic expendability is concerned and serves as a ready source of abundant calories.[1] Fat provides nine calories per gram whereas protein and carbohydrate supply only four. The quantities of nitrogen and carbohydrate in the body are relatively fixed, and most caloric excesses or deficiencies are reflected by either an increase or a decrease in the body fat.

Carbohydrate, if in excess of current needs, can be transiently retained in an expanded glycogen pool; however, since the glycogen stores are usually already optimal in normal man, the excess calories are rapidly converted into fat and stored in adipose tissue.

Many of the changes in fat metabolism after trauma are due to the effects of catecholamines. Catecholamines cause increased triglyceride breakdown, increased concentration of free fatty acids (FFA), glycerol and ketone bodies in the blood, increased esterification of FFA, accumulation of lipid in the liver, and increased oxidation of fatty acids. These effects are mediated by the cyclic nucleotide 3,5-AMP, which is produced in increased amounts by catecholamine-induced activation of the enzyme adenyl cyclase.[12] This same mechanism can also cause increased glycogenolysis, insulin secretion and stimulation of gluconeogenesis.

FUEL CHANGES DURING STARVATION AND FOLLOWING TRAUMA

Brief Starvation

A patient receiving no caloric intake for one or two days loses approximately 10 to 15 gm of nitrogen daily in the urine; however, 100 gm of carbohydrate will reduce this daily nitrogen loss to approximately 3 gm.[1,10,13] The major source of glucose during starvation comes from gluconeogenesis from amino acids, derived from muscle protein. The administration of 100 gm of glucose replaces the need for most of this gluconeogenesis and spares, therefore, much of the muscle catabolism that would otherwise occur. Consequently, the patient receiving I.V. fluids should be given at least two liters of 5% glucose daily in addition to his electrolyte requirements.

The increased glucose concentration caused by glucose infusion triggers an insulin release which, even in small amounts, inhibits amino-acid release from muscle, amino-acid extraction by the liver, and gluconeogenesis from amino acids.[1] High insulin levels which are achieved from ingestion or infusion of a large load of carbohydrate facilitate glucose uptake into peripheral tissues, especially muscle and fat.

Following Trauma

Trauma creates a set of added and unique problems stemming from altered utilization of glucose. If large amounts of glucose are administered to a traumatized individual, there is little, if any, effect on the rate of protein catabolism beyond that achieved by the first 100 to 200 gm.[1] In fact, the capacity of traumatized patients to secrete the extra insulin needed to metabolize exogenous glucose is so markedly decreased that this response has been called the "diabetes of trauma." Since only the brain and reparative tissue can utilize glucose without insulin, glucose in excess of that which these tissues can use accumulates in the blood.

The metabolism of trauma, therefore, is fixed. The catabolism of trauma, unlike that in normal starvation, is relatively free of insulin control and is resistant to feedback suppression by carbohydrate. Even the patient who produces enough insulin to prevent the severe hyperglycemia of trauma still has an increased nitrogen catabolism.[1] In the severely injured patient who is totally dependent on parenteral alimentation for a prolonged period of time, allowance must be made for additional metabolic changes.

Prolonged Starvation

If an individual were totally fasted, and the rate of nitrogen catabolism continued at 10 to 15 gm daily, survival would be limited. Even if only small amounts of glucose were required daily over a prolonged period, the quantity available from glycogen and protein would be completely inadequate. In prolonged starvation keto acids produced by the liver apparently cross the blood-brain barrier as glucose does and progressively displace glucose as the fuel used by the brain. The net effect of this utilization of keto acids instead of glucose is to spare nitrogen, and urinary nitrogen decreases progressively to about 3 to 4 gm daily.[1]

SPECIAL METABOLIC PROBLEMS
AFTER TRAUMA

Some of the more complicated metabolic problems which may develop after trauma are related to diabetes mellitus, adrenal insufficiency and hyperthyroidism.

Diabetes Mellitus

Any previous absolute or relative deficiencies of insulin are magnified after trauma; as a consequence, the release of amino acids from muscle, fatty acids from adipose tissue, and glucose from the liver and muscle may be greatly increased. As the liver glycogen is depleted, the liver tends to produce more and more keto acids. Since glucose cannot enter muscle or adipose tissue unless adequate insulin is present, glucose levels rise rapidly in the blood, exceed the tubular maximum for reabsorption in the kidneys and spill over into the urine causing glycosuria and an osmotic diuresis. In addition, the elevated levels of keto acids in blood can result in a significant ketosis and metabolic acidosis.

Diabetics who have had surgery or trauma and require I.V. fluids may be controlled in a number of ways. One simple method is to add 10 to 15 units of regular insulin to each liter of 5% glucose. The urine sugar is then followed at four- to six-hour intervals and covered with a sliding scale of insulin. Four-plus urine glucose is covered with 10 to 15 units of regular insulin and three-plus urine with 5 to 10 units of regular insulin. If the urine is positive for acetone, 5 additional units of insulin are added. When diabetic acidosis or coma develops, the problems of the trauma patient are greatly compounded. In these circumstances, the major emphasis must be on the administration of sufficient insulin and fluid to correct the acidosis and dehydration. The initial dose of insulin used will vary according to the serum acetone and/or blood glucose. Later, when the glucose begins to be utilized properly and blood levels begin to fall, it is essential to supply extra glucose and potassium.

Serum acetone	Blood glucose (mg/100 ml)	Initial insulin dose (units)
+ Undiluted	300	50
+ 1:1 dil	400	50
+ 1:2 dil	600	100
+ 1:4 dil	800	100
+ 1:8 dil	1000	150

Usually half the insulin is given intravenously and half subcutaneously. If there is any question about the adequacy of tissue perfusion due to hypovolemia or shock, the total dose of insulin may be given intravenously. The response of the blood glucose level and serum acetone should be reappraised hourly.

Since many patients are severely dehydrated, up to two to four liters of fluid may have to be given in the first one to two hours to establish and maintain a reasonable urinary output. The best fluids to administer initially in severely acidotic patients are isotonic saline, isotonic sodium bicarbonate or 0.5 N saline with two ampules of sodium bicarbonate.

PITFALL

IF GLUCOSE AND POTASSIUM ARE NOT ADDED TO THE I.V. FLUIDS OF THE PATIENT WITH DIABETIC ACIDOSIS AS SOON AS THE BLOOD OR URINE GLUCOSE LEVELS BEGIN TO FALL, THE PATIENT MAY DEVELOP INSULIN SHOCK OR A HYPOKALEMIC CARDIAC ARREST.

When the blood glucose falls to less than 300 mg/100 ml or urine glucose becomes less than 3+, this is evidence that the insulin may be starting to work effectively. The blood glucose and potassium levels may then fall abruptly as glucose and potassium enter the cells to be utilized or converted to glycogen. When this occurs, glucose should be added to the I.V. fluids to prevent insulin shock and about 20 mEq KCl should be given each hour to prevent hypokalemia. While the patient is acidotic, the serum potassium levels tend to be normal or elevated; however, when the insulin begins to be effective, the potassium levels may fall abruptly not only because potassium follows glucose into the cells but also because of the fall in pH.

Adrenal Insufficiency

PITFALL

IF OCCULT ADRENAL INSUFFICIENCY IS NOT CONSIDERED AS A POSSIBLE CAUSE OF PERSISTENT SHOCK, PATIENTS MAY DIE FROM RELATIVELY MINOR TRAUMA WHEN THEY MIGHT HAVE BEEN EASILY SAVED BY ADMINISTRATION OF 200 MG HYDROCORTISONE I.V.

Any patient who has been taking steroids for at least several days in the past, especially during the previous six months, may have adrenal insufficiency. Although adrenal function may be minimal or absent, it may not be apparent clinically as long as there is no stress; however, even minor trauma in such individuals may cause severe cardiovascular collapse and shock. Whenever shock occurs or persists during or after surgery or trauma for no apparent reason, the possibility of adrenal insufficiency must be considered, and 200 mg of hydrocortisone given rapidly I.V. may be lifesaving.

The following regimen has been used successfully to manage trauma patients with possible adrenal insufficiency:

On the day of trauma:
100 to 200 mg I.V. hydrocortisone immediately and 100 mg every 6 to 12 hours in the I.V.s and another 100 to 200 mg during any surgery.
Second day:
Hydrocortisone 100 mg I.V. by slow drip in the I.V. every 12 hours.
Third day:
Hydrocortisone 75 mg I.V. by slow drip in the I.V. every 12 hours.
Fourth day:
(Assuming the patient is recovering well) Hydrocortisone 50 mg I.V. by slow drip in the I.V. every 12 hours.
Fifth day:
Steroids discontinued if the patient continues to recover well.

Hyperthyroidism

Rarely, a patient with latent or mild hyperthyroidism will develop a thyroid storm or crisis after trauma or surgery. The clinical picture may be extremely confusing unless the diagnosis is suspected. Treatment must be aggressive and the patient may require steroids, reserpine, iodine, fluids, hypothermia, and propranolol.[14–16]

NUTRITION IN THE TRAUMA PATIENT

In most patients, the metabolic consequences of trauma are not critical. The weight loss and negative nitrogen balance are usually reversed within a few days as the activity of the gastrointestinal tract is resumed and sufficient calories and protein are taken by mouth. However, in the severely traumatized or burned patient, or when complications develop, the negative nitrogen balance may continue for several weeks or longer. If a disorder or dysfunction of the alimentary tract is also present, the weight loss due to depletion of body protein and fat may be considerable, with a significant increase in mortality. Lawson[17] found that an acute loss of 30% of body weight within 30 days in severely ill surgical patients was uniformly fatal. Cahill[1] and Morgan[18] observed that rapid loss of approximately one-third of total body protein, even in normal individuals, was lethal.

Three methods that have been used to improve nutrition in patients with gastrointestinal problems after trauma include intravenous fat, elemental diets and I.V. hyperalimentation.

Intravenous Fat

It was widely felt for many years that it was impractical to supply total caloric requirements intravenously unless fat were included in the infusion. Intensive investigation led to the development of Lipomul. Although extremely beneficial at times, this 15% cottonseed-oil emulsion can, if used in large amounts for more than 10 to 14 days, cause anorexia, loss of weight, vomiting, gastrointestinal bleeding, hyperlipemia, anemia and thrombocytopenia. Prolonged coagulation times may also occur unrelated to the thrombocytopenia. As a result of these side effects the use of Lipomul was discontinued in the United States. Soybean oil emulsion (Intralipid) is better tolerated and is used widely in Europe.

Elemental Diets

In recent years the introduction of the elemental diets has been helpful in the management of patients who have undergone resection of long lengths of bowel or who have difficulties with absorption. Vivonex-100 HN supplies 1 gm of available nitrogen per 150 kcal (the basic formula used in parenteral hyperalimentation) and may be given orally or by tube feeding. Although it is a hyperosmolar solution (844 mOsm/L), it is well tolerated by most patients. All essential nutrients are provided in rapidly assimilated forms, including amino acids, simple sugars, essential fat, vitamins and minerals. Since this is rapidly and almost completely absorbed in the upper intestine, little bulk is presented to the colon—an advantage in selected cases with impaired function in the distal bowel.

Intravenous Hyperalimentation

PATIENT SELECTION. I.V. hyperalimentation is an excellent method for improving nutrition and healing in a wide variety of patients who cannot take an adequate quantity of calories or other nutrients by the usual routes.[19] However, it carries certain potentially lethal hazards that make meticulous supervision mandatory and preclude its routine use. Sepsis and the immediate post-traumatic period pose special problems. Both interfere significantly with the adequate utilization of glucose and increase the incidence of catheter complications. Since hyperosmotic solutions can cause a severe osmotic diuresis, I.V. hyperalimentation should not be started in the hypovolemic patient. Any signs of excessive fluid loss or reduced intravascular volume which develop during treatment should be rapidly corrected.

INTRAVENOUS LINES FOR HYPERALIMENTATION. *Location.* The tip of the intravenous catheter, usually of an 18-gauge size, must be placed in a vessel with a large enough flow rapidly to dilute the intravenous fluid to an osmolarity which is only slightly greater than normal. The veins most frequently used are the subclavian in adults and the external jugular in children. In both instances, the tip of the catheter is advanced until it is in or near the superior vena cava.

Techniques of Insertion.[20] During the insertion of the catheter the patient's head should be lowered and legs elevated (Trendelenburg position) to prevent air embolism and to distend the subclavian veins. Sterility cannot be stressed too strongly. These procedures should be performed with masks, gloves and drapes. A wide area around the proposed puncture site must be shaved, cleaned with soap or detergent, defatted with acetone, and painted with an antiseptic solution.

Once the catheter has been advanced to the desired location, it should be secured in place with a skin suture tied snugly around the catheter several times. All I.V. connections are taped to prevent inadvertent disconnection of the catheter or tubing and consequent air embolism. In children up to three or four years, the catheter is usually brought out through a skin tunnel onto the scalp. A radiopaque catheter should be used so that x-ray confirmation of its position can be readily obtained. A topical antibiotic ointment is then put over the puncture site and the area covered with a dry waterproof dressing. This dressing should be changed every two to three days or more often if it gets wet or dirty. Whenever the dressing is changed, complete sterile precautions must be employed. The skin around the puncture site should be defatted with acetone and new antibiotic ointment applied.

Management of the Catheter. Ideally, the catheter used for hyperalimentation should not be used for anything else, e.g. monitoring of central venous pressure, drawing of blood or delivering of medications or transfusions. In most patients, the catheter can be kept in place and managed for many weeks with meticulous care. We have used simple gravity infusion without a pump in adults and have been satisfied that the infusion rate can be kept relatively constant by checking the drip chamber every 15 to 30 minutes. Since the catheter used in infants is smaller and the need for accuracy of infusion much more critical, a constant infusion pump is often used in children younger than two to three years.

SOLUTION USED. Although different formulas are available, the basic solution used for I.V. hyperalimentation consists of a 5% protein or fibrin hydrolysate· in 5% glucose water with enough 50% glucose added to bring the caloric content up to about one calorie per ml. The amount of KCl and NaCl added will vary according to the electrolyte levels and losses in each patient and may change greatly from day to day. A number of other hyperalimentation fluids for special purposes are now being given.[21]

AMOUNTS USED. There are individual variations in the amount of hyperalimentation fluid metabolized in the early stages. The average amount tolerated initially per day is about 1500 ml in adult females and 2000 ml in adult males, but a period of adjustment may be required. Not uncommonly, the I.V. hyperalimentation will uncover a latent diabetic. If spill of glucose in the urine or diuresis is excessive, the intake can be temporarily reduced by 500 ml per day and insulin added to increase glucose utilization. If the insulin does not reduce the glycosuria to at least 3+, the intake of hyperalimentation fluid must be reduced accordingly. The insulin to cover the glycosuria can be given subcutaneously; however, after several days when the insulin needs have been stabilized, more consistent control may be obtained by adding up to

40 units of regular insulin to each liter of solution.

If the patient does not have excessive glycosuria (3+ or more), hyperglycemia (200 mg/100 ml or more) and/or polyuria, the amount of I.V. hyperalimentation solution given can be advanced about 200 to 300 ml per day. Relatively few problems are encountered while increasing the infusion rate to 3000 calories per day; advances beyond this level, however, are often more difficult.

PATIENT MONITORING. Maximum benefit from hyperalimentation can be obtained only if the patient's response is monitored closely. The most important measurements to follow are urine output, urine and blood glucose levels, weight and serum electrolytes.

Urine Output

PITFALL

IF THE URINE OUTPUT IS NOT MONITORED CLOSELY WHEN THE I.V. HYPERALIMENTATION IS STARTED, SEVERE OSMOTIC DIURESIS, DEHYDRATION, AND HYPEROSMOLAR STATES MAY NOT BE APPRECIATED UNTIL COMA OR HYPOTENSION DEVELOPS.

Osmotic diuresis in some patients may be sufficient to produce dehydration and shock. Fluid intake should usually exceed the measured total output by at least 20 to 30 ml per hour. Not uncommonly, however, there will be an increased urine output in relation to intake for the first few days because of mobilization of previously administered fluid. If this fluid loss is not excessive, the same infusion rate can be continued and insulin added if necessary, until the patient's metabolic and renal systems adapt. If dehydration or hypovolemia begins to develop, large amounts of additional fluid should be given and the I.V. hyperalimentation reduced.

Urine and Blood Glucose. The glucose levels are measured in all urine samples at least every four hours. Glycosuria of 3+

and 4+ may cause excessive osmotic diuresis and should be corrected. A glycosuria of 4+ is of marked significance in that it may reflect a urinary glucose concentration well in excess of 2.0 gm/100 ml and is, therefore, not an accurate gauge. Hyperglycemia is usually not a problem unless it exceeds 300 mg/100 ml.

PITFALL

IF RELIANCE IS PLACED ON THE DEGREE OF GLYCOSURIA TO REGULATE INSULIN COVERAGE IN ELDERLY PATIENTS AND THOSE WITH RENAL DISEASE, DANGEROUS ELEVATIONS OF BLOOD GLUCOSE MAY BE MISSED.

Elderly patients and patients with renal disease not uncommonly have a high renal threshold for glucose and can have rather severe hyperglycemia with little or no glycosuria.

Weight. The patient should be weighed daily, making appropriate corrections for dressings and tubes. A weight loss of up to 0.5 kg per day for the first three to five days can be expected. Greater weight loss than this, however, may indicate a need to reduce the amount of hyperalimentation and/or increase the intake of colloid, blood, or fluids. If the patient gains weight in the first few days, the possibility of fluid overload must obviously be considered.

Electrolytes. Serum and urine electrolyte concentrations must be studied daily for the first week and at least twice a week thereafter. The serum potassium should be observed especially closely, as it tends to fall during I.V. hyperalimentation because of the polyuria and the intracellular binding of potassium as glucose enters the cells. Occasional patients require over 160 mEq KCl a day to maintain normal potassium levels. If the urine sodium concentration falls below 20 to 40 mEq/L, the patient may need additional quantities of a balanced electrolyte or colloid solution, especially if he is oliguric.

FAILURES AND COMPLICATIONS. Results

with I.V. hyperalimentation improve with practice and the physician should not be discouraged by any initial failures or complications. The most important problems include mechanical catheter complications, polyuria, glucose intolerance, and infection.

Mechanical Complications with the I.V. Catheter. Some of the problems which may occur with the introduction of a subclavian vein catheter or its management include pneumothorax, incorrect positioning, puncture of the subclavian artery, catheter embolism, and air embolism.

PNEUMOTHORAX. The incidence of pneumothorax can be reduced by keeping suction on the needle during its insertion parallel to the medial third of the clavicle, with the tip directed toward a point just behind the sternoclavicular junction.

PITFALL

IF A CHEST X-RAY IS NOT TAKEN TO CONFIRM THE ACCURACY OF PLACEMENT OF A CATHETER IN THE SUBCLAVIAN VEIN, PNEUMOTHORAX, HYDROTHORAX, OR INCORRECT POSITIONING WILL BE MISSED.

A radiograph of the chest should always be taken after the procedure to exclude pneumothorax and to confirm the position of the catheter. Any pneumothorax which may have occurred can usually be managed with a small chest tube or catheter inserted into the pleural cavity and attached to a water seal. The technique for insertion has been well described by Wilmore and Dudrick.[20]

INCORRECT POSITIONING OF THE CATHETER. The tip of the catheter must be checked as it may turn up into the internal jugular vein or pass through the vein to lie in the pleural cavity with consequent development of hydrothorax when fluid is given.

PUNCTURE OF THE SUBCLAVIAN ARTERY. The subclavian artery may be entered, but, if this is recognized and the needle withdrawn, complications are exceedingly rare. The chances of entering the artery are reduced by keeping the needle and syringe parallel to the floor during insertion.

CATHETER EMBOLISM. The catheter should never be withdrawn while the needle tip is subcutaneous. Both needle and catheter should be withdrawn as a single unit to prevent transection of the catheter by the sharp needle tip. When catheter embolism is suspected, the catheter should be identified on plain x-ray or angiography and removed.

AIR EMBOLISM. Air embolism is an ever-present hazard if the I.V. tubing is accidentally disconnected. It is, therefore, vital to tape and properly secure the catheter and connecting I.V. tubing. If any disconnection is recognized and corrected immediately, there may be only a temporary shortness of breath; if the problem is not discovered rapidly, sudden death may result.

Air embolism is more likely to be fatal if the patient is sitting or standing when the catheter becomes disconnected because the lower intrathoracic pressure in these positions allows a greater volume of air to enter the open catheter. It has been found that up to 100 ml of air per second may pass through an 18-gauge subclavian catheter if the same venous-atmospheric pressure differential is present as might be expected in an erect patient. If air embolism does occur, the patient should be placed on his left side with his legs elevated[22] and an attempt should be made to aspirate the air by advancing a catheter or a needle into the right ventricle.

Polyuria

PITFALL

IF I.V. HYPERALIMENTATION IS STARTED ON AN ELDERLY, SEPTIC OR DIABETIC PATIENT WITHIN TWO TO FIVE DAYS OF TRAUMA, IT MAY BE EXTREMELY DIFFICULT TO MANAGE THE FLUID INTAKE AND DIFFERENTIATE AMONG THE VARIOUS CAUSES OF POLYURIA.

Not uncommonly, large volumes of urine may be excreted while the patient is on I.V. hyperalimentation, especially during the first few days. This polyuria may be due to hyperosmolar diuresis, fluid overload, or mobilization of previously administered fluid. Osmolality studies of the serum and urine may be of value in diagnosing the cause of the polyuria.

HYPEROSMOLAR DIURESIS. We have had several patients who developed urine outputs exceeding 150 ml/hr when their blood glucose levels rose above 300 mg/100 ml. All these patients responded to slowing of the infusion and/or addition of insulin. Diabetic patients are much more labile and prone to develop hyperosmolar coma. This was well illustrated in a recent dehydrated diabetic with a small bowel fistula, a blood glucose of 1500 mg/100 ml and a serum sodium of 162 mEq/L. She required 12 liters of fluid and large doses of insulin over a 24-hour period before she regained consciousness.

FLUID OVERLOAD. Additional balanced electrolyte solution fluid is usually required at the beginning of I.V. hyperalimentation because of the osmotic diuresis that almost invariably occurs. On the other hand, in the effort to prevent dehydration from this diuresis, too much fluid can easily be given. Under these circumstances, it may be difficult to differentiate the polyuria due to osmotic diuresis from that due to overload. Later, when the patient begins to accommodate to the increased glucose load and the volume of I.V. hyperalimentation fluid is increased, other I.V. fluids must be tapered off to prevent overhydration.

MOBILIZATION OF PREVIOUSLY ADMINISTERED FLUID. During initial treatment, patients with moderate to severe trauma or sepsis often require large amounts of fluid, much of which is retained in an expanded "third space." Between the second and fifth day of recovery, much of this fluid may be rapidly mobilized. When the trauma or sepsis is severe or complications develop, the mobilization may be greatly delayed. If I.V. hyperalimentation is started during or just prior to this mobilization of "third-space" fluid, the resultant polyuria may exceed five to six liters per day for several days. Attempts to correct for this polyuria (because of a mistaken impression that the patient has an excessive osmolar diuresis) can cause serious overloading.

Glucose Intolerance. Although glucose intolerance is unusual when the increase in I.V. hyperalimentation is gradual, problems tend to occur in four groups: diabetics, patients with recent trauma, septic patients, and the elderly. The management of patients with two or more of these factors may be especially troublesome.

DIABETES. In general, diabetics tend to have widely fluctuating levels of blood glucose, glycosuria and an osmolar diuresis which are often difficult to correct. It is often necessary to increase the amount of glucose very gradually and to use large doses of insulin. I.V. fructose has been advised by some authors for the more difficult diabetics;[23] however, fructose is more expensive, requires more elaborate preparation, and in the long run has no advantage over glucose.[24]

TRAUMA. During the first two to four days after moderate to severe trauma, a temporary glucose intolerance is common.[25] We prefer to wait until this phase is over and the patient is fully stabilized before starting I.V. hyperalimentation. If it is considered important to start early, insulin in fairly large doses may be necessary. Furthermore, the rapidly changing glucose tolerance will require daily alteration of insulin and extremely careful monitoring. While the insulin needs are so unstable, we give the regular insulin subcutaneously according to the blood and urine levels rather than adding specific amounts to the I.V. solutions.

SEPSIS. Septic patients may develop significant hyperglycemia and glycosuria on as little as 150 to 200 gm glucose per day. The I.V. glucose tolerance curves are very similar to those found in diabetics. As soon as the sepsis is controlled by drainage of pus or by antibiotics, the blood glucose levels usually come down to more normal levels and large doses of insulin are no longer necessary.

AGE. The elderly develop hyperglycemia easily and, because of this high renal threshold, blood glucose determinations are particularly important in this group. Because of this tendency to hyperglycemia, the I.V. hyperalimentation should be increased in the aged slowly and cautiously.

Infection. If a patient on I.V. alimentation develops a fever above 101 F without evident cause, the I.V. catheter is removed and cultures are taken from the blood, the catheter tip and the fluid in the tubing. Where I.V. hyperalimentation is considered essential for the patient, another I.V. catheter is inserted at a different site.

The problem is much more difficult when the patient is septic before the hyperalimentation is started. A continued febrile course may be due to: (1) the underlying sepsis, (2) an infected sleeve thrombus around the catheter, (3) infection at the site of insertion in the skin and subcutaneous tissue, or (4) contaminated fluid. If doubt exists as to the origin of the continued fever, it may be wise to switch to 10% dextrose in water and watch the patient carefully; if there is no improvement, the catheter should be removed.

Controversy continues about the risk of candidiasis from I.V. hyperalimentation.[26-28] Of 40 recent patients who have had I.V. hyperalimentation under our direct control, two have had positive blood cultures for Candida. Both patients had been on large doses of multiple antibiotics for long periods of time, and Candida was grown from all orifices in addition to the blood. The catheter was removed in both cases; one patient improved rapidly without further therapy but the other, who had been on I.V. hyperalimentation for only three days, died in spite of treatment with amphotericin B. Ellis and Spivak[26] recommend that the central venous catheter be removed as soon as candidiasis is proved by blood culture; if a blood culture on the following

3

day is also positive for C. albicans, amphotericin should be given.

FLUID AND ELECTROLYTE CHANGES IN TRAUMA

Sodium and Water Retention

PITFALL

IF HYPONATREMIA (IN A PREVIOUSLY NORMAL TRAUMA PATIENT) IS ASSUMED TO BE DUE TO A TOTAL BODY DEFICIT IN SODIUM AND IS TREATED WITH NORMAL SALINE, THE PATIENT MAY BE OVERLOADED WITH FLUID VERY RAPIDLY.

Patients tend to retain salt and water after trauma. Water retention is due primarily to increased ADH secretion, while salt retention is caused mainly by an increased secretion of corticosteroids. This may be particularly dangerous in the patient with cardiac, renal or liver disease. Since the retention of water is relatively greater than salt, the trauma patient tends, in spite of a normal or increased total body content of sodium, to develop a dilutional hyponatremia.[10]

The injured tissues may be regarded as a sponge, silently accumulating large quantities of sodium and water which are not available to the rest of the body for at least two to three days. This salt and water retention can be especially difficult to manage in the very young and very old, who are easily overloaded. If the trauma is severe, if complications or sepsis develop, or if the patient is old or debilitated, the mobilization of this fluid may be greatly delayed. Later, when the retained fluid is mobilized from the patient's expanded third space, the fluid intake must be carefully reduced.

Hyperkalemia

Following trauma, there is an extensive release of potassium into the blood which, in spite of hemodilution and an increased excretion of potassium in the urine, usually results in a significant rise in serum potassium levels. Some of the increased potassium comes from cells damaged by trauma or hypoxia, and some is derived from muscle which has been catabolized to meet the energy needs caused by the trauma and fasting.

Since potassium and nitrogen are stored in muscle in a ratio of approximately 3 : 1, catabolism of muscle protein would be expected to result in an excretion of these two substances in a similar proportion. In most studies, however, potassium is excreted in much greater quantities than nitrogen. Some of this excess potassium may be that stored with glycogen and released as the glycogen is metabolized. Similarly, during the subsequent period of repair, potassium is retained by the body in amounts greater than would be predicted on the basis of nitrogen retention. This may reflect the movement of potassium into the cell as glycogen is synthesized.

Fluid and Electrolyte Replacement in Trauma

No rigid formula for fluid replacement can be devised. If basic principles are observed and intelligent interpretation is made of simple laboratory measurements, fluid and electrolyte balance can usually be maintained quite well. Fluid needs should be considered under three separate headings: (1) replacement of basic needs, (2) replacement of current losses, and (3) correction of deficits and prior losses.

REPLACEMENT OF BASIC NEEDS. The basic needs to be replaced include the urinary output and insensible water loss. The urine usually consists of 600 to 1500 ml of fluid with a highly variable content depending on the electrolyte intake, blood volume, renal perfusion, and status of the kidneys. Under most circumstances, however, the urine sodium and chloride concentrations will average 40 to 100 mEq/L. Insensible water loss (as evaporation from the skin and lung) amounts to about 300 to 800 ml of pure water per day. Thus, an intake of 2000 to 2500 of 5% glucose/0.3 normal saline will adequately replace the basic I.V. needs of most adult patients. Since trauma tends to cause a retention of salt and water, the amount of sodium and fluid given should be reduced in older patients, especially in those with cardiac, renal, or hepatic disease. Because of the elevated serum levels, potassium is usually not added to the I.V. fluids until the third day, unless there is excessive diuresis or hypokalemia. In general, we increase the amount of I.V. fluid given to adults if the patient is septic or if the urine output is less than 35 ml/hr, and we will tend to reduce intake if the urine output exceeds 75 ml/hr and the patient is not septic (Chap. 30).

REPLACEMENT OF CURRENT LOSSES. Replacement of continuing losses can usually be calculated readily by measuring the intake and output of the patient in terms of both volume and electrolyte content. It is essential that there be an accurate measurement and recording of all gastrointestinal fluid losses, including drainage from nasogastric tubes, biliary T-tubes, ileostomies, and colostomies. Dressings soaked with drainage from fistulae must be weighed. Nasogastric secretions can be replaced, volume for volume, with 5% glucose/0.5 normal saline solutions, and drainage of biliary and most other body fluids can usually be replaced by 5% glucose in normal saline or Ringer's lactate. All fluid given to replace gastrointestinal fluid losses should contain 20 mEq of potassium per liter of I.V. fluid.

CORRECTION OF DEFICIT AND PRIOR LOSSES. No exact formula can be provided for calculating deficits or prior losses, but if the patient seems to be mildly, moderately, or severely dehydrated we estimate that he has lost about 6, 8, or 10% of his body weight respectively. This fluid should be replaced with saline or Ringer's lactate. At least half the fluid deficit is replaced prior to emergency surgery, about a fourth during the surgery, and a fourth later. A severely dehydrated 80-kg man who needs emergency surgery would usually, there-

fore, be given at least 4 liters of 5% glucose in Ringer's lactate or saline prior to surgery, 2 liters during surgery, and 2 liters after surgery.

Deficits of sodium and chloride are calculated in terms of the extracellular fluid space (20% of body weight) while bicarbonate deficits are calculated in terms of 30% of body weight. Thus, a 70-kg man with a serum sodium concentration of 120 mEq/L, a chloride of 70 mEq/L, a CO_2 content of 15 mEq/L, and an estimated extracellular fluid space of 14 liters (20% × 70 kg) has a calculated total sodium deficit of 280 mEq (14 L × 20 mEq/L), a total chloride deficit of 420 mEq (14 L × 30 mEq/L), and a bicarbonate deficit of 210 mEq (21 L × 10 mEq/L). As a rough guide, 50 to 100 mEq of potassium will raise the serum concentration by 1 mEq/L.

PITFALL

IF CHRONIC SEVERE FLUID AND ELECTROLYTE ABNORMALITIES ARE CORRECTED TOO RAPIDLY AFTER TRAUMA OR PRIOR TO SURGERY, THE SUDDEN CHEMICAL CHANGES CAN CAUSE SEVERE DETERIORATION OR DEATH.

It is extremely dangerous to try to correct chronic electrolyte abnormalities very rapidly in patients with trauma, especially if these changes have developed slowly over periods of months or years. Patients seem to have gradually adjusted to these abnormalities and their homeostatic mechanisms have been reset to operate in a different chemical environment. Thus, the patient who has been on a low salt diet and diuretics for many months or years gradually adapts to sodium levels as low as 105 to 110 mEq/L, which may be fatal if they develop acutely. Rapid addition of concentrated or normal saline to such individuals may cause severe congestive heart failure or pulmonary edema.

In treating multiple fluid and electrolyte deficits, a certain priority for correction is essential. Restoration of blood volume is the most urgent need, followed in importance by correction of pH, potassium, sodium, and chloride in that order. It is better to have the patient live with a chronic imbalance than to have him die with normal electrolyte values.

REFERENCES

1. Cahill, G. F., Jr.: Body fuels and their metabolism. Bull. Amer. Coll. Surg., 20:12, 1970.
2. Rosenberg, J. C., et al.: Studies on hemorrhagic and endotoxin shock in relation to vasomotor changes and endogenous circulating epinephrine, norepinephrine and serotonin. Ann. Surg., 154:611, 1961.
3. Egdahl, R. H.: Pituitary-adrenal response following trauma to the isolated leg. Surgery, 46:9, 1959.
4. Ahlquist, R. P.: A study of adrenotropic receptors. Amer. J. Physiol., 153:596, 1948.
5. Skinner, S. L., McCubbin, J. W., and Page, I. H.: Renal baroceptor control of renin secretion. Science, 141:814, 1963.
6. Davis, J. O., et al.: Evidence for secretion of an aldosterone stimulating hormone by the kidney. J. Clin. Invest., 40:684, 1961.
7. Bartler, F. C., et al.: Studies on control and physiological action of aldosterone. Recent Progr. Hormone Res., 15:275, 1959.
8. Henry, J. P., and Pearce, J. W.: The possible role of cardiac atrial stretch receptors in the induction of changes in urine flow. J. Physiol., 131:572, 1956.
9. Verney, E. B.: The antidiuretic hormone and the factors which determine its release. Proc. Roy. Soc. B, 135:25, 1947.
10. Moore, F. D.: Metabolic Care of the Surgical Patient. Philadelphia, W. B. Saunders, 1960.
11. Kinney, J. M.: Proceedings of a Conference on Energy Metabolism and Body Fuel Utilization. Cambridge, Harvard Univ. Press, 1966.
12. Sutherland, E. W., and Rall, T. W.: The relationship of adenosine 3–5 phosphate and phosphorylase to the action of catecholamines and other hormones. Pharmacol. Rev., 12:265, 1960.
13. Holden, W. O., et al.: The effect of nutrition on metabolism in the surgical patient. Ann. Surg., 146:563, 1957.
14. Harrison, T. S.: The treatment of thyroid storm. Surg. Gynec. Obstet., 121:837, 1965.
15. Hughes, G.: Management of thyrotoxic crisis with a beta-adrenergic blocking agent (Pronetrabe). Brit. J. Clin. Pract., 20:579, 1966.
16. Rosenberg, J. C., and Cushner, G.: Biochemical basis of thyroid crisis. Amer. Surg., 31:354, 1965.
17. Lawson, L. J.: Parenteral nutrition in surgery. Brit. J. Surg., 52:795, 1965.
18. Morgan, A., Filler, R. M., and Moore, F. E.: Surgical nutrition. Med. Clin. N. Amer., 54:1367, 1970.
19. Dudrick, S. J., et al.: Long term parenteral nutrition with growth, development and positive nitrogen balance. Surgery, 64:134, 1968.
20. Wilmore, D. W., and Dudrick, S. J.: Safe long-term venous catheterization. Arch. Surg., 98:256, 1969.
21. Dudrick, S. J., and Ruberg, R. L.: Principles and practice of parenteral nutrition. Gastroenterology, 61:901, 1971.
22. Durant, T. M., Long, J., and Oppenheimer, M. J.: Pulmonary (venous) air embolism. Amer. Heart J., 33:269, 1947.
23. Miller, M., et al.: Intravenous fructose and glucose in normal and diabetics. J. Clin. Invest., 31:115, 1952.
24. Bonerjee, S.: Studies in the comparative utilization of glucose, fructose and galactose in alloxan–diabetes. Indian J. Med. Res., 46:269, 1958.
25. Ross, H., et al.: Effect of abdominal operation on glucose tolerance and serum levels of insulin, growth hormone, and hydrocortisone. Lancet, 2:563, 1966.
26. Ellis, C. A., and Spivak, M. L.: The significance of candidemia. Ann. Intern. Med., 67:511, 1967.
27. Aschcraft, K. W., and Leape, L. L.: Candida sepsis complicating parenteral feeding. JAMA, 212:454, 1970.
28. Curry, C. R., and Quie, P. O.: Fungal septicemia in patients receiving parenteral hyperalimentation. New Eng. J. Med., 285:1221, 1971.

Suggested Reading

1. Yates, F. E., Russell, S. M., and Dallman, M. F.: Potentiation by vasopressin of corticotrophin release induced by corticotrophin-releasing factor. Endocrinology, 88:3, 1971.
2. McNamara, J. J., et al.: Intravenous hyperalimentation: An important adjunct in the treatment of combat casualties. Amer. J. Surg., 122:70, 1971.
3. Travis, S. F., et al.: Alterations of red-cell glycolytic intermediates and oxygen transport as a consequence of hypophosphatemia in patients receiving intravenous hyperalimentation. New Eng. J. Med., 285:763, 1971.
4. Curry, C. R., and Quie, P. G.: Fungal septicemia in patients receiving parenteral hyperalimentation. New Eng. J. Med., 285:1221, 1971.
5. Greenstein, A. J., and Dreiling, D. A.: Nonketotic hyperosmolar coma in the postoperative patient. Amer. J. Surg., 121:698, 1971.
6. Flanigan, W. J., et al.: The surgical significance of hyperosmolar coma. Amer. J. Surg., 120:652, 1970.
7. Stephens, R. V., and Randall, H. T.: Use of concentrated, balanced liquid elemental diet for nutritional management of catabolic states. Ann. Surg., 170:642, 1969.
8. Hakansson, I.: Experience in long-term studies on nine intravenous fat emulsions in dogs. Nutr. Dieta, 10:54, 1968.

9. McNamara, J. J., et al.: Hyperglycemic response to trauma in combat casualties. J.
Trauma, 11:337, 1971.

10. LaBrosse, E. H., and Cowley, R. A.: Tissue
levels of catecholamines in patients with different types of trauma. J. Trauma, 13:61, 1973.

11. Steiger, E., et al.: Postoperative intravenous
nutrition: Effects on body weight, protein regeneration, wound healing, and liver morphology. Surgery, 73:686, 1973.

12. Pindyck, F., et al.: Cardiorespiratory effects
of hypertonic glucose in the critically ill patient. Surgery, 75:11, 1974.

13. Woodruff, P., et al.: Corticosteroid treatment
of major trauma. Arch. Surg., 107:613, 1973.

14. Johnson, W. C.: Oral elemental diet. Arch.
Surg., 108:32, 1974.

5 SHOCK DUE TO TRAUMA

R. F. WILSON
L. P. LEBLANC
A. J. WALT

"When you can measure what you are speaking about . . ., you know something about it, but when you cannot measure it, your knowledge is of a very meagre kind."

LORD KELVIN

DEFINITION

"Shock" is a much abused word, and has been used to describe clinical entities of widely diverse origins and manifestations. Although it is generally defined as a state associated with poor tissue perfusion, shock cannot always be ascribed to poor blood flow alone. It is probably best thought of as a problem related to poor or inadequate cell metabolism.

PITFALL

IF SHOCK IS NOT SUSPECTED OR DIAGNOSED UNTIL THE PATIENT DEVELOPS OVERT HYPOTENSION, CYANOSIS AND A COLD, CLAMMY SKIN, TREATMENT MAY BECOME EXTREMELY DIFFICULT.

Even today, many of the concepts concerning the pathophysiology of shock are tied to ideas which have been discredited by modern clinical investigations. When this is not appreciated, physicians may fail to recognize the syndrome and the need for urgent treatment. For example, patients with septic shock often have a warm, pink skin in contrast to the classic picture of a cold, clammy, cyanotic skin. Patients with severe hypovolemic and cardiac problems usually have a reduced cardiac output and are vasoconstricted while most patients with uncomplicated sepsis have a normal or increased output.[1,2]

While full-blown shock is easily recognized by most laymen, early or impending shock may be missed by even the most experienced clinician. Physicians who may treat patients with severe trauma must train themselves to recognize incipient shock and to forestall by prompt and vigorous therapy any tendency for the changes to become irreversible. If treatment is to be logical, intelligent, and effective, recognition of the problem must occur almost spontaneously and the underlying physiologic responses must be understood clearly.

ETIOLOGY

Hypovolemia

In the early phases following trauma, shock is usually associated with a reduction in the circulating blood volume. The amount of blood or fluid that a patient can lose before he goes into shock varies greatly from individual to individual but depends primarily on the rate at which the loss occurs and the patient's health prior to injury. Nevertheless, an acute blood loss of 1000 to 1500 ml in less than 30 to 60 minutes will cause some degree of shock in most patients.

Massive blood loss externally or into the peritoneal or pleural spaces is usually readily appreciated and corrected. Bleeding into the retroperitoneal spaces, mesentery, muscles, and other tissues, however, is often not recognized; consequently, it may be treated inadequately. A fractured pelvis, for example, may result in a local loss of more than 2000 ml of blood, while bleeding from a fractured humerus or femur may exceed 1000 ml.

Cardiac Shock

Pump failure or cardiac shock following trauma may be caused in two ways. Direct injury to the chest may cause myocardial contusion, pericardial tamponade, septal rupture, or valvular insufficiency. More frequently, however, the myocardial damage following trauma results from hypotension caused by blood loss in a patient with diseased coronary arteries. If the patient has severe coronary-artery narrowing or occlusion, even mild transient hypotension may cause myocardial damage or an infarction and can severely compound what may have previously been relatively mild shock due to blood loss alone.

Sepsis

Shock due to sepsis seldom occurs in the first 24 to 48 hours following trauma unless preexisting infection is present. While atelectasis alone can cause high fever in the early postoperative period, it seldom causes shock by itself except in the most critically ill or injured patients. Massive spillage of gastrointestinal contents, especially from the colon and more especially when driven into the tissues (as may occur with shotgun injuries), can also cause relatively early severe sepsis. Suppurative thrombophlebitis

around I.V. catheters and generalized peritonitis with a leaking gastrointestinal anastomosis should be suspected if the patient suddenly becomes markedly septic three or four days after surgery.

Neurogenic Shock

PITFALL

IF SHOCK IS ATTRIBUTED TO HEAD INJURY, SEVERE BLEEDING ELSEWHERE, ESPECIALLY IN THE ABDOMEN, IS APT TO BE MISSED.

Neurogenic factors are often listed with the more common causes of shock. In our opinion, however, neurogenic shock is an extremely overworked diagnosis; it is rarely encountered in clinical practice except as a very transient phenomenon. Brain damage from direct trauma, ischemia, or hypoxia tends to produce increased intracranial pressure with a resultant reflex rise in blood pressure. It is not until the patient is preterminal that damage to the central nervous system causes hypotension. Any shock resulting from head trauma is usually due to massive blood loss from lacerations of the scalp or face.

PHYSIOLOGIC CHANGES

Early Shock (Fig. 1)

VASOCONSTRICTION AND BLOOD FLOW TO VITAL ORGANS. The physiologic changes which occur in early shock are compensatory mechansims designed to maintain an adequate blood flow to the brain and heart. These changes, mediated mainly through the sympathetic nervous system, consist primarily of arterial and venous vasoconstriction and an increase in the rate and force of myocardial contraction. The vasoconstriction is selective initially, and is greatest in those vessels supplying the tissues most resistant to hypoxia, e.g. the skin and kidneys.

The classical clinical picture of hypovolemic or cardiac shock is that of a nervous,

TRAUMA

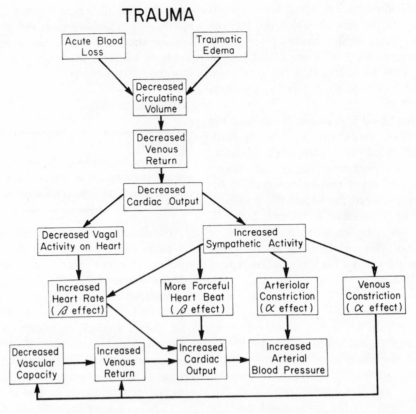

FIG. 1. In early shock following trauma, acute blood loss and edema into traumatized tissue result in decreased venous return which is compensated for primarily by increased sympathetic stimulation of the heart and blood vessels.

anxious patient with a cold clammy skin, a rapid, thready pulse and oliguria. The sympathetic stimulation of the central nervous system causes the nervousness and anxiety. Stimulation of the sweat glands causes the skin to be moist, and the poor blood flow causes it to be cool. Cold clammy skin is a valuable sign to the clinician because, regardless of the blood pressure, it strongly implies that the patient has excessive vasoconstriction and poor tissue perfusion which should be corrected rapidly.

In the normal individual, about 15% of the blood volume is in the pulmonary vascular system. Of the blood in the systemic circuit, about 60% is located in the larger (capacitance) veins.[3] Constriction of the arteries and veins may reduce vascular capacity by as much as 10 to 20% and in-

creases the rate and amount of blood return to the heart. This vascular constriction alone can account for much of the ability to tolerate a loss of up to 15 to 25% of the blood volume with minimal ill effects.

PITFALL

IF A PATIENT WITH ACUTE MULTIPLE TRAUMA IS GIVEN MEPERIDINE, MORPHINE, OR A SIMILAR NARCOTIC BEFORE IT IS ASCERTAINED THAT HIS BLOOD VOLUME IS ADEQUATE, HE MAY DEVELOP SEVERE HYPOTENSION OR SHOCK FROM THE INCREASE IN VASCULAR CAPACITANCE.

Impairment of cardiovascular reflexes seen with the use of morphine, meperidine, chlorpromazine, or other drugs may result in a severe discrepancy between blood volume and vascular capacity in the hypovolemic patient, with a consequent precipitous drop in blood pressure.

In an effort to create a conceptual model to facilitate understanding of some of the hemodynamic changes occurring in shock, it may be helpful to think of the cardiovascular system as having two types of receptors, alpha and beta.[4] This theoretical concept is not demonstrable anatomically but is of great help in formulating a rational physiologic and pharmacologic approach to the neural and hormonal control of the heart and blood vessels. According to Ahlquist,[4] the alpha receptors in blood vessels respond to nerve or blood-borne cathecholamines by vasoconstriction. There are essentially no alpha receptors in the brain and only a few in the heart. These receptors have their greatest concentration in the tissues with the greatest resistance to hypoxia. The beta receptors are stimulated only by blood-borne catecholamines and respond peripherally with a mild arteriolar vasodilation in striated muscle and venous constriction; centrally they cause an increase in the rate and force of myocardial contraction. Whereas isoproterenol (Isuprel) is a pure beta-stimulating drug, epinephrine exercises its effects equally on both alpha and beta receptors, and norepinephrine is predominantly alpha stimulating.

HYPOTENSION. In the previously normal individual, a systolic blood pressure below 80 mm Hg usually indicates shock. The weak, thready pulse often seen in hypovolemic or cardiac shock is frequently associated with a low pulse pressure and is primarily the result of a low cardiac output and stroke volume.

PITFALL

PARADOXICALLY, IF VASOPRESSOR DRUGS ARE INDISCRIMINATELY GIVEN TO PATIENTS WITH AN UNOBTAINABLE (CUFF) BLOOD PRESSURE, DANGEROUS EXCESSIVE VASOCONSTRICTION MAY BE PRODUCED IN A PATIENT WHO IS ALREADY NORMOTENSIVE OR HYPERTENSIVE.

It may be dangerous to assume that a blood pressure unobtainable by a cuff technique is extremely low. The so-called unobtainable blood pressure or pulse may be deceptive, for, while it is usually associated with severe hypotension and systolic pressures less than 50 mm Hg, about 5 to 10% of such patients actually have a normal or increased blood pressure when it is measured directly intra-arterially; one patient on our service had an intra-arterial blood pressure of 260/140. The ease with which the pulse is felt or heard when taking a blood pressure with a sphygmomanometer is directly related to the pulse pressure which, in turn, is usually directly related to the stroke volume. If the stroke volume is too small, the vibrations produced as blood escapes past the portion of artery constricted by the sphygmomanometer are too low in amplitude to be audible, and the expansion of the artery during systole may be too small to produce a palpable pulse. The pulse pressure is of less value in elderly patients because their inelastic aortas and arteries can cause a high pulse pressure even if the stroke volume is very low.

If the blood pressure is unobtainable for more than 5 to 10 minutes in patients who, by all clinical and objective criteria, have had adequate blood-volume replacement, an effort should be made to measure the pressure with an 18-gauge or similar catheter in the radial or femoral arteries. (Although special Teflon catheters are preferable, a regular 18-gauge venous catheter can be used.) We prefer the radial artery because it is more accessible during abdominal surgery. If transducers are available for measuring the pressure, they should be used; however, the arterial pressure can also be measured with a system similar to that used for monitoring the CVP (Fig. 2). This system consists of a series of I.V. tubes connected to make a column extending at least 60 to 80 inches above the midaxillary line of the patient. This tubing is attached to a tall I.V. pole and connected by a three-way stopcock to the arterial

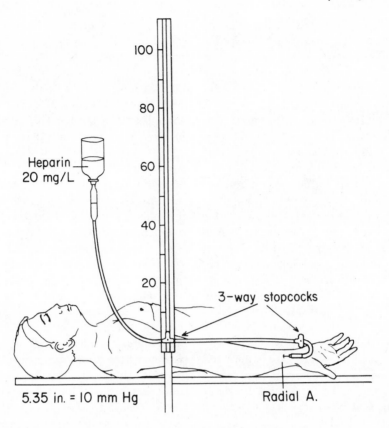

FIG. 2. The arterial blood pressure may be determined directly by a method similar to that used for measuring central venous pressure. 5.35 inches of saline is equivalent to 10 mm Hg pressure.

catheter and to a flush bottle containing normal saline with 20 mg heparin per liter. The measuring column is filled and the stopcock turned so that it is in continuity with the arterial catheter. The column of saline will then fall until its pressure is equivalent to the mean arterial pressure. The measuring column is calibrated, with every 5.35 inches above the midaxillary line representing 10 mm Hg mean arterial pressure. With each heartbeat the height of the column of saline will rise and fall a few millimeters. The mean arterial pressure is usually equal to the diastolic pressure plus about 30% of the pulse pressure. Thus if the systolic/diastolic BP is 120/80, the mean pressure is about 92 mm Hg.

HYPERVENTILATION

Patients in early or mild shock, especially from trauma or sepsis, usually have a mild

---

PITFALL

IF SODIUM BICARBONATE IS GIVEN INDISCRIMINATELY TO PATIENTS IN SHOCK, A SEVERE COMBINED ALKALOSIS WITH RESULTANT ARRHYTHMIAS OR CARDIAC ARREST MAY BE PRODUCED.

---

to moderate respiratory alkalosis, with little or no metabolic acidosis. The severe combined alkalosis which may result if sodium bicarbonate is given can suddenly reduce the concentration of ionized calcium and cause cardiovascular collapse. Respiration tends to be rapid in early shock because of fear, anxiety and stimulation of the respiratory center by catecholamines or endotoxin. This may cause a fairly severe respiratory alkalosis with a Pco_2 of 20 to 30 mm Hg or lower. Later, continued inadequate blood flow to tissues may cause enough anaerobic metabolism and accumulation of lactic acid to produce a metabolic acidosis. At this point, unless the lungs can compensate for the resultant reduction in bicarbonate, the patient may develop a dangerous degree of acidosis, and a drop of pH below 7.20 to 7.25 may interfere with cardiovascular and metabolic function. On the other hand, if the hyperventilation is excessive, the resulting severe respiratory alkalosis may interfere with blood flow to the heart and brain, especially if the Pco_2 falls below 20 to 25 mm Hg.

In our studies on critically ill and injured patients we have found that severe alkalosis can be quite deleterious. As the arterial pH rises above 7.55, the mortality rate also increases until at a pH of 7.65 or higher it exceeds 80%.[5] Accordingly, if a patient has a metabolic alkalosis and is on a respirator, we are careful to keep the Pco_2 above 30 to 35 mm Hg by reducing the respiratory rate and adding up to 300 ml of external dead space to the respirator. The metabolic alkalosis may also be partially corrected with fluids containing potassium chloride, arginine hydrochloride, and saline.

OLIGURIA. One of the homeostatic attempts by the body to increase or maintain an adequate blood volume consists of reducing urine formation by decreasing renal blood flow and increasing tubular reabsorp-tion. The urine output during hypotension is usually closely related to the amount of renal blood flow. Of all the organs of the body, the kidney has the most alpha receptors and, except for the skin, suffers the greatest degree of vasoconstriction during shock. As a consequence, the kidney can be considered as the "window of the viscera." If the kidney is excreting more than 35 to 50 ml urine per hour without the artificial stimulation of a diuretic drug, the perfusion of all other organs is probably also adequate.

FLUID SHIFTS FROM THE INTERSTITIAL SPACE (FIG. 3)

PITFALL

IF ONLY THE INITIAL HEMOGLOBIN AND HEMATOCRIT ARE USED TO DETERMINE THE NEED FOR TRANSFUSIONS IN PATIENTS WITH ACUTE SEVERE HEMORRHAGE, THE AMOUNT OF BLOOD LOSS AND NEEDED REPLACEMENT WILL USUALLY BE GROSSLY UNDERESTIMATED.

When hypovolemia or shock develops, there is an accelerated movement of fluid from the interstitial space, including thoracic-duct lymphatic flow into the vascular space.[6] In young healthy individuals this fluid shift may be rapid and proceed at a rate of up to 500 to 1000 ml per hour for the first hour or two. The shift usually continues

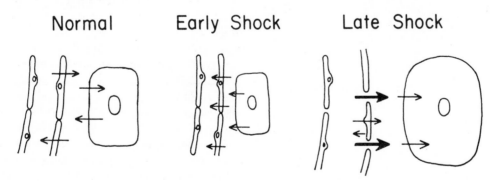

Normal   Early Shock   Late Shock

FIG. 3. Normally there is a fairly equal movement of fluid back and forth between the vascular space and the interstitial and cellular spaces. In early hypovolemic shock, fluid moves rapidly out of the cells and interstitial space into the constricted vascular space. In late shock, increased capillary permeability and impaired cell-membrane function result in a movement of fluid into the interstitial and cellular spaces.

at a progressively slower rate until either the blood volume is adequate or approximately half the interstitial fluid has been lost. The interstitial-fluid space is about 16% of the body weight and, in an average adult male, up to 5 to 6 liters may move from it into the vascular space within 6 to 48 hours.

It is important to remember that it takes at least several hours for enough fluid to move into the vascular space to dilute the remaining red cells significantly. Consequently, hemoglobin and hematocrit levels obtained soon after blood loss may still be deceptively normal and give little evidence of the actual amount of hemorrhage.

FLUID SHIFTS FROM THE INTRACELLULAR SPACE. As fluid leaves the interstitial space to enter the vascular compartment, a concomitant but much slower movement of fluid occurs from the intracellular space into the extracellular compartment. This probably does not exceed 50 to 200 ml per hour. Although this fluid shift is not of much value in compensating for acute massive blood or fluid deficits, it can be extremely important in patients with subacute or chronic blood or fluid loss.

Prolonged Shock

PROLONGED VASOCONSTRICTION AND PERIPHERAL CELL DEATH. Although selective vasoconstriction in the organs resistant to ischemia may be temporarily beneficial by maintaining blood flow to vital organs, it can, if prolonged, ultimately cause damage or death to the poorly perfused tissues. The longer shock persists, the greater the amount of cell death distal to the vasoconstriction. In addition to dysfunction in the poorly perfused organs and alterations in cell and capillary-membrane permeability, lysosomal breakdown releases vasoactive substances, especially kinins and histamine, from the cells and blood. These vasoactive substances can, in turn, aggravate and complicate any changes in the microcirculation.

CAPILLARY DAMAGE

Alteration or damage to the capillary walls can increase their permeability, re-

PITFALL

IF ONLY CRYSTALLOIDS (RATHER THAN BLOOD AND COLLOIDS) ARE GIVEN TO PATIENTS WITH ADVANCED SEPSIS OR SHOCK, THE FLUID CAN INCREASE THE CHANCES OF LATER RESPIRATORY FAILURE WITHOUT EFFECTIVELY EXPANDING THE BLOOD VOLUME.

sulting in a greatly increased loss of protein and fluid from the vascular into the interstitial space. This reduces the net intravascular osmotic pressure and further increases the movement of fluid out of the vascular compartment into the tissues. Clinically this "capillary leak" may be manifested by a tendency for the patient to become grossly edematous and yet remain hypovolemic in spite of the administration of large quantities of crystalloids. Under these circumstances, the patient may gain excessive weight while the blood pressure, CVP and cardiac output change only slightly.

CELL-MEMBRANE CHANGES AND INTRACELLULAR EDEMA. Ischemic, hypoxic, chemical, or physical damage impairs the selective permeability of cell membranes. As a consequence, there is an increased tendency for potassium to leave the cell and sodium to enter. Water tends to follow the sodium and, as fluid enters the cells, the volume of the interstitial and intravascular fluid spaces are correspondingly reduced. This shift of fluid into the damaged cells can occur in spite of a reduced extracellular fluid volume and may greatly aggravate any tendency to hypovolemia.

INAPPROPRIATE OR OBLIGATORY POLYURIA

PITFALL

IF IT IS ASSUMED THAT PATIENTS WITH URINARY OUTPUTS EXCEEDING 50 TO 100 ML/HR ARE OVERLOADED AND IF THE PHYSICIAN THEN REDUCES THEIR FLUID INTAKE RAPIDLY AND SUBSTANTIALLY, SOME PATIENTS WITH SEPSIS AND "OBLIGATORY POLYURIA" MAY BECOME HYPOTENSIVE AND DEVELOP OLIGURIC RENAL FAILURE.

Occasionally a peculiar renal problem develops in which septic patients have a very high urine output at a time when they have an apparently normal or expanded blood volume but a disproportionately increased vascular capacitance. The relatively normal blood pressure, CVP, and cardiac output may encourage a decrease in the fluid administered to such a patient on the assumption that he is overhydrated. This reduction in fluid intake can result in a severe relative hypovolemia, hypotension, and oliguria.

EFFECTIVE BLOOD-VOLUME CHANGES

PITFALL

IF RELIANCE IS PLACED ON BLOOD-VOLUME DETERMINATIONS WITHOUT UNDERSTANDING OF THE TECHNICAL AND PHYSIOLOGIC COMPLEXITIES INVOLVED, GRAVE ERRORS MAY RESULT WHEN THIS IS USED AS AN INDEX OF FLUID NEEDS, ESPECIALLY WHEN THE VASCULAR CAPACITY IS ABNORMAL.

Effective blood volume is reduced in advanced shock by any tendency for red blood cells to clump or clot within the capillaries. In the early phases of shock, tissues suffer from an "ischemic anoxia" because of the proximal arterial constriction; later, however, the proximal arterial vasoconstriction may relent while the postcapillary sphincters remain relatively constricted, producing a pooling of blood in the capillaries and "stagnant anoxia."[7]

The degree to which the effective circulating blood volume may be reduced in shock is often not fully appreciated. Ordinarily, the tracer used for blood-volume determinations, whether RISA or ^{51}Cr tagged red blood cells, tends to equilibrate with the entire blood volume in less than ten minutes. In shock, however, the time required for equilibration may be considerably prolonged and the tagged red cells may disappear from the circulation at an increased rate. Obviously the presence of a large quantity of slowly circulating blood

would significantly interfere with tissue perfusion, especially if cardiac output is already reduced because of cardiac or hypovolemic problems.

PLATELET EMBOLI. The tendency for platelets to aggregate in the capillary beds of damaged or hypoxic tissues not only interferes with local blood flow but also results in the formation of emboli which can travel to the lungs and liver.[8] These platelets may mechanically occlude portions of the microcirculation, act as a nidus for red-cell and fibrin deposition, and liberate vasoactive substances, especially serotonin.

VASOACTIVE SUBSTANCES. Damaged cells or tissue tend to produce or bring about the release of vasoactive substances such as histamines and kinins. "Induced histamine" in contrast to "preformed histamine," which is stored in mast cells and is inhibited by antihistamines, is produced directly in the damaged or anoxic cells.[9] Proteolytic enzymes or proteases released from the lysosomes of damaged cells may, on escaping into the bloodstream, convert inactive kininogens to active kinins. These kinins, especially bradykinin, are extremely potent vasodilators and may account for many of the abnormal vascular responses seen in shock.

THE TRANSLATION OF THEORY INTO THE PRACTICAL MANAGEMENT OF THE PATIENT

Treatment

Treatment of acute shock may be outlined under the following headings:

1. Correction of the initiating cause of the shock
2. Ventilation and oxygenation
3. Insertion of intravenous catheters
4. Infusion of blood and fluid
5. Correction of acid-base abnormalities
6. Antibiotics
7. Digitalis
8. Diuretics
9. Vasoconstrictors and vasodilators
10. Steroids
11. Heparin.

The appropriate steps should be carried out as rapidly as possible. The longer the patient is in shock, the greater is the incidence of complications and the less is the chance for recovery.

CORRECTION OF INITIATING CAUSE. Unless the cause of the shock is corrected rapidly, all other treatment may be of no avail. In the initial phases after trauma, most shock is due to hemorrhage. If internal bleeding is so massive that the administration of blood and fluid cannot keep up with the loss, the patient should be operated upon as soon as possible, even if he is in shock. If blood and fluid can be given faster than they are being lost, the patient should be brought into the best condition possible before he is given an anesthetic.

VENTILATION AND OXYGENATION. Ventilation in the patient with shock or severe trauma or sepsis must be maintained at levels greater than normal to compensate for the impaired pulmonary function. On clinical examination alone, it is extremely difficult to detect early respiratory failure in these patients; accordingly, it is essential to obtain frequent blood gas determinations. Measurements of the physiologic shunting in the lung and alveolar-arterial oxygen differences are especially valuable. All patients in shock should probably be given oxygen, and where there is any doubt about the ventilatory exchange the patient should be given respiratory support.

INTRAVENOUS CATHETERS. Depending on the severity of shock, two or three large I.V.s should be started, using 18- or preferably 15-gauge catheters. One of these catheters should be advanced into the superior vena cava to be used for constant monitoring of the CVP. Blood is drawn at this time for typing and cross-matching; in addition, a complete blood count is ordered and electrolyte and blood gas measurements are obtained. If there is any suggestion of diabetes, renal disease, or pancreatic trauma, blood should also be drawn for determinations of glucose, creatinine, and amylase respectively.

Several locations for inserting CVP catheters are available, but we prefer to pass the catheter up the basilic vein through a cut-down just anterior and proximal to the medial humeral epicondyle. It is often difficult to get the catheters past the axilla or first rib when the cephalic and brachial veins are used. Alternatively, an Intracath or similar catheter can be passed percutaneously into the external jugular vein, but such catheters often dislodge easily and the position of the patient's head may greatly influence the I.V. and CVP function. Insertion of catheters percutaneously into the subclavian vein by an infraclavicular approach has been written about extensively.[10] This maneuver is useful if no other veins are readily available and is especially valuable for long-term intravenous hyperalimentation. Before a CVP catheter can be considered to be properly placed and functioning, fluid should run through it rapidly, the fluid level should fluctuate well with respiration, and blood should be drawn back readily. A chest x-ray should be obtained routinely after inserting all subclavian catheters, checking for pneumothorax and the catheter position. If there is still any question about the accuracy of its position, a chest x-ray should be obtained while 10 ml of Renovist or a similar intravenous contrast agent is injected.

ADMINISTRATION OF FLUID. *Types of Fluid.* CRYSTALLOIDS. The all-purpose fluid begun on most patients with trauma tends to be 5% glucose in Ringer's lactate. If the patient is in very severe shock or has moderate to severe liver disease, the lactate may not be readily metabolized to bicarbonate; under these circumstances, we prefer to use 5% glucose in normal saline with two ampules (89.2 mEq) sodium bicarbonate added to each liter. After two to three liters of crystalloid are given, additional fluid should consist roughly of half crystalloid and half colloid or blood.

COLLOIDS. The colloids most frequently used are albumin, plasma, and low-molecular-weight dextran (L.M.W.D.). When shock is prolonged or severe, capillary permeability is increased and the substances most apt to remain in the vascular space are those with a high molecular weight. Although L.M.W.D. is a readily available colloid in most emergency rooms, it may cause increased bleeding, problems with cross-matching and occasional anaphylactic reactions. Therefore, L.M.W.D. should not be started until a cross-match is obtained and should usually not be given in quantities greater than 1000 ml in 24 hours. We prefer to use 25 to 50 gm of albumin in each liter of normal saline or Ringer's lactate. Plasma can also be useful; fresh frozen plasma will not only help expand the intravascular volume but can also supply needed clotting factors.

BLOOD. In an emergency, type-specific blood can usually be made available without a cross-match in 5 to 15 minutes. A saline cross-match may require another 5 to 10 minutes. If even the wait for type-specific blood is too long, low-titer O-positive blood may be used in male patients and low-titer O-negative in females still in the childbearing age. Although there is a general tendency for blood-bank directors to persuade physicians to use specific blood components wherever possible and to avoid use of blood which is not thoroughly cross-matched, there is probably nothing as beneficial to the critically ill or injured patient as the rapid early administration of whole fresh blood.

PITFALL

IF THE INITIAL HEMOGLOBIN ALONE IS USED AS A GUIDE FOR THE ADMINISTRATION OF BLOOD, THE AMOUNT OF BLOOD LOSS MAY BE GREATLY UNDERESTIMATED AND SEVERE HYPOVOLEMIA OR ANEMIA MAY RESULT.

If the patient is given large amounts of fluid and blood for several hours, the hematocrit should be measured every 1 to 2 hours and kept between 35 and 40%. In acute severe injuries with massive blood loss, 3000 to 4000 ml of crystalloids and colloids may be given initially; after that, blood becomes essential, the amount depending upon the rapidity of the bleeding (Chap. 10).

Rate and Amount of Fluid. The rate and amount of fluid given will depend upon the patient's response. The immediate objective is to correct the shock as rapidly as possible without overloading the heart and lungs. Once adequate blood flow and pressure are obtained the amount of fluid administered should be reduced to that needed to cover the basic needs and current losses, with further allowance made for 500 to 1500 ml of blood-volume deficit which may still be present. If shock persists, the main guidelines to the volume and rate at which further fluid is given are the blood pressure, pulse, central venous pressure, pulmonary-wedge pressure, auscultation of the lung bases, and urinary output.

BLOOD PRESSURE. In shock, we are primarily concerned with the blood flow throughout the body, especially to the brain and heart. Unfortunately, an extremely poor or negative correlation often exists between blood flow and blood pressure. This is especially true when vasopressor drugs are used to raise the pressure.

In the average patient, the blood volume must often be reduced by 15 to 25% before the systolic blood pressure begins to fall below 80 to 90 mm Hg. Blood-volume deficits of 30 to 35% usually cause moderate to severe shock, and deficits exceeding 45% are often fatal. Thus, the margin between the onset of hypotension and death may be only 20% of the blood volume or about 1.0 liter in the average 70-kg adult male. It is the defense of this margin which is critical in the treatment of traumatic shock.

It is important to remember that even when the systolic blood pressure is restored to normal there may still be a reduction of 15 to 25% in the blood volume and even larger interstitial-fluid deficits. If the shock has been severe or has persisted for more than an hour or two, the blood volume can be maintained at normal levels only if the concurrent intracellular and intercellular deficits have also been corrected. We attempt to maintain the arterial blood pressure 10 to 20 mm Hg above the minimal level needed to provide satisfactory cerebral, cardiac, and renal function. If the patient is alert and has a normal EKG and urine output (at least 35 to 50 ml per hour), the systolic pressure is probably adequate, even if it is less than 80 mm Hg. If the patient was hypertensive previously, he may need a systolic pressure of 120 mm Hg or more.

The pulse pressure can be a helpful guide to the adequacy of fluid therapy. In general, the diastolic pressure is determined by the degree of arteriolar constriction present, and the pulse pressure reflects the stroke volume. In many respects a B.P. of 80/40 is preferable to one of 120/100. The higher diastolic pressure is usually due to severe arterial vasoconstriction and, therefore, is apt to be associated with poor tissue perfusion. Continued coldness and clamminess of the skin in the presence of an otherwise adequate systolic blood pressure also indicates excessive vasoconstriction and poor tissue perfusion. Even at systolic pressures less than 100 mm Hg a patient with a high pulse pressure often has a better blood flow, a warmer, drier skin, and a fuller, more easily palpable pulse than one with a higher systolic pressure and a lower pulse pressure.

PULSE RATE. Although the pulse rate is a relatively poor guide to the adequacy of fluid therapy, there is a general tendency to tachycardia if the cardiac output is low. As the blood volume and flow improve, the pulse rate usually begins to slow toward a more normal range. Anxiety, fright, or pain, however, may cause the pulse rate to exceed 120 to 130 per minute even if the blood flow is adequate. It is also not uncommon for elderly patients, especially those with arteriosclerotic coronary-artery disease, to maintain deceptively low pulse rates in the presence of a rather severe

hypovolemia and low cardiac output. This is usually a bad prognostic sign; however, once the blood volume has been restored, isoproterenol, which works best when the pulse is slow, may greatly improve cardiac output.

CENTRAL VENOUS PRESSURE (CVP). Fluids should never be given indiscriminately; the physician must strive to administer the optimal amount, which provides adequate tissue perfusion and yet does not aggravate any tendency to cardiac failure or pulmonary insufficiency. Overall, the best single guide to the rate and volume of fluid administration is the CVP *response*. It has been shown that there may be no correlation between the initial CVP *level* and the blood volume in patients with shock.[11,12] The CVP should be monitored almost constantly whenever fluid is being given rapidly to patients with severe shock, trauma, or sepsis. If 200 ml of fluid given over ten minutes cause the CVP to rise more than 2 cm H_2O and this rise is persistent, further fluid administration should be reduced or slowed until the CVP begins to fall again (Fig. 4). Even in the face of fairly severe hypovolemia, a high CVP may be found in straining hyperactive patients, those with

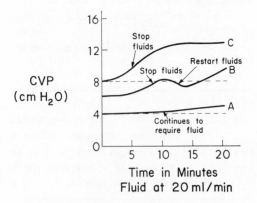

FIG. 4. If I.V. fluid causes only a slight rise in CVP (A) in the patient in shock, further fluid should be given. (One should also be listening to the lungs.) If the CVP rises abruptly but falls back after the fluid is stopped (B), more fluid can be given. If the CVP rises abruptly and does not fall again within 5 to 10 minutes (C), little or no additional fluid should be given.

cardiopulmonary disease, during general anesthesia, and while vasopressors are being given.

Whenever the CVP seems unusually high, the CVP line must be checked to see that it is open adequately, positioned correctly and read accurately. A good CVP fluctuates widely with respiration and blood can be drawn through it readily. Although the zero level should be at the center of the tricuspid valve, which is near the midaxillary line in most normal patients, adjustments must be made for abnormal configurations of the chest or heart. Although we tend to give fluids somewhat more slowly and cautiously when the CVP approaches or exceeds 12.0 to 16.0 cm H_2O, some patients, especially those with cardiopulmonary disease, may show little or no improvement until enough blood and fluid have been given to raise the CVP above 16.0 to 20.0 cm H_2O.

PULMONARY-WEDGE PRESSURE

PITFALL

IF LARGE AMOUNTS OF FLUID ARE GIVEN RAPIDLY TO A PATIENT WHO HAS HAD A RECENT MYOCARDIAL INFARCTION OR CARDIAC ARREST, HE MAY DEVELOP PULMONARY EDEMA EVEN THOUGH THE CVP IS LESS THAN 5 CM H_2O.

Although the CVP usually reflects the filling pressure of both sides of the heart fairly well, there are a few notable exceptions. For at least several hours after a recent myocardial infarction or cardiac arrest, the patient may have an isolated left ventricular failure. Under these circumstances, the left atrial pressure may be very high while the CVP or right atrial pressure is much lower. We have had several instances in which patients with this problem went into pulmonary edema with a CVP less than 5.0 cm H_2O. The reverse can also occur. If the patient has mitral disease, sepsis, severe lung disease or cor pulmonale, he may have an isolated right ventricular fail-

ure with a high CVP (in spite of severe hypovolemia) and a very low left atrial pressure; failure to give adequate blood or fluids to such an individual may be fatal, especially after cardiac surgery.

In an effort to obtain more accurate information about the filling pressure of the left heart, pulmonary-artery pressures may be measured in patients who might have isolated right or left ventricular failure by the use of the Swan-Ganz catheter, which is soft and has a balloon near its tip. The catheter is introduced through a venous cut-down in the arm and passed into the superior vena cava or right atrium. After the balloon is inflated with 1 to 2 ml of air and advanced slowly, it is usually carried by the blood flow into the pulmonary artery. If the catheter can be passed into a wedge position, the resultant pressure will reflect the left atrial pressure fairly accurately. In patients with isolated left ventricular failure, the pulmonary-wedge pressure will often rise more rapidly than the CVP as fluid is administered. In daily practice, however, measurement of pulmonary-wedge pressure has not produced clinical dividends to recommend it except in cases with suspected isolated right or left ventricular failure.

AUSCULTATION OF THE LUNGS. In those instances of isolated right or left ventricular failure where the CVP may not properly reflect the left atrial pressure, it is extremely important to listen to the bases of the lungs for any evidence of increasing congestion. If, while fluid is being administered rapidly, the patient develops increasing rales in spite of adequate ventilation and coughing, the infusion must be reduced or stopped, even if the CVP is low. It is impossible to overemphasize the importance of frequent auscultation of the lung bases posteriorly in the patient who is in shock, has myocardial failure or is receiving large amounts of fluid. Rales at the lung bases are often the first signs that the pulmonary or cardiovascular systems are being overloaded.

URINARY OUTPUT. If the urinary output can be increased to 35 to 50 ml/hr without a diuretic, we can usually be assured that perfusion of the rest of the body is also adequate. Conversely, when the urinary output and urine sodium are low and the specific gravity and osmolarity are high, the kidneys are still inadequately perfused and further fluids or inotropic agents should be given. If oliguria persists but urinary specific gravity and osmolarity are low and urinary sodium concentration is high, the patient probably has some degree of renal failure and the quality of renal perfusion is uncertain.

Problems of Overloading. The importance of meticulous monitoring of the quantity and composition of intravenous-fluid replacement lies in the fact that excessive administration of fluid during the initial resuscitation may result in an increased congestion of pulmonary capillaries, interstitial pulmonary edema, and transudation of fluid into the alveoli. These factors seem to contribute to the development of a progressive respiratory failure. This has become an increasingly frequent and difficult problem in patients who are now kept alive for at least a few days with injuries which previously would have been immediately lethal. This pulmonary insufficiency has been seen so frequently in critically injured patients that it can almost be regarded as part of a "post-resurrection syndrome."

ACID-BASE BALANCE. *Respiratory Alkalosis.* It is often assumed that the characteristic acid-base problem in shock is a metabolic acidosis. Although this is true of moderately advanced shock when there is significant interference with tissue perfusion and metabolism, in early shock respiratory alkalosis is the usual problem. The acid-base changes may be monitored easily and accurately by measuring arterial pH, P_{CO_2}, and standard bicarbonate. When these measurements are not available, the CO_2 content of the venous blood in patients with fairly normal lungs may provide some useful information. If the lungs are functioning adequately, the patient can usually blow off enough carbon dioxide to maintain a fairly reasonable bicarbonate-carbonic acid ratio, and an approximation of the arterial bicarbonate present can be calculated by subtracting 1.0 to 2.5 mEq/L from the CO_2 content.

PITFALL

IF A PATIENT WITH SHOCK, SEPSIS, AND HYPERVENTILATION IS GIVEN SODIUM BICARBONATE BECAUSE IT IS ASSUMED THAT A METABOLIC ACIDOSIS IS PRESENT, A SEVERE AND DANGEROUS COMBINED ALKALOSIS MAY DEVELOP.

Hyperventilation in many disease states is an expression of the body's attempt to compensate for a metabolic acidosis; in shock, however, the hyperventilation can occur with a normal or even elevated standard bicarbonate, especially when associated with sepsis. The cause of this hyperventilation is not clear but is probably related to stimulation of the respiratory center by endotoxin or vasoactive substances released from ischemic, infected, or necrotic tissue. The administration of sodium bicarbonate to a patient who already has a high pH from a respiratory alkalosis can cause a severe (combined) alkalosis with a resultant precipitous drop in ionized calcium and a possible cardiac arrest or arrhythmia.

Correcting Metabolic Acidosis. Metabolic acidosis of a moderate degree will often correct itself when the cardiac output is improved by I.V. fluids or inotropic agents such as digitalis, isoproterenol, or dopamine. More severe acidosis, especially if associated with poor cardiac, renal, or pulmonary function, may require additional treatment and sodium bicarbonate is usually the drug of choice. Sodium bicarbonate should be used carefully, if at all, in the presence of respiratory acidosis because, unless the CO_2 produced from the combination of hydrogen ion and bicarbonate can be blown off, the respiratory acidosis will get much worse. The sodium in the sodium bicarbonate may also cause a problem because it can overload the circulation in patients who have a tendency to congestive heart failure, cirrhosis, or renal disease. When a combined metabolic and respiratory acidosis is present, or if sodium bicarbonate cannot be used, THAM (tris buffer) may be useful; it is an extremely powerful alkalinizing agent and must be used with great care, especially since it can cause apnea. Although it can correct severe acidosis effectively, it did not improve our survival figures, and we have not used it for several years now.

The dose of bicarbonate or THAM is calculated by multiplying the base deficit or reduction in CO_2 content by 30% of the body weight in kilograms. Usually only half the deficit is corrected at any one time. Sodium bicarbonate or THAM should not ordinarily be given faster than 2.5 to 5.0 mEq per minute except after a cardiac arrest.

Acidity of Stored Bank Blood. Although normal patients can readily tolerate and buffer the acidity in banked blood, the patient with poor tissue perfusion has an impaired ability to maintain a normal pH; therefore, whenever massive transfusions are given to patients in severe shock, an ampule of sodium bicarbonate should probably be given with every two units of blood.

ANTIBIOTICS. In severe persistent shock, the epithelial and reticuloendothelial barriers to bacteria and their products in the lungs and intestinal tract are impaired and there appears to be an increased susceptibility to infection. As a consequence, massive broad-spectrum intravenous antibiotics should be given to such individuals. If there is any hint that sepsis may already be present, three separate blood cultures and cultures of the urine, throat, sputum, and wounds should be obtained. Several different antibiotic combinations are useful (Chap. 29).

PITFALL

IF LARGE DOSES OF I.V. AQUEOUS POTASSIUM PENICILLIN ARE GIVEN RAPIDLY, THE SUDDEN RISE IN SERUM POTASSIUM LEVELS MAY CAUSE A CARDIAC ARREST.

DIGITALIS. Controversy still surrounds the use of digitalis and inotropic agents in trauma and shock. We feel, however, that since patients with severe persistent shock usually have some impairment of cardiac function, they may benefit from digitalis. Other indications include any history or evidence of congestive heart failure, an abnormally elevated CVP, or a severe persistent atrial tachycardia above 130 to 140, especially in patients over 65 years of age.

The usual I.V. digitalizing dose of digoxin, our favorite digitalis preparation, averages about 1.25 to 1.75 mg. The dose required to obtain an optimal effect when shock is present, however, may be extremely variable because of changes in acid-base balance, electrolyte abnormalities, and altered cell metabolism. A frequent dose schedule used is 0.5 to 0.75 mg digoxin I.V. stat followed by 0.25 mg every two hours $\times$ 2, then 0.125 mg every two hours $\times$ 4 or until there is evidence of a digitalis effect. An EKG strip is taken before each dose is given. If any changes in rate, rhythm, or S-T segments develop which indicate digitalis effect or toxicity, no further drug is administered until the maintenance doses are required. A new inotropic agent, dopamine, started as a slow I.V. drip of 200 mg in 250 ml 5% G/W, may rapidly raise both blood pressure and cardiac output. Isoproterenol may be helpful in patients with a slow weak heart. To maintain levels of ionized calcium which are optimal for cardiac function, a gram of $CaCl_2$ should be given after every 4 units of blood.

DIURETICS. In patients in shock, urinary output should be closely monitored with an indwelling Foley catheter. If the urinary output is less than 25 ml per hour in spite of all the treatment described above, we give diuretics such as mannitol, furosemide, or ethacrynic acid. Before any diuretic is given, however, hypovolemia should be eliminated as the cause of the oliguria. The fluid load described earlier in this chapter usually corrects and continues to correct any fluid deficits. Nevertheless, if the specific gravity is above 1.020 or if the urine sodium is below 20 mEq/L in the presence of oliguria, this usually indicates an inadequate renal blood flow which might improve either with further fluid or with cardiotonic drugs. If there is any question about the need for further fluid, a fluid load of 500 ml 5% glucose in water may be given carefully over 15 to 30 minutes. If the oliguria is from inadequate fluid, this will usually increase the urinary output.

Mannitol. If oliguria persists, in spite of adequate fluid loading and a normal blood pressure, 25 gm of mannitol are given I.V. over 15 to 30 minutes. If there is any response to this osmotic diuretic, the dose is repeated as needed to maintain a urine output of at least 35 ml and preferably 50 ml per hour. No more than 100 gm of mannitol is given in any 24-hour period. One disadvantage of mannitol is that, at least temporarily, it expands the intravascular volume and can overload a patient with borderline cardiac function.

Ethacrynic Acid and Furosemide. If there is an inadequate response to the mannitol or if the patient is too overloaded to risk the use of an osmotic diuretic, an I.V. dose of 25 mg of ethacrynic acid or 10 to 20 mg of furosemide is given rapidly. If there is some response, this dose is repeated as needed to maintain a urinary output of at least 35 ml per hour. If there is no response, the dose is doubled every 15 to 30 minutes. We have successfully given up to 200 mg every 4 to 6 hours to maintain this amount of urine flow. When a large diuresis has been felt to be desirable, we have added 5 to 20 mg of furosemide to each I.V. to maintain urine outputs of 200 to 500 ml/hr; with this degree of polyuria, it is essential to replace the urine potassium losses, which may exceed 60 to 80 mEq/L.

Peritoneal Dialysis. If there is an inadequate response to the diuretics, the patient is treated for renal failure with fluid restriction and/or peritoneal or hemodialysis. Obviously, fluid restriction places severe limitations on our ability to treat shock. Although peritonitis has been considered a contraindication to peritoneal dialysis in the past, a combination of dialysis and irrigation of the peritoneal cavity has been used effectively in some of our patients with renal failure and peritonitis or pancreatitis.

VASOCONSTRICTORS AND VASODILATORS. Vasoconstrictors and vasodilators are of limited value in the treatment of shock. If all the steps outlined above fail to bring the patient out of shock, his prognosis is extremely poor.

Possible Value of Vasoconstrictors. The use of vasopressor drugs such as Levophed and Aramine is often condemned. There may, however, be some circumstances in which these drugs can be of value, e.g. in patients who have been on antihypertensive drugs and in those with significant atherosclerosis. In contrast to young patients with little or no vascular disease, who can often tolerate hypotension well, older patients with more than a 75 to 85% occlusion of the coronary or cerebral vessels may require increased blood pressure to maintain an adequate flow through the diseased arteries. If the arterial blood pressure falls below the critical closing pressure of an important part of the coronary or cerebral circulation, a myocardial or cerebral infarct may result.

Although increased vasoconstriction may be needed to maintain adequate coronary and cerebral circulation in the severely hypotensive patient, it should be remembered that the vasoconstrictors do this by diverting blood from other areas. Fortunately, the tissues which develop the greatest degree of vasoconstriction happen to be able to tolerate hypoxia and poor blood flow for relatively long periods, but even these tissues will eventually die if the vasoconstriction is excessively severe or prolonged. Furthermore, the increased coronary blood flow produced by vasoconstriction and rise in blood pressure may not compensate for the increased needs of the myocardium as it pumps against increased pressure and resistance.

In these tenuous circumstances, the essential problem is determination of the blood pressure required to provide acceptable tissue perfusion with as low a dosage of vasopressor as possible. One useful technique for doing this is to raise the pressure above normal levels and to note the patient's renal, cerebral, and cardiovascular function. The blood pressure is then allowed to fall slowly. The pressure at which any deterioration in the state of consciousness, the urinary output, or the EKG is noted is the minimal pressure needed, and the pressure then aimed at is 10 to 20 mm Hg higher.

Vasoconstrictors Combined with Vasodilators. Animal and clinical experiments have shown that Levophed by itself can be lethal and can cause tissue necrosis, especially in the hypovolemic animal or where the drug extravasates into the tissue around a vein. If vasodilators, even in small quantities, are used with the vasoconstrictor, however, the lethality and tissue necrosis are greatly reduced or abolished. The vasoconstrictor-vasodilator combination most frequently used now at Detroit General Hospital is four ampules (16 mg) Levophed and two ampules (10 mg) Regitine in 500 ml 5% glucose in water. Although this amount of Regitine experimentally reduces the tissue necrosis and the extremes of vasoconstriction caused by Levophed alone, it does not produce any significant clinical vasodilation; to do this, doses in the range of 0.5 to 2.5 mg per minute are needed.

Vasodilators Alone. If severe vasoconstriction persists in spite of all attempts at treatment, vasodilator therapy is warranted provided certain potential hazards are recognized. It is important to remember that vasodilators not only reduce blood pressure by arteriolar vasodilation but also produce a severe relative hypovolemia by dilatation and increase in the volume of the capacitance veins. Consequently, before any vasodilator is given, any existing hypovolemia should be corrected and preparations made to infuse up to two to three liters of blood or fluid rapidly if hypovolemia or severe hypotension should develop.

Currently chlorpromazine (Thorazine) appears to be one of the safest and most effective clinical vasodilators. It is given in 1- to 2-mg I.V. increments at 1- to 2-minute intervals until the skin becomes warmer, drier, and pinker or until the blood pressure begins to fall. Although 2 to 5 mg of chlorpromazine may produce the desired effect for 2 to 4 hours or longer, occasionally 10.0 to 15.0 mg or more are needed. Regitine may also be used, but the dosage required is high and expensive, and the drug has a much lower margin of safety.

STEROIDS. *"Physiologic" Doses.* Adrenal insufficiency due to disease or previous treatment with adrenal cortical hormones must always be considered as a possible cause of an otherwise unexplainable persistent hypotension. Patients with a deficiency of hydrocortisone often have little or no difficulty unless they are under some sort of stress. Even minimal illnesses, injuries, or operations, however, can cause these individuals to develop severe hypotension which may be unresponsive to anything except hydrocortisone. An otherwise unexplained hyponatremia and/or hyperkalemia may also suggest this problem. Even where there is no evidence of adrenal insufficiency, it seems prudent to give at least 100 to 200 mg of hydrocortisone rapidly I.V. to any patient with persistent unexplained hypotension. If the hypotension is due to adrenal insufficiency alone, the improvement may be quite dramatic. Consequently all patients with persistent unexplained hypotension should be given at least 100 to

200 mg hydrocortisone I.V. on an empiric basis. Maintenance doses during or following trauma usually total about 200 to 300 mg daily.

"Pharmacologic" Doses. "Massive steroids" in doses equivalent to 50 to 150 mg of hydrocortisone per kg of body weight are being used with increasing frequency in the treatment of severe or prolonged shock. The exact mechanism of action of massive steroids is not clear, but some investigators have felt that they may stabilize lysosomal and cell membranes,[13] act as vasodilators or "normalize" cardiovascular activity,[14] and improve pulmonary function. Massive steroids may also be beneficial by reducing certain detrimental inflammatory or antigen-antibody reactions. Our technique for giving massive steroids is to administer 6 mg of Decadron or 30 mg of Solu-Medrol per kg of body weight I.V. as a bolus over a 5- to 10-minute period followed by another bolus in 4 to 6 hours or a continuous infusion over 12 to 24 hours. If the patient improves, the infusion or bolus dose may be repeated.

HEPARIN. Although heparin probably has little or no place in the treatment of acute traumatic and/or hemorrhagic shock, it may be of benefit if there is laboratory or clinical evidence of a clotting disorder due to disseminated intravascular coagulation (D.I.C.). D.I.C. not only interferes with blood flow and reduces the effective circulating blood volume but also causes a reduction in the platelet count and the concentrations of Factor V, Factor VIII, and fibrinogen. Once this syndrome is established, successful treatment requires complete heparinization of the patient for at least 24 to 72 hours. Heparinization is best achieved by giving 50 mg of heparin rapidly I.V. followed by 10 to 15 mg per hour by constant infusion (Chap. 34). With the patient heparinized, the clotting factors are restored with fresh frozen plasma or platelet-rich fresh blood. While the clotting factors are being restored, the process which began the intravascular clotting must also

be corrected or the D.I.C. will recur when the heparin is stopped.

Persistent Acute or Unexplained Shock

If shock persists in spite of all the steps outlined above, some other factors must be considered or reviewed. These include:

1. continued and/or hidden loss of blood or fluid;
2. acid-base imbalance;
3. hypothermia;
4. hypocalcemia;
5. previous treatment with antihypertensive drugs;
6. cardiac contusion or tamponade;
7. pneumothorax;
8. anesthesia;
9. "vascular fatigue."

CONTINUED LOSS OF BLOOD OR FLUID. Probably the most common cause of severe persistent hypotension in the patient with trauma is a continued loss or inadequate replacement of blood or fluid. Unfortunately the bleeding sites may not be immediately obvious. Lacerations which were not bleeding preoperatively may begin to bleed again when the blood pressure improves and may be hidden by the surgical drapes. Hemorrhage into the chest or abdominal cavity may be extensive before it is recognized, but it still is usually easier to pinpoint than the blood loss associated with hematomas in the mesentery, retroperitoneal spaces, traumatized muscle, and around fractures. Blood return to the heart can be reduced by packs or hematomas which compress or occlude large veins, especially the inferior vena cava; this may also aggravate the blood loss from the area drained by the occluded vein.

ACID-BASE IMBALANCE. Although every effort is made to correct blood volume and electrolyte abnormalities prior to surgery, it is not uncommon for the acid-base status of the patient to become grossly abnormal during the operation. The combinations of anesthetic medications, positive-pressure ventilation, massive blood loss, and rapid blood and fluid replacement, especially if shock is present, may cause sudden, severe changes in pH. By far the most common problem in severe, persistent shock is metabolic acidosis resulting from poor tissue perfusion and inadequate cellular metabolism. If facilities are not available for frequent monitoring of arterial blood gases and acid-base balance, treatment must be largely empiric. If the patient is in severe persistent shock in spite of adequate blood replacement, two ampules of NaHCO$_3$ can be given over a 10- to 20-minute period and the patient's response carefully noted. If the patient does improve, the NaHCO$_3$ should probably be slowly repeated as often as necessary to maintain or continue the improvement.

Patients in severe shock receiving massive transfusions may be unable adequately to buffer the acidity (pH 6.4 to 6.8) of the stored blood. Since it generally takes at least half an ampule of NaHCO$_3$ to restore the pH of bank blood to the normal range, we recommend giving this amount with each unit transfused to patients in severe persistent shock.

HYPOTHERMIA. If the temperature of the body falls below 30 to 32 C, cardiovascular function may be severely impaired. Long operations and the administration of large amounts of cold blood or fluid may contribute to this problem. Unless the rectal and esophageal temperatures are monitored, the degree of hypothermia may not be recognized or appreciated. Prevention and treatment of this problem can be facilitated by having a hypothermia-hyperthermia blanket under the patient and warming the blood or fluid while it is being given.

HYPOCALCEMIA. Reduction in the concentration of ionized calcium in the blood during shock is infrequent except with massive blood transfusions or following the rapid administration of large amounts of sodium bicarbonate or THAM. Very little calcium is needed for clotting, and a bleeding or clotting problem should never be blamed on a calcium deficit. Much more calcium is needed to maintain adequate cardiovascular function, and the patient would die on the basis of hypocalcemic cardiovascular failure long before any coagulation abnormality developed. If tissue perfusion is adequate, there is probably little or no need for the administration of calcium chloride or calcium gluconate during or following blood transfusions; however, if the patient is in severe shock, calcium mobilization may be inadequate and 1.0 gm of calcium chloride I.V. after every four units of blood is usually given. The calcium should be given slowly I.V. over at least a 10-minute period and through tubing completely separate from that used for transfusing blood.

PREVIOUS TREATMENT WITH ANTIHYPERTENSIVE DRUGS. Previous treatment with antihypertensive drugs, especially reserpine, may result in significant hypotension following trauma and particularly during general anesthesia. Reserpine depletes the concentration of catecholamine granules at the sympathetic nerve endings, thereby reducing the ability of the sympathetic nervous system to bring about the vasoconstriction needed to maintain an adequate blood pressure.[15] A dilute infusion of norepinephrine (1 to 2 ampules per liter of I.V. solution) is usually sufficient to maintain reasonably normal vasomotor tone in such patients.

CARDIAC CONTUSION OR TAMPONADE. In patients with severe blunt trauma or penetrating injuries to the chest or upper abdomen, cardiac contusion or tamponade, which may not be apparent initially, can significantly reduce cardiac output and cause cardiogenic shock. The presence of an elevated CVP or of distended neck veins in a patient with hypotension is often associated with an intrathoracic problem such as hemopneumothorax, cardiac injury, tamponade, vena caval occlusion, or mediastinal hematoma. Preoperative x-rays and EKG and continuous monitoring with a cardioscope are essential in all seriously injured patients where the trauma has involved the chest or in whom there is evidence of previous cardiopulmonary disease.

If there is a reasonable chance that tamponade is present, careful pericardiocentesis should be performed. If the problem develops during a laparotomy, a small incision through the pericardial portion of the diaphragm will readily show the presence or absence of any tamponade.

PNEUMOTHORAX. An air leak from an injury to the lung or a spontaneous rupture of a bleb, especially during anesthesia, may occasionally result in an enlarging pneumothorax which can cause persistent shock and/or cardiac arrest. An elevated CVP or distended neck veins combined with hypotension, or increasing difficulty ventilating the lungs, should raise the suspicion of this complication. If the drapes are arranged so that the breath sounds can be auscultated bilaterally, the involved side can often be identified clinically and a large needle can be inserted to confirm the diagnosis and to aspirate the air. Needles may have to be placed bilaterally if the diagnosis is not clear or if the improvement is only temporary. Once a pneumothorax is identified, a chest tube should be inserted and connected to water-seal drainage, with or without suction depending on the severity of the air leak.

ANESTHESIA. Severe or persistent shock may be aggravated by the type or amount of anesthetic used. Fluothane in large doses is especially apt to cause hypotension. If all treatment fails to correct the shock during surgery, anesthesia should be reduced, stopped or changed, depending upon the patient's response. A local anesthetic may have to be used. In general, the less anesthetic used and the more oxygen given, the better the cardiovascular system will function. Of the general anesthetics used, light cyclopropane in experienced hands may be valuable for patients with frank or impending shock.

"VASCULAR FATIGUE." After the patient has been in severe prolonged shock, he may continue to show profound hypotension until and unless a vasopressor such as norepinephrine is given. Occasionally, even though the vasopressor is stopped after 15 to 30 minutes and essentially no other treatment is given, the patient will subsequently maintain an adequate blood pressure. It is somewhat difficult to explain this rather infrequent phenomenon, but it may possibly be related to an unusual form of "vascular fatigue" or catecholamine depletion at the sympathetic nerve endings.

Cardiac Shock

If cardiac shock supervenes, the management is much the same as with other types of shock. Although there may initially be a problem only with pump failure, if the hypotension persists some degree of hypovolemia may develop, and the administration of fluid and/or blood may greatly improve the blood pressure and cardiac output. This fluid loading may be beneficial in about 10 to 20% of those who go into shock following a myocardial infarction. It is important in such individuals to differentiate between rales caused by fluid overload and those caused by inadequate ventilation.

In about 5% of cases with cardiac shock the patient appears to have a weak, slowly beating heart. Under these circumstances an infusion of 0.2 mg of Isuprel in 100 ml of glucose and water at a very slow drip, just enough to raise the pulse rate to between 90 to 110 beats per minute, has been of great benefit. By increasing the pulse rate in this manner, we have been able to increase the cardiac output by 50% or more in some patients with bradycardia and hypotension. In individuals with tachycardia, I.V. infusion of dopamine, digitalis and/or glucagon may be helpful. If an arrhythmia is the cause of the poor perfusion and can be corrected, the prognosis may be quite good. It is in the management of arrhythmias and the prevention of ventricular fibrillation that coronary-care units have their greatest benefit.

In the remaining 30 or 40% of patients with persistent shock, the problem is considered to be "pump failure." If this "pump failure" is unresponsive to inotropic drugs, and the shock persists for more than two hours, the mortality rate is virtually 100%. In these individuals, new modes of therapy such as intra-aortic balloon pumping,[16] counterpulsation, partial cardiopulmonary bypass, and membrane oxygenators may be of value. It is also in this small number of individuals that direct surgery for proximal coronary-artery occlusions, as demonstrated by arteriograms, may be of value.

REFERENCES

1. Wilson, R. F., et al.: Hemodynamic measurements in septic shock. Arch. Surg., 91:121, 1965.
2. MacKenzie, G. J., et al.: Circulatory and respiratory studies in myocardial infarction and cardiogenic shock. Lancet, 2:17, 1964.
3. Shires, T., et al.: Distributional changes in extracellular fluid during acute hemorrhagic shock. Surg. Forum, 11:115, 1960.
4. Ahlquist, R. P.: A study of the adrenotropic receptors. Amer. J. Physiol., 153:586, 1948.
5. Wilson, R. F., et al.: Severe alkalosis in critically ill surgical patients. Arch. Surg. in press.
6. Moore, F. D., et al.: The effects of hemorrhage on body composition. New Eng. J. Med., 273:567, 1965.
7. Lillihei, R., et al.: Hemodynamic alterations and results of treatment on patients with gram-negative septic shock. Surgery, 67:377, 1970.
8. Robb, H. J., and Jabs, C. S.: Distortion and dynamics of cellular elements in the microcirculation. Angiology, 19:602, 1968.
9. Schayer, R. W.: Relationship of stress-induced histidine decarboxylase activity in histamine synthesis to circulatory homeostasis and shock. Science, 131:226, 1960.
10. Phillips, S. J.: Technique of percutaneous subclavian vein catheterization. Surg. Gynec. Obstet., 127:1079, 1968.
11. Borow, M., and Escaro, R.: The reliability of central venous pressure monitoring and errors in its interpretation. Surg. Gynec. Obstet., 127:1288, 1968.
12. Wilson, R. F., Sarver, E., and Birks, R.: Central venous pressure and blood volume determinations in clinical shock. Surg. Gynec. Obstet., 132:631, 1971.
13. deDuve, C.: *Lysosomes: A New Group of Cytoplasmic Particles, Subcellular Particles.* New York, Ronald Press, 1959.
14. Wilson, R. F., and Fisher, R. R.: The hemodynamic effects of massive steroids in clinical shock. Surg. Gynec. Obstet., 127:769, 1968.
15. Dale, H. H., and Richards, A. N.: Vasodilator actions of histamine and other substances. J. Physiol., 52:100, 1918.
16. Kantrowitz, A., et al.: Current states of the intra-aortic balloon pump and initial clinical experience with an aortic patch auxiliary ventricle. Transplantation Proc., 3:1459, 1971.

Suggested Reading

1. Shoemaker, W. C.: Cardiorespiratory patterns in complicated and uncomplicated septic shock. Physiologic alterations and their therapeutic implications. Ann. Surg., 174:119, 1971.
2. Dietzman, R. H., et al.: Corticosteroids as effective vasodilators in the treatment of low output syndrome. Chest, 57:440, 1970.
3. Mueller, H., et al.: Hemodynamics, coronary blood flow, and myocardial metabolism in coronary shock; response to 1-norepinephrine and isoproterenol. J. Clin. Invest., 49:1885, 1970.
4. Schumer, W., and Nyhus, L. M.: Corticosteroid effect on biochemical parameters of human oligemic shock. Arch. Surg., 100:405, 1970.
5. Gunner, R. M., et al.: The hemodynamic effects of myocardial infarction and the results of therapy. Med. Clin. N. Amer., 54:235, 1970.
6. Loeb, H. S., et al.: Acute hemodynamic effects of dopamine in patients with shock. Circulation, 44:163, 1971.
7. Siegel, J. H., Greenspan, M., and Deb Guercio, L. R. M.: Abnormal vascular tone, defective oxygen transport and myocardial failure in human septic shock. Ann. Surg., 165:504, 1967.
8. Siegel, J. H., et al.: The effect of glucagon infusion on cardiovascular function in the critically ill. Surg. Gynec. Obstet., 131:505, 1970.
9. Shoemaker, W. C., et al.: Hemodynamic patterns after acute anesthetized and unanesthetized trauma. Arch. Surg., 95:492, 1967.
10. Udhoji, V. N., et al.: Hemodynamic studies on clinical shock associated with infection. Amer. J. Med., 34:461, 1965.
11. Wilson, R. F.: Current concepts in the monitoring and treatment of shock. J. Mount Sinai Hosp., 20:65, 1972.
12. Kones, R. J.: Pathogenesis of cardiogenic shock II. N.Y. State J. Med., 73:1793, 1973.
13. Misra, S. N., et al.: Hemodynamic effects of adrenergic stimulating and blocking agents in cardiogenic shock and low output state after myocardial infarction. Amer. J. Cardiol., 31:724, 1973.
14. Moss, G. S., and Spleha, J.: Traumatic shock in man. New Eng. J. Med., 290:724, 1974.
15. Stahl, W. M., Jr.: Shock and metabolism. Surg. Gynec. Obstet., 136:210, 1973.
16. Rosenbaum, R. W., et al.: Efficacy of steroids in the treatment of septic and cardiogenic shock. Surg. Gynec. Obstet., 136:914, 1973.

6 SPECIAL PROBLEMS OF TRAUMA IN THE AGED, ADDICTED, AND ALCOHOLIC

J. R. KIRKPATRICK
R. L. KROME
A. J. WALT
R. F. WILSON

"Years, indeed, taken alone are a very fallacious mode of reckoning age: it is not the time but the quality of a man's past life that we have to reckon. . . . The old people who are thin and dry and tough, clear voiced and bright eyed, with good stomachs and strong wills, muscular and active are not bad; they bear all but the largest operations very well; but very bad are they, who are feeble and soft skinned, with little pulses, bad appetites, and weak digestive powers."

SIR JAMES PAGET, 1877

THE AGED

The tendency to treat old patients less vigorously than young ones, or to withhold needed surgery on the grounds of a projected short life expectancy or an inability to withstand major operation, should be avoided. The life expectancy for individuals above the age of 60 is greater than many physicians recognize:[1]

Age	Average Life Expectancy		
	Male	Female	All
60	15.8	20.0	17.9
65	12.8	16.2	14.6
70	10.3	12.8	11.6
75	8.2	9.7	9.0
80	6.2	7.1	6.7
85	4.5	4.8	4.7

However, while old age in itself is not a contraindication to surgery, operations in older patients are definitely associated with an increased mortality and morbidity. This higher mortality rate is directly related to deterioration of specific organ systems and, in some cases, to the presence of superimposed chronic diseases. Recognition of this fact is essential in evaluating the traumatized aged patient.

The preoperative assessment should be as thorough as possible under the circumstances which prevail at the time of injury. This evaluation may lead to critical decisions on the need for digitalization, the importance of establishing and maintaining a high urinary output, special pulmonary support, or antidiabetic therapy. An important part of understanding the elderly patient is realizing that a fine balance exists between his "normal" function and what would be considered disease in a younger patient. It must be remembered also that the likelihood of preexisting chronic disease is great, and the examiner must be diligent and perceptive in distinguishing the "physiologic changes of aging" from actual disease.

Cardiovascular System

The heart in the absence of specific disease undergoes little anatomic change with aging. However, although its weight is remarkably constant after age 25,[2] physiologic changes are numerous and well documented. Cardiac output and stroke volume decrease 30 to 40% between the ages of 25 and 65 years. Myocardial conduction and contraction times are increased, limiting the heart's ability to increase its rate in response to added work loads. Consequently, changes in cardiac output may be dependent upon changes in stroke volume, especially in the presence of a preexisting tachycardia. To complete this vicious circle, peripheral resistance increases markedly with age. Because of these changes, the cardiovascular system is particularly susceptible to pump failure in response to increased work and, as a result, cardiac complications are the most common cause of postoperative death in the elderly. The probability of myocardial deterioration can be directly correlated with the cardiac status at the time of injury. As older patients frequently have significant narrowing of important vessels, arterial flow is primarily pressure dependent; the likelihood of cerebral or myocardial infarction increases markedly if significant hypotension occurs.

PITFALL

IF SERIAL EKGS AND ENZYME STUDIES ARE NOT OBTAINED IN ELDERLY PATIENTS WHO HAVE BEEN HYPOTENSIVE, MANY SILENT MYOCARDIAL INFARCTIONS WILL BE MISSED.

The arteriosclerotic narrowing and inelasticity of the arteries and arterioles in elderly patients alter their ability to compensate for blood loss and hamper homeostatic responses to subsequent events.

Other important cardiovascular factors contributing to an increased risk include angina pectoris (especially if it is increasing), recent myocardial infarction, cardiac arrhythmias, and unstable hypertension. A myocardial infarction during the previous three months greatly increases the risk of operation; if the infarct is more than six months old, however, the risk is only slightly increased, especially if there are no other signs or symptoms of coronary-artery disease. Congestive heart failure or arrhythmias, especially when resistant to treatment, greatly increase the operative risk. Multiple premature contractions are of particular concern.

The cardiovascular system is extremely brittle and fluid overload is a constant hazard. Many patients with chronic cardiac failure who have been treated with diuretics for months or years develop severe deficiencies in serum sodium, potassium, chloride, magnesium, and calcium. These electrolyte abnormalities may have wide-ranging effects manifested clinically by weakness, hypotension, lethargy, and abnormal responses to many drugs, especially anesthetics and myocardial stimulants.

Massive transfusions of blood and the persistence of prolonged hypotension can cause wide swings in pH, acid-base balance, and serum electrolyte concentrations, altering not only the excitability of the myocardium and its conducting system but also the patient's response to some drugs, especially digitalis. During massive blood transfusions, a large bolus of cold blood may reduce the cardiac temperature below 32 to 34 C, thus further impairing cardiac performance and predisposing toward the development of arrhythmias.

Patients with a long history of hypertension may require arterial pressures higher than normal to maintain adequate perfusion of essential organs. If systolic blood pressure falls below 140 mm Hg, signs of overt renal failure may develop. In these patients it is vital to anticipate the physiologic effects of general anesthesia and blood loss, as both of these tend to produce hypotension. We have found that general anesthesia can reduce effective cardiac output by as much as 33%. The vascular system in the aged, by virtue of the established arteriosclerosis, is significantly less responsive to changes in flow and pressure, necessitating meticulous monitoring and constant support.

Genitourinary System

Reduction in renal mass,[3] number of glomeruli,[4] and filtration rates[5] in the aged is well documented. Of these changes, those affecting filtration and perfusion are the most significant. The glomerular filtration rate decreases by 46% between the third and the tenth decade.[6] Effective renal blood flow also decreases dramatically with aging (Fig. 1).

Within a narrow range, the kidney in the older individual is capable of maintaining normal acid-base balance as long as adequate perfusion is maintained and the metabolic load is not excessive.[7] The ability to compensate for a metabolic acidosis or alkalosis is closely related to the deterioration of renal function with aging, and is decreased even further if preexisting renal disease is present.

The osmolality of the urine is determined by the composition of the plasma, the integrity of the renal tubules, and the adequacy of perfusion. In a healthy young kidney this is reflected by the ability, in the face of dehydration, to concentrate to a specific gravity of 1.035 and a maximum osmolality of 1400. With aging, this ability to concentrate urine decreases so that specific gravities greater than 1.024 and osmolalities greater than 750 are rarely achieved after age 70.[7] As a result, older individuals usually need a much larger urine volume to clear the plasma of quantities of waste which might pose no problem for a younger patient even if he were slightly oliguric.

This decrease in renal function in conjunction with a loss of cardiac reserve causes a double problem. In the elderly traumatized patient, increased amounts of fluids must often be given to maintain an adequate urinary output at a time when even minimal overloading can cause severe heart failure or pulmonary edema.

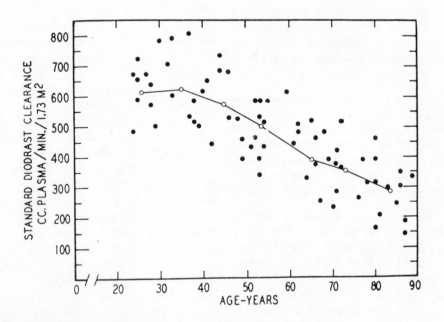

FIG. 1. Change in standard Diodrast clearance or effective renal plasma flow with age. 0—0 = Average values ml plasma/min/1.73 sq m body surface area. (After Shock, N. W.: In *Cowdry's Problems of Ageing*, 3rd ed. (Lansing, A. E., Ed.). Baltimore, Williams and Wilkins, 1952.)

Respiratory System

A number of classic changes in respiratory function have long been associated with aging. An increase in anterior-posterior diameter of the thoracic cage is common, and this, together with the kyphosis which results from bone and soft-tissue changes, can cause a severe loss of thoracic-cage compliance. Even though total lung capacity may not be decreased, residual volume tends to increase from a normal of 20 to 25% to 35 to 45% with a corresponding decrease in vital capacity (Fig. 2). Dramatic decrease can also occur in the timed

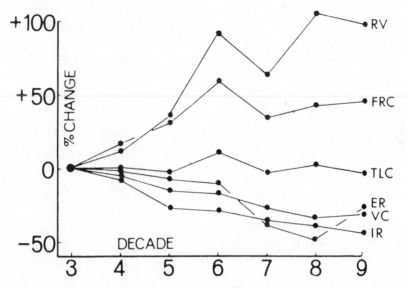

FIG. 2. Percentage changes in static lung volumes in normal subjects at various ages compared to values found in the third decade of life. All data are expressed as volume per sq m of body surface area. RV = Residual volume, FRC = functional residual capacity, TLC = total lung capacity, ER = expiratory reserve, VC = vital capacity, IR = inspiratory reserve. (From Mithoefer, J. C., and Karetzky, M. S.[9])

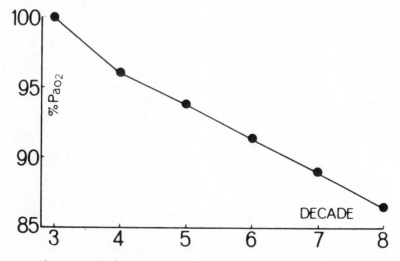

FIG. 3. Percentage change in partial pressure of oxygen (P_{AO_2}) with age in normal subjects. For calculation of absolute values, 90 mm Hg can be assumed to be normal in the third decade. (From Mithoefer, J. C., and Karetzky, M. S.[9])

forced expiratory volume. Although the ratio of the $F.E.V._{1.0}/T.V.C.$ in a young patient is often 0.8 to 0.9, in elderly patients the gradual increase in airway obstruction can reduce the ratio to 0.6 to 0.7 or lower.

The ability of the lungs to function as an effective membrane oxygenator also decreases with age. There is almost a linear decline in the partial pressure of oxygen with aging (Fig. 3). This change in oxygenation potential may represent changes in the diffusion capacity of the lung or ventilatory-perfusion derangements. Little change is noted in the Pco_2 in normal subjects as a result of aging; however, if the patient has had a chronic hypercapnia, the Pco_2 must not be reduced too rapidly because of the severe combined alkalosis which may result.

PITFALL

IF AN ELDERLY PATIENT WITH CHRONIC SEVERE RESPIRATORY DISEASE IS VENTILATED AGGRESSIVELY, THE SUDDEN REDUCTION IN Pco_2 CAN CAUSE A SEVERE COMBINED ALKALOSIS WITH RESULTANT ARRHYTHMIAS OR HYPOTENSION.

The arterial pH in patients with chronic severe respiratory disease and hypercarbia is maintained at approximately normal levels by a compensatory rise in the plasma bicarbonate levels. Under ordinary circumstances, bicarbonate levels change much more slowly than Pco_2. Thus, if the Pco_2 and serum carbonic acid are suddenly and rapidly reduced by hyperventilation, the bicarbonate/carbonic acid ratio and pH will rise abruptly and dangerously. Chronic acid-base and electrolyte abnormalities should not be corrected rapidly except under very unusual circumstances.

Clinically these pulmonary changes may have little effect on the healthy aged patient; however, most elderly patients have some chronic bronchitis from smoking or some degree of emphysema, and these problems combined with severe chest

trauma can be devastating. Characteristically, the elderly are poor coughers; this, together with the emphysema and bronchitis, not only interferes with gaseous exchange but also dramatically increases the chance of postoperative atelectasis and pneumonia. At least 50% of elderly patients undergoing thoracic surgery develop postoperative complications, and of these two thirds are pulmonary.[10] Vigorous application of pulmonary toilet and ventilatory support in the elderly postoperative patient cannot be overemphasized.

Other Organ Systems

Although the changes seen in the cardiovascular, respiratory and renal systems have the most pronounced effects on the survival of the elderly trauma patient, it should be noted that other systems also manifest definite yet often subtle deterioration with aging. The elderly patient with decreased gastrointestinal motility is often dependent on cathartics and is prone to develop a prolonged postoperative ileus.

PITFALL

IF UNEXPLAINED DIARRHEA OCCURS AND A DIGITAL RECTAL EXAMINATION IS NOT PERFORMED, FECAL IMPACTIONS WILL BE MISSED.

Fecal impaction, which often manifests itself as diarrhea, is a frequent event in the hospital course of elderly patients. The use of stool softeners may help to prevent this complication.

Metabolic changes in the aged include the development of an abnormal glucose tolerance in 50% of patients over 70 years of age.[11] It is not clear whether this should be considered merely a physiologic change of aging or actual diabetes mellitus, but it can occasionally cause severe problems, especially during I.V. hyperalimentation. Although several laboratory studies of the steroid response to stress have shown that the adrenal glands in the aged respond normally,[12,13] many elderly patients act clinically as if they have some adrenal insufficiency. There is a precipitous fall in estrogen in females after menopause and a more gradual decrease in testosterone in males. Significant decreases in androgen production with aging as measured by urinary 11-deoxy-17-ketosteroids[14] probably reflect some decrease not only in gonadal but also in adrenal function. This results in a precarious anabolic-catabolic balance which may be easily tipped to catabolism by trauma or surgery.

The elderly are frequently dependent on a variety of drugs, and the physician must be careful to inquire about them fully. When a patient is unable to give a clear history, special attempts must be made to elicit the pertinent data from friends or family. It is also not uncommon for patients to take excessive or inadequate doses of their medications; this can result in severe problems, such as electrolyte abnormalities from diuretics, gastrointestinal disturbances and arrhythmias from digitalis, and clouding of the sensorium from tranquilizers, sedatives, or other drugs.

PITFALL

IF IT IS ASSUMED THAT CONFUSION IN AN ELDERLY PATIENT IS DUE TO SENILE BRAIN CHANGES, EASILY CORRECTABLE HYPOXIA OR RESPIRATORY DYSFUNCTION CAN BE MISSED.

Restlessness and disorientation must not be mistaken for senile brain changes when in fact they may be caused by hypoxia. The surgeon should approach every patient who demonstrates cerebral dysfunction as though these changes were correctable, and his demeanor must be such that the patient senses his interest and concern. Oftentimes transient nocturnal confusion can be successfully treated with reassurance and a light within the room. Tranquilizers and barbiturates should be used with special care for elderly patients, since their effects often cause or potentiate confusion.

Satisfaction of the psychologic demands of elderly patients is important not only to improve their sense of well-being but also to elicit their cooperation, especially in areas of respiration, ambulation and feeding. Finally, since many of these patients are easily depressed, it is essential that optimism and good cheer be included among the medications administered.

THE ADDICTED

The special considerations of trauma in addicted patients are becoming increasingly important. In New York City the most common cause of death in the 18- to 35-year age group is overdosage or other drug-related problems.[15] During 1969-1970 over 200 patients were admitted to the surgical ward at Detroit General Hospital with problems resulting directly or indirectly from heroin addiction.[16] At least 8% of the patients treated in our emergency department have problems related to drug abuse. It has therefore become mandatory for the physician to be able to recognize drug-related symptoms and to deal effectively with the problems posed by addiction. It is important for the physician to recognize that failure to manage the addiction as well as the injury may precipitate serious problems in patient care (Table 1).

Illicit drug use produces difficulties primarily from either "too little" or "too much." The "too little" produces withdrawal symptoms whereas the "too much" causes

TABLE 1. THE MOST FREQUENT ERRORS IN MANAGING DRUG-ADDICTED PATIENTS WITH TRAUMA

Failure to recognize drug abuse in a trauma patient.

Failure to treat drug withdrawal prior to the induction of anesthesia.

Failure to know the common contaminants of street drugs and their effects.

Attributing the patient's low level of consciousness to drugs and not searching for head injury.

Failure to treat the addiction and stabilize the patient.

---

physiologic changes related to the side effects and toxicity of the drug. Associated problems such as infection and thrombosis at sites of injection must also be considered.

The diagnosis of addiction, not always a simple matter, is vital. The compelling reason for establishing an early diagnosis centers around the fact that the patient's abuse may involve drugs which are synergistic, antagonistic, or additive to other drugs needed to maintain homeostasis. Secondly, many of the signs and symptoms produced by addiction are likely to be confused with those resulting from the patient's injuries. It is prudent, therefore, for the physician to search out and treat the drug-related problem with the same speed and effort that he employs in managing the trauma itself.

PITFALL

IF THE DIAGNOSIS OF DRUG USAGE IS OVER-LOOKED PREOPERATIVELY, WITHDRAWAL MAY OCCUR UNDER ANESTHESIA WHEN IT IS MUCH MORE DANGEROUS AND DIFFICULT TO DIAG-NOSE AND TREAT.

Not infrequently it may be difficult to obtain an adequate history after trauma because the patient is under the influence of drugs at the time, has organic brain damage, or is in shock. Failure either to elicit a history of drug ingestion or to obtain laboratory evidence confirming usage may lead to disastrous results. For this reason, the physicians at Detroit General Hospital maintain a liaison with community-action groups intimately involved with many drug users. These centers conduct regular analyses of available street drugs and furnish us with this and other related information. In addition, we attempt to interview the friends or family who accompany the patient to the emergency department.

Confirmation of drug use is difficult to obtain. The physician should check specifically for "needle tracks" (indicative of repeated intravenous injections), nasal ulcerations (seen with intranasal cocaine and

---

PITFALL

IF THE PHYSICIAN IS UNAWARE OF THE CON-TAMINANTS IN STREET DRUGS, HE MAY BE UNABLE TO TREAT THE PATIENT ADEQUATELY AND UNEXPLAINED DEATH MAY OCCUR.

---

heroin usage), cardiac murmurs, or retinal changes. Unexplained respiratory difficulty should make the physician suspicious of a narcotic or barbiturate overdose.[18,19] Although a rapid pulse is usually indicative of hypovolemia, tachycardia associated with a normal or elevated blood pressure may be an early clue to the ingestion of amphetamines or hallucinogens. In contrast, patients with bradycardia and hypotension may have taken large doses of depressants such as narcotics, barbiturates or tranquilizers. Patients with sluggish but widely dilated pupils and with no evidence of head injury should be suspected of having taken excessive doses of barbiturates or tranquilizers.

PITFALL

IF A PATIENT'S POOR LEVEL OF CONSCIOUS-NESS IS CASUALLY ATTRIBUTED TO THE IN-GESTION OF A DRUG, A SIGNIFICANT HEAD INJURY MAY BE OVERLOOKED.

No change in the mental status of a trauma patient should be considered as drug related until all other causes (subdural hematomas, skull fractures, and contusions) are excluded and the diagnosis of drug use is firmly established. Every trauma patient must have a thorough neurologic examination which includes palpation of the scalp for penetrating wounds. Small penetrating wounds of the skull are easily overlooked and their significance is often underestimated. Although vague generalized signs or symptoms are often caused by drugs, unconsciousness associated with localizing signs is rare. X-rays and blood glucose, barbiturate, salicylate and alcohol levels should also be obtained to aid in the differentiation of traumatic and drug-induced coma.

For practical purposes, all the narcotic drugs, including heroin, morphine, Demerol, and codeine can be considered in one group. Paregoric and elixir terpin hydrate with codeine (ETH-C) are grouped with the narcotics but also contain a relatively large volume of alcohol. The barbiturates and tranquilizers may be placed in a secondary category since they produce similar symptoms of addiction and withdrawal. The hallucinogens, the third important category of drugs, include LSD, mescaline, peyote, and STP. The final group (adulterants) includes drugs and inert substances frequently mixed with "street drugs" either to potentiate the effect of the primary drug or to dilute the amount of drug required. Strychnine, atropine, belladonna, talcum powder, quinine and sugar are the major offenders in this group.

Specific symptom complexes and addiction management vary with each drug; however, general guidelines are available for each major category.

Group I (Narcotics)

Narcotic addiction is now recognized as one of the most important causes of violent behavior. The addict's attempts to procure funds to support his habit can result in gunshot wounds, stabbings, or occasionally blunt injuries from beatings. Different problems result from the addiction itself. Included among these are abscesses, septicemia, hepatitis, endocarditis and, rarely, pneumothoraces. Knowing that there is an increased incidence of these diseases among addicts may help the physician recognize the coincident drug problem.

Occasionally, young heroin addicts will exhibit a bizarre type of cardiac and respiratory difficulty characterized by mental confusion, x-ray evidence of pulmonary congestion, and progressive cardiac failure. This type of cardiac failure, resistant to the usual forms of therapy, is typical of the so-called heroin-toxicity death.[20] At autopsy, these patients frequently have edematous congested lungs similar to the "wet lungs" seen in other diseases. Patients with this difficulty should be given narcotic antagonists, but these must be administered slowly and in small doses (3 to 5 mg) with close scrutiny of the pupillary reflexes, the level of consciousness, and respiration.

Another confusing situation encountered with some frequency in emergency departments is the appearance of an unconscious patient without evidence of trauma. If this patient has respiratory difficulty and pinpoint pupils, a narcotic overdose should be suspected; after ventilatory support has been provided, a small dose of an antagonist (either Nalline or Narcan) should be injected while pupillary and respiratory changes are observed. Too rapid or too large a dose may potentiate the depressant effects of the narcotic. If there is no response, and if serum levels for barbiturates, salicylates, alcohol and sugar are within normal limits, we assume that the patient's obtunded state is not related to an overdose of a drug, and extra care must be taken to determine an organic cause.

Withdrawal from narcotic addiction can be a frightening experience for both physician and patient, especially if it occurs during the postoperative period. It is important to realize that rarely, if ever, is death due to the cardiorespiratory effects of withdrawal alone. The withdrawal syndrome (rhinorrhea, lacrimation, confusion, sweating, cramping, and diarrhea) can, however, produce severe dehydration and electrolyte imbalances similar to those seen with excessive vomiting and diarrhea. With the current popularity of methadone, the physician must also be aware that withdrawal from methadone can occur but may not start until 24 hours after the last dose; in some instances the physiologic changes due to methadone withdrawal may be dangerous. At least one instance of hypotension and death has been reported in a patient withdrawing from large doses of methadone while undergoing anesthesia.

4

Talwin should not be administered to the narcotic addict during withdrawal since it is a mild narcotic antagonist and can potentiate the effects of nalorphine.

Whenever possible, narcotic addicts should be stabilized prior to surgery.[21] If the patient has not previously taken methadone, oral or intramuscular methadone may be administered in doses of approximately 10 mg every four to six hours unless signs of an overdose (nystagmus, pinpoint pupils, drowsiness) appear. The dose is repeated during the second 24 hours; subsequently, the dose may be reduced by 5 to 10 mg every second or every third day so that the patient is kept comfortable. Patients receiving oral methadone from treatment programs should be maintained on their usual doses. Methadone is rapidly absorbed from the stomach and small intestine and may be given by mouth even if a nasogastric tube is in place, provided the tube is clamped for 30 minutes following ingestion. It may be prudent to delay surgery for an hour or so after oral methadone administration so that absorption is complete and the patient can be protected from withdrawal. It is important to remember that the trauma patient in shock who is immediately taken to the operating room will often not manifest withdrawal symptoms until he is under anesthesia or until he reaches the recovery room.

During the postoperative period, the patient should be started or continued on methadone. As long as it does not complicate his treatment, the drug may be given orally. The use of tranquilizers or barbiturates to aid in the treatment of withdrawal is usually not necessary if the patient is obtaining an adequate narcotic or methadone dose; however, if additional medication is required for comfort or sleep, we rely upon antihistamines such as Benadryl rather than barbiturates. This has been safe and successful in our hands. If narcotic withdrawal symptoms are managed without methadone, it may be necessary to rely on antiemetics such as Tigan and antispasmodics such as Donnatal for relief of the gastrointestinal symptoms.

PITFALL

IF THE PHYSICIAN FAILS TO CARE FOR THE ADDICT'S NARCOTIC NEEDS WHILE HE IS IN THE HOSPITAL, THE ADDICT MAY SEEK TO OBTAIN DRUGS FROM NONMEDICAL SOURCES, LEADING TO SUDDEN UNEXPLAINED RESPIRATORY DIFFICULTIES AND/OR DEATH.

Sudden deterioration or exacerbation of an addict's symptoms in the hospital without explanation should alert the physician to the possibility that the patient is receiving heroin from friends or family. It is important for the trauma surgeon to remember that illicit narcotics are readily available to patients in most urban hospitals. On several occasions visitors have injected heroin into the I.V. lines of critically ill patients; in at least two patients, this may have been a cause of otherwise unexplained death.[22]

Group II (Barbiturates, Tranquilizers)

The common pharmacologic action of these drugs is depression of the central nervous system with resultant lethargy, slurred speech, inability to solve simple mental problems, and confusion. As previously noted, severe overdoses may also produce bradycardia and hypotension.

Treatment of barbiturate or tranquilizer intoxication varies with the severity of the symptoms and depression. Gastric lavage, if feasible, should be carried out as soon as possible with a large 40 to 50 F Ewald tube to remove any drug still retained in the stomach. If the patient is reasonably alert and unlikely to aspirate, the stomach can be filled with warm saline and the patient encouraged to vomit. It may take two, three, or more liters of saline to clear the stomach adequately.

If there is severe respiratory depression, an endotracheal tube should be inserted and a respirator used to maintain adequate ventilation. If the patient becomes hypotensive, large volumes of fluid may be needed to fill the dilated vascular space and provide an adequate cardiac output. Occasionally, inotropic drugs or norepinephrine (Chap. 5) may be needed to maintain a satisfactory blood pressure and tissue perfusion.

Short-acting barbiturates such as Nembutal and Pentothal are metabolized primarily by the liver while long-acting barbiturates are excreted with little or no change by the kidneys. Since the excretion of both types of barbiturates, especially the long-acting group, is increased by alkalinizing the serum and urine and maintaining a high urine output, large volumes of intravenous fluid and bicarbonate should be given. Diuretics in small amounts should be given as needed to achieve urinary outputs of at least 100 to 200 ml/hr. If treatment is begun within a reasonable period of time, hemodialysis or peritoneal dialysis is rarely required.

Barbiturate withdrawal may produce a variety of symptoms and signs, including seizures, delirium, hyperpyrexia, tachycardia, and coma. Symptoms occurring in the postoperative period may be especially severe and can cause death. Of all the drugs which may be abused, the barbiturates are the most likely to cause death as a result of acute withdrawal.

The problems during anesthesia may be especially great. If Pentothal sodium is used to induce anesthesia, the barbiturate addict may have a sudden reexacerbation of his respiratory crisis. The administration of large doses of these barbiturates will reintoxicate the patient, and when the anesthetic wears off he may redevelop the withdrawal syndrome. Barbiturate withdrawal in the postoperative period requires intramuscular injection of short-acting barbiturates, repeated in doses of 100 mg every hour until the patient appears intoxicated. This dose is then reduced over a period of several weeks at a rate of no more than 100 mg each day.

Group III (Hallucinogens)

Patients under the influence of the hallucinogens often have wild visual and, rarely, auditory images; perceiving these as reality, they act accordingly. The hallucinations may, as a consequence, precipitate self-inflicted wounds and suicidal gestures. This type of addiction should always be suspected when the physician is confronted with a bizarre suicide attempt.

Excitability, disorientation, inappropriate verbiage, and occasional fits of rage can characterize a "bad trip"; overdoses can produce death, seizures, or unconsciousness. A "good trip" results in euphoric states, tranquility, or mere vagueness. In selected cases, physical findings can include mydriasis, hyperthermia, pilo-erection, hyperglycemia and bradycardia. The psychiatric effects of the hallucinogens are often more dangerous than the trauma itself.

The physician should assume that the history is not valid unless he can document that the reported "street drug" is in fact the same as the patient thinks he has taken. As with narcotic users, we rely upon local referral centers to ferret out much of this information. It should also be remembered that the patient is incompetent to sign his own operative permit while under the influence of drugs.

Preoperative medication should not include drugs such as atropine since these may potentiate the anticholinergic effects of some of the hallucinogens. Generally, we have found the safest drug for control of the hallucinogenic experience is intramuscular Valium in doses of 5 to 10 mg every 2 to 4 hours as needed. Since these patients often are experiencing active hallucinations and are very susceptible to visual and auditory stimuli, they should be placed in a quiet room and managed by either a physician or a nurse who can appreciate the subjective sensations experienced by the patient.

Group IV (Adulterants)

The three most important drugs in this group are atropine, strychnine, and quinine. Any of these drugs may produce symptoms more lethal and incapacitating than the primary narcotic with which they are mixed.

Classic cases of atropine toxicity are occasionally encountered in heroin addicts (this is a common drug combination). Tachycardia, fever, cutaneous blushing, dilated pupils, and extreme dryness of the skin and mucous membranes are characteristic. Recognition is vital, especially in conjunction with preoperative medications. Atropine toxicity represents an obvious contraindication to the use of anticholinergic drugs. If the toxicity is mild, time alone will solve the problem. Severe overdoses should be managed with short-acting barbiturates, hypothermia, intravenous fluids and eye patches to prevent blinding from the excessive light which may reach the retina through the dilated pupils. Cholinergic drugs such as methacholine and Urecholine are of no therapeutic value, but may be useful in substantiating the diagnosis of atropine toxicity. Administration of 10 to 20 mg of methacholine subcutaneously will produce rhinorrhea, lacrimation, salivation, sweating and cramps in a normal person. Since atropine will prevent these symptoms, a negative response to methacholine stimulation is diagnostic of atropine toxicity.

Strychnine is a popular adulterant and many compounds have been produced containing it as an active ingredient. Although toxicity is easily recognized when far advanced, early changes may include nothing more than reflex hyperexcitability. The chronic user does not develop tolerance or manifest cumulative effects. Sudden overdosage produces muscle spasms which progress to seizures and true opisthotonos. Abdominal cramps and constricted facial muscles are diagnostic of acute toxicity. Treatment is directed toward respiratory support; control of seizures can generally be managed with short-acting barbiturates, but occasionally paralysis with curare is required.

Quinine overdosage (anchorism) is difficult to distinguish from salicylate poisoning. Early symptoms include tinnitus, headache, nausea, and blurred vision. Either chronic poisoning or acute toxicity can produce photophobia, dyslogia, blindness, cramps, vomiting, and a characteristic papular scarlatina-like rash. Death can occur from respiratory failure. A subtle clue to the identification of the chronic user of quinine is the presence of an unexplained hemolytic anemia. Treatment is symptomatic and survival after 24 hours is usually assurance of complete recovery.

THE ALCOHOLIC

The combination of alcoholism and severe trauma provides the surgeon and emergency physician with some of their most difficult problems. A relationship with alcoholism is found in industrial accidents, and recently a correlation with home accidents has also been established.

The usual difficulties faced by the physician are those associated with acute alcoholic intoxication; however, he must also be prepared to contend with complications of acute alcoholic withdrawal or of chronic alcoholism, usually in the form of cirrhosis.

Acute Alcoholism

The main problems in treating acute alcoholism, especially with trauma, include management of the acute intoxication and prevention of diagnostic errors and respiratory complications.

ACUTE INTOXICATION. Alcoholic "overdose" (acute intoxication) is often manifested by: a change in mental state, nystagmus, slurred speech, and a staggering gait. Not uncommonly patients may also have a slow pulse, slow respiratory rate, and orthostatic hypotension completely unrelated to the trauma. Many of these patients are extremely loud, belligerent, and uncooperative. Frequently those with minimal injuries will loudly insist on extensive care while those with severe trauma often cannot be made to appreciate fully the seriousness of their injuries and will want to leave without definitive care.

PITFALL

IF IT IS NOT APPRECIATED THAT ACUTE ALCOHOLIC INTOXICATION CAN SERIOUSLY IMPAIR A PATIENT'S JUDGMENT, SERIOUSLY INJURED UNCOOPERATIVE OR UNWILLING PATIENTS MAY BE ALLOWED TO LEAVE THE HOSPITAL WITHOUT ADEQUATE CARE.

Since the emergency-department personnel are often happy to be rid of these uncooperative or obnoxious patients, especially if they are "repeaters," cool professional judgment is essential. Rapidly available psychiatric help may also be extremely valuable.

MISTAKEN DIAGNOSES. Because of an absent or unreliable history and a physical examination which is often incomplete because of poor patient cooperation, mistaken or delayed diagnoses in acutely intoxicated patients are quite frequent.

PITFALL

IF ALCOHOLICS ARE NOT ROUSED FREQUENTLY AND CHECKED AFTER THEY HAVE FALLEN INTO DRUNKEN SLEEP, SERIOUS NEUROLOGIC LESIONS MAY NOT BE REVEALED UNTIL TOO LATE. THE MEDICOLEGAL IMPLICATIONS ARE OBVIOUS.

Although many patients are hyperactive and may even have to be restrained initially, they later tend to fall asleep and become extremely difficult to arouse. Under these circumstances a subdural hematoma can easily be missed unless the patient is examined completely at frequent intervals.

Although significant neurologic lesions in the acutely intoxicated patient may be overlooked, the stupor of intoxication will occasionally mimic an intracranial lesion and lead to overtreatment. Both of these unfortunate errors can usually be avoided by following certain basic rules with all acutely intoxicated patients who have had head trauma or are unconscious:

1. Obtain complete vital signs at least every 30 minutes.
2. Do a neurologic examination, which includes pupillary size and reaction and deep tendon reflexes, at least every 30 minutes while the patient is unconscious.
3. Obtain skull films on all alcoholics with head trauma and all unconscious patients.
4. Observe patients who are acutely intoxicated and have skull fractures for subdural hematoma.
5. Remember that acute alcoholic intoxication per se never produces lateralizing neurologic signs.
6. Do not accept alcoholism as a cause of unconsciousness if the blood level of alcohol is less than 150 mg/100 ml.

Injuries to the chest or abdomen in unconsciousness patients are best diagnosed by objective means such as x-rays and peritoneal lavage. Alcoholism should not be accepted as a cause for unstable vital signs, and a careful search should be made for possible sources of bleeding.

Mistakes in diagnosis can be avoided if it is appreciated that acutely intoxicated patients are unreliable historians and that lack of pain or tenderness has little significance. In short, these patients must be investigated completely before accepting the happy drunk's frequent evaluation of his problem: "I'm all right."

RESPIRATORY COMPLICATIONS. Almost all grossly intoxicated patients who are lying down will tend to "snore" because of partial airway obstruction from a flaccid overly lax tongue falling into the pharynx. This problem can be readily handled by turning the patient on his side, if this position does not aggravate his other injuries. Alternatively, an oral airway may be necessary. Occasionally the respiratory depression is so severe that an endotracheal tube and respiratory assistance are required.

Chronic smoking very frequently accompanies alcoholism and the resultant chronic bronchitis and emphysema produce many of the respiratory problems seen in these patients. Alcoholics are also prone to develop cervical spinal fractures, aspiration, and severe acute respiratory infections, including lung abscesses. This not uncommonly is the result of aspiration of vomitus. Aspiration, especially if combined with severe trauma, sepsis or shock, can produce a severe progressive pneumonitis with respiratory failure. Evidence of aspiration should be looked for carefully and treated vigorously with bronchoscopy, tracheostomy, respirator assistance, and steroids as needed.

Acute Withdrawal (Delirium Tremens)

Delirium tremens (DTs) is the most dramatic of the complications of alcoholism and may be fatal in 10 to 15% of cases. The usual patient with DTs has been recently and acutely deprived of alcohol after having been an excessive and steady drinker for many years. Trauma is a common mechanism by which this deprivation occurs, and DTs under these circumstances are especially lethal.

The full-blown syndrome in the trauma patient usually does not become manifest for at least 24 to 48 hours, but in some instances it may be delayed for four to five days or more. The first indications of the approaching attack are restlessness and mental irritability. The patient becomes "shaky," anorexic and has a strong desire for alcohol. In severe untreated form, delirium tremens is characterized by a disoriented, disheveled patient who is constantly moving, rearranging bedclothes, tugging at his restraints, and often incontinent. The obvious tremor is so grossly disorganized that even simple chores become impossible. The patient actively hallucinates and characteristically engages in imagined conversation. He may shout or scream in anguish to ward off the people or animals who threaten to imprison or destroy him. Vomiting, dehydration, hyperthermia, hypovolemia, severe electrolyte imbalances and aspiration pneumonitis can occur and if untreated progress to death.

Efforts should be begun immediately to prevent the above sequence of events in all patients deprived of alcohol and especially in those with impending DTs. These patients should be well hydrated with a balanced electrolyte solution administered intravenously, as they are apt to vomit and aspirate if oral fluids are given.

Trace elements, especially magnesium and calcium, and multivitamins, including liberal amounts of thiamine and nicotinic acid, should be added to the I.V.s routinely. Isolation or restraint of the patient should be avoided if possible at this point, as these measures only increase both anxiety and metabolic demands. Sedation is mandatory, but oversedation is injurious and increases the likelihood of aspiration, atelectasis or pneumonia. Various drugs have been used to sedate acute alcoholics, including the perennial standbys chloral hydrate and paraldehyde. If paraldehyde is chosen, 10 ml should be administered orally or rectally every 4 to 6 hours. Tranquilizers, including Librium, Thorazine, and Valium, have also been used. Valium is a safe, reliable drug and has the advantage that it can be given orally, intramuscularly, or intravenously with a fairly wide margin of safety.

If the patient is admitted with or develops full-blown delirium tremens, treatment must be especially intense. It is vital to closely monitor his vital signs, intake, output, and serum electrolytes. The patient may need 6 to 8 liters per day of balanced electrolyte solution to reverse the dehydration and electrolyte imbalance. Nasogastric suction is usually necessary to control vomiting. Large quantities of sedatives or tranquilizers, restraints, and a reasonably quiet environment are often required to control agitation. If there is fever, this should be treated by a hypothermia blanket rather than aspirin.

Many patients with delirium tremens or

acute withdrawal symptoms may also develop seizures, gastrointestinal bleeding or pneumonia. The convulsions should be controlled or prevented with intravenous or intramuscular Valium or Dilantin, after hypoglycemia has been eliminated as a possible etiologic factor.

Gastrointestinal bleeding can usually be controlled with iced saline gastric lavage although occasionally surgical intervention is required. Bleeding from esophageal varices is fraught with an appalling mortality if the patient has concurrent delirium tremens, regardless of the mode of therapy. The recent technique of pharmacotherapy through an intra-arterial catheter may be the initial approach of choice in these special circumstances. It should be stressed that establishment of an accurate diagnosis in gastrointestinal bleeding is of paramount importance. One of the safest, most reliable ways to accomplish this is to utilize the fiberoptic esophagogastroscope and the skill of an experienced endoscopist.

Chronic Alcoholism

Chronic alcoholism is the most frequent cause of cirrhosis in the United States. Patients suffer a wide variety of changes to many different organ systems, all of which must be considered in the alcoholic patient with multiple trauma.

NEUROLOGIC CHANGES. The neurologic changes of chronic alcoholism can make it extremely difficult to obtain an adequate or reliable history, to follow the neurologic changes caused by head trauma, and to get the patient ambulating postoperatively. Korsakoff's syndrome or similar problems can result in medical histories which are extremely misleading. Wernicke's syndrome can cause severe central neurologic changes which unfortunately are not usually localized. The peripheral neuropathy may cause the patient to lose peripheral sensation, coordination, and strength.

CARDIOVASCULAR PROBLEMS. The cardiovascular changes of advanced cirrhosis include a reduced ability to tolerate hypotension and an increased tendency to congestive heart failure. In spite of the tendency of cirrhotics to a high cardiac output, persistent shock in these patients is associated with an extremely high mortality rate.[23] Cardiomyopathies are common. In the past it was thought that most of these cardiac problems were due to a thiamine deficiency and were identical to those seen in beri-beri heart disease. Many of these patients, however, respond only partially to large doses of thiamine. Furthermore, the lesions make the patient overly sensitive to digitalis, especially when acidosis and hypotension are also present. Since the resultant cardiac failure is difficult to manage, extra care must be taken to avoid fluid overload. Conversely, even though severe uncorrected ascites may produce some respiratory distress, complete removal of the fluid at laparotomy is dangerous and can cause severe hypotension unless adequate fluids and protein are administered as the ascites reaccumulates.

COAGULATION PROBLEMS. Severe coagulation problems, especially prothrombin deficiencies, can also be encountered in chronic alcoholics. The injection of vitamin K is mandatory prior to surgery. If transfusions are needed, fresh whole blood and fresh frozen plasma should be used. If at all possible, surgery should be delayed until the prothrombin time is within five seconds of the normal (control) values.

ANESTHETIC CONSIDERATIONS. After initial resuscitation of the traumatized cirrhotic and correction of coagulation defects if possible, critical decisions are required as to the type of anesthetic agents to be utilized. In general, we should choose an agent such as ether or nitrous oxide which does not require detoxification by the liver; Fluothane is avoided. It is probably more important, however, to keep the patient normotensive and well oxygenated than to argue the merits of any particular agent so long as the agent is not primarily hepatotoxic.

PROBLEMS DURING SURGERY. During surgery, especially in the abdomen, excessive bleeding must be anticipated almost in direct proportion to the degree of portal hypertension and coagulation abnormalities. Although the bleeding may be extensive and hypotension is common, care must also be taken not to overhydrate the patient, especially with salt and crystalloids. Fresh whole blood or frozen plasma should be insisted upon as the main fluids for volume replacement.

Direct injuries to the cirrhotic liver are especially difficult to manage. Minor tears and lacerations may bleed profusely, sutures may not hold well, and exposure is often difficult. There is no easy solution to this problem, and at our institution several patients have bled to death from this lesion despite heroic attempts at hemostasis.

POSTOPERATIVE RESUSCITATION. The postoperative management of the chronic alcoholic is often extremely demanding. At best only general rules can be stated: (1) Supply trace elements and vitamins liberally. (2) Transfuse as needed, utilizing fresh blood as often as possible. (3) Avoid excess water and salt. (4) Administer salt-poor albumin as needed. (5) Control ascites with diuretics, particularly aldactone. (6) Avoid ammonia intoxication by cleansing the gastrointestinal tract of blood. (7) Administer intestinal neomycin in selected cases.

The most important postoperative problems in cirrhotics include bleeding, ascites, heart failure, respiratory failure, ammonia intoxication, gastritis, and impaired wound healing. Continued postoperative bleeding all too often is assumed to be caused by coagulation abnormalities. However, usually such bleeding occurs from open vessels which must be controlled directly at surgery. Although the reduction of ascites formation with salt restriction and diuretics is important, overzealous treatment can cause severe hypotension and increased liver failure. Excessively aggressive attempts to correct the hypovolemia caused by continued bleeding and ascites forma-

tion may rebound and result in congestive failure; monitoring of all vital signs, including CVP, is therefore essential.

General debility, poor resistance to infection, chronic respiratory infections, an increased tendency to aspiration, and elevation of the diaphragm by ascites all increase the chances of postoperative pneumonitis and respiratory failure. Complete gastrointestinal decompression, early respirator assistance, and vigorous bronchial toilet are mandatory.

The incidence of ammonia intoxication is greatly increased in the cirrhotic patient with trauma. Liver function is reduced, and this, coupled with the protein load resulting from blood transfusions and absorption of blood from the gastrointestinal tract and peritoneal cavity, sets the stage for hepatic encephalopathy. Cleansing of the gastrointestinal tract of blood with enemas and cathartics as soon as possible and the use of parenteral and intestinal antibiotics may help to reduce ammonia formation by intestinal bacteria. Upper gastrointestinal bleeding may also be increased because of portal hypertension and possibly impaired mucus production. Complete removal of all gastric acid is essential and irrigation with iced saline should be begun as soon as any blood is seen in the nasogastric aspirate.

WOUND HEALING. Alcoholics tend to have poor wound healing and an increased incidence of wound rehiscence. These problems are often attributed to multiple dietary deficiencies which contribute to the development of wasting, hypoproteinemia and alcoholic nutritional cirrhosis. Many chronic alcoholics—even those without documented cirrhosis—will manifest similar metabolic derangements, including magnesium, zinc, and vitamin deficiencies, hypoproteinemia, salt retention, and failure to metabolize adrenal steroids properly. It is thus extremely important to supply increased quantities of glucose, vitamins, and trace metals.

METHANOL. An unusual complication caused by ingestion of methyl alcohol, most frequently encountered in severe alcoholics, is acute pulmonary distress with supraclavicular cyanosis. This respiratory distress is associated with very severe metabolic acidosis and an arterial pH approaching 7.0, but with no evidence of airway obstruction. In such a patient, especially if he is a victim of trauma, the natural tendency of the uninitiated physician is to perform a tracheostomy. If the lungs are examined carefully, however, it will be noted that there is good air exchange; acid-base studies will show that the hyperventilation is an attempt to compensate for the severe metabolic acidosis.

REFERENCES

1. *Mortality*. Vital Statistics of the United States, Vol. 2, Part A, 1966.
2. Korenchevsky, V.: *Physiological and Pathological Aging*. New York, Hafner, 1961.
3. Roessle, R., and Roulet, F.: *Mass and Zahl in der Pathologie*. Berlin, Springer, 1932.
4. Arataki, M.: On the postnatal growth of the kidney, with special reference to the number and size of the glomeruli (albino rat). Amer. J. Anat., 36:399, 1926.
5. Davies, D. F., and Shock, N. W.: Age changes in glomerular filtration rate, effective renal plasma flow and tubular excretory capacity in adult males. J. Clin. Invest., 29:496, 1950.
6. Miller, J. H., McDonald, R. K., and Shock, N. W.: Age changes in the maximal rate of renal tubular reabsorption of glucose. J. Geront., 7:196, 1952.
7. Adler, S., et al.: Effect of acute acid loading on urinary acid excretion by the aging human kidney. J. Lab. Clin. Med., 72:278, 1968.
8. Lindeman, R. D., et al.: Influence of age, renal disease, hypertension, diuretics and calcium on the antidiuretic response to suboptimal infusions of vasopressin. J. Lab. Clin. Med., 68:206, 1966.
9. Mithoefer, J. C., and Karetzky, M. S.: The cardiopulmonary system in the aged. In: *Surgery of the Aged and Debilitated Patient* (Powers, J. D., Ed.). Philadelphia, W. B. Saunders, 1968.
10. Niesenbaum, L.: Problems of pulmonary disease in the aged. Geriatrics, 23:127, 1968.
11. Andres, R.: Diabetes and aging. Hosp. Pract., 2:63, 1967.
12. Solomon, D. H., and Shock, N. W.: Studies of adrenal cortical and anterior pituitary function in elderly men. J. Geront., 5:302, 1950.
13. Duncan, L. E., Jr., et al.: The metabolic and hematologic effects of the chronic administration of ACTH to young and old men. J. Geront., 7:351, 1952.
14. Pinkus, G.: Aging and urinary steroid excretion. In: *Hormones and the Aging Process* (Engle, E. T., and Pinkus, G., Eds.). New York, Academic Press, 1956.
15. Richter, R. W., Baden, M. N., and Pearson, J.: Medical news. JAMA, 212:967, 1970.
16. Kirkpatrick, J. R., and Krome, R. L.: Surgical manifestations of heroin addiction. JACEP, 2:24, 1973.
17. Atlee, W. E.: Talc and cornstarch emboli in eyes of drug abusers. JAMA, 219:49, 1972.
18. Bodzin, L. J., and Krome, R. L.: Drug overdose. Med. Opinion, 2:34, 1973.
19. Brill, H.: Death and disability in drug addiction and abuse. Ann. Intern. Med., 67:205, 1967.
20. Helpern, M., and Rho, Y.: Deaths of narcotism in New York City. N.Y. State J. Med., 66:2391, 1966.
21. Mark, L. C., et al.: Hypotension during anesthesia in narcotic addicts. N.Y. State J. Med., 66:2685, 1966.
22. Krome, R. L., Ledgerwood, A., and Lucas, C. E.: The hazards of drug addiction on a trauma ward. Mich. Med., 70:603, 1971.
23. Wilson, R. F., and Krome, R.: Factors affecting prognosis in clinical shock. Ann. Surg., 169:93, 1969.

Suggested Reading

1. Auerbach, O., et al.: Relation of smoking and age to findings in lung parenchyma: A microscopic study. Chest, 65:29, 1974.
2. Webster, I. W.: The age-prevalence of cardiovascular abnormalities in relation to the aging of special sense function. J. Amer. Geriat. Soc., 12:13, 1974.
3. Mitialic, M. J. and Fishh, C.: Electrocardiographic findings in the aged. A review. Amer. Heart J., 87:117, 1974.
4. Hant, M. J., and Cowan, D. H.: The effect of ethanol on hemostatic properties of human platelets. Amer. J. Med. 56:22, 1974.
5. Weyman A. E., et al.: Accidental hypothermia in alcoholic population. Amer. J. Med., 56:13, 1974.
6. Eichner, E. R.: The hematologic disorders of alcoholism. Amer. J. Med., 54:621, 1973.
7. Becker, C. E.: Changing medical complications of illicit drug use. Calif. Med., 119:69, 1973.
8. White, A. G.: Medical disorders in drug addicts: 200 consecutive admissions. JAMA, 223:1469, 1973.

Part 3

GENERAL CONSIDERATIONS OF TRAUMA AND ITS PROBLEMS AND TREATMENT

7 THE INITIAL EVALUATION AND MANAGEMENT OF THE SEVERELY INJURED PATIENT

R. F. WILSON
C. E. LUCAS

"A stitch in time saves nine."

The severely injured patient should be brought to the emergency room rapidly and in the best possible condition if optimal results are to be obtained. To achieve this, we must depend on the first aid provided by trained laymen or paramedical personnel and on well-planned communication and transportation systems (including the use of helicopters, particularly in rural areas). There is obviously a great need for vigorous educational programs for ambulance attendants and the public.

AT THE SCENE OF THE ACCIDENT

Notification of the Accident or Injury

The treatment of the severely injured patient begins at the scene of the accident, with the simple but critical procedure of notifying someone, usually the police, that an accident or injury has occurred. Until this has been done, none of the community health resources can begin to operate. Under ideal circumstances, it should take only a few minutes for the initial telephone or radio call to be made to the dispatch center. The extensive use of freeways has, however, created some delay in this critical period because of the unwillingness of some witnesses to stop, leave the freeway and find a telephone. A system of telephones placed on the freeways at regularly spaced intervals might help to circumvent this problem.

During a prospective evaluation by the Department of Transportation of emergency medical services in Detroit in 1968, it was found that it took an average of 15 minutes for police, firemen, or a private ambulance service to deliver a patient to an emergency room after being notified of an accident (Table 1). This response time was similar for all three groups despite the differences in their modes of operation. The time was rather evenly divided among: (1) dispatch to arrival at the scene of the accident, (2) time at the scene, and (3) time from the scene to the nearest qualified emergency center. The time from accident to notification of the accident could not be precisely determined, but was usually about five minutes. Thus, getting an injured patient to a qualified emergency center in Detroit took an average of 20 minutes.

Central Dispatch Units

Ideally, there should be a central dispatch unit well known to the public and to everyone involved in emergency medical care: firemen, policemen, ambulance drivers, hospitals and telephone operators. This unit, to be effective, must have immediate

TABLE 1. TIME DELAYS* FROM NOTIFICATION OF AN ACCIDENT UNTIL ARRIVAL AT THE HOSPITAL

Time (min.)	Police ambulance	Fire department	Commercial ambulances
From notification until arrival at scene	4.7 ± 2.7	4.2 ± 1.8	4.2 ± 3.2
At the scene of the accident	5.5 ± 5.4	4.1 ± 2.8	4.9 ± 4.7
From scene to hospital	7.3 ± 4.3	4.9 ± 2.2	5.2 ± 3.1

* Average ± S.D.

access to all information concerning the availability and location of emergency vehicles. Such a dispatch center will usually by necessity be integrated with either the police or fire department. The dispatch officer, by knowing the location of all emergency vehicles at all times, should be able to send the nearest available vehicle(s) to the scene.

The quality of care available in the local hospital emergency rooms must be considered in deciding where the patient with multiple injuries is to be taken. In most instances, even if it requires an extra 5 to 10 minutes, the patient should be taken to a hospital which is well equipped to handle severely injured patients. If critically injured patients are to be given adequate care, the physicians, nurses, and paramedical personnel at all levels must be experienced in treating such patients as a matter of daily routine. Obviously, the emergency room must be backed up by an operating-room team prepared to receive within minutes a patient with any type of severe trauma.

PITFALL

IF THE CENTRAL DISPATCH UNIT DOES NOT KEEP TRACK OF THE WORK LOAD AT EACH HOSPITAL, THE CRITICALLY INJURED PATIENT MAY BE SENT TO A HOSPITAL WHICH IS SO OVERWORKED AND CROWDED THAT GOOD CARE MAY BE DELAYED.

The dispatch officer must know the case loads at the various emergency treatment centers. In some circumstances, it may be preferable to send the patient to a small but capable hospital rather than to a large center which is already overloaded.

Emergency Transportation

PITFALL

IF THE AMBULANCE TEAM IS CONCERNED ONLY WITH GETTING THE PATIENT TO THE HOSPITAL AS SOON AS POSSIBLE, THEY MAY GIVE INADEQUATE ATTENTION TO URGENT BUT EASILY HANDLED PROBLEMS, AND THIS MAY MEAN THE DIFFERENCE BETWEEN SEVERE COMPLICATIONS AND A SUCCESSFUL RECOVERY.

All personnel responsible for transporting the injured should have adequate training in the proper initial evaluation and management of the patient. The importance of this may be demonstrated by the following example:

A 33-year-old man was assaulted, robbed and stabbed in the left neck after leaving a theater. The crime was witnessed and the police dispatcher was notified of the injury within three minutes. An emergency vehicle was immediately sent to the scene and arrived four minutes later. The officer noted a large pool of blood beside the victim, who was quite weak but still talking. The victim was placed in the station wagon immediately and arrived at the hospital within another four minutes. The total time elapsed from injury to arrival at the hospital was only 13 minutes. As the patient was being brought from the station wagon, he stopped breathing and was rushed into the "trauma room" where resuscitation was unsuccessful. After the blood was cleared from the wound, a single 1.5-cm laceration was seen to be communicating with the common carotid artery. The police officer was convinced that he had done his best but failed to realize that digital pressure on the wound at the scene and during the trip to the hospital might have saved the patient's life.

It is apparent from this and similar cases that a massive educational effort is needed for all individuals who may be required to give emergency care at the scene of an accident. Unfortunately, the training of police as ambulance attendants is an expensive and extensive undertaking. This is especially true in urban areas where many patients requesting ambulances are not facing true medical emergencies. It is likely that future ambulance service will be increasingly provided by specially trained individuals who have no other responsibility while on duty.

First-aid Treatment

The ambulance personnel must have an organized approach to treatment at the scene of the accident, which follows a list of established priorities.

MAINTENANCE OF AIRWAY AND VENTILA-TION. The attendant must be taught quickly to determine if respiratory obstruction is present and how to treat it. If ventilatory assistance is needed, the attendant should be able to use the rubber face mask with the Ambu-bag to provide manual respiratory support. In addition, all ambulance attendants should be proficient in mouth-to-mouth and mouth-to-nose ventilation.

CONTROL OF HEMORRHAGE. The importance of efficient local compression rather than hazardous tourniquet control of external bleeding cannot be overstressed. Probably the only situation in which a tourniquet may be useful is with a traumatic amputation of an arm or leg. Massive internal bleeding is best treated by safe rapid transit to the nearest qualified emergency room. If the transit time from the scene of the accident to the emergency room is more than 15 minutes, intravenous fluids of a balanced electrolyte type should be given en route.

SPLINTING FRACTURES. Proper splinting provides an effective means of decreasing pain, blood loss and late morbidity following many long-bone fractures. The technique of splinting fractures is easily taught, especially with the modern splints now available.

MOVEMENT OF THE PATIENT

PITFALL

IF A PATIENT IS MOVED WITHOUT CONSIDERING THE POSSIBILITY OF FRACTURES OF THE SPINE, PARALYSIS MAY RESULT FROM COMPRESSION OR TEARING OF THE SPINAL CORD OR NERVES.

Education is needed in the techniques of safely removing patients from disabled vehicles into ambulances. Few attendants know the benefit of, or how to use, the halfback board, with which a patient with neck or back injury can be easily extricated from an automobile seat. The long back board is somewhat more cumbersome and rarely used by emergency medical service personnel, but is helpful in handling the patient with multiple injuries involving both upper and lower extremities.

EXTERNAL CARDIAC MASSAGE

PITFALL

IF A CARDIAC ARREST IS NOT DIAGNOSED AND TREATED WITHIN THREE MINUTES, DEATH OR SEVERE BRAIN DAMAGE OFTEN RESULTS.

The fundamentals of diagnosis and treatment of cardiac arrest must be taught to the ambulance attendant during his training program. The patient will die if the attendant fails to recognize a cardiac arrest. However, if a cardiac arrest is incorrectly diagnosed and external cardiac massage is given to a patient whose primary complaint is severe respiratory difficulty with fractured ribs and perhaps a hemothorax, the result can be equally disastrous. Nevertheless, basic principles can be taught with careful instruction, and the yield from these efforts may be spectacular. Recently two Detroit police officers received departmental recognition for saving two citizens by a combination of simultaneous external cardiac massage and mouth-to-mouth respiration, taught to them during a 20-hour training course.

EVALUATION OF THE PATIENT IN THE EMERGENCY ROOM

To treat the patient with trauma as effectively as possible, evaluation of the patient and his injuries must be accomplished quickly and thoroughly. While ideally a systematic approach should be adopted, it is often necessary that evaluation and treatment be conducted simultaneously. As soon as any immediate threat to life has been averted, further examination and investigation may proceed.

History

The history should include detailed information on the accident and present symptoms. Items from the past history which are especially important include previous illnesses or injuries, the response to previous surgery, and any drugs the patient may have been taking, such as insulin, steroids, digitalis, diuretics, and antihypertensive agents.

PRESENT SYMPTOMS. All the patient's complaints should be listed. Unfortunately physicians often direct their attention to the main or most serious problems and ignore secondary complaints which may be very important later. Initially, many patients may have relatively few symptoms, even with serious injuries, but may suddenly deteriorate hours or even days later.

Therefore new or changing symptoms should be continuously looked for, especially if the trauma was severe and the initial symptoms and apparent tissue damage are minimal.

CIRCUMSTANCES UNDER WHICH THE INJURY OCCURRED. In automobile accidents, it is important to know where the patient was sitting, what part of the car was damaged, how fast the cars were going, how badly the cars were damaged, how seriously the other passengers were injured, and whether or not a seat belt was worn.

PITFALL

IF THE PATIENT HAS BEEN IN A SEVERE ACCIDENT AND IS NOT OBSERVED CLOSELY IN THE HOSPITAL FOR AT LEAST 12 TO 24 HOURS, HIS CONDITION MAY SUDDENLY DETERIORATE AFTER HE HAS BEEN PREMATURELY DISCHARGED.

Patients who have been involved in accidents which demolished the cars or seriously injured the other passengers should be observed especially carefully for at least 12 and preferably 24 hours, even if their initial symptoms are minimal. Not uncommonly, tears or fractures of the spleen, liver, pancreas or bowel may suddenly begin to bleed or leak hours after the initial injury. Many of these patients look and feel deceptively well when first seen.

Although seat belts and shoulder harnesses are usually of great value in reducing the severity of many injuries in auto accidents, they can themselves cause special injuries.[1]

PAST HISTORY. The patient's medical condition prior to the injury and any drugs that he was taking may greatly influence subsequent surgery or medical therapy. It is important to know if the patient has had any serious complications following previous surgery or injuries, if he has had any problems with bleeding or with his respiratory, cardiovascular, renal, or hepatic systems.

ALLERGIES. Drugs to which the patient has an allergy, especially if he has had angioneurotic edema or anaphylactic shock, should never be given. If a patient has one known allergy, he possibly also has a number of others, and the physician should therefore use the least allergic drugs possible. In many instances, however, patients have assumed that gastrointestinal symptoms following certain medications were due to allergic reactions, and this is often not the case.

Physical Examination

In many instances of extremely severe or critical injuries, the physician may have to be totally dependent on the initial physical examination—especially in comatose or confused patients.

PITFALL

NO MATTER HOW MINOR THE INJURY APPEARS INITIALLY, IF A COMPLETE PHYSICAL EXAMINATION IS NOT DONE SIGNIFICANT INJURIES MAY NOT BECOME APPARENT UNTIL THEIR TREATMENT BECOMES DIFFICULT OR IMPOSSIBLE.

Unless the injured part or parts require immediate emergency treatment, it is usually best to examine the patient systematically, leaving the obviously injured part for last. All too often, a complete neurologic examination is omitted during the turmoil of the initial resuscitation, and then completely forgotten until a severe deficit becomes apparent.

PITFALL

IF IT IS FORGOTTEN THAT A PATIENT HAS A BACK AS WELL AS A FRONT, IMPORTANT WOUNDS MAY BE MISSED.

Bullets may take bizarre courses, and the absence of an exit wound should not be assumed without first examining the patient meticulously, especially in the skin creases, in the scalps of long-haired individuals and around the anus.

If the patient has sustained blunt trauma, the physical examination may be especially deceptive. Special attention should be directed to all points which may have received the weight of the fall or impact. The victim of a pedestrian accident with injuries involving both upper and lower extremities should be suspected of also having an abdominal or chest injury between these two areas. Complete examination of a patient with blunt abdominal or pelvic trauma must include a rectal examination and a careful examination of the urine. Blood on rectal examination may indicate trauma to the rectum or colon.

Laboratory Studies

Any patient who may have had significant blood loss or who may require surgery should have serial hemoglobin or hematocrit determinations, a type and cross match and a urinalysis. If he has had any cardiovascular symptoms, has had moderate to severe chest trauma, or is over 45 years of age, he should also have an electrocardiogram.

Other laboratory studies which might be advisable in patients with previous medical problems include:

1. In diabetics: blood glucose.
2. In patients with renal disease: blood creatinine.
3. In patients with liver disease: bilirubin, serum proteins, and prothrombin times.
4. In patients with any bleeding tendency: partial thromboplastin time, prothrombin time, platelets, type and cross match.
5. In malnourished or dehydrated patients: serum sodium, potassium, chloride, and CO_2 content.

X-rays

The specific x-rays ordered are determined by the type, severity, and location of the injury and are discussed more fully in Chapter 13. In general, however, any area which may have a fracture should have a radiologic examination. If the patient has abdominal pain, upright films of the abdomen and chest should also be obtained. All patients except those requiring urgent operation for exsanguinating hemorrhage should have chest x-rays prior to admission to the hospital. With all severe trauma, however, the proper priority of x-rays in overall patient management must be considered with the need for constant surgical attendance.

PITFALL

IF AN X-RAY IS TAKEN BUT IS NOT EXAMINED BY SOMEONE COMPETENT, AN ERRONEOUS INTERPRETATION MAY CAUSE MORE HARM THAN IF NO X-RAY WERE TAKEN AT ALL.

Observation

Continued careful repeated observation and examination of the patient with any potentially serious injury are often more important than the initial evaluation. It is not uncommon for the signs and symptoms of shock or abdominal injury to be delayed for several hours. Continued bleeding or air leak into an initially small pneumothorax may be missed if the patient is sent home after an examination made soon after the trauma. Patients seldom suffer from 24 hours of careful observation, but may die if they are sent home too soon.

TREATMENT IN THE HOSPITAL

The main principles in the treatment of all types of trauma, in order of importance, are: (1) preservation of life, (2) preservation and restoration of function, and (3) restoration of appearance (cosmetic).

Preservation of Life

Preservation of life in the injured patient depends primarily upon the maintenance of adequate pulmonary and cardiovascular function.

VENTILATION. A quick look at a patient by a trained observer is often all that is needed for a reasonable estimate of the adequacy of air exchange. Patients who

have had trauma tend to hyperventilate; if their ventilation is even slightly less than normal they often need oxygen and respiratory support. If the patient does not appear to be breathing satisfactorily, the cause must be identified and corrected rapidly. The questions to be asked are:

Is the Patient Trying to Breathe? Weak or absent ventilatory effort can be a result of neurologic damage either from trauma to the skull or cervical spine or from advanced hypoxia or shock. Drugs, particularly narcotics, can cause motor impairment or severely depress the respiratory or neuromuscular systems. Regardless of the etiology, inadequate air exchange demands prompt effective ventilatory support by any of several techniques: mouth-to-mouth, mouth-to-nose, mask-to-mouth (preferably with an oral airway in place) or endotracheal tube.

PITFALL

IF AN ENDOTRACHEAL TUBE CANNOT BE INSERTED ACCURATELY WITHIN 30 TO 60 SECONDS, BUT CONTINUED ATTEMPTS ARE MADE TO PLACE IT, THE HYPOXIA WHICH DEVELOPS MAY BE LETHAL.

For most emergency situations, it is better to continue mouth-to-mouth or mask-to-mouth respiration until someone experienced with endotracheal intubation is available. The details of handling this problem are discussed more fully in the chapter on respiratory failure (Chap. 31).

Is the Airway Obstructed? If the patient is trying to breathe but little or no air is moving, airway obstruction is usually present. Whereas obstruction of the upper airway is characterized by inspiratory stridor, obstruction of the lower airway is most pronounced during expiration and is often not readily apparent. In severely depressed, drunk, or comatose patients, an upper-airway obstruction can be caused by the tongue falling back to occlude the pharynx. This can be readily corrected by turning the patient on his side, pulling the jaw forward and extending the neck, and inserting an oral airway or a nasopharyngeal or endotracheal tube. False teeth and foreign bodies in the mouth and pharynx should be removed with the fingers. Excessive secretions or vomitus should be aspirated until the mouth, nose, pharynx and larynx are clear. Emergency tracheostomies are seldom needed in immediate management; orotracheal or nasotracheal tubes are preferable, and these allow subsequent tracheostomies to be performed in a safe unhurried manner. Further details on tracheostomy can be found in Chapter 19.

Excessive bleeding into the mouth or pharynx is one of the few situations in which insertion of an endotracheal tube may be impossible, necessitating an emergency tracheostomy in desperate circumstances. When an endotracheal tube cannot be inserted, especially in a patient with a short fat neck, a cricothyroid puncture (coniotomy) may be lifesaving.[2] When the patient's general condition permits, this cricothyroidostomy opening should be converted to a standard tracheostomy.

Is the Chest Wall Intact? Sucking wounds of the chest must be covered immediately, preferably with a sterile airtight dressing, and a chest tube should be inserted to drain any fluid or air that may have accumulated in the pleural cavity. Later, after the patient's condition has stabilized, the chest wound can be debrided and closed properly in the operating room (Chap. 20).

Fractures involving multiple ribs or the sternum frequently cause a "flail chest." The presence of eight or more fractured ribs, significant preexisting pulmonary disease, or obvious flail on the initial examination, especially in a patient with multiple severe injuries, should be regarded as an indication for early internal stabilization of the chest using a volume respirator.[3] As a temporary measure, a well-placed sandbag can be used to control a large flail. External stabilization with towel clips, wires,

screws or other mechanical devices are not usually as effective as internal stabilization with a respirator.

Does the Patient Have a Pneumothorax or Hemothorax? Compression or collapse of one or both lungs by collections of fluid or air in the pleural cavities can severely impair ventilation. This is most accurately diagnosed with a chest x-ray taken with the patient upright, but auscultation and percussion can also be informative. Decreased breath sounds with dullness suggest fluid, and decreased breath sounds with normal or increased resonance suggest a pneumothorax. Tracheal deviation is usually not remarkable unless a tension pneumothorax is present. Aspiration of the pleural cavity with a long 15- to 18-gauge needle attached to a 50-cc glass syringe with a moistened and partially removed plunger may confirm the presence of intrapleural air or fluid. A tension pneumothorax will push out the plunger quite vigorously. Blood in the pleural cavity should be drained with a chest tube attached to a water seal; if the hemothorax or air leak is large, evacuation of the pleural cavity may be improved by applying 10 to 20 cm H_2O suction to the water-seal bottle.

Whenever possible, a chest x-ray should be obtained before a chest tube or needle is inserted to drain any suspected hemo- or pneumothorax, but if the patient's condition is critical an attempt at aspiration should be made without waiting for the x-ray.

PITFALL

IF A PHYSICIAN BLINDLY INSISTS ON A CHEST X-RAY IN EVERY PATIENT BEFORE INSERTING A CHEST TUBE FOR A HEMOTHORAX OR PNEUMOTHORAX, HE MAY ACCUMULATE A FINE COLLECTION OF CHEST X-RAYS OF CADAVERS.

Other Questions. If, after all the above, the patient is still having difficulty breathing, other questions that should be answered include:

1. Is the difficulty due to excessive chest pain that can be safely controlled with intercostal blocks or mild analgesics?
2. Does the patient have abnormal elevation of the diaphragm because of excessive fluid or bowel distension below the diaphragm?

Many patients with abdominal or retroperitoneal injuries may develop gastric dilatation and may have a severe ileus which can persist for 10 to 14 days. In these patients, it is important to provide early and complete nasogastric decompression.

PITFALL

IF THE STOMACH IS NOT EMPTIED OF AIR AND FLUID PRIOR TO A GENERAL ANESTHETIC, THE CHANCES THAT THE PATIENT MAY VOMIT AND ASPIRATE GASTRIC CONTENTS DURING THE OPERATION ARE GREATLY INCREASED.

Aspiration of gastric contents into the lungs during and after trauma or anesthesia (with the resultant severe respiratory complications) is often unappreciated but remains one of the most common causes of death after an otherwise successful initial resuscitation.

3. Could the patient have a diaphragmatic hernia compressing the lungs? This may on occasion be difficult to determine except with x-rays following passage of an opaque Levin tube and, when necessary, the instillation of some Gastrografin.
4. Is the dyspnea due to shock or cardiac damage?

CARDIOVASCULAR FUNCTION. *Cardiac Massage.* While ensuring adequate ventilation, the physician must assess cardiac function; if necessary he should begin external cardiac massage (Chap. 11). If external cardiac massage is inadequate or if the patient has a penetrating wound of the chest, the physician should be prepared to open the left chest anteriorly through the fifth interspace for internal cardiac massage.

Not only is open cardiac massage usually more effective than external massage, but with the chest open the descending thoracic aorta can be clamped just above the diaphragm. This not only improves blood flow to the heart and brain but may also reduce any continuing intra-abdominal hemorrhage. There should be no hesitancy in performing a thoracotomy in the emergency room when necessary, if the physician has experience with this procedure. It is crucial to remember that cardiac massage must be done in conjunction with adequate respiratory support and correction of any coexistent hypovolemia or hemorrhage. Paradoxically, few of these emergency thoracotomy incisions become infected even though performed with little or no concern for sterility.

Controlling Hemorrhage. External bleeding is usually obvious, except occasionally from the scalp and back, and generally can be readily controlled with direct pressure over the wound. Hemostats are rarely necessary, except perhaps in long slashing wounds, and if improperly used may cause severe injury to tissues and vessels, making later vascular repairs difficult or impossible.

Internal hemorrhage, especially into the peritoneal cavity, may be difficult to diagnose at times and is often suspected only after other causes of hypotension have been excluded. Four-quadrant paracentesis may be helpful and should be considered positive even if only a drop of blood is obtained in the aspirating syringe or needle. If no blood is obtained, peritoneal lavage should be performed. Saline, 500 to 1000 ml, is infused into the peritoneal cavity through a plastic needle. After 10 to 20 minutes, the fluid is allowed to drain out by gravity. This technique is 90 to 95% accurate in diagnosing intra-abdominal bleeding.[4] Bleeding into the chest may be suspected on physical examination and can be confirmed by x-ray of the chest or needle aspiration. Blood loss around fractures of the pelvis may exceed 1000 to 2000 ml with minimal or no local evidence of the loss. Hematomas around fractures of the femur may exceed 1000 ml (Table 2).

Intravenous Lines. Depending on the extent and location of the blood loss and injuries, two or three large (15-gauge) intra-

TABLE 2. ANTICIPATED BLOOD LOSS FROM FRACTURES

	Blood loss
Pelvis—Bilateral	2000 cc
Pelvis—Unilateral	1000–1500 cc
Femur	1000 cc
Tibia	500 cc
Humerus	350 cc
Ribs	125 cc/per rib

venous catheters should be inserted, percutaneously or by cut-down, and one of these should be advanced centrally into the superior vena cava or right atrium for continuous measurement of the central venous pressure (CVP). The basilic vein just proximal and anterior to the medial condyle at the elbow is an excellent site for a cut-down; other readily available sites include the large veins in the antecubital fossa, the cephalic vein as it runs up over the biceps brachii muscle, and the superficial or external jugular vein in the neck. If arm veins are thrombosed, too small, or not available, leg, neck or subclavian veins will have to be used. If a line has to be inserted in the leg, it is best placed in the greater saphenous vein just proximal to the anterior superior border of the medial malleolus. Whenever possible, however, the leg veins should be avoided because catheters in the lower extremities are difficult for the anesthetist to control in the operating room and they increase the chances of later thromboembolic complications.

PITFALL

IF FLUID IS INFUSED INTO A VEIN WHICH IS DAMAGED OR COMPRESSED DURING SURGERY, THE FLUID MAY NOT ENTER INTO THE GENERAL CIRCULATION AND SEVERE HYPOVOLEMIA MAY DEVELOP OR PERSIST IN SPITE OF MASSIVE INFUSIONS.

In the excitement of an emergency situation, I.V.s are sometimes started in the first available veins on the arms without considering the possibility that the vein may be damaged proximally. For example, an I.V. should not be started in the left arm if the left axillary, left subclavian, or left innominate veins or superior vena cava might be injured.

The "subclavian stick" has become popular over the past few years and is especially valuable in the patient who has poor arm and leg veins. Like many surgical procedures, however, it can cause several complications, especially if performed by inexperienced personnel. Pneumothorax is not uncommon; if the patient is on a respirator, the danger of lung puncture is especially great because of the increased likelihood that the pneumothorax will be large and under tension. A chest x-ray should therefore always be taken soon after any subclavian stick is attempted to ascertain catheter position and to rule out a pneumothorax. If a pneumothorax is present, it should be treated with a small chest tube.

A more serious potential complication is that of air embolization, which may occur if the I.V. tubing accidentally comes apart in patients who are hypovolemic or standing or sitting up. The amount of air that can enter through the tubing is remarkable. Air can move through a 17-gauge needle at 100 ml per second with a pressure differential of only 5 mm Hg, and as little as 50 ml of air injected into the superior vena cava of a 10-kg dog in one second can block the pulmonary artery and cause death. Although air embolization has been reported only rarely, it may be rapidly fatal.[5] Leaving the catheter open for as short a time as two seconds in a patient making a maximal inspiratory effort can cause significant air embolization and death. Certain precautions can be taken to prevent air emboli, particularly in the hypovolemic patient who characteristically hyperventilates (Chap. 4). Putting the patient in the Trendelenburg position during insertion of the subclavian catheter will raise the pressure in the subclavian veins so that blood will flow out of instead of being sucked into the catheter. The needle used for the subclavian stick should be connected to a syringe as a further precaution against air embolus and, after the I.V. is established, all connections should be well taped.

Blood Volume Expanders. The initial fluid used for blood volume expansion should be a balanced electrolyte solution, either lactated Ringer's or normal saline. If the patient appears to be severely acidotic, two ampules of $NaHCO_3$ may be added to each liter. Lactate should probably be avoided in patients who are in severe shock or who have severe liver disease, because such patients may not be able to metabolize lactate adequately. Ringer's lactate has a pH of about 4.8 to 6.5, and unless the lactate is metabolized to bicarbonate it may make the patient more acidotic.

Continued volume needs after rapid infusion of two to three liters of crystalloid solution generally indicate continued severe bleeding requiring whole blood replacement and surgery. As a general guideline, subsequent infusions should consist of one half blood and plasma and one half balanced electrolyte solution (Chaps. 5 and 10). One unit of fresh frozen plasma is often given after every four to five transfusions to help maintain normal coagulation and assist in maintaining intravascular oncotic pressure. Dextran may facilitate the maintenance of oncotic pressure but its use has been associated with bleeding difficulties, problems with type and cross-matching and anaphylaxis; therefore, its role in the immediate resuscitation period is questionable. Likewise, albumin infusion may facilitate intravascular expansion but has little value as a blood substitute. The amount of fluid and/or blood given (as mentioned in Chap. 5) will depend largely on the response of the patient's CVP, blood pressure, pulse, lung and urine output.

URINARY OUTPUT. Foley-catheter drainage and monitoring of the hourly urine output are extremely important in the early evaluation of the severely injured patient and his response to treatment. If possible, a spontaneously voided urine specimen

should be obtained before insertion of the Foley catheter, because any manipulation of the lower urinary tract can cause microscopic and occasionally gross hematuria. Once the catheter is inserted, the hourly urine output is correlated with the patient's vital signs and CVP to regulate the rate and volume of fluid administration.

SEVERE BURNS. The problems with severe burns are mainly hypovolemia initially and sepsis subsequently. The admitting officer should also be aware of the potential hazards of burns to the upper respiratory tract and of the chemical pneumonitis and carbon monoxide poisoning which may occur from smoke inhalation. In some instances the pulmonary changes from smoke inhalation may not become apparent for 12 to 48 hours.

PITFALL

IF TRACHEOSTOMIES ARE PERFORMED ON ALL PATIENTS WITH SEVERE FACIAL BURNS ON THE ASSUMPTION THAT THEY WILL ALL DEVELOP RESPIRATORY DIFFICULTY, MANY NEEDLESS TRACHEOSTOMIES WILL FURTHER COMPLICATE BURN THERAPY, ESPECIALLY IN INFANTS.

Most patients with burns to the head and neck can be given adequate respiratory support without tracheostomies. Infants and young children rarely need tracheostomies and, furthermore, tracheostomies in children less than two years of age can be difficult to manage and may occasionally cause fatal complications. A nasotracheal or endotracheal tube may be used to maintain ventilation in the early postburn period. Any need for tracheostomy will be apparent by the second or third day.

Fluid replacement should be begun immediately and can be based initially on various burn formulas (Chap. 28). These formulas provide rough guides to the volume of fluid needed, but the physician should be guided primarily by the blood pressure, pulse, central venous pressure, hemoglobin or hematocrit, and hourly urine output. Following stabilization of the cardiovascular system, consideration can be given to the initial debridement and dressings. Later, when good granulation tissue is present, skin grafts should be applied.

Preservation of Function

Once resuscitation has proceeded successfully to the point where survival is fairly well assured and the patient's condition is stable, increasing attention can be given to the preservation of individual organs and limbs.

EXTREMITIES. *Blood Vessels.* Interruption of the blood supply to a limb for more than two to three hours may seriously jeopardize its viability and later function. The seriousness of the vascular injury will depend upon its location, the status of the collateral vessels, the overall cardiac output, and the concomitant tissue injury to the limb itself. The classic symptoms and signs of pain, paresthesia, pallor, paralysis, and lack of pulse should immediately alert the physician to the probability of severe vascular injury. Rapid localization of the vessel damage and its correction are imperative. If there is a concomitant fracture or dislocation, prompt reduction and stabilization may relieve pressure on the vessels and restore the blood supply. In no case should it be assumed that the vascular problem is due to spasm; to do so is to ignore an obvious mechanical problem which may later cause loss or irreversible damage to the limb. Angiography frequently provides valuable information in these circumstances (Chap. 26).

Bones. All fractured extremities should be splinted as soon as possible. Although usually no attempt is made to correct any deformities before the x-rays are examined, closed fractures or dislocations causing vascular or neurologic impairment should be reduced as soon as they are recognized clinically. A more complete discussion of musculoskeletal injuries is given in Chapter 17.

Nerves. Lacerated nerves do not have to be repaired immediately, but primary repair may be attempted if the wound is clean and adjudged likely to heal without complications.

Muscles and Tendons. Muscle edges can usually be approximated if the wound has not been contaminated and if the muscle is definitely viable. Tendons, like nerves, however, are not usually repaired unless the wound is clean and promises to heal without infection or other complications. Flexor tendon repair is often delayed even in clean wounds if the injury is in the no-man's-land between the distal palmar crease and the insertion of the flexor sublimis tendon at the base of the middle phalanx.

VISCERAL INJURIES. *Lungs.* Optimal respiratory function in the severely injured patient is best accomplished by maintaining adequate tissue perfusion, inflating the lungs well, removing excessive secretions (preferably by having the patient cough) and preventing fluid overloads. Patients with severe trauma often cannot tolerate even mild degrees of hypoxia or hypercarbia for more than a few hours. The emphasis in the management of the lungs after severe trauma must be on prevention of respiratory failure rather than on treatment. Once respiratory failure is established and becomes obvious on gross clinical examination, the mortality rate rises precipitously[6] (Chap. 31).

Heart. Optimal cardiac activity is obtained primarily by maintaining adequate blood volume, blood pressure, pulse, and central venous pressure. Various inotropic agents such as digitalis, Isuprel, and dopamine may be required if congestive failure or shock develops (Chaps. 5 and 32).

Kidneys. There appears to be some value in maintaining a slightly increased urine output of 50 to 75 ml/hr after injury, especially if the patient has been in shock, has severe muscle damage, or has had multiple blood transfusions. If the urinary output is low in spite of an adequate blood volume, blood pressure, cardiac output, and acid-base balance, diuretics such as mannitol, ethacrynic acid, or furosemide should be given in the smallest possible effective dose.

PITFALL

IF IT IS MISTAKENLY ASSUMED THAT THE OLIGURIA IN AN INJURED PATIENT IS DUE TO RENAL FAILURE WITHOUT COMPLETELY RULING OUT THE POSSIBILITY OF HYPOVOLEMIA, THE USE OF DIURETICS MAY CAUSE AN EVEN WORSE HYPOVOLEMIA OR SHOCK.

Although overinfusion of fluids may aggravate any tendency to respiratory failure, the most common cause of oliguria after trauma, at least initially, is inadequate blood or fluid replacement. Nephrotoxic drugs such as kanamycin should be avoided or kept to a minimum. If the patient has gross or microscopic hematuria, he should usually have an emergency intravenous pyelogram followed by a cystogram or cystourethrogram as soon as possible. The physician, however, should recognize priorities before obtaining these studies and not allow the patient to get lost in a morass of investigations by various services while his condition deteriorates.

Liver. Preservation of hepatic function requires an adequate blood flow, blood pressure, and glucose. Potentially hepatotoxic drugs such as Fluothane should be avoided, especially if there has been direct liver damage or previous hepatic disease such as cirrhosis.

CENTRAL NERVOUS SYSTEM. Preservation of CNS function is based primarily on maintenance of adequate respiratory and cardiovascular function. Brain swelling or cerebral edema due to trauma, ischemia or hypoxia may be partially reduced by hypothermia, fluid restriction, diuretics, steroids, and mild hyperventilation. Convulsions must be vigorously treated with Valium, Dilantin, and/or phenobarbital. Keeping the head elevated may help reduce cerebral edema but may also aggravate any tendency to hypovolemia.

Although clamping of the descending thoracic aorta may improve perfusion of the upper part of the body in the hypovolemic patient who has an injury below the arch of the aorta, it may also occlude the arteria magna which usually provides the major blood supply to the middle and lower spinal cord and which usually comes off the aorta between the sixth and tenth thoracic vertebrae. Aortic occlusion proximal to the arteria magna for more than 20 minutes is associated with an increased risk of paraplegia and subsequent renal failure.

Preservation of Appearance (Cosmetic Considerations)

Clean soft-tissue injuries should be repaired as soon as possible. Wounds which are older than 8 to 12 hours or are contaminated should usually be left open for two to five days until clean and granulating. Certain exceptions may be made for facial wounds if proper debridement has been performed and if there is a good local blood supply. The physician who does the primary or first repair generally has the best chance of getting good results. The plastic surgeon performing secondary repairs or reconstruction, regardless of his expertise, seldom has the opportunity to achieve as cosmetically pleasing a scar as the initial surgeon.

IMPORTANCE OF A TEAM CAPTAIN

PITFALL

IF A PATIENT WITH MULTIPLE INJURIES DOES NOT HAVE HIS OVERALL CARE COORDINATED BY AN IDENTIFIABLE AND EXPERIENCED PHYSICIAN, THE CORRECT PRIORITIES OF CARE MAY NOT BE RECOGNIZED AND FOLLOWED.

The multiply injured patient's general condition is subject to rapid changes, requiring a dynamic and cooperative team approach. Many things are happening at the same time and, in the midst of all this activity, it is important that one person be recognized as the patient's physician. He must supervise resuscitation and direct the efforts of the various consulting services. Unfortunately, this "team-captain" approach occasionally breaks down. An example of this is described below:

A 53-year-old man involved in a pedestrian accident was brought unconscious to the emergency room approximately 20 minutes after injury. At the time of admission his pressure and pulse were reasonably stable, so that after I.V. fluids and appropriate blood specimens were drawn he was sent to the x-ray department. Multiple injuries were present: a severely fractured pelvis, multiple rib fractures on the left side, a laceration of the scalp and arm, and a Colles' fracture of the right wrist. In addition, he had microscopic hematuria. At this time he was able to communicate although he was still confused. By the time his x-rays were completed, he had developed a tachycardia which improved with more intravenous balanced electrolyte solution. Consultation was then requested from the urologist for the hematuria, from the neurosurgeon for the concussion and disorientation, and from the orthopedist for the fractures of the wrist and pelvis. The orthopedist was the first to arrive and he promptly applied a short arm cast for the wrist fracture. At the end of this procedure, noting that the patient was more disoriented, he urged the neurosurgeon to see the patient quickly. When the neurosurgeon arrived the patient was almost unconscious and had a tachycardia of approximately 140 with a blood pressure of 80/60 mm Hg. He completed his neurologic examination and decided that the patient was suffering more from hypovolemic shock than from increased intracranial pressure. A general surgeon was called. Approximately five minutes later the patient had a cardiac arrest and external and internal massage were unsuccessful.

The error in this case can be found in the fact that the physician in the emergency department who first saw the patient did not fully realize the critical nature of his condition and the need for an experienced surgeon to coordinate therapy. Unfortunately, this type of error occurs frequently, even in large emergency departments.

REFERENCES

1. Williams, J. S., and Kirkpatrick, J. R.: The nature of seat belt injuries. J. Trauma, 11:207, 1971.
2. Edgerton, M. T., Jr.: Emergency care of maxillofacial and neck injuries. In *The Management of Trauma* (Ballinger, W. F., II, Rutherford, R. B. and Zuidema, G. D. Eds.). Philadelphia, W. B. Saunders, 1968.
3. Sankaran, S., and Wilson, R. F.: Factors affecting prognosis in patients with flail chest. J. Thorac. Cardiov. Surg., 60:402, 1970.
4. Olsen, W. R., and Hildreth, D. H.: Abdominal paracentesis and peritoneal lavage in blunt abdominal trauma. J. Trauma, 11:824, 1971.
5. Lucas, C. E., and Irani, F.: Air embolus via subclavian catheter. New Eng. J. Med., 281:966, 1969.
6. Wilson, R. F., et al.: Clinical respiratory failure after shock or trauma: Prognosis and methods of diagnosis. Arch. Surg., 98:539, 1969.

Suggested Reading

1. Williams, J. S., and Kirkpatrick, J. R.: The nature of seat belt injuries. J. Trauma, 11:207, 1971.
2. DeMuth, W. E., Jr.: The mechanisms of shotgun wounds. J. Trauma, 11:219, 1971.
3. Clark, D. W., and Morton, J. H.: The motorcycle accident: A growing problem. J. Trauma, 11:230, 1971.
4. Kirkpatrick, J. R., and Youmans, R. L.: Trauma index. An aid in the evaluation of injury victims. J. Trauma, 11:711, 1971.
5. Waddell, J. P., and Drucker, W. R.: Occult injuries in pedestrian accidents. J. Trauma, 11:844, 1971.
6. Steichen, F. M.: The emergency management of the severely injured. J. Trauma, 12:786, 1972.
7. Boyd, D. R.: A symposium on the Illinois trauma program: A systems approach to the care of the critically injured. Introduction: A controlled system approach to trauma patient care. J. Trauma, 13:275, 1973.
8. Cowley, R. A., et al.: An economical and proved helicopter program for transporting the emergency critically ill and injured patient in Maryland. J. Trauma, 13:1029, 1973.
9. Lowe, R. J., and Baker, R. J.: Organization and function of trauma care units. J. Trauma, 13:285, 1973.
10. Meyer, P. R., Jr., and Raffensperger, J. G.: Special centers for the care of the injured. J. Trauma, 13:308, 1973.
11. McSwain, N. E., Jr.: On site trauma management. Surg. Gynec. Obstet., 137:581, 1973.

8 GENERAL PRINCIPLES OF WOUND CARE

R. F. WILSON
A. J. WALT

Strict adherence to the general principles of wound care is important to reduce the incidence of wound infections and increase the chances of optimal healing. The most important underlying principles are reduction of contamination, proper surgical technique, support of the patient's general condition, and appropriate use of antibiotics, antitoxins and toxoids.

REDUCING CONTAMINATION

All traumatic wounds are contaminated; efforts must, therefore, be directed both toward preventing further contamination and controlling that which is already present. In the emergency department all wounds should immediately be covered with sterile dressings until they can be properly treated. Most bleeding, even from fairly large vessels, can be controlled by direct pressure accurately applied over the sterile dressing for 10 to 30 minutes. Bleeding from large arteries may rarely require a temporary proximal tourniquet, direct ligation, or occlusion with a vascular clamp before repair in the operating room.

PITFALL

IF TOURNIQUETS ARE APPLIED INDISCRIMINATELY TO CONTROL BLEEDING FROM EXTREMITIES, THEY CAN CAUSE INCREASED BLEEDING AND SEVERE TISSUE NECROSIS.

Tourniquets are seldom needed except above major amputations and, if used incorrectly, can cause much harm. A tourniquet should ideally be at least 2 to 3 inches wide so that the pressure is evenly distributed (a blood-pressure cuff makes an excellent tourniquet). The pressure applied must be high enough to prevent arterial inflow. With lower pressures, blood will enter the extremity but is prevented from returning to the heart and the resulting rise in venous pressure distal to the tourniquet causes additional bleeding from the open veins. If the tourniquet is applied tightly for too long a period, it can cause irreversible ischemic damage distally; consequently, it should be loosened for a short time every 15 to 20 minutes.

Once the bleeding from the wound has been adequately controlled, the surrounding area can be cleaned, with the wound itself still protected by a sterile dressing. An area at least 3 to 6 inches wider than the wound should be thoroughly washed, and the wound should be debrided and cleaned. Harsh chemicals are not needed and vigorous irrigation with copious amounts of sterile saline is usually adequate. Any residual dirt or necrotic tissue left after thorough irrigation is probably best removed by debridement. If the wound is to be primarily repaired, fresh drapes and gloves should be used.

PITFALL

There is a tendency to handle small wounds less conscientiously than larger, more open wounds. Small wounds may give rise to large infections. In fact, dirt and foreign bodies in small wounds are often very difficult to see and are more apt to be incompletely removed than those in larger wounds.

A frequent error in sterile technique during long operations for severe trauma is to continue to use drapes which have become saturated with blood or fluid. Wet drapes no longer represent an effective barrier to bacteria and should be changed as soon as possible.

SURGICAL TECHNIQUE

Debridement

Open contaminated wounds will often heal quite well, but closed contaminated wounds are apt to develop severe infections.

PITFALL

A wound should not be closed if all devitalized tissue and foreign bodies cannot be removed from it. Occasionally, however, facial wounds may be closed with tissue of questionable viability, because of the excellent blood supply of the face and the better cosmetic result that can be obtained during the primary repair. If a wound is excessively contaminated or more than 8 to 12 hours old, by completely excising the wound edges it can be converted to a relatively clean, fresh wound. Although the skin and subcutaneous tissues can be left open, bowel, cartilage, tendons, vessels and bones should be covered with at least one layer of tissue such as peritoneum, fascia, or muscle.

Irrigation

The bacterial population in contaminated wounds can be reduced by irrigating the area thoroughly with large amounts of saline under moderate pressure. Use of antibiotics such as 1% neomycin in the irrigating solution may also help reduce the local bacteria count. Since chemicals such as Merthiolate, Mercurochrome, or alcohol may damage cells in the wound and interfere with healing, they should not be applied directly into wounds.

Foreign Bodies

In grossly contaminated wounds, not only must debridement be complete but careful consideration must also be given to keeping the introduction of foreign bodies, including suture materials, to a minimum; certainly prosthetic grafts or other materials should never be used in grossly contaminated wounds. Nonabsorbable sutures such as silk and cotton should be used as little as possible, because they may act as foreign bodies and perpetuate infection with resultant chronic draining sinuses. If absorbable sutures are used for tying off small vessels, Dexon is usually preferable to catgut as it causes less local inflammatory response while being absorbed.

The increased ease with which infections occur in the presence of foreign bodies has been demonstrated by experiments showing that a single silk suture reduces the minimal pus-forming dose of bacteria by a factor of 1/10,000.[1] The infective dose is even further reduced if the suture contains a minute piece of tissue. Consequently, the surgeon should use the finest possible suture material and incorporate the smallest amount of tissue needed to accomplish the suture's purpose.

PITFALL

IF IT IS ASSUMED THAT A FOREIGN BODY IS
NOT PRESENT IN A WOUND BECAUSE IT DOES
NOT SHOW UP ON X-RAY, RETAINED GLASS,
WOOD OR PLASTIC MAY BE LEFT BEHIND TO
CAUSE SEVERE LOCAL INFECTION AND DAMAGE.

It is difficult for physicians treating traumatic wounds to exclude with certainty the presence of a foreign body in small, deep punctures or lacerations. Even extensions of the wound may not permit completely satisfactory exploration. If the suspected foreign body is radiopaque, an x-ray of the area provides a simple solution to the question. Where the foreign body is wood or nonleaded glass, however, it usually cannot be seen on the roentgenogram. Under such circumstances, thorough careful local exploration is mandatory.

Whether or not to use drains is a recurrent controversy. Drains represent a two-way street. While in situ they encourage the drainage of pus, bile, and leaking intestinal contents, they also permit the ingress of bacteria, especially if the wound area is carelessly dressed or handled. Consequently, drains should be used only for specific definable reasons: the obliteration of dead space, oozing, or to provide egress for bile, pancreatic juice or intestinal contents.

Sutures

Finer sutures create less foreign-body reaction, especially if they are monofilament wire or one of the plastic sutures such as Tevdek, nylon or Mersilene. The outer skin sutures can be especially fine (5-0 or 6-0) if the wound edges are already well approximated by deeper sutures. The sooner the skin sutures come out, the less scarring or cross-hatching will be caused by the sutures themselves. If the underlying tissues are closed properly, sutures on the face can be removed in 3 to 5 days. Sutures in the skin of the abdomen or chest can usually be removed in 7 days, while sutures on the

hands, feet, or legs should often be left in place for 10 to 14 days. If the sutures are in an area which is subject to much movement, or if the patient is apt to heal poorly, the sutures may have to be left in place for an additional one to two weeks. Adhesive strips or tape have been used enthusiastically for several years by a number of physicians and may be of special value in wounds which will have relatively little tension or movement.

Hematomas

A hematoma is an ideal culture medium for bacteria and, acting as a foreign body, it also prevents or inhibits the delivery of phagocytic cells to the area. Meticulous hemostasis is, therefore, an absolute requirement before closing any deep wound. When all the oozing cannot be stopped, hematoma formation should be prevented with a pressure dressing or a suction catheter or Hemovac.

Dead Space

During closure of any wound, all tissue must be carefully approximated; any residual dead space is soon filled with tissue fluid which, like a hematoma, can act as an excellent culture medium for bacteria. In some circumstances it may be necessary to rotate adjacent muscle into the area. Where all dead space cannot be obliterated, the wound should be left open or drained.

Delayed Closure

In heavily contaminated wounds, or in wounds from which all foreign material or devitalized tissue cannot be satisfactorily removed, delayed closure will minimize the development of serious infection. Some physicians working in emergency departments have been deterred from delayed closure because of a false belief by them or the patients that an unsightly scar will result. In actual practice, the final result often will be virtually indistinguishable from that achieved by a primary closure.

Wound Configuration

A jagged, irregular wound running perpendicular to the "wrinkle lines" is likely to give a wide unsightly scar. Not only will such a wound have a poor cosmetic result but healing will be retarded and the scar is likely to be painful. Wherever possible, wound edges should be straight, sharp and parallel to the wrinkle lines (which are not the same as Langer's lines). If the wound must be debrided or lengthened to achieve this, it should be done without hesitation. Whenever possible, the wound edges should be slightly everted or elevated to compensate for the tendency for the scar to sink in slightly as it heals. This can usually be achieved with fine vertical mattress sutures.

Wound Tension

Wound edges should come together with little or no tension. Relaxing incisions or freeing of more tissues at the level of the superficial fascia may help to bring wound edges together with less tension, but there are limits to the degree of undermining permissible without danger of producing ischemia. Except for the face and scalp, it is generally unwise to undermine more than 2 to 3 cm from the wound edge. If some tension is needed to pull the wound edges together, it is better to apply the tension to the underlying tissue and leave the skin itself "approximated, but not strangulated."

Skin Loss

Treatment when there has been a significant loss of skin will depend on the type and size of the defect, its location, and the expertise of the physician.

ABRASIONS. Treatment of partial-thickness skin loss is aimed at protecting the area from infection and mechanical injury. The area must be cleaned thoroughly and all dirt and embedded foreign material removed to prevent tattooing. Bulky dressings may reduce local pain, but they tend to allow exudate to accumulate. Leaving the wound open greatly reduces the chances of infection but may be very uncomfortable initially. Fine mesh gauze impregnated with a water-soluble emollient is probably the best compromise dressing.[2]

FULL-THICKNESS SKIN LOSS. *Direct Closure.* If tissue loss occurs where the skin is relatively loose, the wound can sometimes be closed by approximating the skin edges. Wound tension may be at least partially relieved in such circumstances by undermining the adjacent skin and subcutaneous tissue, taking care not to devitalize the tissue. With greater wound tension, healing is impaired and the chances of infection and unsightly scars increase.

Partial-thickness Skin Grafts. If the tissue loss in a fresh clean wound is too extensive to allow a direct closure, a partial-thickness skin graft can be used as either a temporary or permanent surface repair. The donor site should match the wound area as closely as possible for color and amount of hair. The ulnar side of the index finger or forearm is ideal for repair of avulsed fingertips. The chest and upper back provide a good color match for the face and neck. For most other parts of the body the nonhairy portion of the thigh is quite satisfactory.

No devitalized tissue, infection, or brisk bleeding should be present in the recipient area. The graft should be pressed down firmly to provide uniform complete tissue contact. The fine sutures used to tack the graft down should be left long enough to be tied over a stent pressure dressing. If the wound is on an extremity, a splint should be applied to prevent undue motion at the wound site. After three days, the graft should be examined for removal of devitalized tissue and puncture or aspiration of hematomas or seromas.

In certain wounds with questionable devitalized tissue or contamination, autograft, hemograft, or heterograft partial-thickness skin grafts can be used as temporary biologic dressings. Such grafts are often far superior to the wet soaks usually used to clean up these wounds.

Full-thickness Skin Grafts. Full-thickness skin grafts should seldom be used to treat fresh wounds (except for clean wounds of the head and neck by experienced surgeons). Full-thickness grafts vascularize very slowly and require optimal conditions and postoperative care; however, when they do take, the color and function of the graft are usually better than those achieved with split-thickness grafts.

SKIN AVULSIONS. Completely avulsed tissue, except for fingertips, is usually contaminated and too thick to allow adequate revascularization. Amputated portions of a composite structure such as the eyelid, nose, or ear should be placed in a sterile container and saved in case a plastic surgeon may be able to use them later. Partial or complete avulsions on the face and neck usually heal well if the surrounding tissue is healthy. Partial avulsions on extremities, especially if long and narrow or if pedicled distally, are apt to die; therefore, if the partial avulsion is clean, it should be converted to a fat-free partial-thickness graft.

SIMPLE LOCAL FLAPS. Local skin flaps have certain advantages in that they carry their own blood supply and match the color and contour of the surrounding skin much better than free grafts. Although straight advancement flaps with minimal undermining can be utilized readily by most physicians, complicated transposition and rotation of tissue and z-plasty require much more experience and skill.

SYSTEMIC FACTORS

A number of systemic factors including circulation, nutrition, coincident disease and drugs have an important influence on wound healing.

Circulation

An adequate circulation to the wound is essential to supply the area not only with the oxygen and nutrients needed for local cell growth but also with the leukocytes and immunoglobulins necessary to prevent or fight infection. Shock must be kept to an absolute minimum by rapid aggressive treatment. It has been shown experimentally that epinephrine-induced ischemia, endotoxin shock or hypovolemic shock greatly reduces the minimal dose of bacteria required to produce cutaneous infections.[3]

Hunt has shown that the local Po_2 is important in wound healing. Any interference with circulation or any increased edema fluid in the area can drastically reduce the Po_2 at the wound edges.[4] Anemia or a reduction in the red cell content of 2,3-DPG may also decrease the arterial Po_2 and oxygen availability to the tissues. Wherever possible, the hemoglobin levels in severely injured or burned patients should be kept above 12 gm/100 ml.

Nutrition

By and large, in the ordinary civilian population, the state of nutrition itself does not substantially influence the rate of wound healing. Nevertheless, patients with cirrhosis and certain deficiencies often show signs of poor healing. Some of the deficiencies most apt to impair wound healing include protein, ascorbic acid and zinc.

PROTEIN. Protein deficiencies in themselves seem to have relatively little effect on wound healing unless they cause edema in the wound. If the edema is prevented or corrected by using a nonprotein colloid, wound healing will usually revert toward normal.[5]

ASCORBIC ACID (VITAMIN C). Delayed healing and even breakdown of old healed wounds have been described for hundreds of years in scorbutic sailors. The basic problems are impaired collagen synthesis and increased capillary fragility. More than adequate quantities of vitamin C are available in most diets and can be readily supplied with the usual intravenous vitamin solutions; however, critically injured patients should probably be given much greater amounts of vitamin C than usual, even up to 500 to 1000 mg daily.

ZINC. Zinc deficiencies have been shown to retard wound healing and growth in a number of animals.[6] Human zinc deficiencies are rare except when there is little or no oral intake and an excessive loss, as can occur with alcoholism, cirrhosis, burns, gastrointestinal fistulae, and severe sepsis. About 20% of the patients with severe trauma and sepsis seen at Detroit General Hospital tend to develop reduced plasma zinc levels.

Coincident Diseases

Some common conditions or diseases known to interfere with wound healing are old age, obesity, infection, cancer, cirrhosis, leukemia, uremia, diabetes mellitus and congestive heart failure. Whenever such factors can be identified, appropriate treatment should be instituted. Deficiencies in blood volume or blood constituents are corrected selectively. Unless extraordinarily meticulous care and operative technique are used in these individuals, many problems with wound healing may result.

Drugs

Of the drugs which can interfere with wound healing, those most frequently encountered in clinical practice include steroids, antineoplastic agents and immunosuppressive drugs. Steroids reduce the local inflammatory response while the antineoplastic and immunosuppressive drugs interfere with cell division and growth. Although antineoplastic agents can generally be discontinued for at least 10 to 14 days after any major trauma, the surgeon is often limited in his options with steroids and may be forced to give hydrocortisone throughout the period of stress. If the patient has a transplanted organ, the immunosuppressive drugs must also be continued.

SPECIFIC ANTIBACTERIAL AND ANTIVIRAL THERAPY

Prophylactic Antibiotics

The question of the use of prophylactic systemic antibiotics has been and remains controversial. Indiscriminate use of antibiotics is always to be discouraged because it may lead to toxic side effects or hypersensitivity reactions. In patients with trauma, the need for selective usage is doubly important because inappropriate administration may lead rapidly to the development of superinfection with secondary antibiotic-resistant organisms. Furthermore, the antibiotics may mask or alter the usual signs and symptoms of established infections, making diagnosis more difficult and treatment less effective.

There are two broad areas where the use of "prophylactic" antibiotics may be considered: contaminated (but not infected) wounds and clean wounds in patients with a tendency to infection. It would appear that antibiotics are most effective in local wounds when given within three hours of injury; later, their ability to prevent infection diminishes rapidly.[7] Consequently, if a patient has a wound which is judged to be grossly contaminated, antibiotics should be started shortly after the patient is admitted to the emergency department. Secondly, in the patient with extensive clean wounds and severe injury—especially when there has been severe hypotension or previous disease—there may be a greatly reduced resistance to infection; under such circumstances antibiotics should probably be started immediately and continued for at least three days.

Antibiotics in critically injured patients are preferably given intravenously to provide high levels in the blood and wounds. Under most circumstances, we recommend large doses of aqueous penicillin (1 to 5 million units in each liter of I.V. fluids) with tetracycline (not to exceed a total dose of 1000 mg I.V. in any 24-hour period).[8] Where there is extensive gastrointestinal spillage, gentamicin is the most effective antibiotic and may be used in place of tetracycline, paying strict attention to renal function when administering subsequent doses. With extensive damage to the distal small bowel or colon, where infection by anaerobic organisms, particularly Bacteroides fragilis, is likely, clindamycin is advocated. Where staphylococci are apt to be involved, Staphcillin or Keflin is added (Chap. 29).

In summary, antibiotics are recommended in the following cases:

1. All contaminated dirty wounds.
2. All surgery or wounds allowing spillage from organs that may contain bacteria, especially if these organs are obstructed. This would apply primarily to injuries or surgery involving the lung, intestine (especially the colon), and the genitourinary tract.
3. Patients with clean wounds but in whom infection would be especially dangerous. This includes those who have had neurosurgical or cardiovascular procedures, especially when prosthetic materials are implanted.
4. Patients who have an increased chance of infection. This includes those with shock, large areas of traumatized tissue, massive transfusions, obesity, diabetes mellitus, hematologic disorders, and drug therapy with steroids or immunosuppressive drugs. Old age, debility, and prolonged surgery may also be indications for prophylactic antibiotics.

Although the administration of penicillin in burn patients has been effective in preventing early infection by streptococci and pneumococci, the indications for other systemic antibiotics in these patients are questionable, especially since the topical antimicrobial agents such as Sulfamylon and silver nitrate are very effective.

Antitoxins and Toxoids

Active immunity developed by exposing the patients to specific antigens (toxoids) is generally preferred to passive immunity produced by administering preformed anti-bodies (antitoxins). The main advantage of the antitoxins is the rapidity with which they can help the patient who has not had previous immunization. Antitoxins do, however, have the disadvantage of a greatly increased incidence of allergic reactions, especially if the serum is obtained from nonhuman sources. Tetanus, gas gangrene, and rabies are three types of infections in which immunotherapy with antitoxins and toxoids has been used.

TETANUS. Although tetanus could be almost completely eliminated by universal active immunization during infancy and childhood, approximately 500 cases of clinical tetanus, with a mortality rate of about 20%, are reported in the United States each year.[9] Prevention of tetanus involves proper surgical management of the wound, use of antibiotics, and immunization.

Surgical Management of the Wound. All wounds should be carefully debrided, cleaned, and irrigated. In an injury likely to lead to tetanus (a deep puncture wound, a wound associated with much muscle damage or impregnation with foreign material) the debridement and irrigation must be especially thorough, and the skin and subcutaneous tissue should be left open. It should be stressed, however, that we have recently seen a few cases of tetanus occurring with small, relatively superficial lacerations.

Antibiotics. If the status of immunization of a patient is in doubt or if the wound has a reasonably good chance of becoming infected with clostridial or other organisms, it may be wise to give penicillin and tetracycline or other antibiotic(s) in an effort to prevent or control the infection (Chap. 29).

Immunization. It is important to remember that tetanus antitoxin does not prevent the actual infection with Clostridium tetani organisms, but it does inactivate the toxin they produce. Most people in the United States have had tetanus immunization; however, we cannot take this for granted and consequently we give 0.5 cc tetanus toxoid subcutaneously to all patients with lacerations unless they have been completely immunized and have had a booster within the past six months.

If there is any doubt about previous immunization, an immunization program should be begun consisting of the initial injection followed by two booster injections of toxoid a month apart. If the patient has been immunized previously but has a severe wound which has a good possibility of developing tetanus, he should also be given 0.5 cc tetanus toxoid and 400 to 500 units of human tetanus immune globulin at a different site than the toxoid.

GAS GANGRENE. Gas gangrene antitoxin and toxoid are now generally considered to be contraindicated, as they cause an extremely high incidence of allergic reactions and produce little or no benefit. The best prophylaxis for gas gangrene is proper surgical management of the wound. Hyperbaric oxygenation may also be of benefit in selected cases.[10]

RABIES. One of the main concerns with any animal bite is the possibility that rabies might develop. Although this is a rare disease, with an average of only one or two cases reported each year, it is so lethal that until recently only one patient with probable symptomatic rabies has survived.[11] As a consequence, tens of thousands of patients with animal bites are given antirabies vaccine annually.

Local Care. All dog or other animal bites should be irrigated vigorously with saline, swabbed with 1% Zephiran chloride or 40 to 70% ethanol and debrided thoroughly. Antibiotics should also be given except for the smallest, most superficial wounds. Tetanus toxoid is given unless the patient has had a booster within the past 3 to 6 months.

Rabies Immunization. DUCK-EMBRYO VACCINE. If there is any reasonable chance that the animal has rabies, the patient should be started on duck-embryo rabies vaccine immediately.[12] If there have not been any cases of rabies in animals in the area for some time, rabies vaccine or antiserum must be given only if the patient is bitten by a dog which acts or becomes rabid or

by a wild animal such as a wolf, fox, or bat. In all instances, unless it is definitely known that the dog has been properly immunized against rabies, the dog should be closely observed for five days for the purposeless movements, snapping, drooling, or vocal paralysis characteristic of this disease. Although duck-embryo vaccine (DEV) is much safer than the previously used nerve-tissue vaccine (NTV), the nerve-tissue vaccine appears to provoke better antibody levels.

RABIES ANTISERUM. When rabies is strongly suspected or proven in the animal which caused the bite, hyperimmune serum should be administered intramuscularly in a single dose of not less than 40 international units per kg of body weight, with some of this dose infiltrated in the tissue around the wound. If the wound is extensive and involves the head, a larger dose (50 to 100 I.U. per kg) should be given. Since this antirabies serum is prepared from immunized horses, sensitivity tests must be performed prior to its use. In all cases when the serum is used, two supplemental doses should be given 10 to 20 days following the completion of the usual vaccine schedule.

REFERENCES

1. Elek, S. D., and Conen, P. E.: The virulence of Staphylococcus pyogenes for man. A study of the problems of wound infections. Brit. J. Exp. Path., 38:573, 1957.
2. Baker, R. J., et al.: Wound care techniques: When skin is lost, where do you get more? Patient Care, 20, Feb. 1972.
3. Miles, A. A.: Nonspecific defense reactions in bacterial infections. Ann. N. Y. Acad. Sci., 66:356, 1956.
4. Niinikoski, J., Henghan, C., and Hunt, T. K.: Oxygen and carbon dioxide tensions in experimental wounds. Surg. Gynec. Obstet., 133:1003, 1971.
5. Rhoads, J. E., Fliegelman, M. T., and Panzer, L. M.: The mechanism of delayed wound healing in the presence of hypoproteinemia. JAMA, 118:21, 1942.
6. Oberleas, D., et al.: The effect of zinc deficiency on wound healing in rats. Amer. J. Surg., 121:556, 1971.
7. Burke, J. F.: The effective period of preventive antibiotic action in experimental incisions and dermal lesions. Surgery, 50:161, 1961.

8. Todd, J. C.: Wound infection: Etiology, prevention, and management. Surg. Clin. N. Amer., 48:787, 1968.

9. Altemeier, W. A., and Hummel, R. P.: Treatment of tetanus. Surgery, 60:495, 1966.

10. Brummelkamp, W. J., Hogendi, K. J., and Boerema, I.: Treatment of anaerobic infections (clostridial myositis) by drenching the tissues with oxygen under high atmospheric pressure. Surgery, 49:299, 1961.

11. Morbidity and Mortality. Weekly Reports, 19:479, 1970.

12. Plotkin, S. A., and Clark, H. F.: Prevention of rabies in man. J. Infect. Dis., 123:227, 1971.

Suggested Reading

1. Altemeier, W. A., and Fullen, W. D.: Prevention and treatment of gas gangrene. JAMA, 217:806, 1971.

2. Dunphy, J. E., and Udupa, K. N.: Chemical and histochemical sequences in the normal healing of wounds. New Eng. J. Med., 253:847, 1955.

3. Thomson, H. G., and Svitek, V.: Small animal bites: The role of primary closure. J. Trauma, 13:20, 1973.

4. Guldalian, J., et al.: A comparative study of synthetic and biological materials for wound dressings. J. Trauma, 13:32, 1973.

5. Linares, H. A., et al.: On the origin of the hypertrophic scar. J. Trauma, 13:70, 1973.

6. Rosenthal, S. M.: The influence of proteolytic enzyme inhibitors on traumatic swelling. J. Trauma, 13:548, 1973.

7. Furste, W.: The elimination of tetanus: A responsibility not only of physicians but also of nonphysician citizens in all areas of the world (Editorial). J. Trauma, 13:839, 1973.

9 TRAUMA IN INFANTS AND CHILDREN: SPECIAL CONSIDERATIONS

J. R. LLOYD
Y. SILVA
A. J. WALT
R. F. WILSON

Trauma in childhood has gradually increased in significance and for the past three decades has been the leading cause of death and disability in the pediatric age group[1,2] (Table 1). While the basic principles governing the management of major injuries are often the same for both children and adults, many critical differences related to diagnosis and treatment warrant special consideration.* Chief among these

* To avoid repetition of material presented elsewhere in this book, this chapter will be confined to these special considerations in the management of trauma in infants and children.

are the management of fluid and electrolyte problems, the nature and dosage of medications, the mechanics of resuscitation and the need for psychologic support of the injured child.

PITFALL

IF THE SEVERELY INJURED INFANT OR CHILD IS MANAGED AS A SMALL ADULT, THE TREATMENT WILL OFTEN BE INCORRECT OR INAPPROPRIATE AND THE DOSES OF MEDICATIONS WILL OFTEN BE TOO LARGE OR TOO SMALL.

TABLE 1. TRAUMA CASES—CHILDREN'S HOSPITAL OF MICHIGAN 1965-1969

			Total Cases (Deaths)		
	1965	1966	1967	1968	1969
Head injuries	237(7)	182(6)	200(11)	232(5)	215(5)
Fractures—skeletal	148	143	169	149	131
Fractures—cranial	61	50	101	107	86
Chest	7(1)	2	3(2)	7(2)	2(1)
Abdomen	26(2)	23(2)	36(5)	23(3)	22(3)
Abrasions, contusions, lacerations	313	328	410	300	327
Major eye	9	10	11	12	19
Battered child	9(1)	20(2)	16(2)	13(1)	14(1)
Burns	131(4)	105(5)	157(4)	151(5)	123(0)
Total	941(15)	863(15)	1103(24)	994(16)	939(10)

Total No. of Cases—4,840
Deaths—80

FIRST AID AND INITIAL TREATMENT

General Measures

The initial evaluation of any injured patient should include: patency of the upper airway, adequacy of ventilation, and effective cardiac activity and peripheral circulation. If any problem exists related to these vital functions, appropriate resuscitative measures must be instituted immediately. Beyond these obviously life-threatening problems, covered in detail later in this chapter, several aspects of the care given to infants and children before they are transported to a hospital should be stressed. These emergency first-aid measures may make the difference between an uneventful recovery and disability or death. All of these maneuvers can be applied at the scene of the accident by nonmedical personnel with first-aid training.

REASSURANCE OF THE INJURED CHILD. Anxiety, fear, and apprehension are common and not unexpected after any injury. These reactions are much more pronounced in the child than in the adult, who by virtue of age and experience may have some insight into the nature of the situation. The child, on the other hand, may be so severely disturbed that a state of hysteria can ensue which may profoundly influence the clinical picture. Children tend to thrash about in spite of pain, greatly aggravating their injuries. Any attention that produces a calming effect is vitally important.

MAINTENANCE OF NORMOTHERMIA. Environmentally induced hypo- or hyperthermia may be a serious problem in any injured child and is likely to be more pronounced if the patient is unconscious or in shock. Infants under six months of age are especially prone to develop temperature aberrations from the combination of an immature thermoregulatory mechanism and an incompletely developed shivering response. Hypothermia is the more common problem. It can occur in tiny infants with a compromised temperature-regulating mechanism even when the ambient temperature is as high as 85 F. If the body temperature falls below 32 C (89.6 F), severe cardiac arrhythmias or impaired myocardial contractility can result.

Excessive hyperthermia may make the child restless or confused, increase his oxygen and cardiovascular demands and in some instances cause convulsions. Cooling a patient or preventing overheating can be accomplished simply by fanning, providing shade or applying tepid compresses. Not so simply achieved are the tasks of preventing loss of body heat or warming the already hypothermic infant or child. The immediate physical environment must be dry. Damp clothing should be removed or cut away and the patient wrapped in a dry blanket, coat or other garment. Artificial heat from hot-water bags, hot stones or the body of an adult may provide the necessary additional thermal requirement, and the infant or child wrapped in household aluminum foil and then in a blanket will retain his body heat even under very adverse environmental conditions.

APPROPRIATE SPLINTING. The appropriate splinting of any injured part plays a major role in all first aid, especially in children who tend to move about excessively in spite of pain. Although it is usually best to splint the injured part in the position in which it is found, it may occasionally be necessary for a physician immediately to apply traction to an extremity with a fracture or dislocation to relieve obvious circulatory or neurologic embarrassment.

MOVEMENT OF THE PATIENT. Injured infants should not be picked up to cuddle and comfort them until it is certain that they may be safely moved. This is especially important in children with spinal injuries or with displaced fractures when un-

---

PITFALL

IF A CRYING ANXIOUS INFANT IS PICKED UP BEFORE THE EXTENT OF THE TRAUMA IS ASCERTAINED, THE INJURIES MAY BE SEVERELY AGGRAVATED.

---

due motion might cause neural or vascular complications. Movement of a patient under such circumstances can convert a correctable lesion into one with permanent disastrous sequelae.

Ventilation

If the child is making no effort to breathe, artificial ventilation should be started immediately. If he is trying to breathe but is moving little or no air, he may have an upper-airway obstruction. The mouth is opened and the airway is cleared of blood, mucus, vomitus or foreign bodies. If an adequate suction device is not at hand, the face should be turned downward and the oral pharynx mechanically cleared with a finger. The tongue should be pulled away from the posterior pharyngeal wall, which may be accomplished by pulling the mandible forward. The head is tilted backward and mouth-to-mouth ventilation begun, with the force and duration of each breath gauged to the size of the patient. In infants, mouth-to-nose ventilation may be more successful than mouth-to-mouth breathing.

PITFALL

IF A TINY INFANT IS VENTILATED AT THE SAME RATE AS AN ADULT, THE MINUTE VOLUME MAY BE INADEQUATE AND THE TIDAL VOLUME EXCESSIVE.

While 15 to 20 breaths per minute are adequate for an adult, the respiratory rate should be about 30 breaths per minute for children under two years of age and 20 to 25 breaths per minute for children from ages two to six. If oxygen is available, inserting the oxygen line into one corner of the resuscitator's mouth will significantly increase the oxygen concentration of the air delivered to the patient. Auscultation of the patient's chest is essential to make certain that adequate ventilation of both lungs is accomplished.

Foreign bodies may become lodged in the trachea or bronchi and impair ventilation. When a foreign body is suspected, the infant or small child should be placed face down over an arm and several sharp blows delivered to the upper midback. Larger children may be turned on their sides and rapped sharply over the upper midback in hopes of dislodging the foreign body. If there is no improvement, concentrate on moving as much air as possible around the obstructed site by forceful prolonged ventilatory effort.

A properly sized mask and self-inflating bag, when available, offer more efficient means of ventilation; however, the hazard of overventilation is introduced. The smaller the child, the smaller the tidal volume. If the respiratory exchange is inadequate, endotracheal intubation should be accomplished as soon as such equipment becomes available. The selection of a properly sized endotracheal tube for infants and children is critical and intubation must be done with great care. There is a popular belief that any tube that will fit through a nostril will fit the larynx. This rule of thumb may be used as a rough guide, but the size of the patient's larynx is the critical factor at issue; an oversized endotracheal tube should never be forced through the cords no matter how well it fits the nostril.

It must also be remembered that the smaller the child, the shorter the distance between the larynx and carina. The tube should not be permitted to rest on the carina and care should be taken to avoid inserting the tube into one of the main bronchi. When the endotracheal tube has been properly placed, as determined by auscultation of both lungs, it must be well secured. The patient's head should be immobilized to ensure that the tube will remain properly seated. Because of the relatively short trachea in children, movement of the tube more than a few centimeters in either direction may either push the tube into one of the major bronchi or pull it out of the trachea.

PITFALL

IF THE STOMACH IS NOT EMPTIED WITH A NASOGASTRIC TUBE AS SOON AS POSSIBLE IN ALL SEVERELY INJURED CHILDREN, ESPECIALLY THOSE WITH ABDOMINAL TRAUMA OR SEVERE LETHARGY, THEY MAY VOMIT AND ASPIRATE.

Trauma in children is almost always accompanied by an ileus and gastric retention. Not uncommonly, the child has eaten just prior to being injured. Since the frightened child has an increased tendency to vomit, aspiration of gastric contents into the lungs is a serious life-threatening hazard, especially in unconscious or hypotensive children. As soon as practicable, the stomach should be emptied by irrigation through a nasogastric tube and continuous suction maintained. Meanwhile, the child should be positioned so that aspiration will not occur. The unconscious child should never be placed on his back until the hazard of vomiting and aspiration has been eliminated.

Circulatory Resuscitation

If there is no palpable pulse or audible heart beat, cardiopulmonary resuscitation with external cardiac massage must be started immediately. The patient is placed on a flat hard surface; when this is not feasible, the patient's back should be supported with one hand. In infants the flat surface of two fingers and in older children the heel of one hand is placed over the lower half of the sternum.

PITFALL

IF ALLOWANCE IS NOT MADE FOR THE MORE FLEXIBLE CHEST OF THE CHILD, EXTERNAL CARDIAC MASSAGE CAN CAUSE SERIOUS MYOCARDIAL CONTUSION.

The amount of pressure applied should depress the sternum about one inch in infants and progressively farther in larger children. In general, the magnitude of sternal de-

pression should not exceed one fourth of the anteroposterior diameter of the chest but at the same time should be sufficient to produce a palpable femoral, axillary or carotid pulsation. Rapid cardiac massage does not permit adequate ventricular filling during diastole. The most effective massage rate for infants is about 70 to 80 beats per minute; for older children, it is 60 beats per minute.

Cardiorespiratory resuscitation at the scene of an accident may be discontinued if a strong heart beat and spontaneous respiration are obtained within a few minutes.

TABLE 2. CALCULATIONS FOR SURFACE AREA, INFANTS AND CHILDREN*

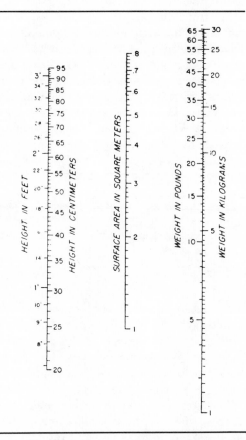

*From Talbot, N. B., Sobel, E. N., McArthur, J. W., and Crawford, J. D.: *Functional Endocrinology from Birth Through Adolescence.* Cambridge, Harvard University Press, 1952.

Otherwise, massage and ventilation should be continued en route to the nearest hospital.

As soon as facilities are available, a dependable venipuncture or cutdown with as large a needle or catheter as possible should be established in an uninjured extremity and in a vein which is not damaged or not apt to be occluded proximally. Blood should be drawn for a complete blood count, electrolyte determination, typing and cross-matching, pH and blood gases. A satisfactory I.V. fluid to use initially is 5% glucose/Ringer's lactate. Since it is extremely easy to overload tiny infants with I.V. fluids, the initial infusion rate should ordinarily not exceed 1500 ml/M²/24 hours except when treating obvious hypovolemia (Table 2).

An EKG machine or an electronic cardiac monitor with recording capabilities should be connected to the child. If an adequate heart beat is not restored promptly by cardiac massage, undiluted 7.5% sodium bicarbonate (0.9 mEq/ml) is rapidly injected into the I.V. tubing in a dose of 1 ml/lb to combat acidosis. If the cardiac monitor demonstrates asystole, massage and ventilation are continued while cardiac stimulants are given in an attempt to initiate heart action. The doses of these drugs must be carefully modified to fit the age and size of the patient (Table 3). Adrenalin, diluted to 1 to 10,000, is injected intravenously in doses of 0.5 to 1.0 ml in infants under two years of age, 1.0 to 2.0 ml in two- to five-year-olds and up to 3 ml in older children. If asystole persists, a second dose of Adrenalin is administered and a search is made for any acid-base, blood gas, or electrolyte abnormality which might be the cause. If there is any question about the adequacy of the intravenous infusion, it is advisable to give the Adrenalin as an intracardiac injection.

Ventricular fibrillation, although less frequently encountered in children than in adults, does occur and is treated by continued massage until electrical defibrillation can be performed. The initial shock in infants under two years of age should not exceed 50 watt-seconds. In children over two years, a current of 100 watt-seconds may be used. If fibrillation persists beyond 20 to 30 seconds, additional bicarbonate (1 ml/lb) is given while ventilation and cardiac massage are continued. Repeated shocks may be used increasing the current strength by increments of 50 watt-seconds up to 250 watt-seconds. Exceeding this current strength is unlikely to arrest fibrillation and may produce a burn. Persistent or recurrent fibrillation should be treated with intravenous lidocaine. One ml of 1% lidocaine is diluted to 10 ml with physiologic saline and 1 ml of this solution is given at intervals of one to two minutes. The total dose used should not exceed 3 mg/lb. Intravenous lidocaine may be employed initially in lieu of electrical shock and can be an effective means of treating fibrillation if a defibrillator is not available.

TABLE 3. DRUGS USED DURING CARDIAC RESUSCITATION IN INFANTS

Drug	Standard solution	Dilution used in children	Amount of diluted solution used
Epinephrine	1:1,000	1:10,000	2 yr age-1 ml; 2-5 yr age-2 ml 5 yr or older—3 ml
Isoproterenol	0.2 mg/ml	0.02 mg/ml	1 ml/20 lb weight
Calcium chloride	10%	1%	2 ml/yr
Xylocaine	1%	0.1%	1 ml q. 1-2 min not to exceed 3 mg/lb

If a good heart beat is obtained, ventilation is continued until adequate spontaneous respirations are established. If the heart starts but the rate remains under 60, intravenous Isuprel is begun; the usual dose is 1 ml per 20 pounds of body weight of a solution containing 0.2 mg Isuprel diluted in 10 ml of physiologic saline. In general, Isuprel is preferable to Adrenalin when dealing with a severe bradycardia. If the rate is adequate but the heart beat is weak, 1% calcium chloride is given intravenously. The initial dose is 2 ml per year of age up to 10 ml in the five-year-old. Larger doses in older children are not likely to be any more effective and may be toxic.

If cardiac activity is present but remains weak in spite of all the above measures, the circulation may be supported with an intravenous solution of 2 mg Isuprel in 500 ml of 5% dextrose in lactated Ringer's (D/L.R.) solution. The blood pressure and heart rate are titrated to the desired levels by regulating the rate of flow of the Isuprel solution.

When closed-chest massage does not produce an adequate response within ten minutes and a volume deficit is suspected, 10 ml/lb of 5% D/L.R., plasma or low-titer O-negative uncross-matched blood should be given rapidly. If all these measures fail and asystole or fibrillation still persists, open thoracotomy with cardiac massage should be carried out in the patient who does not appear to be beyond all hope of survival. It should be kept in mind that, even in the face of cerebral death demonstrated by a flat EEG, preservation of bodily functions can make life-saving transplantable tissues available to someone else.

Hemorrhage

Children have a much lower margin of reserve with respect to blood loss than do adults. The amount of blood loss resulting from hemorrhage in the injured child is not adequately appreciated unless it is considered in relation to his small circulating blood volume. For example, the total blood volume in an 11-lb infant is approximately 400 ml. The rapid loss of 100 ml can produce clinical shock and acute blood loss exceeding 200 ml can cause death. In all instances, hemorrhage must be completely and promptly controlled and volume deficits rapidly corrected.

PITFALL

IF LARGE QUANTITIES OF BLOOD AND FLUID ARE INDISCRIMINATELY ADMINISTERED TO ALL CHILDREN WHO APPEAR TO BE IN A SHOCK-LIKE STATE IMMEDIATELY AFTER TRAUMA, THE CHILD WHOSE INJURIES ARE RELATIVELY MINOR IS LIKELY TO BE SERIOUSLY OVERLOADED.

A transient shock-like picture due to pain, anxiety or fear is not infrequently encountered in children even with mild trauma. The major hazard in such instances is injudicious overtreatment. If the child is unconscious in addition, a severe head injury and active hemorrhage must be ruled out. As in the adult, persistent hypotension immediately after trauma is almost never the result of a closed head injury or sepsis. With the exception of burn shock or shock resulting from persistent vomiting or diarrhea, severe hypotension in a child is virtually always due to hemorrhage.

Blood is the ideal replacement fluid for blood loss but is not always immediately available. Every physician who may be called upon to treat severely ill or injured infants should know his own blood type. In an extreme emergency, a 50-ml syringe full of his own blood immediately given intravenously to a severely hypovolemic infant with the same blood type may be life-saving. If the parents, for religious or other reasons, refuse to allow blood to be given to their child, an appeal can be made to a probate judge to make the child a ward of the court so that he may receive adequate treatment.

Until blood is available, physiologic saline or 5% D/L.R. solutions may be used for volume replacement. In general, 10 ml/lb of a crystalloid can be safely administered as an intravenous push to correct moderate to severe hypovolemia. Volumes exceeding these amounts, except during active hemorrhage, may overload the patient and cause congestive heart failure.

The response of the central venous pressure is often the best guide to volume replacement in shock. If the CVP is less than 4 cm H_2O, fluids may be given at the rapid safe rate of administration (5 ml/lb/hr). If the CVP is higher than 15 cm H_2O, the possibilities of a tension pneumothorax, cardiopulmonary disease, excessive straining, inaccurate placement of the CVP catheter or an inaccurate reading of the CVP must be ruled out.

Should the CVP measurements be at odds with the clinical picture and a reliable cuff blood pressure cannot be obtained, an intra-arterial line should be established and the arterial pressure monitored. This maneuver is not necessary in most shock patients, but in those instances when all other parameters fail to give assurance that an adequate arterial pressure is being maintained it is most helpful.

Patients being treated for hypovolemic shock should have an indwelling urinary catheter. An output of 40 ml per square meter of body-surface area per hour is usually evidence of adequate renal perfusion. It is especially important to maintain a high urine output in patients with severe burns or crush injuries to reduce the hazard of renal tubular obstruction by cellular debris.

EVALUATION OF THE PATIENT

History

The younger the child, the more difficult it becomes to obtain a detailed history; under three years of age, communication is almost impossible. Furthermore, it is not unusual for the child who has experienced major trauma to have retrograde amnesia for the details of the accident for several days or longer. Evasiveness or vagueness is to be expected when the child was injured while involved in forbidden play or conduct. Scrutiny of the postinjury environment may yield valuable information. For example, a battered bicycle, a blood-stained sharp projection on a toy, a missing part of a toy, skid marks on the pavement, an open second-story window with the screen pushed out may give valuable hints on the possible mechanism of injury.

The past history of the child must usually be obtained from his parents or guardian who, if not already present, must be notified as soon as possible. During the process of informing the parents of the situation, especially when significant distance is involved, certain crucial information regarding the status of the child's immunizations and any accompanying metabolic, hematologic or allergic disorders must be obtained. Problems such as diabetes, hemophilia or drug allergies must be noted early in the appraisal and treatment of the patient. The allergic child is not only apt to have significant drug allergies but may also have been taking enough steroids within the past year to impair his ability to withstand the stress of major trauma. Supplemental intravenous steroids may be lifesaving in such situations.

Physical Examination

The child should be completely undressed by cutting the clothing away rather than unnecessarily manipulating injured parts in an attempt to remove garments intact. External hemorrhage should be controlled while continuing the examination. The position of the cervical trachea is determined and the chest is checked for crepitation, stability, symmetry and adequacy of ventilation. The heart rate and rhythm are noted, as is the point of maximum cardiac impulse (PMI). Any significant displacement of the PMI or cervical trachea indicates an intrathoracic problem with mediastinal shift from causes such as pneumothorax, hemothorax or massive atelectasis. Intrapericardial hemorrhage with cardiac tamponade should be suspected when the heart tones sound distant or muffled. During the examination of the abdomen, special attention is given to the abdominal tone, any masses, evidence of increasing abdominal girth, hyperresonance (with obliteration of liver dullness) and penetrating wounds. An unusually scaphoid abdomen may indicate that the intestines have herniated into the chest through a ruptured diaphragm. If there is distortion of the pelvis or evidence of fractures in that area, a digital rectal examination should be performed and a catheter passed into the bladder. The initial neurologic examination should include state of consciousness, pupillary size and reflexes, type and level of paralysis, and any abnormal reflexes. With extremity injuries, variations of the peripheral pulses must be noted and base-line observations of cold or cyanotic areas established.

PITFALL

IF AN INJURED CHILD IS TREATED ON THE BASIS OF AN INITIAL IMPRESSION RATHER THAN ON OBSERVATIONS MADE OVER A PERIOD OF SEVERAL HOURS, HE MAY WELL BE OVERTREATED INITIALLY AND UNDERTREATED LATER.

The child, more so than the adult, is prone to develop a transient state of neurogenic "shock" after trauma which is not necessarily related to the severity of the injury and may be very difficult to differentiate from coma due to cerebral concussion. Although recovery from this condition is usually very rapid, it initially adds an element of confusion and appears to magnify the degree of injury. This state may clear so dramatically that the physician may be deceived into thinking that the injury is relatively minor. This post-traumatic episode is of importance because it can mislead the physician into overtreating early and undertreating later.

During the course of the examination, skeletal injuries are generally readily detected; however, in the face of extensive trauma, especially when the child is rela-

tively immobile and the bone fragments are not displaced, fractures may not be clinically apparent. It is essential that the physical examination be supplemented by comprehensive radiologic evaluation.

Laboratory Studies

In any potentially serious injury, especially when the chest or abdomen is involved, a complete blood count, urinalysis and type and cross-match are essential base-line studies. A marked leukocytosis is a feature of the early post-traumatic period in children and may be misleading since it can occur with contusions in the absence of visceral or skeletal injuries. If the child has been in shock, base-line studies should also include electrolytes and blood gases.

Occasionally a latent or stress diabetes mellitus will become manifest incident to trauma, resulting in a severe acidosis. This should be suspected if the child exhibits glycosuria, persistent hyperventilation, a low CO_2 content, or a persistently elevated blood sugar.

X-rays

PITFALL

IF X-RAYS ARE NOT TAKEN OF ALL INJURED PARTS IN A CHILD, REGARDLESS OF HOW MINOR THE PAIN, TENDERNESS OR SWELLING, IMPORTANT FRACTURES WILL BE MISSED.

Greenstick or incomplete fractures occur more often in children than in adults and are clinically difficult to ascertain. The initial x-rays in a child with moderate or severe blunt trauma should encompass all possible fracture sites including the spine, skull, chest, pelvis and all long bones. Whenever an extremity is x-rayed, the opposite limb must also be examined for comparison because of difficulty in interpreting the position and alignment of the various growth centers. Any child with broken or missing teeth must either have the teeth accounted for or have a chest x-ray to be sure the teeth have not been aspirated.

While radiologic investigation may be an invaluable diagnostic aid, hours of valuable time needed for intensive treatment may be lost in the x-ray department. Whenever a seriously injured child requires numerous x-ray examinations, a physician should be in constant attendance to ensure continuation of treatment and early detection of any deterioration.

In this modern age, nearly all departments of radiology are efficiently air conditioned. While this provides comfortable working conditions for the medical and ancillary personnel, excessive exposure of young infants to this environment can cause dangerous hypothermia.

Paracentesis and Peritoneal Irrigation

Persistent or recurrent hypotension following trauma is almost always due to hemorrhage. Except for bleeding from large scalp or facial lacerations, head injuries rarely cause shock. If there is no obvious external blood loss, hemorrhage is probably occurring into soft tissues at the site of fractures or into one of the body cavities. If there are no fractures of the long bones or pelvis either clinically or radiologically and if a hemothorax is not apparent on upright or decubitis x-rays of the chest, the abdomen is the most likely site of continuing blood loss. When examination of the abdomen fails to demonstrate any evidence of internal injury and all other possible causes for the hypotension have been eliminated, irrigation of the peritoneal cavity with 100 ml of normal saline in infants and up to 500 ml saline in husky teen-agers is performed. The irrigations are accomplished by passing a plastic catheter through a 16- or 18-gauge needle inserted into the peritoneal cavity. Approximately two minutes after instillation of the saline, the fluid is withdrawn and the presence of more than a trace of blood, bile or intestinal content in the aspirate is an indication for surgical intervention. False negatives are infrequent but may occur. In spite of a negative peritoneal irrigation, if there is no other explanation for persistent hypotension and the abdomen continues to be the most plausible source of hemorrhage, exploratory laparotomy is justified.

TREATMENT

Nasogastric Intubation

Children tend to develop a profound ileus following serious trauma even though the gastrointestinal tract may not be involved. Consequently, early nasogastric intubation is essential in all seriously injured children to prevent vomiting and aspiration and to minimize abdominal distension that may further reduce a compromised respiratory reserve. The prevention of gastrointestinal distension is especially important when attempting to determine the presence of intra-abdominal bleeding or leakage of bile, pancreatic or intestinal fluid by serial measurements of abdominal girth.

Head Injuries (Chap. 14)

Cephalohematomas, large collections of blood under the scalp that result from extracranial hemorrhage in the newborn, are occasionally seen following difficult labor. For the most part, these will resorb. Evacuation by needle introduces the hazards of serious infection and should be avoided. Such areas should be x-rayed to determine the integrity of the underlying calvaria.

PITFALL

IF AN ASYMPTOMATIC CHILD WITH A HISTORY OF SEVERE HEAD TRAUMA OR A SKULL FRACTURE IS NOT ADMITTED AND OBSERVED FOR 48 HOURS, SIGNIFICANT NEUROLOGIC DAMAGE DUE TO INTRACRANIAL HEMORRHAGE MAY BE MISSED.

Skull fractures in children without serious brain injury are common. However, observation of the child with a severe head injury, even though asymptomatic, must be maintained for at least 24 hours to detect any sudden neurologic deterioration due to intracranial hemorrhage.

If there is a depressed fracture, the fragments should be elevated. The flexibility of the infant's skull permits it to depress and spring back without being fractured. In the process, however, underlying brain tissue may be severely contused or bridging veins may be torn causing intracranial hemorrhage. Decompression of any increased intracranial pressure and control of bleeding in such cases must be accomplished without delay. Because of the flexibility of the infant's cranial bones, well-localized "ping-pong ball" fractures can occur. Such deformities need open reduction since the localized pressure exerted against underlying brain tissue may interfere with its growth and can eventually result in convulsive disorders.

Following any severe trauma which includes a head injury, a thorough neurologic evaluation should be conducted. Lumbar puncture, carotid arteriography, pneumoencephalography, and electroencephalography are diagnostic aids in determining the severity of head trauma if continued confusion, coma or localized neurologic deficits are present (Chap. 14). Scalp lacerations should always be cleansed and explored with the sterile gloved finger to rule out an underlying fracture before the wound is closed.

PITFALL

IF A LETHARGIC CHILD IS PERMITTED ANY FOOD OR FLUID FOR AT LEAST 24 TO 48 HOURS AFTER HEAD TRAUMA, HE MAY VOMIT, MAKING ACCURATE APPRAISAL OF THE INJURY MORE DIFFICULT.

Vomiting after head trauma is an important sign of increased intracranial pressure. Small children with severe trauma or mild injuries sustained under frightening circumstances have an increased tendency to vomit; this is a nonspecific reaction to stress and anxiety. To avoid confusing vomiting due to increased intracranial pressure with this nonspecific reaction, it seems prudent not to feed the child while he is under observation for a possible head injury.

There is a tendency in the child who has incurred a severe head injury to develop peptic ulcers or gastric erosions. The incidence of this complication may be reduced by nasogastric suction with intermittent instillation of milk and antacids. Should bleeding occur, as evidenced by the presence of blood in nasogastric secretions, it can usually be controlled by gastric irrigations with iced saline. Blood loss requiring replacement of 10 ml per pound per 8 hours and which persists beyond two 8-hour periods, in the absence of any coagulation defect, is an indication for surgical intervention.

Injuries to the Thorax (Chap. 20)

AIRWAY OBSTRUCTION. Blood, mucus, vomitus or foreign bodies may acutely obstruct the airway of the injured child. When suction is not available, the child should be kept face down and any foreign material in the mouth should be removed with a finger or a clean cloth or handkerchief. If there are still problems with the airway or if respirator assistance is required, an endotracheal tube should be inserted. If ventilatory support is indicated for an indefinite additional period beyond 72 hours of endotracheal intubation, a tracheostomy is recommended. In a few institutions, however, especially skilled and interested physicians have been able to maintain satisfactory respiratory support via endotracheal tubes for several weeks.

The performance of a tracheostomy in an infant can sometimes be extremely difficult and is far more hazardous than in an adult. Since the pleura comes up much higher and closer to the trachea in children, the incidence of iatrogenic pneumothorax is increased. There is also a tendency to use a small skin incision and suture it tightly around the tracheostomy tube; as a consequence air may be trapped beneath the skin, producing subcutaneous emphysema. Furthermore, since the trachea is extremely mobile, the recurrent laryngeal nerves are more easily injured than in the adult. Management of the tracheostomy in infants demands careful attention to detail and the maintenance of sterile technique. There may be difficulty in weaning the child from the tracheostomy. Progressive reduction in the size of the tracheostomy tube and partial plugging are usually successful but occasionally an infant will require continuation of the tracheostomy for many weeks or months.

PNEUMOTHORAX. Acute tension or simple pneumothorax may be relieved temporarily in infants and children and sometimes definitively in older children by needle aspiration through the second or third intercostal space in the midclavicular line. Because of the delicate structure of the infant's lung, extreme care is advised with this procedure. With evidence of a continued air leak, a small-caliber chest tube is inserted at the aspiration site and connected to a water-seal bottle. Should the lung fail to expand, suction may be applied to the chest tube using the smallest negative pressure needed to bring out the lung.

PITFALL

IF EXCESSIVE NEGATIVE PRESSURE IS APPLIED TO CHEST TUBES IN TINY INFANTS, SEVERE MEDIASTINAL SHIFT MAY OCCUR, GREATLY INTERFERING WITH VENOUS RETURN AND CARDIOVASCULAR ACTIVITY.

The mediastinum in infants is very mobile and will move to one side or the other with small unilateral changes in intrapleural pressure. Little or no suction on a chest tube is needed to expand the lung under most circumstances. If negative pressure in excess of 20 cm H_2O is required to effect expansion and hold the lung out, bronchoscopy is indicated to rule out any tracheal or bronchial injury or obstruction.

HEMOTHORAX. While air leaks without bleeding may be controlled with a relatively small chest tube, the presence of blood in the chest requires a tube of at least 20 French caliber in the infant and 24 to 28 French in the older child. The underwater seal or suction apparatus employed should provide a means for measuring the amount of blood lost per unit time. Bleeding through the tube of 2 ml/lb/hr or less with evidence of slowing suggests that the hemorrhage will cease without operation. Blood loss continuing at this rate beyond eight hours with no evidence of slowing indicates a need for surgical intervention.

FLAIL CHEST. The smaller the child, the more flexible the chest cage and the more difficult it becomes to stabilize by external means without dangerously inhibiting respiration. If there is any difficulty in obtaining adequate ventilation and maintaining normal blood gases, endotracheal intubation and a respirator should be used without hesitation. If intubation appears to be needed for longer than 72 hours, a tracheostomy should be considered.

Injuries to the Abdomen (Table 4) (Chaps. 22, 23)

In the injured child, an apparently normal abdomen may harbor unsuspected serious internal trauma while the severely contused, ecchymotic abdominal wall may enclose normal intact viscera. As a consequence, abdominal injuries in childhood frequently tax the diagnostic acumen of the physician and the absence of external signs of trauma may impose undesirable delays in management while a badly bruised abdominal wall may precipitate unnecessary surgical intervention.

CONTUSIONS. Severe contusion of the abdominal wall in children is often associated with sufficient pain and rigidity to suggest major internal injuries. The white blood cell count, which is almost always elevated in these instances, further confuses the picture. If the child's condition is stable, careful observation is recommended. Tenderness and rigidity due to abdominal-wall

TABLE 4.   ABDOMINAL TRAUMA—CHILDREN'S HOSPITAL OF MICHIGAN 1965-1969

Site	1965	1966	1967	1968	1969	Total
Liver	1(1)	1	4(3)	1	1	8(4)
Spleen	1(1)	0	1	0	1	3(1)
G.U.	8	6(1)	4(1)	5(1)	7(1)	30(4)
Pancreas	1	0	1	0	0	2(0)
G.I.	4	2(1)	5(1)	2(1)	3(1)	16(4)
Contusions	11	14	21	15(1)	10(1)	71(2)
Total	26(2)	23(2)	36(5)	23(3)	22(3)	130(15)

contusion are usually transient and tend to subside after a few hours. Conservative or nonoperative management is permissible as long as shock does not develop, the serial blood counts remain stable and the x-rays are normal.

INTRA-ABDOMINAL HEMORRHAGE. If internal bleeding is suspected, a nasogastric tube should be inserted and attached to suction. The abdominal girth should then be measured at a designated mark every 30 to 60 minutes. Increasing abdominal girth can be caused by free intraperitoneal air, blood, ileus with distension, edema of the abdominal wall secondary to contusion or retroperitoneal extravasation of urine. Peritoneal irrigation employed in such instances is an aid to differential diagnosis.

The most likely causes of massive, intraperitoneal hemorrhage are rupture of the liver or disruption of the mesenteric vessels at the base of the mesentery. The injured spleen can also bleed massively; however, the hemorrhage is usually much less apt to be exsanguinating and there is usually some warning of impending disaster. An enlarged spleen secondary to infectious mononucleosis or a hematologic disorder may be ruptured by forces so light that they may not leave any mark or may not have caused any significant discomfort at the time of injury. Pain over the top of the left shoulder and radiologic evidence of displacement of the gastric air bubble are aids to the diagnosis. Conservative management of splenic trauma has been employed in a

few institutions on an investigational basis.[3] In general we do not recommend conservative management of intra-abdominal hemorrhage and favor surgical exploration with evidence of persistent blood loss.

Detecting abdominal masses depends to a large extent on a cooperative patient. Tears in omental vessels, for example, may produce a palpable hematoma of the mesentery. When examination of the abdomen is crucial in determining the necessity for surgical intervention in an uncooperative but otherwise stable patient, he may be sedated with 2 mg/lb of intramuscular Seconal or Nembutal. This will relax a fearful, apprehensive child within 20 to 30 minutes and will not mask true tenderness caused by peritoneal irritation. Obviously this sedation should be used only with great caution if the child is being simultaneously observed for head injury.

INTESTINAL INJURIES. Penetrating wounds of the abdomen are less frequently seen in children than in adults, but when demonstrated the patients are immediately explored. While most adults will permit an adequate examination of an abdominal laceration to determine its depth, the child will usually resist such maneuvers unless adequately sedated.

Nonpenetrating injury to the gastrointestinal tract of the child must be suspected when there is persistent abdominal tenderness following a closed injury. Injuries may range from contusion with ecchymosis of the gut through lacerations, intramural hematomas, transections, and gangrene secondary to loss of the blood supply from injuries involving primarily the mesentery. Symptoms and signs may include tenderness, distension due to ileus or obstruction, edema of the abdominal wall, a palpable mass, obliteration of liver dullness due to free air, a doughy abdomen due to bleeding, increased abdominal girth, leukocytosis and hyperthermia.

Flat and upright abdominal films are essential. In the unconscious child, cross-table posteroanterior left decubitis films are the best means for demonstrating free air and air fluid levels. Peritoneal lavage may be useful when the x-rays are not diagnostic.

Intramural hematomas, most often involving the second or third portion of the duodenum, usually produce symptoms of high intestinal obstruction. When such lesions are suspected and the child is otherwise stable, a study of the upper gastrointestinal tract is diagnostic. About 50% of these lesions will resolve in six to eight days on conservative management. Post-traumatic duodenal obstruction persisting beyond seven days should be investigated surgically and in many instances evacuation of the hematoma is curative.[4] Tears or transections of the gastrointestinal tract most commonly occur in the upper jejunum or terminal ileum where there is relative fixation of the bowel adjacent to a freely mobile portion. Early diagnosis and prompt surgical intervention are the best means for avoiding severe complications and mortality. Small tears may be closed but extensive injury associated with any possible vascular compromise is best managed by resection and end-to-end anastomosis.

Perforation of the rectum by a thermometer occasionally occurs in newborn nurseries. Such perforations are usually not detected until severe peritonitis has developed. Infants are usually toxic and hypovolemic by the time the diagnosis is established. In our experience, this injury has a 50% mortality rate. Because of this hazard, rectal temperatures are no longer routinely taken at the Children's Hospital of Michigan.

PANCREATIC TRAUMA. Blows to the upper abdomen in a child may severely damage the pancreas and cause significant retroperitoneal hemorrhage. Amylase levels of 200 to 250 Somogyi units are occasionally seen with abdominal injuries without major pancreatic trauma.[5] Amylase levels over 500 units with ileus and generalized pain suggest significant pancreatic injury and are usually an indication for surgery. Pancreatic pseudocysts not uncommonly are found in children who survive conservative management of significant pancreatic trauma. Surgical resection of the distal fragment of a severely crushed or transected pancreas is recommended. Adequate drainage is essential in the presence of pancreatic contusion or edema.

UROLOGIC INJURIES. Urinalysis is essential in all patients who have had abdominal trauma. When spontaneous micturition is not possible, judicious catheterization is done and an immediate urinalysis obtained. Clear urine with no microscopic hematuria may rule out damage to the lower urinary tract but does not exclude major renal trauma. Urethral damage that does not permit catheterization should be approached from above and adequate drainage established by suprapubic cystostomy. Retrograde catheterization of the urethra is often possible from above and may be important in maintaining urethral continuity. When there is blood in the urine obtained by catheterization, the catheter should be left in place and a pyelogram performed. Massive extravasation of dye around a kidney or nonvisualization of a kidney in the absence of any known upper genitourinary anomalies is an indication for renal exploration. Moderate extravasation of dye with an apparently intact kidney is not an indication for urgent surgery. Careful observation of renal lacerations is replacing emergency exploration in most pediatric centers. Many torn kidneys will heal or can be reconstructed if the vascular pedicle is intact.

If intravenous pyelography is not diagnostic, selective renal arteriography is recommended.

Burn Injuries (Chap. 28)

INCIDENCE OF THE BURN PROBLEM. Of the approximately 2,000,000 burns that occur in the United States each year, about half involve children. Burn injuries are now one of the first five causes of death in children. Scalds and grease burns occur most commonly (Table 1). Direct flame burns are less frequent but are much more apt to be lethal.

Over 80% of burn injuries in children are avoidable accidents; 50% are due to the child's own actions, 15% are the result of carelessness or neglect and 15% involve innocent bystanders. In 10% of burn injuries, the child is an intended victim, and three fourths of this latter group are "battered children" with evidence of previous abuse such as scars or x-ray findings of healed fractures. Two percent of the burn patients are rescuers, 3% have prior illnesses such as paralytic conditions or seizures, and in about 5% the cause cannot be determined.

PITFALL

IF CHILDREN WITH AS LITTLE AS 15% SECOND-DEGREE BURNS ARE NOT GIVEN INTRAVENOUS THERAPY, SEVERE SHOCK MAY DEVELOP WITHIN 18 TO 24 HOURS.

CRITERIA FOR ADMISSION. Burns in infants and young children involving more than 15% of the body surface can produce life-threatening shock. All these patients should receive intravenous therapy. When the extent of involvement is over 10% total burn and 5% third-degree burn, admission is advised and intravenous fluids are administered if careful observation suggests that oral intake is inadequate or if the child starts vomiting. Regardless of the extent of the burn, any child with burns of the hands, face or genitalia is admitted. Minor burns of the trunk or extremities may be treated on an outpatient basis.

GENERAL MEASURES. Where appropriate, the early application of cool compresses or immersion in cool water at approximately 55 F is the most effective method for relieving pain. Ointments or home remedies such as butter or Vaseline should not be applied. Upon arrival at the hospital the patient should be divested of all clothing, weighed and wrapped in a sterile sheet. Intravenous therapy is started with 5% G/L.R. at the rate of 10 ml/kg/hr without delaying to evaluate the extent of the burn and/or to calculate the fluid requirements according to any one of several formulas.

Copious amounts of cool physiologic saline are used to irrigate the burn areas. Blisters are gently debrided, whether intact or collapsed. Cleansing of the burn must not be done with solutions containing hexachlorophene, which has been reported to be neurotoxic.[6]

TOPICAL AGENTS. Several topical agents such as Sulfamylon, Betadine and Silvadene (silver sulfadiazine) creams are effective in reducing bacterial invasions. Silvadene, which has a low incidence of hypersensitivity, has been used at Children's Hospital of Michigan since August 1968. Comparison with other topical agents over a 2-year period demonstrated the effectiveness and advantages of silver sulfadiazine, and it has been used almost exclusively ever since. No metabolic or electrolyte disturbances are associated with its use. The cream is relatively painless on application and dressing changes are remarkably atraumatic. In conjunction with vigorous local wound care, bacterial control is excellent and Candida albicans is effectively suppressed. The eschar is softer and more pliable, permitting more rapid debridement.

Dressings are changed once every 24 hours and are accompanied by a 30- to 40-minute tubbing in warm water containing two pounds of common table salt, one half cup of Pink Dreft and 20 ml of Clorox bleach per 50 gallons of water.

Although 0.5% silver nitrate compresses are effective for controlling burn infection, we have abandoned their use because of severe associated electrolyte disturbances and the excessive work load necessitated by two to three dressing changes each day. One half percent silver nitrate in a water-soluble cream can be made up in most hospital pharmacies and is also an effective topical agent. Staining is still produced but electrolyte disturbances are minimized.

Topical agents may be used with or without dressings and equally good results have been reported with either approach. We have tried both and prefer dressings because of our impression that children who have their burns covered are usually physically more active and psychologically less withdrawn.

After the initial evaluation, the extent of the burn injury is mapped out on a special surface-area chart to permit accurate determination of the extent of the burn.

CALCULATIONS OF FLUID AND ELECTROLYTE REQUIREMENTS. On the first day, the formula used is: percent burn $\times$ body weight (kg) $\times$ 2 = ml 5% D/L.R. Half this volume is administered within the first eight hours after the burn. Maintenance fluids consisting of 5% D/L.R. are calculated on the basis of 1500 ml/M²/day. If the burn exceeds 40% of the body surface, 50 mEq NaHCO₃ are added to each liter of resuscitation fluid, and, if the burn exceeds 60%, 100 mEq NaHCO₃ are added to each liter. CVP monitoring is usually not necessary for burns under 50% unless there has been a delay in intravenous therapy and the patient is in shock. A Foley catheter is inserted and the hourly urine output is monitored in all infants with burns over 20% and in all older children with burns over 30%. Sufficient fluids should be given to maintain a urinary output of at least 40 ml/M²/hr. Essentially the same volume of fluid is given through the second day, modified only on the basis of the patient's responses assessed by electrolyte levels, urinary output, and vital signs.

Oral fluids should be administered only in small amounts and with great caution. Severe thirst usually indicates persistent hypovolemia and necessitates "reevaluation" of crystalloid requirements. In spite of all precautions, occasionally an infant or child will inadvertently be given, or take on his own, large amounts of water. This can result in severe dilutional hyponatremia, water intoxication and/or congestive failure.

NUTRITION. As in other forms of trauma, the infant or child who incurs serious burns tends to develop an ileus. In patients with over 20% burns, in spite of complaints of severe thirst, no attempt is made to provide an oral intake during the first 48 hours to avoid the hazards of vomiting and water intoxication. After this initial period of restricted intake, feedings are gradually increased to a high-protein, high-caloric diet. By the fifth day, most patients can sustain themselves by the oral route and intravenous fluids can be discontinued.

A marked acceleration of metabolism occurs in nearly all patients with third-degree burns in excess of 50% of the body surface, and the nutritional needs imposed by this hypercatabolic state frequently cannot be met by the oral route alone. Transfusions of whole blood (5 ml/lb) are administered with sufficient frequency to maintain hemoglobin levels at or above 12 gm/100 ml. Serum albumin 5 ml/lb/day is infused as needed during the period that the open wound exceeds 10% of the body surface to maintain plasma protein levels at or above 5 gm/100 ml. In addition to these measures, hyperalimentation has proved to be a valuable nutritional adjunct for the severely burned patient.

PITFALL

IF CIRCUMFERENTIAL THIRD-DEGREE BURNS OF THE EXTREMITIES OR CHEST ARE NOT INCISED LONGITUDINALLY, THE ESCHAR CAN SERIOUSLY INTERFERE WITH CIRCULATION AND RESPIRATION.

CIRCULATORY EMBARRASSMENT—ESCHAROT-
OMY. Full-thickness thermal injury of the
skin destroys its elasticity and third-degree
burns of extremities will produce a tourniquet effect which interferes with the blood
supply to the distal portions of the extremity. Cyanosis of the hands or feet is an indication for performing escharotomy. Three
or four longitudinal incisions are made
throughout the length of the eschar, thereby interrupting its tourniquet effect and
restoring the distal circulation. Care must
be exercised to incise only through the eschar; incisions carried into the subcutaneous tissue will result in troublesome bleeding when the circulation improves.

Escharotomies are frequently needed in
circumferential burns of the chest to permit
adequate ventilation. An inelastic circumferential eschar of the abdomen can result
in elevation of the diaphragm in the presence of an ileus or distension.

SMOKE INHALATION. Patients who are
burned in a closed area will usually have
some degree of smoke inhalation. The actual burn of the skin may be relatively
minor but the pulmonary insult may be
life-threatening. Such patients should be
observed for at least 24 hours since clinical
evidence of chemical pneumonitis may be
delayed. Rich concentrations of well-hu-
midified oxygen should be provided and, if
blood gases reflect inadequate respiratory
exchange, massive doses of steroids and
ventilatory assistance via an endotracheal
tube may be required for 72 hours or
longer. In general, tracheostomies in burn
patients, especially infants, are to be avoided since they provide an additional route
for the development of sepsis.

IMMUNIZATION AND ANTIBIOTICS. All
burned patients should receive a booster
shot of tetanus toxoid if previously immunized and immune human globulin if not.
Because the primary bacterial invaders of
the burn wound are usually endogenous
streptococci, penicillin or ampicillin is given
for the first four to five days. After this
period, colonization of the burn surface will

ensue with a variety of organisms and subsequent antibiotic therapy is based on cultures obtained from the burned tissues.
Within seven to ten days after the burn,
coliform and Pseudomonas organisms appear. It may be useful to quantitate the
severity of infection; 100,000 organisms per
cm^2 of burn surface is the level of infection
considered to be associated with invasive
burn wound sepsis.[7] If methods are not
available for accurate colony counts, quantitation of bacteria should be reported in
terms of light, moderate and heavy growth.
A decidedly heavy growth of an organism
should alert the physician to the possibility
of invasive infection and appropriate antibiotic therapy should be instituted and
local care intensified. Any suspected purulent subeschar accumulation should be unroofed. The use of silver sulfadiazine on
the burn unit of the Children's Hospital of
Michigan has all but eliminated Pseudomonas as a serious threat. Organisms of the
genus Klebsiella and Aerobacter are emerging in the place of Pseudomonas but thus
far have not demonstrated a significant
lethal potential.

DEBRIDEMENT. Since the introduction of
effective topical agents in the management
of burns, eschar separation has been markedly delayed. The clean eschar which is not
harboring bacteria will persist for long periods of time in the absence of bacterial necrosis and must be mechanically removed.
Tangential excision of the eschar has now
become an essential adjunct to effective
early debridement of devitalized tissue.
Using a modified hand-held dermatome as
advocated by Monafo,[8] those areas of the
burn that appear to be full thickness or
deep second degree are tangentially excised without anesthesia to a depth that results in either pain or bleeding. Skin autografts immediately applied over these areas
will "take," greatly reducing total healing
time. Moderate sedation with local infiltration anesthesia may be employed for obtaining autografts in lieu of general anesthesia.

The exposed granulating wound is a potential site for infection and early permanent closure is desirable. In the absence of adequate autograft skin, homografts or heterografts provide satisfactory temporary closure. The availability of fresh or freeze-dried porcine xenografts through several commercial sources at reasonable cost has greatly facilitated the use of this technique. These grafts are used primarily as a physiologic dressing and are changed every fourth or fifth day. They help control fluid loss, infection and vaporizational heat loss until the limited supply of the patient's own skin can be utilized to effect permanent coverage of the burn.

In extensive burns where a limited donor site must provide multiple crops of autografts, care must be taken to avoid converting the donor site to a full-thickness defect. General anesthesia at frequent intervals is poorly tolerated by burn patients and local anesthesia becomes essential when five or more graftings are contemplated. A simple technique successfully used at Children's Hospital consists of injecting 0.1% Xylocaine (1.0 mg/ml) into the subcutaneous tissue of the donor site, being careful not to exceed 4 mg/lb of Xylocaine. Utilizing the Castroviejo keratatome, strips of skin are obtained from the anesthetized area and are employed as 2 × 4 cm postage-stamp grafts applied 1.5 to 2 cm apart. By not exceeding a depth of 0.25 mm or 10/1,000 of an inch thickness, the donor site may be reharvested within nine or ten days.

REHABILITATION. Successfully covering the burn wound in the young child by no means completes his rehabilitation. The release and skin grafting of contractures involving the neck or joint surfaces are frequently necessary, and the younger the child the greater the problem. Since the burn scars will not grow with the child, disabling contractures may eventually develop as a result of growth in spite of excellent healing. Support and assistance from the occupational therapist, physiotherapist and psychiatrist are essential to the successful rehabilitation of the severely burned child.

The "Battered-child Syndrome"

PITFALL

IF INJURIES IN CHILDREN ARE ALWAYS ASSUMED TO BE ACCIDENTAL, THE "BATTERED CHILD" WILL NOT BE RECOGNIZED AND THUS WILL BE UNPROTECTED FROM FURTHER ABUSE.

The battered-child syndrome, with its wide spectrum of injury, is usually the result of hostile action on the part of a member of the child's immediate family. One or both parents are the most frequent offenders, but older siblings, other relatives, and people such as baby-sitters may be involved.

The problem of the battered child is being recognized with increasing frequency. Statistically, this is a relatively new source of trauma but, in all likelihood, the apparently increased prevalence of child abuse reflects a more frequent recognition of the problem.[9] During the past five years, the social service department of the Children's Hospital of Michigan has observed a tenfold increase in requests to investigate homes in which it is suspected that a child has been deliberately injured.

Formerly, when child abuse was suspected, physicians were reluctant to pursue the problem because of concern over litigation, inadequate investigative mechanisms and a general apathy toward the problem on the part of law-enforcement bodies. Recently, the seriousness of the problem has gained widespread recognition and legislation has been enacted to protect the physician in the event his suspicions are not correct. At the same time the law makes mandatory the disclosure of any information or physical findings that suggest child abuse or neglect. All hospitals in which children are seen should have a mechanism for expediting investigation into any family situation which appears suspicious. In most states the social service department is the primary investigative agency.

The spectrum of trauma is broad and includes severe contusions, lacerations, burns, sprains, fractures, concussion, and intra-thoracic and intra-abdominal injuries. Occasionally, a concerned member of the family or an interested neighbor will disclose information that relates the child's injuries to frequent or excessively harsh punishment, drunken rages, or uncontrollable anger associated with emotional disturbances in a specific person or persons. More often, a history of trauma is absent or denied. Often the child is accused of being careless or of having injured himself while at play. Usually the victim is either too young or too frightened to relate a meaningful history and suspicion on the part of the examining physician should be aroused when the nature and alleged mechanism of the injury are incompatible. For example, we have seen children who were said to have fallen into a tub of scalding water where the distribution of their burns could have been caused only by purposeful immersion.

Unusual scars or deformities, resolving ecchymoses not adequately explained, strap marks or burn scars should be viewed as possible evidence of previous child abuse until proved otherwise. X-ray examination of these children is vitally important and, when the nature of the injury is suspect, full-body x-rays should be obtained. The presence of one or more healed or healing fractures not logically or adequately explained is nearly always evidence of previous abuse.

The problem is compounded in the child who is comatose at the time of admission, especially if the parents seem to be genuinely solicitous of the child's welfare. A misleading history can direct attention away from parts of the body that may be harboring life-threatening injuries. A careful examination of the entire surface of the body is essential and any evidence of trauma, no matter how minor, that cannot be related to the site of alleged injury should be regarded with suspicion and calls for a thorough diagnostic evaluation.

Abdominal distension, tenderness and ileus are the most frequently encountered signs and symptoms of significant intra-abdominal injury. In approximately 20% of such patients, a mass may be palpated. Peritoneal lavage may be helpful when the physical findings are not diagnostic. Tenderness alone suggests contusion of the abdominal wall without significant internal injury but careful observation for the development of additional findings is mandatory.

Sixteen cases of abdominal trauma in battered children have been seen during the period 1963-1972 at Children's Hospital of Michigan. There were no splenic or renal injuries in these patients. The major findings included two instances of lacerations of the liver, two instances of perforation of the small bowel, one patient with an intramural hematoma involving approximately two feet of small intestine, two patients with segmental gangrene of the small intestine due to tears in the mesentery with segmental disruption of the blood supply, one large retroperitoneal hematoma, one lesser sac hematoma, and one case of exsanguinating hemorrhage from a torn mesentery. The remainder had multiple contusions of the viscera and scattered hematomas of the mesentery and omentum.

In some instances, family counseling or psychiatric help may significantly improve the environmental situation but, in general, it is not considered safe for the child to be returned to the home; investigations have frequently brought to light evidence of abuse of other children in the family. Foster homes are provided in nearly all battered-child cases.

SUMMARY

In general, the basic principles of management of patients with major injuries are the same regardless of age. There are, however, certain refinements of these principles related to the age, size and relatively immature physiology of the child that must be observed to ensure optimal results of treatment. Ten cardinal features of management that must be adapted to the infant and child involve: (1) the volume and rate of administration of intravenous fluid, electrolytes, and colloids, (2) dosages and routes of administration of medication, (3) mechanical factors pertaining to cardiopulmonary resuscitation where overzealous efforts may result in serious harm, (4) communication with the injured child, (5) psychologic support of the injured child, (6) an awareness of certain transient physiologic, neurologic and metabolic reactions to trauma that make the proper assessment of the degree and severity of the injury difficult, (7) the relation of the amount of hemorrhage to the relatively small circulating blood volume of the infant or small child, (8) the difficulty in maintaining normothermia following trauma, especially in infants, (9) the necessity for employing carefully controlled sedation to permit adequate examination of the frightened and injured child, and (10) an awareness that not all trauma occurring in childhood is accidental.

The magnitude of the problem is exemplified by the fact that trauma has become the major cause of death and disability in the under-14 age group and that 15,000,000 of our children are injured each year. Childhood injuries may be further dramatized by the fact that the results of inept, inadequate or improper management impose a lifetime of suffering and disability on the victim. The fact that accidents are theoretically avoidable for the most part requires the profession to publicly emphasize prevention as well as to achieve expertise in the salvage of the injured patient.

REFERENCES

1. Nelson, W. E.: *Textbook of Pediatrics.* Philadelphia, W. B. Saunders, 1969.
2. Izant, J., Jr., and Hubay, C. R.: The annual injury of 15,000,000 children. J. Trauma, 6:65, 1966.
3. Douglas, G. J., and Simpson, J. S.: The conservative management of splenic trauma. J. Pediat. Surg., 6:565, 1971.
4. Kakos, G. S., et al.: Small bowel injuries in children after blunt abdominal trauma. Ann. Surg., 174:238, 1971.
5. Welsh, K., et al.: Abdominal and thoracic injuries. In: *Pediatric Surgery.* Chicago, Yearbook Medical Publishers, 1969.
6. James, L. S.: Hexachlorophene (commentaries). Pediatrics, 49:492, 1972.
7. Bretano, L., et al.: Bacteriology of large human burns treated with silver nitrate. Arch. Surg., 93:456, 1966.
8. Monafo, W. W., Aulenbacher, C. E., and Pappalardo, C.: Early tangential excision of the eschars of major burns. Arch. Surg., 104:503, 1972.
9. Ebbin, A. J., et al.: Battered child syndrome at the Los Angeles County General Hospital. Amer. J. Dis. Child. 118:660, 1969.

10　BLOOD REPLACEMENT

R. F. WILSON
A. J. WALT

Although prompt correction of severe blood-volume deficits in the critically injured patient may be lifesaving, the blood and fluids used for replacement can, in themselves, cause significant complications, especially if used inappropriately. Methods for guiding the rate and volume of fluid and blood administration have been discussed in Chapters 5 and 7. This chapter will deal primarily with the characteristics of stored (bank) blood and other blood substitutes and the complications associated with their use.

CRYSTALLOIDS

Clinically speaking, the term *crystalloid* applies to any of several solutions containing electrolytes or carbohydrates of low molecular weight which can readily diffuse through normal capillary membranes. The carbohydrate solution used most frequently is 5% glucose (dextrose) which has approximately the same osmotic pressure as plasma. More concentrated solutions of 10%, 20%, 30% or 50% glucose are used occasionally for their nutritional value or osmotic effect but are much more irritating, especially to small peripheral veins.

The electrolyte solutions used most frequently are sodium chloride and Ringer's lactate. Normal or 0.9% sodium chloride has 150 to 155 mEq of sodium and a similar amount of chloride. When half- and third-normal salines are used, 5% glucose is added to bring the osmolarity of the solution to or above that of normal plasma. Hyperosmotic solutions may be irritating to the vein but are not apt to cause dangerous red-cell damage. Because of the hemolysis which they may produce, hypo-osmotic solutions are used only to treat patients with severe hyperosmotic problems. Ringer's lactate is slightly more physiologic than normal saline because its electrolyte concentrations (sodium 130 mEq/L, chloride 109 to 110 mEq/L, lactate 25 to 30 mEq/L, potassium 4 to 5 mEq/L, and calcium 3 to 4 mEq/L) are closer to those of normal serum.

Crystalloids are of greatest value in patients who require I.V. fluids but have a relatively stable cardiovascular system. Glucose is usually added to the I.V. infusion to increase the osmolarity of hypotonic electrolyte solutions or to supply enough calories (400 to 600 per day) to reduce the excessive nitrogen loss that would occur with a lesser caloric intake.

In an emergency 5% glucose in normal saline or 5% glucose in Ringer's lactate can be used for the initial replacement of lost blood. These solutions have the advantage of being convenient, easily stored, and stable for long periods of time, even at room temperature.

PITFALL

IF CRYSTALLOIDS ALONE ARE USED TO RE-
PLACE MASSIVE BLOOD LOSS IN PATIENTS WITH
SEVERE SHOCK, EXCESSIVE AMOUNTS OF FLUID
MAY BE REQUIRED TO PRODUCE EVEN TEMPO-
RARY IMPROVEMENT AND THE RISK OF LATER
RESPIRATORY FAILURE MAY BE GREATLY IN-
CREASED.

Although crystalloids can expand the intravascular volume temporarily, they dilute the remaining red cells and protein, reducing the oxygen-carrying capacity, buffering ability, and colloid osmotic pressure of the blood. In disease states such as severe trauma, sepsis or shock, in which the capillaries may have a greatly increased permeability, these solutions may leave the intravascular space so rapidly that only transient volume expansion is provided. Although correction of an extravascular fluid deficit can be important in these situations, excessive administration of such fluids can cause interstitial edema in the lungs and interfere with movement of oxygen and nutrients to tissue cells, increasing the likelihood and severity of later respiratory failure.

Because we have had so many complications from excessive hemodilution by crystalloids, we pay close attention to the hemoglobin and protein levels in the blood. It is our practice to maintain the hemoglobin concentration above a minimum level of 10.0 gm/100 ml and preferably above 12.5 gm/100 ml. The serum albumin level is kept above a minimum level of 2.5 gm/100 ml and preferably above 3.0. Consequently, after the initial 2000 to 3000 ml of crystalloids are given to a critically injured patient, one quarter to one half of any additional fluid should be colloid or blood.

PITFALL

IF LARGE QUANTITIES OF RINGER'S LACTATE
OR OTHER LACTATE SOLUTIONS ARE GIVEN TO
PATIENTS WITH SEVERE CIRRHOSIS OR SHOCK,
AN INCREASING LACTIC ACIDOSIS MAY DEVELOP.

Because lactate may be metabolized very slowly when liver function or perfusion is severely impaired, we prefer, in patients with advanced cirrhosis or shock, to use normal saline with 1 to 2 ampules of sodium bicarbonate in each liter of fluid. Recently studies by Shires, however, suggest that even in advanced shock lactate metabolism by the liver may be adequate.[1]

COLLOIDS

Clinically the term *colloid* refers to solutions containing substances of high molecular weight (usually at least 10,000) which cannot readily diffuse through normal capillary membranes. The colloids used most frequently in patients with trauma include plasma, albumin, Plasmanate, and dextran.

Plasma

Plasma is the liquid fraction of unclotted whole blood remaining after the red blood cells have been removed. The two main types of plasma preparations used are "pooled plasma" and "fresh-frozen plasma." The former usually consists of plasma pooled from a number of donors. Although storage at a mean temperature of 31.6 C for six months is said to eliminate the chances of developing serum hepatitis in the recipient,[2] the incidence of this complication is still very high.[3]

Pooled plasma has relatively few of the factors needed for clotting. It contains no functioning platelets and has little or no Factor V, Factor VIII, prothrombin or clottable fibrinogen. The albumin and globulin present, however, can increase colloid osmotic pressure and provide significant blood-volume expansion for 24 to 48 hours or longer.

Each unit of fresh-frozen plasma is removed from only one individual, thereby greatly reducing the risk of hepatitis. Because it is kept frozen until just prior to use, it may have almost normal concentrations of many of the substances (Factor V, Factor VIII, prothrombin, and fibrinogen) needed for clotting. Thus, the fresh-frozen plasma given to the patient with severe trauma not only provides significant blood-volume expansion and increased colloid osmotic pressure but may also help correct certain clotting deficiencies. However, since it does not contain any functioning platelets, bleeding problems due to thrombocytopenia can still occur.

Albumin

This concentrate of human serum albumin is usually marketed as a salt-poor solution in 50-cc ampules containing 12.5 gm of protein. It does not provide any clotting factors but can be of value in providing blood-volume expansion and increased colloid osmotic pressure for 4 to 24 hours.

PITFALL

IF ALBUMIN ALONE IS USED TO RESTORE PLASMA VOLUME OR COLLOID OSMOTIC PRESSURE, THE IMPROVEMENT, ESPECIALLY IN PATIENTS WITH SHOCK OR SEPSIS, MAY BE TRANSIENT.

Radioiodinated serum albumin (RISA) is normally destroyed or leaves the vascular space at about 8% per hour. During or following shock, trauma, or sepsis, the RISA disappearance rate is greatly increased and may exceed 30 to 35% per hour.[4] At the end of 24 hours only 5 to 10% of the albumin given to critically ill or injured patients can still be found in the bloodstream. In patients with acute trauma, a half-colloidal or colloidal solution can be readily prepared merely by adding 2 to 4 ampules of albumin respectively to each liter of I.V. fluid.

Plasmanate

Plasmanate is a commercial I.V. solution containing 5 gm/100 ml selected plasma proteins, including normal human albumin (88%), alpha globulin (7%), and beta globulin (5%). Its main electrolytes are sodium (100 mEq/L) and chloride (50 mEq/L). It can expand the blood volume for up to 48 hours, and a maximum of 2000 ml may be given each day at a rate which ordinarily should not exceed 8 ml/min.[5] We have had no experience with Plasmanate at Detroit General Hospital because of the ready availability of albumin and plasma.

Dextran

Dextran is a branched polysaccharide composed of glucose units formed by the action of the bacterium Leuconostoc mesenteroides on sucrose. The two dextrans used most frequently in clinical practice are Dextran-70 and Dextran-40.

DEXTRAN-70. Dextran-70 (Macrodex) is a 6% solution, in either normal saline or 5% glucose in water. The dextran fraction has an average molecular weight of 70,000 with more than 90% of the molecules within the range of 25,000 to 125,000. The colloidal properties of Macrodex are similar to those of plasma and result in expansion of the plasma volume slightly in excess of the volume infused. Approximately 40% of the dextran with a molecular weight below 50,000 is excreted in the urine within 24 hours. The larger molecules are enzymatically degraded to glucose at a rate of about 70 to 90 mg/kg body weight per day.[6] Thus, about half the Dextran-70 is gone in 24 hours and little remains after 72 hours.

PITFALL

IF DEXTRAN IS GIVEN WITH MULTIPLE BLOOD TRANSFUSIONS, IT MAY BE DIFFICULT TO DETERMINE THE CAUSE OF REACTIONS OR INCREASED HEMORRHAGE, AND PROBLEMS WITH CROSS-MATCHING MAY OCCUR.

The most frequent problems seen with dextran include allergic reactions, impaired coagulation, and difficulties with typing and crossing blood. The allergic reactions may be manifested as urticaria, nausea, vomiting, hypotension, or anaphylaxis, which may develop immediately or after a delay of 30 minutes or more. The impaired coagulation is due to an interference with platelet aggregation and may be impossible to detect with the standard in vitro coagulation tests.

Type and cross-match problems arising after dextran administration are related to an increased tendency to rouleaux formation. Red blood cells from patients receiving dextran should be washed in saline prior to performing the type and cross-match.

The total amount of Dextran-70 used during the first 24 hours is usually only 500 ml and generally should not exceed 20 ml/kg. We have not used Dextran-70 clinically except to attempt to reduce the transcapillary leak of fluid into the interstitial spaces in patients with sepsis.

DEXTRAN-40. Dextran-40, also known as low-molecular-weight dextran (L.M.W.D.) and Rheomacrodex, is a 10% solution marketed either in normal saline or in 5% glucose in water. The dextran fraction has an average molecular weight of 40,000, with more than 90% of the molecules within the range of 10,000 to 80,000. Since this 10% solution has 2 to 2½ times the colloid osmotic pressure of normal plasma, it can produce a rapid expansion of the intravascular volume. After 500 ml of Dextran-40, the plasma volume expands by about 1000 ml and gradually decreases over the next 12 to 24 hours.

The dextran molecules with a molecular weight of less than 50,000 are rapidly excreted in the urine, raising the specific gravity of the urine in proportion to the amount of dextran present. In these circumstances, urine osmolality may help in the evaluation of renal function.

The main value of low-molecular-weight dextran is its ability to improve tissue perfusion by a combination of an expanded intravascular volume and decreased blood viscosity.[7] The decreased viscosity is due largely to a lowered hematocrit and a reduced aggregation of platelets and red cells. When hemostasis has been established after vascular surgery, L.M.W.D. infused at a rate of 40 ml/hr may help to prevent intravascular thrombosis and occlusion of the vessel or graft.

The complications of Dextran-40 are similar to those of Dextran-70. Although L.M.W.D. may help correct hypovolemia in the patient with recent trauma, its tendency to reduce platelet aggregation may also cause increased hemorrhage or hematoma formation. Its use is usually contraindicated if there is any tendency for the patient to bleed, if there is any reduction in the concentrations of the various factors needed for clotting, or if there is severe oliguria. Since it can rapidly expand the vascular system, dextran is also contraindicated in patients who are overhydrated or are in congestive heart failure.

BLOOD

Massive acute blood loss is best replaced by properly typed and cross-matched fresh whole blood. Whole blood provides not only plasma with its proteins and some clotting factors but also red blood cells; if it is very fresh, it also supplies viable functioning platelets. Although hemoglobin levels below 3 to 4 gm/100 ml can be tolerated if the blood loss occurs slowly and the intravascular volume is maintained at normal or high levels, sudden severe loss of an equivalent number of red cells can be fatal.

Acute severe blood loss results in a loss
of intravascular volume and red cells. It
takes at least several hours for normal compensatory hemodilution to reduce the hemoglobin and red-cell concentrations to levels
which reflect the amount of blood lost. Although reductions in intravascular volume
are much more critical than red-cell deficits, sudden severe reductions in hemoglobin concentration can greatly impair the
patient's ability to tolerate severe stress,
even if the blood volume is kept in a relatively normal range.

The hemoglobin in the red cells is needed to carry oxygen to the tissues, to help
buffer the blood, and to carry carbon dioxide back to the lungs. If the hemoglobin
concentration is less than 10.0 gm/100 ml,
oxygen transport may be seriously impaired, especially if the cardiac output and/or the 2,3–diphosphoglycerate
(2,3–DPG) levels in red cells are reduced.
Since stored red cells tend to have reduced
quantities of 2,3–DPG,[8] it is even more important to maintain adequate hemoglobin
levels in patients receiving massive transfusions.

Technical Aspects of Transfusing Blood

CROSS-MATCHING. The World War II concept of the "universal donor" (group O)
and "universal recipient" (group AB) is
now considered obsolete and unsafe. Since
then, many other blood groups have been
found to be capable of causing serious
transfusion reactions. Although type-specific, properly cross-matched blood or blood
components are always the first choice for
any transfusions, certain emergency situations may force the physician and blood

bank to administer blood under less than
ideal conditions.

Group-O Uncross-matched Blood. Even
under the best of circumstances, it usually
takes 30 to 45 minutes to type and cross-
match blood properly. If the need for
blood is extremely urgent, uncross-matched
group-O blood may be given. Low-titer O-
negative whole blood is the least dangerous
of the uncross-matched blood, but if none
of this is available nontitered O-negative
can be used. At Detroit General (Receiving) Hospital, there is a frequent need for
group-O uncross-matched blood. If only a
small amount of O-negative whole blood is
available, it is generally saved for emergency transfusions of uncross-matched
blood to girls or young women; O-positive
uncross-matched blood is usually given
only to males and women past the childbearing age.

Some of the drawbacks to using group-O
uncross-matched blood include: "immediate" or "delayed" incompatible transfusion
reactions, the possibility that the patient
might be group AB, and the great risk of
returning to the patient's type-specific blood
after 4 to 5 units of group-O are given. Because of the risks involved, the physician
requesting such blood has to sign an "acceptance of responsibility" at some hospitals.

Type-specific Uncross-matched Blood. If
a 5-minute delay in giving the patient
whole blood is tolerable, the blood bank
should be able to deliver uncross-matched
whole blood of the same ABO and Rh(D)
type as the recipient. This is much preferable to using whole blood which is not

type specific. It greatly reduces the hazards of reactions, especially in patients who have not had any prior transfusions, and eliminates the cross-match problems that occur if more than 4 to 5 units of group-O blood are given to a patient with group A, B, or AB.

Type-specific Incompletely Cross-matched Blood. If a 15-minute delay in giving the patient whole blood is tolerable, the blood bank should be able to deliver type-specific incompletely cross-matched whole blood. An immediate-spin Coombs' test can be done, and if no incompatibility is demonstrated the blood can be released. If an incompatibility is found when the final Coombs' test is completed, the unused incompatible blood is returned to the blood bank, and treatment for a possible transfusion reaction should be begun.

ROUTES OF ADMINISTRATION. In patients with severe trauma and/or acute blood loss, it is important to insert at least 2 or 3 large I.V. catheters so that fluids and blood can be administered as rapidly as needed. Catheters are preferable to needles because they are less likely to become dislodged or penetrate the vein with extravasation of the fluid into the tissues. Fifteen-gauge needles or catheters are the preferred size and, in some instances, large tubes such as sterile pediatric feeding tubes have been utilized to great advantage when extremely rapid transfusion of large quantities of blood was needed. Although there has been much discussion of the advantages of subclavian catheters, we still generally prefer cut-downs in upper-extremity veins for severely injured patients; large-sized catheters can be used and the risk to the patient of complications from catheter insertion is reduced (Chap. 4).

Hazards or Side Effects Due to Transfused Blood

MISMATCH. *Recognition.* Although the typical signs and symptoms of a transfusion reaction are usually readily discernible in a convalescing patient, they may be extremely difficult to identify in a patient who is anesthetized, especially if he is in shock. Under these conditions, the first sign of a transfusion reaction may be the sudden onset of urticaria, increased oozing from open wounds or hypotension.

PITFALL

IF THE USUAL SIGNS OF INCOMPATIBILITY ARE WATCHED FOR ONLY DURING THE FIRST FEW MINUTES OF A TRANSFUSION, RECOGNITION OF SIGNIFICANT REACTIONS MAY BE DELAYED OR MISSED ENTIRELY.

Transfusion reactions seldom declare themselves clinically until at least 50 to 100 ml of blood have been given. Most reactions, such as chills, urticaria and fever, occur in spite of a satisfactory type and cross-match. Dyspnea, pain, nausea, hematuria and shock are less common, but are apt to be related to transfusion incompatibilities. In a series of 624 transfusion reactions studied at Detroit General Hospital, only 35 were found to involve a factor that might have been predicted by the cross-matching or prevented with more care. These included a positive Coombs' test in 9 patients, bacterial contamination in 7, transfusion with wrong blood in 5, incompatible major cross-match in 5 and nonspecific agglutinins in 2.[9]

Management. If a reaction is suspected, the transfusion should be stopped immediately and the remainder of the stored blood, with a sample of the patient's blood, should be sent to the blood bank for repeat cross-match and analysis. Benadryl (50 mg) is given I.M. or I.V. immediately and every six hours as needed for urticaria, itching or other allergic phenomena. If the patient is not in danger of being overloaded, I.V. fluids should be administered rapidly with 12.5 to 25.0 gm of mannitol to ensure a copious urine output. One to two ampules of sodium bicarbonate may also be added to each I.V. to alkalize the urine. If shock occurs, Adrenalin and hydrocortisone should be administered. If the hypotension is mild, the Adrenalin can be given subcutaneously as 0.2 to 0.5 cc of a 1:1000 solution. If severe shock develops, 1.0 cc of 1:1000 Adrenalin should be given intravenously in 50 to 100 ml of 5% glucose in water over a 5- to 20-minute period. If the pulse is irregular or faster than 120 per minute, Adrenalin is usually contraindicated. Hydrocortisone can be given as a 200-mg I.V. bolus.

MASSIVE TRANSFUSIONS. The hazards or side effects caused by transfused blood itself are more likely to occur in patients receiving massive transfusions. Some of the more serious complications seen in these patients include hypothermia, electrolyte and acid-base abnormalities, coagulation defects, overtransfusion, and serum hepatitis.

Hypothermia. Massive transfusions of cold blood can cause severe hypothermia, especially if the patient has a low cardiac output and poor tissue perfusion. If large quantities of blood are administered very rapidly into large intrathoracic veins, the temperature of the heart may drop abruptly to levels below 30 to 32 C, with resultant impaired cardiac function and an increased tendency to arrhythmias. Satisfactory blood warmers are available and should be used if a massively injured patient will require rapid transfusion of more than 2 to 3 units of blood. In addition, warming blankets or mattresses should be placed under any patient who may receive massive transfusions as an additional method for preventing hypothermia. Although body temperature seldom changes significantly during elective surgery in adults, close monitoring of the patient's temperature with a rectal or, preferably, an esophageal probe in the operating room may be extremely informative in a critically injured patient receiving massive transfusions.

Hypocalcemia. The citrate present in stored blood binds ionized calcium and thereby prevents clotting during storage. When transfused into the patient, the excess citrate present complexes with some of the patient's ionized calcium. If more than four units of bank blood are given rapidly, especially to a patient who is in shock and has impaired calcium mobilization, the citrate may cause a significant drop in the concentration of ionized calcium. Although only minute amounts of ionized calcium are needed for clotting, normal or near-normal levels of ionized calcium are needed for proper function of the neuromuscular and cardiovascular systems. Therefore, if massive transfusions are required in a critically injured patient, 10 cc of 10% calcium chloride or calcium gluconate should be given after every 2 to 4 units of blood. Obviously, calcium should not be given through I.V. tubing containing stored blood because the calcium would cause clots to form in the line. Calcium should also be used with great caution in patients receiving digitalis preparations. In general, the sensitivity of the heart to digitalis is increased by calcium and decreased by potassium.

Hyperkalemia. The potassium level in bank blood rises approximately 1 mEq/L per day, and at 21 days the potassium concentration may exceed 20 to 25 mEq/L. Much of this hyperkalemia is due to red-cell hemolysis, but a large portion is related to movement of potassium out of the red blood cells as the plasma becomes more acidotic. After the blood is administered and its pH is corrected back to normal, some of the potassium will leave the plasma and reenter the red cells. If perfusion is poor, the pH may not be corrected rapidly and the patient may develop a dangerous hyperkalemia with impaired cardiovascular function.

PITFALL

IF IT IS ASSUMED THAT ALL PATIENTS WHO HAVE HAD RECENT MASSIVE TRANSFUSIONS ARE HYPERKALEMIC, SERIOUS ERRORS IN THE ADMINISTRATION OF ELECTROLYTES AND DIGITALIS PREPARATIONS MAY BE MADE.

It is often assumed that patients who are given massive transfusions are almost necessarily hyperkalemic. Our studies on 402 patients receiving massive transfusions, however, revealed that within 24 hours after massive transfusions only 10% had a hyperkalemia; 80% had normal potassium levels, and 10% were hypokalemic.[9] Thus it is extremely important to obtain frequent electrolyte determinations in these patients, especially if they are to be given or are receiving digitalis-like drugs.

Acid-base Abnormalities. Stored blood has a pH of 6.4 to 6.8. Much of this acidosis is due to an accumulation of carbon dioxide. Under ordinary circumstances most of the acid load is rapidly buffered by the patient after it is transfused. If there is any difficulty with respiratory function and/or tissue perfusion, however, the transfusions may lower the patient's pH to levels (below 7.1 or 7.2) which may interfere with cardiovascular function. It has been found in our own laboratory that usually about 20 to 45 mEq of sodium bicarbonate are required to restore the pH of bank blood to 7.4. Although we do not ordinarily give bicarbonate or THAM with transfused blood, if the patient is in severe shock and has been receiving massive transfusions we administer a half ampule (25 ml) of 7.5% sodium bicarbonate after or with each unit of blood.

Recently we have noted an increasing incidence of severe alkalosis in critically injured patients.[10] At least a portion of their alkalosis appears to be related to the metabolism of citrate present in blood that was given 24 to 48 hours earlier.

Coagulation Defects. Special efforts should be taken to obtain meticulous hemostasis and to rapidly correct any clotting abnormality which develops during or after massive transfusions. CPD blood stored at 4 C for more than 24 to 48 hours has essentially no functioning platelets. Although platelets may be recognized microscopically, they have lost the adhesiveness and aggregability which are essential to the first phase of clotting. Other clotting factors also disappear when blood is stored.

Within a few days, the activities of Factor V and Factor VIII fall to less than 20% of control, and the concentrations of prothrombin and fibrinogen are reduced at a slightly slower rate. In view of these problems with old stored blood, efforts should be made to obtain fresh whole blood (preferably less than 24 hours old) for any patient likely to need massive transfusions. Optimally, as a prophylactic measure, we would like to give a unit of fresh whole blood after every three units of older bank blood, especially if the patient has had recent massive hemorrhage or severe shock.

PITFALL

IF EXCESSIVE OPERATIVE BLEEDING IN A CRITICALLY INJURED PATIENT IS ASSUMED TO BE DUE TO A COAGULATION DEFECT, THE TIME AND EFFORT NEEDED TO OBTAIN COMPLETE HEMOSTASIS WILL BE NEGLECTED.

By far the most frequent cause of excessive bleeding at surgery is inadequate effort by the surgeon in tying, suturing, or coagulating open bleeding vessels. When the bleeding seems to occur from multiple small vessels, especially after a long operation in a poor-risk patient, the surgeon may attribute the bleeding problem to some clotting defect; therefore, he may attempt to terminate the anesthetic as soon as possible, hoping that hemostatic agents, packs and drains will control the bleeding or prevent hematoma formation. Certainly, if excessive or abnormal bleeding appears to have developed, transfusion reactions and coagulation defects should be considered; under these circumstances, however, there is even greater need for increased time and effort to obtain complete hemostasis.

If a coagulation problem does develop or is suspected, the physician should have a definite and practical plan of management. We believe that the initial coagulation tests in such a patient should include a Lee-White clotting time, a platelet count, and observation for clot lysis (Table 1).

TABLE 1.   SIMPLE INITIAL INVESTIGATION AND TREATMENT OF EXCESSIVE BLEEDING DURING OR FOLLOWING MASSIVE TRANSFUSIONS

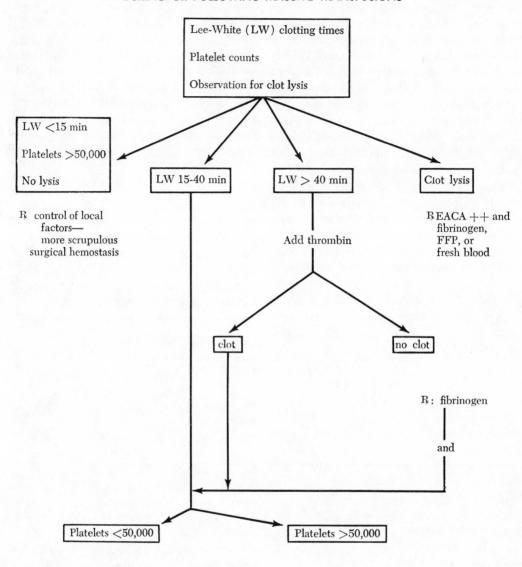

FFP + = Fresh frozen plasma
EACA ++ = Epsilon-aminocaproic acid

More sophisticated tests include partial thromboplastin times, thrombin times (for fibrinogen split products), euglobulin lysis times and direct measurement of fibrinogen and other individual clotting factors. Unfortunately these are often not readily available to the hard-pressed surgeon, especially on weekends and at night. A reasonable approach to immediate therapy may be obtained, however, from these simple tests, all of which may be done in or close to the surgical suite.

If the blood clots normally in the test tube, it is unlikely that there is a significant deficit of platelets or other clotting factors. The test tube with the clot should then be taped to the bed or wall so that the clot can be observed for retraction and lysis. If the clot lyses rapidly, excessive fibrinolysis can be assumed; this may be treated with epsilon-aminocaproic acid (Amicar) if D.I.C. can be ruled out (Chap. 34).

If the blood does not clot properly in the test tube, a deficit of platelets or other clotting factors should be considered. Bleeding rarely occurs from a platelet deficiency unless the count is below 30,000 to 50,000/mm^3. Occasionally, however, excessive bleeding may occur with larger numbers of aged, damaged, or otherwise ineffective platelets. If there is a platelet deficit, platelet concentrates or fresh warm blood less than six hours old should be given. If there is no platelet deficit, the clotting defect may be due to low levels of Factor V, Factor VIII, or fibrinogen, all of which may be restored with fresh frozen plasma or fresh whole blood.

It must be stressed that the excessive bleeding found in acutely injured patients is often attributed to clotting abnormalities; it is more likely, however, that it is due to inadequate or incomplete efforts by the surgeon to control bleeding vessels. Meticulous hemostasis and rapid complete correction of any hypovolemia or impaired tissue perfusion are the best prophylaxis and treatment for coagulation abnormalities during an operation.

OVERTRANSFUSION. It is often extremely difficult to determine the optimal amount of blood to be given to a critically injured patient.

PITFALL

IF IT IS ASSUMED THAT A CRITICALLY INJURED HYPOTENSIVE PATIENT WITH A HIGH CVP IS OVERLOADED, SOME PATIENTS MAY REMAIN SERIOUSLY HYPOVOLEMIC.

There is a poor correlation between blood volume and central venous pressure in critically ill and injured patients.[4] Intrathoracic trauma or disease, positive-pressure ventilation, straining by the patient, and cardiac tamponade are only a few instances in which hypovolemia can occur concurrently with a high CVP. As mentioned in Chapter 5, the status and response of skin, lungs, blood pressure, pulse, central venous pressure, and urine output must all be followed closely. The response of the central venous pressure, as the blood and fluid are administered, is the best overall guide to the adequacy and rate of fluid replacement. If the CVP is above 16 cm H_2O, if the CVP rises more than 1.0 cm H_2O for each 100 ml of fluid given, or if rales develop in the lungs, the infusions should be given very cautiously.

PITFALL

IF AN INJURED PATIENT HAS HAD A RECENT MYOCARDIAL INFARCTION OR CARDIAC ARREST, ADMINISTRATION OF LARGE QUANTITIES OF BLOOD AND FLUID, IN SPITE OF A LOW CENTRAL VENOUS PRESSURE, MAY SERIOUSLY OVERLOAD THE CARDIOVASCULAR SYSTEM.

For at least several hours after a cardiac arrest or acute myocardial infarction, the patient may have an isolated left ventricular failure with a high left atrial pressure and low CVP. Continued transfusions to such a patient can cause pulmonary edema while the CVP is still low.[4,11] Pulmonary-wedge pressures in such patients are more apt to reflect the filling pressures on the left side of the heart than the CVP (Chap. 5).

In spite of these precautions, it is still possible, especially during general anesthesia, to overtransfuse patients. Ordinarily mild overtransfusion is not harmful, but in older individuals with borderline cardiac reserve and/or prolonged shock, even a slight fluid overload may result in frank congestive heart failure with pulmonary edema. Once the overtransfusion is recognized, further blood or fluid administration should be stopped; subsequent measures will depend on the severity of the overtransfusion and/or heart failure. If pulmonary edema occurs, positive-pressure ventilation should be maintained and blood return to the heart should be reduced. This may be accomplished by elevating the head, lowering the legs, applying rotating tourniquets to the extremities and/or performing a phlebotomy. Drugs that may also be used include digoxin or Cedilanid, ethacrynic acid or furosemide, aminophylline, morphine, and chlorpromazine. Rapid digitalization may be accomplished with 1.0 to 1.6 mg of digoxin or Cedilanid given I.V. in divided doses over 2 to 6 hours. Ethacrynic acid or furosemide can be given in initial doses of 20 to 50 mg I.V. and repeated every 15 to 60 minutes as needed to produce a rapid profound diuresis.

PITFALL

THE ADMINISTRATION OF LARGE QUANTITIES OF FUROSEMIDE OR ETHACRYNIC ACID TO A CRITICALLY INJURED PATIENT WHO DEVELOPS CONGESTIVE HEART FAILURE MAY CAUSE EVEN GREATER CARDIOVASCULAR PROBLEMS FROM HYPOVOLEMIA.

The critically injured patient with poor cardiac reserve can develop severe congestive heart failure with only a mild fluid overload. Under such circumstances, powerful diuretics such as furosemide can, within 15 to 60 minutes, cause the kidneys to excrete several hundred ml of urine; this can result in severe hypovolemic shock. Use of smaller quantities of these diuretics, e.g. 5 to 10 mg every 30 minutes as needed, in patients with known severe cardiac problems may be prudent.

Aminophylline given in doses of 250 to 500 mg slowly I.V. over 5 to 20 minutes may help relieve wheezing and bronchospasm. Morphine given in small doses (1 to 2 mg) I.V. every 5 to 10 minutes, with careful observations for any tendency to hypoventilation or hypotension, can also reduce patient anxiety and decrease the fluid overload by increasing vascular capacity. Chlorpromazine in similar doses also increases vascular capacity but is apt to cause hypotension. Any sudden severe drop in blood pressure after morphine, Demerol, or any analgesic, sedative, or anesthetic should be considered due to hypovolemia until proven otherwise.

SERUM HEPATITIS. Serum hepatitis must always be considered as a possible hazard whenever blood or blood products, especially multiple-donor plasma or fibrinogen, are given. Blood or blood products from blood banks using professional donors are especially apt to be contaminated with the virus of serum hepatitis. Careful assay for Australian (hepatitis-B) antigen and avoidance of any blood in which it is found should greatly reduce the incidence of hepatitis from blood transfusions.

In a prospective study involving 14 university hospital centers,[3] transfusion of 4984 patients having cardiovascular surgery with an average of 7.7 units of blood resulted in hepatitis in 3.2% and death from hepatitis in 0.1%. Hepatitis developed in 82 (2.5%) of 3284 patients receiving 2 to 8 units of blood, 50 (3.8%) of 1323 receiving 9 to 15 units, and 23 (6.1%) of 377 receiving more than 15 units.

PITFALL

IF POOLED PLASMA OR FIBRINOGEN IS USED, THE RISK OF SERUM HEPATITIS IS GREATLY INCREASED.

TABLE 2.   OUTLINE OF MANAGEMENT OF PATIENTS RECEIVING MASSIVE TRANSFUSIONS

1. Maintain adequate or increased ventilation by whatever means necessary. Do not hesitate to use respirator assistance.

2. Monitor the patient closely
   A. EKG
   B. Central venous pressure
   C. Urine output
   D. Rectal and/or esophageal temperature

3. Blood
   A. Insert 2 or 3 large polyethylene catheters
   B. Fresh blood or fresh frozen plasma: 1 unit for every 3 units of stored blood greater than 48-72 hours old
   C. Continue the use of type O if three or more units of uncross-matched type O blood have been given
   D. Warm the transfused blood

4. Drugs
   A. Sodium bicarbonate (22.3-44.6 mEq) for each unit of blood while the patient is in severe shock
   B. Mannitol and/or furosemide if urine output remains below 25 ml/hr in spite of adequate fluid and blood replacement
   C. Calcium chloride 1.0 gm I.V. slowly for every 2 to 4 units of blood if the patient is in severe shock
   D. Digitalis if present evidence or past history of congestive cardiac failure
   E. Steroids (equivalent to 150 mg/kg hydrocortisone I.V.) in severe persistent shock when blood volume, acid-base balance and calcium needs appear to have been satisfied

Of 136 patients receiving multiple-donor plasma, 16 (12%) developed hepatitis. Of an estimated 80 patients given fibrinogen (multiple donor), 15 (19%) developed hepatitis and 3 (4%) died of their hepatitis. Some physicians have used gamma globulin to reduce the hazard of hepatitis in patients receiving massive transfusion. The incidence of hepatitis in randomized patients receiving I.M. immune serum globulin (gamma globulin), however, was essentially the same as in patients given a placebo.[3]

Hepatitis occurring within 15 days of surgery was noted only among those patients who received halogenated inhalation anesthetics such as halothane or methoxyflurane. With rare exceptions, cytomegalovirus appears to survive only in fresh blood[12] and may cause the splenomegaly, fever, and lymphocytosis which is sometimes referred to as the "postperfusion syndrome."

MANAGEMENT OF PATIENTS RECEIVING MASSIVE TRANSFUSIONS

The hemostasis of any patient receiving massive transfusions is invariably disrupted.

Under these circumstances efforts must be directed toward prompt restoration of the various physiologic parameters to as close to normal as possible. This has led us to adopt a special plan of management which takes into account the unique changes in this group of patients (Table 2). It is especially important to maintain an adequate ventilation, particularly in those with severe metabolic acidosis due to poor tissue perfusion. If the patient retains a combined metabolic and respiratory acidosis for any substantial length of time, the mortality rate approaches 100%.

REFERENCES

1. Canizaro, P. C., and Shires, G. T.: The infusion of Ringer's lactate solution during shock. Changes in lactate, excess lactate, and pH. Amer. J. Surg., 122:494, 1971.
2. Allen, J. G.: Blood transfusions and related problems. In: Surgery, Principles, and Practice, 3rd ed. (Moyer, C. A., Rhoads, J. E., Allen, J. G., and Harkins, H. N., Eds.). Philadelphia, J. B. Lippincott, 1965.
3. Grady, G. F., and Bennett, A. J. E.: Risk of post-transfusion hepatitis in the United States. A prospective cooperative study. JAMA, 220:692, 1972.

4. Wilson, R. F., Sarver, E., and Birks, R.: Central venous pressure and blood volume determinations in clinical shock. Surg. Gynec. Obstet., 132:631, 1971.

5. How to administer Plasmanate. Package information supplied with Plasmanate by Cutter Laboratory, Berkeley, California.

6. Langsjoen, P. H.: Observations on the excretion of low molecular dextran. Angiology, 16:148, 1965.

7. Evarts, C. M.: Low molecular weight dextran. Med. Clin. N. Amer., 51:1285, 1967.

8. McConn, R.: The respiratory function of blood: Transfusion and blood storage. Anesthesiology, 36:119, 1972.

9. Wilson, R. F., Mammen, E., and Walt, A. J.: Eight years of experience with massive blood transfusions. J. Trauma, 11:275, 1971.

10. Wilson, R. F., et al.: Severe alkalosis in critically ill patients. Arch. Surg., 105:197, 1972.

11. Rapaport, E., and Scheinman, M. M.: Rationale and limitations of hemodynamic measurements in patients with acute myocardial infarction. Mod. Conc. Cardiov. Dis., 38:55, 1969.

12. Henle, W., et al.: Antibody to the Epstein-Barr virus and cytomegaloviruses after open-heart and other surgery. New Eng. J. Med., 282:1068, 1970.

Suggested Reading

1. Gallie, B. L., et al.: Correction of the interstitial diffusion defect in hemorrhagic shock by balanced salt solution. Surg. Forum, 22:21, 1971.

2. Broennle, A. M., et al.: Oxygen transport and massive transfusion: The unsteady state. Surg. Forum, 21:52, 1970.

3. Wilson, R. F.: In: Overview on Massive Transfusions in Modern Surgery (Egdahl, R. H., and Mannick, J. A., Eds.). New York, Grune & Stratton, 1970.

4. Hutchin, P.: History of blood transfusion. A tercentennial look. Surgery, 64:685, 1968.

5. Churchill-Davidson, H. C., Burton, G. W., and Bennett, P. J.: Massive blood transfusion. Proc. Roy. Soc. Med., 61:681, 1968.

6. Wilson, W. B.: Emergency management of unexpected defects of hemostatic function in surgical patients. JAMA, 201:123, 1967.

7. Cuello, L., et al.: Autologous blood transfusion in cardiovascular surgery. Transfusion, 7:309, 1967.

8. Collins, V. J., and Winnie, A. P.: Pharmacologic adjuncts to the management of shock. J. Nat. Med. Assoc., 59:183, 1967.

9. Takaori, M., and Sofar, P.: Treatment of massive hemorrhage with colloid and crystalloid solutions. Studies in dogs. JAMA, 199:297, 1967.

10. Tullis, J. L., and Lionetti, F. J.: Preservation of blood by freezing. Anesthesiology, 27:483, 1966.

11. Vogel, J. M., and Vogel, P.: Transfusion of blood components. Anesthesiology, 27:373, 1966.

12. Editorial: Warm blood for massive transfusions. Lancet, 1:1193, 1966.

13. Kliman, A.: Complications of massive blood replacement. New York J. Med., 65:239, 1965.

14. Howland, W. S., Schweizer, O., and Boyan, C. P.: Massive blood replacement without calcium administration. Surg. Gynec. Obstet., 118:814, 1964.

15. Baker, R. J., et al.: Low molecular weight dextran therapy in surgical shock. Arch. Surg., 89:373, 1969.

16. Allen, J. G., and Sayman, W. A.: Serum hepatitis from transfusions of blood—epidemiologic study. JAMA, 180:1079, 1962.

17. Gelin, L. E., Solvell, L., and Zederfeldt, B.: Plasma volume expanding effort of low viscous dextran and Madrox. Arch. Chir. Scand., 122:309, 1961.

18. Swan, H., and Schechter, D. C.: The transfusion of blood from cadavers: A historical review. Surgery, 52: 545, 1962.

11 CARDIOPULMONARY RESUSCITATION

R. F. WILSON
N. THOMS
A. ARBULU
Z. STEIGER

Cardiac arrest may be defined as a sudden cessation of effective cardiac action. It may be due to asystole, ventricular fibrillation, or any other arrhythmia that reduces cardiac output to a negligible level.

PITFALL

IF A PHYSICIAN, CONFRONTED BY A PATIENT WITH A POSSIBLE CARDIAC ARREST, DELAYS RESUSCITATION EFFORTS BECAUSE OF UNCERTAINTY ABOUT THE DIAGNOSIS OR TREATMENT, FEW, IF ANY, PATIENTS WILL SURVIVE WITHOUT NEUROLOGIC DAMAGE.

Every physician must have a clear idea of how cardiac arrest is diagnosed and how it is treated. In many aspects of medicine there is enough time for a relatively casual examination of the patient and discussion of the diagnostic possibilities and therapeutic maneuvers. When a cardiac arrest occurs, however, recognition and treatment must almost be reflex in nature. With early and aggressive management, over 20% of patients with a cardiac arrest can go home alive. The long-term prognosis on these patients is also good; three fourths of those who go home will survive to one year and half will survive to three years.[1]

The most common conditions leading to cardiac arrest are coronary-artery disease

PITFALL

IF THE BASIC CAUSE OF A CARDIAC ARREST IS NOT RECOGNIZED AND CORRECTED IMMEDIATELY, SUCCESSFUL RESUSCITATIVE EFFORTS ARE APT TO BE INFREQUENT AND ONLY TEMPORARY.

and pulmonary insufficiency (Table 1). Unless the myocardial ischemia, electrical instability, and hypoxemia associated with these diseases are rapidly corrected, the resultant tissue changes become progressively irreversible. It is extremely difficult to prevent or correct ventricular fibrillation once severe metabolic acidosis has developed.

PATHOPHYSIOLOGY

The two most frequent types of electrical disorganization of the heart causing cardiac arrest are ventricular fibrillation and ventricular asystole.

Ventricular Fibrillation

Ventricular fibrillation is an uncoordinated irregular twitching movement of the myocardium. After an acute myocardial infarction there appears to be an enhanced automaticity of myocardial cells,[2] especially at the junction of ischemic and nonischemic tissue, caused by local biochemical changes

TABLE 1. CARDIAC ARRESTS: ALLEN PARK V.A. HOSPITAL
(JANUARY 1, 1968–DECEMBER 31, 1971)

Etiology of cardiac arrest	Total # of patients	# of Initially resuscitated	# Dying later	# Leaving hospital alive	% Leaving hospital alive
Heart disease	75	13	8	5	6.7%
Chronic pulmonary insufficiency	25	7	3	4	16.0%
Hepatic insufficiency	22	0	0	0	0
Convulsive disorder	13	2	0	2	15.4%
Metabolic or electrolyte imbalance	11	2	0	2	18.2%
Sepsis	6	1	0	1	16.7%
Gastrointestinal hemorrhage	5	4	0	4	80.0%
Cerebrovascular accident	5	1	0	1	20.0%
Intraoperative	4	4	0	4	100.0%
Renal insufficiency	4	0	0	0	0
Aspiration	4	2	0	2	50.0%
Massive hemoptysis	4	2	1	1	25.0%
Other	21	2	1	1	4.8%
Total	199	40	13	27	13.5%

and leading to ventricular ectopic beats. Reentrant mechanisms[3] may also be facilitated by myocardial changes at the edges of the infarct, resulting in earlier repolarization of the ischemic tissues. Bradycardia, because of the long diastolic intervals, also increases the chances of ventricular ectopic beats and tachyarrhythmias.

PITFALL

IF ACID-BASE BALANCE AND ARTERIAL BLOOD GASES ARE NOT MONITORED CLOSELY IN THE PATIENT WITH TRAUMATIC OR ISCHEMIC MYOCARDIAL DAMAGE, VENTRICULAR FIBRILLATION MAY OCCUR SUDDENLY AND BE VERY DIFFICULT TO REVERSE.

The myocardial fibrillation threshold is reduced by increased circulating norepi-nephrine, especially if arterial hypoxemia and metabolic acidosis are present. Drugs which can further increase the incidence of ectopic beats and tachyarrhythmias include digitalis, quinidine in toxic doses, diuretics, and isoproterenol. Ventricular fibrillation caused by implanted pacemaker impulses falling in the vulnerable portion of the electrical cycle is rare, but the chances of this occurring are reduced by proper positioning of the pacemaker tip and the use of demand pacemakers, low-voltage currents, and strict electrical isolation.

Ventricular Asystole

Ventricular asystole usually has a much graver prognosis than ventricular fibrillation. For ventricular asystole to occur and persist, not only must supraventricular impulse formation and/or conduction pathways fail but the myocardial damage must also be so extensive that the ventricular escape mechanisms are not activated or are ineffective. Not uncommonly, asystole is preceded by sinus-node dysfunction and varying degrees of A-V nodal or bundle branch block. The chances of asystole are furthered by factors such as excessive pain or fear, which increase vagal tone.[4]

DIAGNOSIS

The cardinal signs of cardiac arrest include lack of a palpable or audible pulse, blood pressure or heart beat. Although these signs are generally reliable when considered together, taken individually they can be misleading. If the stroke volume is low, it may not produce a palpable expansion of the artery during systole or create audible vibrations as the blood is pumped through the portion of the artery narrowed by the BP cuff. If a cardiac arrest is suspected during an operation, the surgeon should immediately palpate the largest vessel in the field. If it is an abdominal operation, the aorta or the diaphragm under the heart can readily be felt to ascertain whether or not the heart is still beating.

In many instances, a cardiac arrest is not suspected until severe cyanosis develops and/or the patient stops breathing. Unfortunately, respirations do not always stop immediately; the patient may continue to breathe or gasp for 20 or 30 seconds or longer after the heart has stopped. If the patient is anemic, cyanosis may not develop until blood flow or ventilation has stopped for more than 30 to 60 seconds; if sudden severe cyanosis does develop, it can be assumed that a cardiac arrest either has occurred or is imminent.

PITFALL

IF THE DIAGNOSIS OF A CARDIAC ARREST IS MADE ONLY AFTER THE PATIENT HAS HAD A CONVULSION, SEVERE BRAIN DAMAGE HAS ALREADY OCCURRED.

Not infrequently a cardiac arrest is noticed only after the patient has had a convulsion, and then it is often assumed that the convulsion caused the cardiac arrest. In many instances, it is not possible to determine whether the convulsion was a result of cerebral anoxia caused by the cardiac arrest or whether the convulsion itself caused enough hypoxia to produce the cardiac arrest. In general, however, the convulsion is due to the cardiac arrest and not vice versa. Although dilatation of the pupils is usually a late sign of a cardiac arrest, a few patients with temporarily dilated and fixed pupils have been resuscitated.

PITFALL

IF CRITICALLY ILL OR INJURED PATIENTS UNDERGOING SURGERY OR EXPERIENCING ARRHYTHMIAS ARE NOT CONTINUOUSLY MONITORED WITH A CARDIOSCOPE, THE DIAGNOSIS AND TREATMENT OF PREMONITORY CHANGES OR A CARDIAC ARREST MAY BE SERIOUSLY DELAYED.

By far the most accurate method for early diagnosis of a cardiac arrest, except for looking at the heart directly during surgery, is continuous monitoring with a cardioscope. If a suspected cardiac arrest occurs and a cardioscope or EKG is not immediately available, the physician must guess whether a cardiac arrest actually has occurred and whether it is due to ventricular fibrillation, asystole, or some other arrythmia.

Patients likely to have a cardiac arrest or develop an arrhythmia should be monitored with a cardioscope; such patients are those who may develop sudden severe hypoxia, hypotension, or metabolic or electrolyte changes. In the trauma patient these changes are most apt to occur during the initial resuscitation in the emergency department, during general anesthesia and surgery, and in the immediate postoperative period. The risk of ventricular fibrillation is especially great if the patient has an acute myocardial infarct and develops multiple ventricular ectopic beats, A-V node or bundle branch blocks, or tachyarrythmias.

TREATMENT

PITFALL

IF CARDIOPULMONARY RESUSCITATION IS DE-LAYED UNTIL A SUSPECTED CARDIAC ARREST IS CONFIRMED, THE CHANCE OF SUCCESSFUL RESUSCITATION DECREASES AND THE RISK OF IRREVERSIBLE CEREBRAL AND MYOCARDIAL DAMAGE INCREASES.

Treatment must not be delayed until the diagnosis of cardiac arrest is confirmed. Resuscitative efforts should begin immediately, even if the diagnosis is only suspected. It is far more dangerous to wait for conclusive evidence of cardiac arrest than to begin treatment, even if a cardiac arrest has not occurred. The goal is to restore blood flow, especially to the brain, as soon as possible. The cerebral circulation ordinarily cannot stop for more than three to four minutes without causing irreversible brain damage. Furthermore, efforts to restore effective cardiac action are less apt to be successful if the myocardium becomes ischemic, hypoxic, and acidotic.

Assistance

As soon as a cardiac arrest is suspected, cardiopulmonary resuscitation should be initiated and assistance summoned. Successful resuscitation usually requires the cooperation of several well-trained individuals and certain emergency equipment. All hospitals must have a well-rehearsed practical plan for bringing the necessary personnel and equipment to the patient's bedside in the shortest possible time. A special telephone number should be assigned for use when there is a cardiac arrest, and the operator must answer these calls immediately. She, in turn, depending on the time of day, etc., announces the cardiac arrest (using a special code known to the responsible individuals) and its location over the hospital loudspeaker and/or calls certain offices and/or personnel.

PERSONNEL. At many teaching hospitals, the optimal number of individuals for treating a cardiac arrest is four to six. Too many people get in the way and make the resuscitation efforts inefficient. At least one individual should concentrate on ventilating the patient and one should begin external cardiac massage. Another can start one or more I.V.s (using a percutaneous needle or catheter or a cutdown) and administer needed medications. A nurse should be available to prepare medications. One or two other assistants can attach EKG leads, draw blood for laboratory studies, and alternate ventilating the patient or performing external massage.

At least one person involved in the resuscitation effort should be skilled in inserting endotracheal tubes; this will usually be an anesthesiologist or anesthetist. Another individual, usually an internist or cardiologist, should have expertise in interpreting EKGs and administering cardiac drugs. In the event that an I.V. is difficult to start, or if internal cardiac massage or a tracheostomy is needed, a surgeon should also be immediately available.

Imperative for the optimal functioning of the resuscitation team is a leader. In most instances the most experienced physician assumes leadership automatically. Everyone's role should be clearly outlined prior to the emergency, and it should be remembered that the best results are obtained when everyone cooperates as a team. Teamwork is developed by practice and critical review of each attempt at resuscitation.

EQUIPMENT

PITFALL

IF A DEFIBRILLATOR, CARDIAC MONITOR AND OTHER RESUSCITATION EQUIPMENT CANNOT BE BROUGHT TO THE PATIENT'S BEDSIDE IN LESS THAN FOUR MINUTES AFTER THE CARDIAC ARREST HAS OCCURRED, THE CHANCES OF SUCCESSFUL RESUSCITATION ARE GREATLY REDUCED.

Ideally the equipment needed for cardiopulmonary resuscitation should be available on each floor and in all special-care areas. If this is not possible or practical, a well-rehearsed plan must be developed for notifying individual(s) in the areas where the equipment is stored and maintained, and these people must have an elevator key to provide immediate vertical mobility.

The resuscitation equipment which must be on the emergency cart includes: standard ventilation apparatus, emergency drugs, a venous cutdown tray, an EKG machine or oscilloscope, a defibrillator, an I.V. pacemaker, and intracardiac needles. The standard ventilation equipment includes oral airways, endotracheal tubes, laryngoscope, a mask, a hand respirator (Ambubag), and suction equipment for aspirating secretions or blood from the larynx, pharynx, or tracheal bronchial tree. A mechanical respirator, preferably of the volume-cycled type, should also be immediately available if prolonged ventilatory assistance is needed.

DRUGS. Emergency drugs that may be needed for cardiac resuscitation and which should be present on the emergency carts *and* on the wards include:

epinephrine (Adrenalin 1:1000 solution)
sodium bicarbonate (50 ml of a 7.5% solution)
isoproterenol (Isuprel 1:5000 solution)
calcium chloride (10 ml of 10% solution)
furosemide and/or ethacrynic acid
Xylocaine (lidocaine 1% and 2%)
atropine
norepinephrine (Levophed)
digoxin and Cedilanid (lanatoside-C)
potassium chloride.

At the first hint of a cardiac arrest, epinephrine and sodium bicarbonate should be drawn up into syringes. One cc of 1:1000 epinephrine should be diluted with 9 cc of saline to make a 1:10,000 dilution. Intracardiac needles 18 to 20 gauge and 4½ inches long should be immediately available. Two ampules of sodium bicarbonate should be drawn up into 50-cc syringes.

Sharp Blow to the Chest

The first step in treatment should be one or two sharp blows to the precordium. This in itself may restore circulation in some individuals, especially if it is done immediately after the arrest. After striking the chest with a clenched fist, listen to the heart and feel for a femoral or carotid pulse to determine if the blow has restored an adequate heart beat. Very little time— only a few seconds—should be spent on this particular maneuver. If a cardioscope or EKG is attached to the patient, the electrical responses can be seen immediately. If there is any question about the adequacy of cardiac action, ventilation and cardiac massage must be begun immediately.

Techniques of Cardiopulmonary Resuscitation

A mnemonic frequently used in teaching the techniques of cardiopulmonary resuscitation are the letters A, B, C, D; these stand for airway, breathing, circulation, and definitive therapy.[5]

AIRWAY. The airway to the lungs must be opened. This may be accomplished by hyperextending the head and pulling the mandible forward. An oral airway or Resuscitube (S tube) helps to hold the tongue forward and allow suction of secretions from the mouth and pharynx; it also prevents the patient from clamping his jaws shut.

PITFALL

IF AN INEXPERIENCED INDIVIDUAL ATTEMPTS TO INSERT AN ENDOTRACHEAL TUBE DURING CARDIOPULMONARY RESUSCITATION, THE PROLONGED INTERRUPTION OF VENTILATION AND CARDIAC MASSAGE MAY BE FATAL.

Although an endotracheal tube provides much better ventilation than mouth-to-mouth or mask-to-mouth techniques and prevents gastric regurgitation into the lungs, a significant amount of expertise is needed to insert it rapidly, especially if the patient has a short "bull" neck, stiff jaws, or excessive secretions. Unfortunately it sometimes becomes a matter of pride for the endoscopist to insert the tube. If the tube cannot be inserted within 5 to 10 seconds, the attempt at intubation should stop and the patient should be ventilated with 100% oxygen for a minute or two before trying again. If the endotracheal tube is soft, a stylus often is of great assistance in angling it anteriorly between the vocal cords. If the airway cannot be established with an oral airway or endotracheal tube, an emergency tracheostomy or coniotomy (cricothyroidotomy) may be needed (Chap. 7).

VENTILATION. Most patients can be adequately ventilated with mouth-to-mouth respiration. With the head hyperextended, jaw pulled forward, and nose pinched (if patient is adult), air is forced into the mouth. The chest should rise perceptively with each breath. If the chest does not seem to inflate, but the abdomen does, the airway is probably not open properly and the head and mandible should be adjusted. Mouth-to-mouth breathing may not be as effective as ventilation through an endotracheal tube, but it can be started immediately; it is far better to do this than to waste time while an inexperienced individual attempts to intubate the patient.

Mouth-to-nose ventilation can also be effective, especially in small children. The Resuscitube (S tube) is constructed so that the airway is maintained with one end and the rescuer ventilates the patient through the other end. If an endotracheal tube is in place, it can be breathed into until an Ambu-bag or respirator becomes available.

If cardiopulmonary resuscitation must be started by one individual, he should breathe or blow into the mouth, airway or endotracheal tube rapidly and deeply three or four times and then begin external cardiac massage. The patient is then ventilated rapidly with two or three puffs every 12 to 15 seconds, and external massage is continued between the respirations until additional help arrives. One member of the

team can then give external massage while another maintains ventilation.

MAINTENANCE OF CIRCULATION. *External Cardiac Massage.* The principle of external cardiac massage involves intermittent compression of the heart between the sternum and spine; lateral expansion of the heart is limited by the pericardium. Proper direction of the blood flow is maintained by the cardiac valves. If the chest wall, pericardium or valves are abnormal, or if the patient is hypovolemic, the effectiveness of external cardiac massage is greatly reduced.

IMPORTANCE OF A FIRM SURFACE. It is important that the patient lies on a firm surface while external cardiac massage is being applied, for it is virtually impossible to compress and empty the heart adequately if the patient bounces on a mattress each time pressure is applied to the sternum. For this reason, all wards and emergency carts should be provided with a backboard which can be placed under the patient when external massage is needed. It should be big enough to support the entire back and to reach the metal frame on either side of the bed. In an emergency a food tray may provide some support. Although it is not desirable to move the patient out of bed to the floor, if nothing else is available the floor does provide a readily available firm surface for external massage. Obviously the patient must be lowered gently and, if he is in traction or has chest tubes in place, this maneuver may be very impractical.

COMPRESSION OF THE CHEST. To perform external cardiac massage, the heel of one hand, not the palm, is placed over the lower half of the sternum. The other hand is placed on top of the first hand. In the adult the sternum is then pressed inward about 3 to 5 cm with each compression.

The ideal rate for cardiac massage in most adults is about 60 times per minute. Inexperienced personnel tend to massage too rapidly, thereby reducing the time for the heart to fill between compressions. A

PITFALL

IF THE CARDIAC MASSAGE IS PERFORMED TOO RAPIDLY OR IF THE PRESSURE ON THE HEART IS NOT RELEASED RAPIDLY AFTER EACH COMPRESSION, THE DIASTOLIC FILLING OF THE HEART AND THE CARDIAC OUTPUT AND CORONARY BLOOD FLOW WILL REMAIN EXTREMELY LOW.

rate of 60 per minute can be maintained fairly well by counting "one thousand one, one thousand two, one thousand three," etc., or by watching the second hand of a clock or watch. If the pressure is not released rapidly after each compression, diastolic filling of the heart may be impaired. Other causes of poor ventricular filling include cardiac tamponade, hypovolemia, and pneumothorax.

In the Shock Unit of Detroit General Hospital patients usually have intra-arterial catheters for continuous pressure monitoring. If they have a cardiac arrest, we try to monitor blood pressure and cardiac output closely. There is often a poor correlation between the recorded intra-arterial pressures and the impression obtained by palpation of the carotid and femoral pulses. We have found that most house officers usually provide a systolic pressure of only about 40 to 60 mm Hg during their external massage. However, if they see the pressures they produce with their efforts, they usually adjust their technique to increase the intra-arterial pressures by 50 to 100%.

Since a fairly significant amount of force and stamina is needed to depress the sternum 3 to 5 cm in the adult for more than a few minutes, the person performing external cardiac massage should position himself to use the weight of his upper body. To accomplish this, he can stand on a chair at the bedside or kneel on one leg next to the patient. If proper help is available, individuals can alternate every 5 to 15 minutes, depending on their strength and endurance. Mechanical devices for performing external massage may be of great value if they can

be applied rapidly and are monitored closely, especially if the massage has to be continued for more then 30 to 60 minutes.

PITFALL

IF EXTERNAL CARDIAC MASSAGE IS INTERRUPTED FOR MORE THAN FIVE SECONDS AT A TIME, ADDITIONAL ISCHEMIC DAMAGE TO THE BRAIN, HEART, AND OTHER VITAL ORGANS WILL OCCUR.

Under no circumstances should cardiac massage be interrupted for more than five seconds at a time, since at best it seldom supplies more than a quarter or half of the patient's normal cardiac output. As a consequence flow to the vital organs is already compromised, leaving little or no oxygen reserve. Even minimal additional interference with blood flow under such circumstances may be fatal. As the individuals performing the cardiopulmonary resuscitation become increasingly tired, they seem to spend more time watching the patient's response to each drug and each attempt at defibrillation. Even if reasonably normal electrical activity is restored, cardiac massage *must* be continued until the patient can achieve a definitely palpable carotid or femoral pulse without manual assistance.

COMPLICATIONS. It is estimated that external cardiac massage, even done properly, will cause potentially lethal complications in about 1% of cases.[4] Some of the more frequent serious complications include damage to the heart, lungs, liver, spleen, or adrenals, gastroesophageal tears, intestinal hemorrhages, and pulmonary fat emboli. In older individuals with severe emphysema and/or a very stiff chest wall, fractures of the ribs and/or sternum may be unavoidable. Although a fractured sternum under other circumstances often temporarily causes a severe flail chest, very few patients who have this complication during cardiopulmonary resuscitation require respirator assistance for more than 24 to 48 hours as a result of the fracture.

DETERMINING THE EFFECTIVENESS OF THE RESUSCITATIVE EFFORTS. To evaluate the effectiveness of the resuscitative efforts, the pulse, blood pressure, pupils, return of spontaneous respiration, skin color, state of consciousness, and electrocardiographic changes should be closely monitored. Unless cardiac massage produces a palpable carotid or femoral pulse, it is probably not effective. This is, however, often difficult to determine because the movement of the patient caused by the external massage can easily be mistaken for a femoral or carotid pulsation. If a definite good pulse cannot be felt, it is probably not present. If no pulse is palpable and the patient is not improving, a surgeon may, under certain circumstances, consider open cardiac massage.

Open Cardiac Massage. At the present time there is some disagreement among physicians about the value and indications of open cardiac massage. On the surgical wards of Detroit General Hospital and in the Shock Unit, open cardiac massage has often been far more effective than the closed technique. Not only have higher arterial pressures and cardiac outputs been achieved but the direct observation of the heart's response to various drugs and attempts at defibrillation has proven informative for guiding further therapy.

PITFALL

IF A PATIENT WITH AN OTHERWISE GOOD PROGNOSIS HAS A CARDIAC ARREST AND DOES NOT RESPOND TO CLOSED CARDIAC MASSAGE, FAILURE TO PERFORM OPEN MASSAGE MAY GREATLY REDUCE HIS CHANCES FOR SURVIVAL.

In spite of the increased morbidity and mortality of a thoracotomy in any patient who has had a cardiac arrest, we do not hesitate to perform or switch to open cardiac massage if the patient has a penetrating chest wound, if external massage cannot produce a palpable pulse, or if there is no improvement after using the closed technique for 5 to 10 minutes. Two other prerequisites are a well-functioning endotracheal tube and a surgeon experienced in performing a thoracotomy and direct cardiac massage. In general we are reluctant to perform open cardiac massage on patients with an acute myocardial infarction; however, cardiopulmonary bypass has recently been used by some surgeons to keep the patient alive while coronary arteriograms and saphenocoronary-artery bypass and/or infarctectomies have been performed.

Intravenous Catheters. As soon as proper help is available, two intravenous catheters at least 18 gauge in size should be inserted percutaneously or by a cutdown. One should be long enough to be advanced into the superior vena cava for monitoring the central venous pressure. The CVP catheter can also be used for giving drugs which should be delivered into the coronary circulation rapidly without much dilution. Because most patients will have a tendency to develop congestive heart failure, fluids should be given very slowly unless there is evidence of hypovolemia.

If the patient remains hypotensive after an otherwise successful resuscitation, a pulmonary-artery catheter of the Swan-Ganz type should be considered. After a cardiac arrest or acute myocardial infarction an isolated left ventricular failure may persist for several hours or longer, allowing the left atrial pressure to rise rapidly and pulmonary edema to develop in spite of a low CVP.[6] Under these circumstances, the pulmonary-artery or wedge pressures reflect left atrial pressure much better than the CVP.[7] In such patients, frequent auscultation of the lungs posteriorly at the bases is essential.

DEFINITIVE THERAPY. Once the airway is opened, breathing is provided, and circulation is established by cardiac massage, definitive therapy based on an accurate diagnosis and utilizing drugs and/or a defibrillator may be provided. Of the problems requiring specific treatment during or after a cardiac arrest the most important are ventricular fibrillation, asystole, bradycardia, other arrhythmias, hypotension, and congestive heart failure.

Ventricular Fibrillation

PITFALL

IF THERE IS ANY DELAY IN DEFIBRILLATING THE HEART ONCE VENTILATION AND CARDIAC MASSAGE HAVE BEEN STARTED, THE CHANCES OF SUCCESSFUL RESUSCITATION ARE REDUCED.

Ventricular fibrillation is the most common cause of cardiac arrest, especially after an acute myocardial infarction, and the chances of successful conversion depend largely on the speed with which the electrical shock is delivered. During a cardiac arrest, there is a rapid, progressive deterioration of the vital organs. Factors such as ischemia and acidosis, which cause electrical instability of the heart, also tend to increase. If a patient suffers a sudden cardiac arrest and the defibrillator is present and ready to be used, it may be wise to defibrillate immediately, without waiting to ascertain by EKG or cardioscope the precise nature of the arrest. If ventricular fibrillation is not present, few untoward effects are noted. Although defibrillators in the past were used almost exclusively to reverse ventricular fibrillation, they are also now being used with increasing frequency in the management of ventricular tachycardia, atrial fibrillation and other tachyarrhythmias.

The two basic types of defibrillators used are the AC (alternating current) and the DC (direct current) defibrillators. The DC type is preferred, especially in the management of arrhythmias other than ventricular fibrillation. One defibrillator paddle is placed over the left lateral chest at about the fifth or sixth intercostal space between the midclavicular and anterior axillary lines and the other is placed over the upper sternum near the clavicles. A liberal amount of electrode jelly is applied to each paddle, but without allowing a "bridge" of electrode jelly to extend between the two paddles. If electrode jelly is not available, saline-soaked 4 × 4 dressings can be placed under the paddles. No one should be touching the patient or the bed when the current is applied; however, defibrillators are now available which negate the need for this precaution.

The amount of energy required to defibrillate the heart varies greatly. The usual starting dose is 75 watt-seconds. If the fibrillation is not terminated by the first attempt, the patient should be hyperventilated for 10 to 15 seconds with 100% oxygen while external massage is continued. Two shocks in rapid succession can then be applied. If the heart is still fibrillating, the energy can be gradually increased to 400 watt-seconds.

PERSISTENT VENTRICULAR FIBRILLATION

PITFALL

IF SEVERE METABOLIC ACIDOSIS OR HYPOXEMIA IS ALLOWED TO PERSIST, IT MAY BE IMPOSSIBLE TO DEFIBRILLATE THE PATIENT.

One of the most frequent causes for persistent ventricular fibrillation is a severe metabolic acidosis; it is not uncommon for the arterial pH to fall below 7.0 within 2 to 3 minutes of the cardiac arrest. This is usually best prevented or corrected with sodium bicarbonate ($NaHCO_3$). Each 50-cc ampule of 7.5% $NaHCO_3$ contains 44.6 mEq of bicarbonate. We generally give 2 to 3 ampules of $NaHCO_3$ during the first 5 minutes of ineffective cardiac action and 1 to 2 ampules every 5 to 10 minutes thereafter. Although $NaHCO_3$ is occasionally given by the intracardiac route, we usually give it intravenously, preferably through a large CVP catheter.

RECURRENT FIBRILLATION. If the ventricular fibrillation is terminated by electric shock but quickly recurs, lidocaine or procainamide may be used to reduce the irritability of the heart.

Lidocaine (Xylocaine) has found increasing use in the management of ventricular arrhythmias because of its ability to reduce the irritability of the myocardium without greatly reducing its contractility. Ventricular fibrillation, ventricular tachycardia, and frequent premature ventricular contractions may respond dramatically to this drug. We usually start with a bolus I.V. injection of 50 to 100 mg (5 to 10 cc of a 1% solution). If little or no response is noted, the loading dose may be repeated two or three times. Once an adequate response has been obtained, lidocaine is continued as an I.V. infusion of 1 to 4 mg per minute to keep the premature ventricular contractions less than 4 to 6 per minute.

PITFALL

IF LARGE AMOUNTS OF LIDOCAINE ARE GIVEN TO A PATIENT WHO IS SLIGHTLY HYPOVOLEMIC, SEVERE HYPOTENSION MAY OCCUR.

It is not uncommon for critically injured patients to have some degree of hypovolemia which is at least partially compensated for by increased arteriolar and venous vasoconstriction. Many drugs, including lidocaine, morphine, Demerol, and Thorazine, can produce significant vasodilation, thereby increasing vascular capacity. In the hypovolemic patient, the resultant discrepancy between the increased vascular capacity and reduced blood volume can cause a sharp drop in blood pressure.

Procainamide (Pronestyl) has an action somewhat similar to that of lidocaine. Its use is reserved for lidocaine-resistant arrhythmias because it has a greater myocardial depressant effect and can cause severe hypotension. The usual dose of procainamide is 500 mg I.V. over a 3- to 10-minute period. depending on the EKG response, with 25 to 50 mg given each minute thereafter until the appropriate effect is obtained (but not exceeding 1000 to 1500 mg). If excessive hypotension is produced, the drug must be slowed or stopped. Subsequent doses will vary with each patient, but may average 500 mg every six hours.

Asystole. If the heart is in asystole or has persistent low-amplitude fibrillation, the prognosis is much worse than with a coarse ventricular fibrillation. Lidocaine, procainamide, quinidine, and potassium should be avoided. Under these circumstances, epinephrine is probably the best drug available for stimulating the heart. Calcium may also be used to increase the rate and force of contraction. If neither of these drugs corrects the asystole, or if a heart block is present, a cardiac pacemaker should be used.

EPINEPHRINE (ADRENALIN). Epinephrine increases the contractility and irritability of the heart and may convert asystole to ventricular fibrillation; it can also increase the strength or amplitude of ventricular fibrillation and make it more susceptible to conversion. It should be used if there is no satisfactory response within one to three minutes after artifical ventilation and external massage are begun. The usual intracardiac dose is 3 to 5 ml of a 1:10,000 solution. For intracardiac injections the ideal needle is 4½ inches long and 18 to 20 gauge in diameter. Spinal needles are often very good. The quickest technique is to insert the needle in the fourth intercostal space about an inch lateral to the sternum, directing it medially and posteriorly.

PITFALL

IF ADRENALIN IS INJECTED INTO THE MYOCARDIUM RATHER THAN THE VENTRICULAR CHAMBER, IT CAN CAUSE PERSISTENT VENTRICULAR FIBRILLATION.

Epinephrine injected into any tissue can cause such severe vasoconstriction and ischemia that local tissue necrosis may occur. Such a damaged area in the heart can act as a focus for persistent or recurring ventricular fibrillation. If a CVP or pulmonary-artery catheter is present, a slightly larger dose of Adrenalin given through it can be almost as effective, and is certainly safer, than intracardiac Adrenalin. Furthermore, the hazards of tearing the anterior coronary artery or anterior myocardium with the intracardiac needle are eliminated.

CALCIUM. Calcium, acting primarily through its ionic fraction, can increase the force of myocardial contraction. This drug can be especially useful if the patient has a low-amplitude ventricular fibrillation or a weakly beating heart in regular sinus rhythm. Trauma patients who have been hypotensive and have received multiple transfusions of stored CPD blood are especially apt to develop cardiovascular problems from or related to ionic hypocalcemia (Chaps. 5 and 10).

Calcium chloride and calcium gluconate are both stocked as a 10% solution in 10-ml ampules. The calcium chloride, however, contains more calcium than calcium gluconate (18 mEq versus 4.7 mEq) and is more rapidly and completely ionized, especially if the patient is in shock or has liver disease. When calcium chloride is given during cardiac resuscitation it can be administered by intravenous (5 to 10 cc of the 10% solution) or intracardiac (2 to 3 cc of a 1.0% solution) injection.

PITFALL

IF DIGITALIS HAS BEEN GIVEN, INTRAVENOUS OR INTRACARDIAC CALCIUM CAN CAUSE SEVERE DIGITALIS TOXICITY, ESPECIALLY IF THE PATIENT IS HYPOKALEMIC.

Calcium opposes the effects of potassium and increases the effects or toxicity of digitalis preparations. Therefore, the administration of calcium to patients who have been given digitalis must be undertaken with caution.

PACEMAKERS. If adequate ventilation, effective cardiac massage, and the various drugs are unsuccessful in correcting asystole, a cardiac pacemaker should be inserted intravenously. The pacemakers are especially useful if there is evidence of heart block or drug toxicity.

A pacing catheter can often be passed blindly into the right ventricle through a cutdown on the antecubital, cephalic, basilic, or external jugular veins. If such an attempt is unsuccessful, a direct percutaneous puncture of the heart with a needle electrode can be performed as a last resort.

Bradycardia. Persistent severe bradycardia is apt to be associated with poor myocardial contraction and an increased chance of recurrent cardiac arrest. This problem may be managed with isoproterenol, atropine and/or a pacemaker.

ISOPROTERENOL (ISUPREL). Isoproterenol is a pure beta-adrenergic stimulator and, as such, increases the rate and force of myocardial contraction, causes some arteriolar vasodilation in vessels in skeletal muscles, and tends to constrict capacitance veins.

PITFALL

IF ISOPROTERENOL IS ADMINISTERED IN THE PRESENCE OF A TACHYCARDIA OR AN IRRITABLE HEART, THE CARDIAC OUTPUT IS NOT LIKELY TO BE INCREASED AND THE PATIENT IS APT TO DEVELOP A SEVERE TACHYCARDIA OR ARRHYTHMIA.

The main value of isoproterenol is its ability to increase the rate and force of myocardial contraction in a weak, slowly beating heart. Under these circumstances, it can produce a significant increase in cardiac output. If too much is given, however, it can cause ventricular tachycardia which may be followed by ventricular fibrillation. Because of its tendency to cause arrhythmias in rapidly beating hearts, its use is generally contraindicated in patients with frequent extrasystoles or pulse rates exceeding 120 to 130 per minute.

If the patient has persistent asystole, an ampule (0.2 mg) may be diluted in 10 ml of saline and 1 ml of this 1:50,000 solution can be injected directly into the ventricular chamber. If the heart is beating, but the contractions are slow and weak, the cardiac output can usually be improved by a slow

I.V. infusion of one ampule (0.2 mg) diluted in 50 to 100 ml of 5% glucose in water.

ATROPINE. Atropine is an anticholinergic drug which may be extremely useful if bradycardia persists following resuscitation and the heart is irritable or isoproterenol has been ineffective. The usual dose is 0.4 to 1.0 mg I.V. The effect of atropine may last for 24 hours or longer. Subsequent doses, usually not to exceed a total of 1.0 mg in 24 hours, will depend on the degree and duration of the response. This drug should not be given to patients with glaucoma or bladder-outlet obstruction.

PACING. Cardiac pacemakers can be used to treat bradycardia in much the same fashion described above for persistent asystole.

Other Arrhythmias. The incidence of primary ventricular fibrillation, occurring in the absence of cardiac failure, can be reduced by an aggressive approach to premonitory arrhythmias, especially premature ventricular contractions and ventricular tachycardia. Lidocaine, as mentioned earlier, is the drug of choice for these arrhythmias. If it is not possible to give I.V. lidocaine immediately when it is needed, and if the patient is not in shock, 300 mg I.M. can maintain a therapeutic blood level for 45 to 60 minutes.[5] Procainamide and quinidine are reserved for lidocaine-resistant arrhythmias. Quinidine in doses of 200 mg every 4 to 8 hours is used primarily for atrial tachyarrhythmias after the patient has been digitalized.

Dilantin, propranolol, and potassium may be especially useful in managing tachyarrhythmias caused by digitalis intoxication. Dilantin should not be given faster than 50 mg per minute and should not exceed an initial total dose of 150 to 250 mg. A subsequent dose of up to 150 mg may be given 30 minutes later.

If digitalis toxicity is suspected, the serum electrolytes should be checked immediately. Low potassium and high calcium levels tend to increase digitalis effect and toxicity. We usually infuse potassium chloride in a solution of 10 mEq of KCl in 50 ml of 5% glucose in water in 30 to 60 minutes, depending on the severity of the problem and the EKG response.

Propranolol is a beta-adrenergic receptor blocking agent which is extremely useful in managing a wide variety of supraventricular tachyarrythmias. The usual initial I.V. dose is 1 to 3 mg given at 1 mg per minute. Depending on the response of the EKG and vital signs, a second dose may be repeated in two minutes. Additional propranolol should not be given in less than four hours. If excessive bradycardia develops after propranolol, 0.5 to 1.0 mg of atropine should be given I.V.

PITFALL

IF PROPRANOLOL IS GIVEN TO A PATIENT WHO HAS A LOW CARDIAC OUTPUT CAUSED BY POOR MYOCARDIAL CONTRACTILITY, THE RESULTANT MYOCARDIAL DEPRESSION CAN CAUSE IRREVERSIBLE CARDIOGENIC SHOCK.

Propranolol is contraindicated in the presence of bronchial asthma, second- or third-degree heart block, bradycardia, cardiogenic shock, and congestive heart failure (unless the failure is due to severe tachyarrhythmia that is treatable with propranolol).

Hypotension. If a regular cardiac rhythm is restored, but the patient is hypotensive, cardiac massage should be continued until the blood pressure is restored spontaneously or maintained with vasopressor and/or inotropic agents. Some of the drugs we have found useful under these circumstances include dopamine, isoproterenol, norepinephrine, metaraminol, and hydrocortisone (Chap. 5).

Dopamine can often produce a dramatic improvement in cardiac output and blood pressure. We begin with a slow I.V. infusion of a solution containing 200 mg of dopamine in 250 ml 5% G/W and increase it as needed.

Isoproterenol, as mentioned earlier, can be extremely useful if the pulse rate is less than 80 per minute. The usual I.V. infusion rate is 1 to 5 μg per minute (0.25 to 1.25 ml per minute of a solution containing 2 mg of isoproterenol in 500 ml of I.V. fluid).

Norepinephrine (Levophed) may be useful as a vasopressor for short periods of time if the heart beat is strong but the patient remains hypotensive. Unless the systolic pressure is raised above 60 mm Hg, cerebral and coronary blood flow may be inadequate. The usual dose of norepinephrine is four ampules (16 mg) in 500 ml of 5% glucose in water. Addition of two ampules (10 mg) of phentolamine (Regitine) to the same bottle reduces the toxicity of the norepinephrine and decreases the chance of its causing a skin slough if it extravasates. The I.V. drip rate is controlled to keep the BP above 80 mm Hg systolic or at the level needed to maintain adequate cerebral, cardiac, and renal function (Chap. 5).

Metaraminol (Aramine) is similar to norepinephrine, but is more of a vasoconstrictor, is usually not as effective as norepinephrine, and is more apt to seriously lower cardiac output. Mild degrees of hypotension may be controlled with a slow I.V. infusion of a solution containing 20 to 100 mg of metaraminol in 500 ml of I.V. fluid.

Steroids—either as a rapid "physiologic" infusion of 200 mg of hydrocortisone I.V. to rule out hypotension from adrenal insufficiency or in much larger "pharmacologic" doses (equivalent to 50 to 150 mg/kg body weight)—may be of some value in combating hypotension, especially if severe sepsis is also present (Chap. 5).

Congestive Heart Failure. If the patient is in severe congestive heart failure or has rapid atrial fibrillation or flutter following the cardiac resuscitation, a digitalis-like drug may be extremely beneficial. We have generally preferred digoxin over lanatoside-C because its onset of action is almost as fast and yet its effect is prolonged enough for long-term maintenance digitalization. The usual total I.V. dose is 1.0 to 1.5 mg given in divided doses over 2 to 8

hours. It is important to examine an EKG strip for any evidence of digitalis effect or toxicity before every dose of digoxin.

Diuretics. If the patient is in congestive heart failure or if he remains oliguric in spite of adequate hydration, a diuretic should be used. In the patient with only mild oliguria without congestive heart failure, 12.5 to 25.0 gm of mannitol may be given over a 10- to 30-minute period. If this increases the urine output only slightly or transiently, additional mannitol, up to 100 gm in 24 hours, may be given to maintain an output of at least 35 to 50 ml/hr.

If congestive heart failure is present, 40 mg of furosemide or 50 mg of ethacrynic acid may be given rapidly I.V. Additional doses, up to 400 to 500 mg in 24 hours, can be given as needed.

PITFALL

IF THE RESPONSE TO THESE DIURETICS IS EXCESSIVE, FAILURE TO CORRECT THE SUDDEN LARGE FLUID LOSS MAY LEAD THE PATIENT TO DEVELOP SEVERE HYPOVOLEMIC SHOCK.

Special Situations. GASTRIC DILATATION. If the initial resuscitative attempts have included mouth-to-mouth or mask-to-mouth ventilation, it can be assumed that substantial amounts of air have been forced into the stomach. The resulting gastric dilatation can be especially dangerous if the patient has recently eaten. During or following the cardiac arrest, the esophageal sphincters and vocal cords tend to relax, and the gastric contents can then be easily regurgitated into the mouth, pharynx, larynx, and lungs. Thus, if there is any evidence or suspicion that gastric dilatation may be present, the stomach should be aspirated with a Levin tube as soon as possible.

HYPERKALEMIA. If there is evidence of severe hyperkalemia, emergency treatment may include I.V. sodium bicarbonate, hypertonic glucose with insulin and/or calcium chloride.

PULMONARY EMBOLISM. If there is evidence of pulmonary embolism, 100 to 200 mg of heparin should be given rapidly I.V. The blood pressure should be maintained with norepinephrine as needed. If the cardiac arrest or shock is persistent, circulatory assistance with cardiopulmonary bypass and possible pulmonary embolectomy should be considered.

PERSISTENT COMA. If the patient has persistent coma following the resuscitation, it is usually due to hypoxic cerebral edema. Although this is a difficult process to reverse, hypothermia (maintaining the rectal temperature at 32 to 35 C or 90 to 95 F) for 48 to 72 hours may be helpful. Diuretics, especially mannitol, may be of value by reducing the amount of brain swelling. Steroids, 4 to 10 mg of dexamethasone every four to six hours, may also help reduce the brain swelling. Slight hyperventilation may reduce cerebral vascular congestion, and elevation of the head and chest may improve venous return from the brain.

WHEN TO STOP ATTEMPTS AT CARDIAC RESUSCITATION

The only contraindication to cardiac resuscitation is terminal disease in which the patient's suffering would be prolonged.

Cardiac resuscitation normally should not be continued if there is apparent brain death as demonstrated by fixed dilated pupils and absence of all reflexes for more than 20 to 30 minutes. Even without these signs, however, if adequate myocardial function cannot be restored after 30 to 60 minutes of effective massage, it is extremely unlikely that further attempts will be successful. Occasionally, however, surgery and cardiopulmonary bypass can correct a mechanical problem, such as a massive pulmonary embolus or an occluded major coronary artery, which might otherwise be fatal.

REFERENCES

1. Lemire, J. G., and Johnson, A. L.: Is cardiac resuscitation worthwhile? A decade of experience. New Eng. J. Med., 286:970, 1972.
2. Hoffman, B. F.: The genesis of cardiac arrhythmias. Progr. Cardiov. Dis., 8:319, 1966.
3. Han, J.: Mechanisms of ventricular arrhythmia associated with myocardial infarction. Amer. J. Cardiol., 24:800, 1969.
4. Mascarenhas, E., and Schoenfeld, C. D.: How we treat cardiac arrest following acute myocardial infarction. Resident and Staff Physician, pp. 62–71, March 1972.
5. Ad Hoc Committee on Cardiopulmonary Resuscitation of the Division of Medical Sciences, National Academy of Sciences—National Research Council: Cardiopulmonary resuscitation. JAMA, 194:373, 1966.
6. Wilson, R. F., Sarver, E., and Birks, R.: Central venous pressure and blood volume determinations in clinical shock. Surg. Gynec. Obstet., 132:631, 1971.
7. Rapaport, E., and Scheinman, M. M.: Rationale and limitations of hemodynamic measurements in patients with acute myocardial infarction. Mod. Conc. Cardiov. Dis., 37:55, 1969.

Suggested Readings

1. Bellet, S., et al.: Intramuscular lidocaine in the therapy of ventricular arrhythmias. Amer. J. Cardiol., 27:291, 1971.
2. Cosbey, R. L.: Cardiopulmonary resuscitation. JAMA, 217:79, 1971.
3. Skinner, D. B., Leonard, L. G., and Cooke, S. A. R.: Resuscitation following prolonged cardiac arrest. Ann. Thorac. Surg., 11:301, 1971.
4. Stiles, O. R., et al.: Evaluation of an active resuscitation program. Amer. J. Surg., 122:287, 1971.
5. Zoll, P. M.: Rational use of drugs for cardiac arrest and after cardiac resuscitation. Amer. J. Cardiol., 27:645, 1971.
6. Brown, C. S., et al.: Cardiopulmonary resuscitation: A review of 184 cases and some applications for future improvements. Canad. Anaesth. Soc. J., 17:565, 1970.
7. Fillmore, S. J., et al.: Serial blood gas studies during cardiopulmonary resuscitation. Ann. Intern. Med., 72:465, 1970.
8. Pantridge, J. F.: Mobile coronary care. Chest, 58:229, 1970.
9. Adgey, A. A., et al.: Management of ventricular fibrillation outside hospital. Lancet, 1:1169, 1969.
10. Aleman, P. J.: Organization of clinical resuscitation. Acta Anaesth. Scand., 29:293, 1968.

12 ANESTHESIA FOR THE TRAUMA PATIENT

M. L. NORTON

"And the Lord God caused a deep sleep to fall upon Adam, and he slept; and He took one of his ribs, and closed up the flesh instead thereof."

GENESIS 2:21

Anesthetic management of the patient with recent trauma[1,2,3] often requires subordination of anesthesiologic needs to the urgency of surgical intervention. Although minimal time may be available, the preoperative evaluation and preparation must be as thorough as possible, even for "minor" cases.

AXIOM

THERE IS NO SUCH THING AS "A LITTLE BIT OF ANESTHESIA."

Minor and major surgery merit equal attention. The anesthetic management for a closed reduction of a dislocated shoulder has the same inherent hazards as that for any major procedure: aspiration, airway management, shock, postanesthetic respiratory and sensory depression, etc.

PREANESTHETIC CONSIDERATIONS

The integrity of the airway, the functional reserve of the cardiovascular system, a history of drug or alcohol intake, a recent ingestion of solid food and liquids, and the degree of pain produced by the injury all merit special emphasis.[4] The level of consciousness after injury and any later changes, the urinary output, and the possibility of preexisting diabetes, epilepsy, or other syndromes all may affect anesthetic decisions.

The anesthesiologist and the surgeon should discuss their respective needs and work together as a team preoperatively, during induction of the anesthetic, intraoperatively, and in the recovery room. If the surgeon wishes to use cautery and other electrosurgical instrumentation, for example, this certainly limits the anesthesiologist in his choice of agents and technique. Ether and cyclopropane certainly cannot be used with electrocautery or defibrillation equipment.

PITFALL

IF THE POSITION OF THE PATIENT ON THE OPERATING TABLE IS DETERMINED BY THE NEED FOR SURGICAL EXPOSURE ALONE, SEVERE CARDIOVASCULAR OR RESPIRATORY PROBLEMS MAY DEVELOP.

Under most circumstances the surgeon will attempt to position the patient to provide maximum exposure with his incision; however, the cardiorespiratory effects of the Trendelenburg, kidney, lithotomy, and prone positions must be recognized.[5] Com-

163

promises may be necessary, especially in patients with severe hypotension or chest injuries. The devices needed to position patients for neurosurgical procedures tend to increase the likelihood of complications. Arm positions must also be considered; excessive abduction, extension, or external rotation, as during thoracic operations or with the patient in a prone position, may cause brachial-plexus stretch palsy. Shoulder braces further increase this risk.

Preoperative Evaluation

Some of the more important factors or systems requiring attention prior to anesthesia include ventilation, cardiovascular function, acid-base balance, and the gastrointestinal tract.[6]

VENTILATION. If there is any question about the adequacy of ventilation, special efforts must be made to determine depression of the respiratory center due to trauma or drugs, obstruction of the upper or lower airway, or hemopneumothorax. Any dentures and excess secretions must be removed. Since any air leak from the lung tends to be increased by the positive-pressure ventilation applied during general anesthesia, all pneumothoraces, even those of small size, should be preoperatively relieved with a chest tube. Moderate to large collections of blood should be removed with a large-caliber chest tube; small hemothoraces can be aspirated with a needle, but the patient must be watched carefully for continued bleeding or an iatrogenic pneumothorax.

CARDIOVASCULAR FUNCTION. Whenever possible, blood pressure, blood volume and tissue perfusion should be normal before the anesthetic is given.

PITFALL

IF EFFORTS ARE NOT MADE TO CORRECT OR PREVENT HYPOVOLEMIA PREOPERATIVELY, SEVERE HYPOTENSION, WHICH MAY BE DIFFICULT TO CORRECT, MAY DEVELOP DURING THE MANAGEMENT OF ANESTHESIA.

Some drop in blood pressure and cardiac output after induction of anesthesia may be due to myocardial depression, arteriolar vasodilation, and increase in vascular capacity. If the patient has been in shock or has had severe trauma, he may require large amounts of fluid and blood, not only to replace actual blood loss but also to compensate for continued movement of fluid into traumatized tissue. Although every effort should be made to correct hypovolemia before induction of the anesthetic, sometimes this is impossible. Under such circumstances, when blood is being lost faster than it can be replaced, immediate surgery and rapid control of the bleeding site are vital.

Patients with arrhythmias or suspected coronary insufficiency should have a preoperative EKG and be seen by a cardiologist. These patients must be monitored constantly with a cardioscope. Where applicable and available, an esophageal or precordial stethoscope can also provide valuable information.

Administration of digitalis and other cardiac drugs prior to the anesthetic should be done after consultation between the anesthesiologist and a cardiologist. Dose and route will vary with the seriousness of the cardiovascular problem, the time available, and the type and duration of the proposed surgery. If the patient has not been taking digitalis and has a tachyarrhythmia or congestive heart failure, we would partially digitalize him with 0.75 to 1.0 mg of digoxin I.V. at least an hour before surgery.

PITFALL

IF ACID-BASE OR ELECTROLYTE ABNORMALITIES ARE CORRECTED WITHOUT REGARD FOR THEIR DURATION OR THE RESULTANT CHANGES IN BLOOD VOLUME, THE PATIENT'S COMPENSATORY MECHANISMS MAY BE SERIOUSLY COMPROMISED.

ACID-BASE BALANCE AND ELECTROLYTES. If possible, serum electrolyte and arterial acid-base studies should be performed before all emergency surgery. Under most circumstances abnormalities should be corrected prior to anesthetic induction; in some instances, however, it is best to compromise. Patients with chronic electrolyte abnormalities have usually adapted quite well to their altered internal environment, and any sudden severe change may cause serious physiologic disturbances (Chap. 4). For example, the patient with chronic congestive heart failure treated with diuretics and a low salt diet for many months may have severe hyponatremia with serum sodium concentrations as low as 105 to 110 mEq/L; attempts to raise the serum sodium level rapidly are apt to result in severe overloading of the cardiovascular system. If blood volume is proper, the hyponatremia can be corrected slowly over a period of several days. Chronic deficiencies should be corrected slowly. With multiple abnormalities, the priorities are generally blood volume, pH, potassium, calcium, sodium and chloride, in that order.

PITFALL

IF THE STOMACH IS NOT EMPTIED BEFORE A GENERAL ANESTHETIC IS GIVEN, THE HAZARD OF REGURGITATION OF GASTRIC CONTENTS INTO THE LUNGS DURING INDUCTION AND IN THE IMMEDIATE POSTOPERATIVE PERIOD IS GREATLY INCREASED.

GASTROINTESTINAL TRACT. If the patient has eaten within four to six hours of the trauma, he may still have a large amount of food or fluid in his stomach. General anesthesia in such instances should be delayed or the stomach should be emptied with a nasogastric tube. If large quantities of solid food were eaten very recently, it may be wise occasionally to empty the stomach completely with an Ewald tube.

Preanesthetic Medications

The choice of preanesthetic medications includes a wide array of vagolytic drugs, narcotic and non-narcotic analgesics, hypnosedative barbiturates, and tranquilizers.[7] Although successful anesthesia may require several of these agents, the patient-doctor rapport is still the best hypnotic-sedative yet devised and may obviate the need for many preanesthetic pharmacologic agents with their inherent undesirable side effects. The dosage and timing of preanesthetic medications should be individualized, especially in patients requiring emergency surgery. We have found, as a rule of thumb, that no more than 50% of the usual dose used for elective surgery, as calculated by body size or weight and physiologic status, should be given to the patient requiring emergency surgery for trauma.

Of the various preanesthetic medications, atropine and scopolamine are by far the most commonly used.[8] Traditionally they have been given in doses of 0.4 to 0.6 mg I.M. about 30 to 60 minutes preoperatively to reduce bronchopulmonary secretions and the chance of vagovagal reflexes. However, the cardiovascular responses to trauma and anesthesia can often be evaluated better without the influence of these vagolytic drugs. If these agents are required on short notice, they can be given intravenously. If some relief of pain is considered mandatory preoperatively, the smallest dose of analgesic possible should be used after any hypovolemia has been corrected. In patients with multiple or severe trauma, it is occasionally difficult to differentiate between the confusion caused by CNS damage or hypoxia and that caused by drugs, especially if large doses have been used.

Intravenous Lines

It is a truism that the safety of an anesthetic procedure is often directly related to the functioning of the intravenous lines. In the severely injured patient, two or more I.V. needles or catheters of at least 18 gauge should be inserted and well secured with sutures and/or tape. If possible, one of the catheters should be advanced into the superior vena cava for measuring the

CVP response to fluid administration. Ideally one I.V. should be started in each arm. If adequate arm veins cannot be found, even by cutdowns, percutaneous catheterization of the external jugular or subclavian veins may be possible. If these veins are also unobtainable or if they are damaged proximally, leg veins will have to be used. We try to avoid using leg veins, except in infants, because of their relative inaccessibility to the anesthetist during surgery and the possible later complications of phlebothrombosis. If they must be used, cutdowns are usually performed on the greater saphenous veins at the ankles.

Preparation of Anesthetic Equipment

PITFALL

IF PERSONNEL AND EQUIPMENT ARE NOT CONSTANTLY PREPARED FOR OPERATION AT A MOMENT'S NOTICE, THE DELAY AND CONFUSION IN PERFORMING EMERGENCY SURGERY MAY BE DISASTROUS.

The patient with severe trauma is often rushed directly to surgery, with little or no forewarning to the operating-room personnel. In the rush to begin the procedure, a proper review of equipment, blood availability and drugs may not be carried out. Changing the soda-lime absorbent and checking gas-tank volumes, laryngoscopy blades and bulbs, inflation of endotracheal-tube cuffs, availability of proper respirators, suction facilities and many other tasks may be neglected or inaccurately performed. The solution lies in having the operative and anesthetic facility constantly and completely set up and checked out.

An important factor often neglected under emergency conditions is the sterility of anesthetic equipment. The absence of documented instances of infection transmitted from anesthetic and inhalation equipment is amazing; however, Lerner[9] has demonstrated not only the existence of such infection but also the specific pathogenesis. The methods used to clean and sterilize equipment need increased attention. "Nothing substitutes for elbow grease" is still the basic premise. Thorough mechanical cleansing with copious amounts of soap and water remains the foundation for later sterilization and wrapping of equipment. Disposable masks, endotracheal tubes and delivery tubes are the only absolute guarantees of cleanliness and sterility; the practice of reusing these "disposables" must be condemned as dangerous.

Blood-pressure Cuffs and Intra-arterial Lines

Use of the Riva-Rocci blood-pressure cuff is common practice; however, if the patient is moved or if the surgical assistants lean against the arm it may be impossible to check the blood pressure accurately. A second cuff on the opposite arm can be of value under such circumstances. A simple system involving an intra-arterial cannula (I.V. catheter, Cournand or Reilly needle, or even a scalp-vein needle) attached to a column of heparinized saline or Ringer's lactate has proven practical in our institution. This intra-arterial line is also invaluable for obtaining frequent blood gas and acid-base studies.

CONSIDERATIONS DURING ANESTHESIA

PITFALL

IF THERE IS A LACK OF COMMUNICATION BETWEEN THE SURGEON AND THE ANESTHETIST, NEITHER IS FULLY AWARE OF THE OTHER'S PROBLEMS, AND CANNOT ADJUST HIS TECHNIQUES OPTIMALLY TO HELP THE OTHER.

The interaction of the surgical and anesthetic teams must be cooperative and smooth; the concept of teamwork must be more than a mere cliché. The operating room is no place for a power struggle. Every individual on each team must not only perform his task with skill but must also assist his colleague wherever possible. Both the surgeon and anesthesiologist must keep each other informed as to the progress of the case and their needs.

The duration of an anesthetic can be an important prognostic factor, especially in the aged. Although the necessary surgery must be accomplished accurately and carefully, it should be done without undue delay. The idea that a patient can be kept under anesthesia safely for an indefinite period is a fallacy. Whenever possible the best and most experienced surgeon should perform the surgery in critically injured patients; this is not the time and place for a junior resident to perform a particular procedure for the first or second time.

Choice of Techniques

If the patient has eaten recently, the best anesthetic for procedures limited to the lower abdomen or lower extremities is a subarachnoid, lumbar-epidural, or caudal-epidural regional technique. Under such circumstances a regional anesthetic, such as a brachial-plexus block, might also be considered for surgery on the upper extremities.

Although regional anesthesia may be extremely useful in poor-risk patients, certain problems can develop from the pyschic effects of surgery during the conscious state coupled with the known propensity of the trauma patient to metabolize anesthetic agents poorly. An inadequate regional technique with later additions of general anesthetic agents can be far more dangerous than a general anesthetic alone given properly from the start. The risk of aspiration during induction of general anesthesia under the former circumstances is especially high. Although the choice of anesthetic technique is often a matter of individual judgment, general endotracheal anesthesia is generally our choice for surgery on the head, neck, chest and abdomen.

Choice of Agents

The specific anesthetic of choice is the one with which the anesthesiologist is most familiar and confident. The advantages and disadvantages of some of the more common agents are listed below.

NITROUS OXIDE AND THE HALOGENS. Nitrous oxide and the halogens, such as halothane (Fluothane) and methoxyflurane (Penthrane), are nonflammable and thus may be used in the presence of electrosurgical apparatus. Nitrous oxide by itself is a relatively weak general anesthetic. As a single agent, it must be given in such high concentrations to obtain proper depth of anesthesia that adequate oxygenation of the patient may be extremely difficult. For this reason, it is usually supplemented with other agents such as Pentothal and the muscle relaxants. In addition, because of its diffusion properties, nitrous oxide can cause pronounced gaseous intestinal distension.

The halogens are popular with many anesthesiologists. They can, however, depress catecholamine release and cause bradycardia. Induction with methoxyflurane is slow and may require significant amounts of other agents, with all their side effects. The question of hepatic cellular damage with the halogens has still not been completely settled; however, it seems prudent to avoid these agents in patients with known liver or biliary-tract disease or trauma, especially if halothane has been given during the previous 6 to 12 months. Renal damage has also been reported after deep methoxyflurane anesthesia.

ENFLURANE (Ethrane), 1-chloro-1,1,2-trifluoroethyl difluoromethyl ether. This halogenated hydrocarbon is a recent addition to our armamentarium. It produces significant muscle relaxation and potentiates the effects of pancuronium bromide. It does, however, have a tendency to produce tachycardia which may be significant enough to mask the early signs of blood loss. This agent is unique in that it may, in the presence of a low Pco_2, produce CNS stimulation leading to a disorientation pattern including convulsive manifestations. Like Penthrane, it must be used with great caution in patients with renal disease or renal transplants.

ETHER. Ether, a flammable and explosive agent, generally requires an induction agent such as a short-acting barbiturate to avoid a significant excitement phase. It stimulates increased catecholamine release, and can cause excessive sialorrhea and bronchorrhea that may be troublesome during induction and in the postoperative period. The nausea and regurgitation following the use of this agent are disturbing to the patient and may increase the risk of aspiration. Nevertheless, this drug is of particular value for the patient who cannot be intubated and in situations where the anesthetist desires to maintain spontaneous respirations and still provide good relaxation. Its irritating effect on the tracheobronchial tree can be profitably used to stimulate respiration.

CYCLOPROPANE. Cyclopropane approaches most closely the properties of an ideal anesthetic. It is rapid acting and supports the circulation better than most other anesthetics. Adequate oxygenation, even in the deepest stages of anesthesia, is easily maintained. Probably the greatest drawback is its explosiveness, which precludes the use of electrocautery and certain monitoring equipment. One of its other disadvantages is the increased catecholamine release which it can stimulate. In the presence of exogenous epinephrine or hypercarbia or other factors which stimulate epinephrine release, there may be an increased incidence of cardiac arrhythmias.

INNOVAR. Innovar, a combination of fentanyl and droperidol, can provide excellent narcotic and tranquilizing effects.[10] In practiced hands, this drug given by slow I.V. infusion gives safe effective anesthesia for minor operations and endoscopy. Dosage varies greatly from one individual to the next, but 1.0 cc for every 25 pounds of body weight given slowly over a 5- to 10-minute period is usually adequate initially. Its main side effects, respiratory depression and hypotension, can be prevented by close attention to dosage and the patient's response to the drug. Since minute volume may be somewhat depressed, it is wise to administer 100% oxygen by mask during and for at least a short time after administration of the drug.

KETAMINE. Intravenous ketamine hydrochloride (Ketaject, Ketalar) produces a "dissociative anesthesia" which may be of value for diagnostic and minor procedures. There is no muscle relaxation, and if large doses are given respiratory depression and other adverse effects may occur. Initially the blood pressure, pulse, and pharyngeal and laryngeal reflexes may temporarily be increased. Emergence hallucinations and tonic and clonic seizures will occasionally occur.

SHORT-ACTING BARBITURATES. The main advantage of the short-acting barbiturates (thiopental, methohexital, and methitural) lies in their remarkable smoothness of induction and ready acceptance by the patient. Usage, however, should be limited to supplementing other agents during the induction phase of general anesthesia and to producing drowsiness and sedation when a regional anesthetic is employed. Side effects are hypotension caused by myocardial depression and peripheral vasodilation. Correction of any hypovolemia prior to or during their use and with careful regulation of the dosage is essential.

PITFALL

IF SHORT-ACTING BARBITURATES ARE ACCIDENTALLY GIVEN INTRA-ARTERIALLY OR IN HIGH CONCENTRATIONS, THEY MAY CAUSE SEVERE VASCULAR SPASM AND THROMBOSIS WITH RESULTANT GANGRENE.

Because of the alkaline pH of these agents and their severe local vasospastic effects, concentrations of thiopental in excess of 2.5% should not be used. If intra-arterial injection or vasospasm is noted, immediate sympathetic blockade should be instituted with acidification of the region with local injections of procaine hydrochloride. In some instances an emergency thromboendarterectomy may be required.

Muscle Relaxants

These agents facilitate endotracheal intubation during anesthetic induction and provide good muscle relaxation without deep levels of general anesthesia. They do, however, have a number of side effects which must be considered, especially in patients with severe trauma.[11]

CURARE. Curare is a generic name for a number of arrow poisons obtained from tropical vines and used by South American Indians. These agents act by blocking the transmission of impulses at the myoneural junctions of skeletal muscle so that, although the muscle can respond to direct electrical stimulation and certain chemical agents, it does not respond to nerve stimulation.

PITFALL

IF CURARE IS GIVEN TO A HYPOTENSIVE OR HYPOVOLEMIC PATIENT, SEVERE CIRCULATORY COLLAPSE MAY OCCUR.

Some of curare's side effects include ganglionic blockade and histamine release, both of which can cause hypotension and circulatory collapse. The histamine release may occasionally also cause bronchospasm. Patients with myasthenia gravis are extremely sensitive to curare and respond excessively to very small doses. Neostigmine methylsulfate (Prostigmin) and edrophonium chloride (Tensilon), which inactivate cholinesterase and thereby permit acetylcholine to be built up, can be used to treat excessive or prolonged curariform effects.

FLAXEDIL. Gallamine triethiodide (Flaxedil) is a synthetic compound similar to the curare drugs but with certain advantages. It has no ganglionic blocking effect, does not cause bronchospasm and has a rapid onset and short duration of action. It may, however, cause allergic reactions in patients sensitive to iodine. Also, since its acetylcholine blocking action in the myocardium tends to cause a marked tachycardia, it is not the relaxant of choice in patients with cardiovascular disease.

Flaxedil has been used with increasing frequency to counteract the bradycardia caused by halothane. It may, however, be difficult to differentiate the tachycardia of Flaxedil from the tachycardia caused by hypovolemia; furthermore, the bradycardia of halothane may be a useful sign of the depth of anesthetic effect.

SUCCINYLCHOLINE. Succinylcholine chloride (Anectine) is an ultrashort-acting myoneural blocking agent which intensifies the depolarizing effect of acetylcholine to such an extent that repolarization of the endplate does not occur. Its short duration is due to its rapid hydrolysis by serum or pseudocholinesterase. Hydrolysis of the drug is increased in alkaline solution and, therefore, it is not mixed with drugs such as Pentothal or sodium bicarbonate.

PITFALL

IF SUCCINYLCHOLINE IS GIVEN TO PATIENTS WITH EXTENSIVE BURNS OR TISSUE DAMAGE, A CARDIAC ARREST MAY OCCUR.

There are relatively few drawbacks to succinylcholine. It does not cause ganglionic blockade or bronchospasm and has relatively few cardiovascular effects. It may, however, cause a sudden release of potassium from tissue. In patients who already have a hyperkalemia because of severe tissue damage, the sudden additional rise in serum potassium levels may result in asystole. A small percentage of patients are deficient in cholinesterase and, therefore, are extremely sensitive to small doses of this drug.[12-15]

PANCURONIUM BROMIDE (Pavulon). This curare-like muscle relaxant also has a tendency to produce tachycardia, but to a lesser degree than Flaxedil. In combination with Ethrane, however, this effect may reach significant levels. Because of this chronotropic effect and because there is no apparent histamine release, hypotension is not produced by this agent. This drug, like other curariform agents, is potentiated by the ethers.

Movement and Positioning

PITFALL

IF AN INJURED PATIENT IS MOVED ABRUPTLY OR HAS HIS POSITION CHANGED SUDDENLY, CARDIOVASCULAR COLLAPSE MAY OCCUR.

Severe falls in blood pressure are sometimes unexpectedly encountered when the trauma patient is moved from the stretcher or operating table or if his position is suddenly changed. The events which occur at these times, and which occasionally result in cardiac arrest, are usually preventable if certain precautions are observed. The trauma patient's central and peripheral cardiovascular compensatory reflexes are often impaired, and a sudden change in position may disrupt his fragile hemodynamic stability. The most common position changes associated with a hypotensive response include sudden, rapid rotation along the longitudinal axis (as in movement from the supine to the prone position) or change from the head-down (Trendelenburg) to the head-up (Fowler's) position.[16] Another marked effect can be provoked by suddenly lowering the patient from one horizontal plane to another.

Use of lithotomy, "kidney," and sitting positions, as mentioned earlier, can also produce cardiovascular and respiratory embarrassment. Elevation of the legs, as in the lithotomy position, forces the abdominal contents against the diaphragm, thereby limiting its excursion. The head-up position reduces venous return to the heart from the dependent portions of the body. If the patient has lost his ability to compensate for this more erect position by peripheral vasoconstriction, the reduced venous return and cardiac output can result in sudden severe hypotension. Extremes of lateral flexion caused by elevation of the kidney rest may not only create pressure on the inferior vena cava but can also produce vagal stimuli which tend to slow the heart and reduce cardiac output.

Airway Management

ENDOTRACHEAL INTUBATION. An endotracheal tube should be inserted in all emergency trauma patients undergoing general anesthesia. Endotracheal intubation provides a dependable airway, decreases dead space, reduces energy needs caused by ventilatory efforts, equalizes intrapulmonary and ambient airway pressures, and ensures a route for suctioning the tracheobronchial tree. If endotracheal intubation is difficult or if excessive tracheobronchial secretions, blood or debris are present, preintubation bronchoscopy may be required.[17] If the stomach cannot be emptied adequately, endotracheal intubation should be performed with the patient awake. In these situations, "twilight sleep" intubation can be employed using Innovar.[18] This technique is valuable because protective gag and cough reflexes remain intact.

PITFALL

IF THE PATIENT IS NOT ADEQUATELY ANESTHETIZED BEFORE THE ENDOTRACHEAL TUBE IS INSERTED, AN INCREASED INCIDENCE OF UNSUCCESSFUL INTUBATION AND COMPLICATIONS WILL RESULT.

The "crash technique" of rapid endotracheal intubation increases the risk of gastric regurgitation and often does not afford the anesthetist an adequate visualization of the larynx. Following trauma, especially if the patient is unconscious, dentures, gum, partially masticated food, or vomitus will frequently be found in the tonsillar fauces or pyriform sinuses.

While total visualization of the larynx is much less frequently obtained with the curved (MacIntosh) blade than with the straight (Eversole) variety, it is easier to use the curved blade, especially if the patient has protruding maxillary teeth or a short bull-neck habitus.

Stylets in endotracheal or endobronchial tubes may be helpful if the intubation is difficult or if the tubes are very soft or flexible; however, such stylets can cause perforation of the larynx, pharynx, or trachea. The endotracheal tube has a tendency to crimp or pull back on the stylet, thus exposing the metal tip. If a stylet must be used, the tip should be withdrawn within the tube a sufficient distance to prevent its protrusion, even with the crimping of the tube. The stylet should be withdrawn as soon as the tip of the endotracheal tube has passed between the vocal cords.

PITFALL

IF THE ENDOTRACHEAL TUBE IS NOT ACTU-
ALLY SEEN TO PASS BETWEEN THE VOCAL
CORDS DURING INTUBATION, ESOPHAGEAL IN-
TUBATION MAY OCCUR.

One of the most frequent and serious hazards of attempting to pass an endotracheal tube is inadvertent esophageal intubation. This will occasionally occur, even in the most experienced hands. Not only can severe hypoxia develop rapidly when this occurs but the resultant gastric distension may cause dangerous vagal reflexes and increase the chances of subsequent regurgitation and severe ileus.[19] Cardiac arrest under such circumstances is frequent. If the chest is watched carefully for bilateral expansion and the lungs are auscultated carefully while ventilating the patient

through the endotracheal tube, improper positioning should be discovered almost immediately. Furthermore, if the color of the blood in the incision is or becomes darker than normal, the position of the tube must be checked again.

Another pitfall of endotracheal intubation, either at the time of insertion or later during anesthesia, is inadvertent passage of the tube down too far into the right or left main-stem bronchus. Because the right main-stem bronchus comes off at a less acute angle from the trachea than the left (25° versus 45°) and is larger, the endotracheal tube is apt to go down to the right. Since transmitted breath sounds anteriorly will occasionally make the ventilation seem equal bilaterally even when the tube is down one side, the lower lobes must be auscultated in the midaxillary line.

Special precautions must be taken if there is the possibility of injury to the trachea. If an apparently well-inserted tube fails to function appropriately, the possibility of the tube having passed out through the lacerated area must be given serious consideration. In such circumstances, a rapid emergency tracheostomy may be lifesaving. The Magill intubating bronchoscope may be of special value in such patients. If a Magill bronchoscope is not available, a well-lubricated 5 or 6 F standard bronchoscope can be inserted into an endotracheal tube and the endotracheal tube passed to the desired location under direct vision.

If the tracheal or bronchial wound lies below the level of the cuff on the endotracheal tube, gases may be forced into the mediastinum. This will ultimately produce a tension pneumothorax which can compress the lungs and other vital structures and interfere with ventilation and venous return. Under such circumstances, either a Carlen's or Gordon-Green tube (which allows separate inflation of the lungs) or deliberate one-lung anesthesia with a standard endotracheal tube may be necessary.

TRACHEOSTOMY. Although endotracheal intubation is generally the safest and quickest method for providing complete airway control for general anesthesia, in some situations a tracheostomy is preferable. Tracheostomy is most apt to be needed if there is severe bleeding or trauma in the pharynx or larynx, preventing adequate visualization of or access to the glottis. Other problems include abnormalities or recent fractures of the cervical vertebrae, which contraindicate or prohibit any flexion of the neck.

In some instances the endotracheal tube can be inserted, but it may be too small to allow proper removal of clots or thick secretions. In addition, with certain types of severe trauma to the jaw or face, the endotracheal tube may restrict or impair efforts at repair or hemostasis. If a tracheostomy has to be performed under such circumstances, however, it is best accomplished over a previously placed endotracheal tube.

ENDOBRONCHIAL TUBES. In some seriously injured patients it may be imperative that the airway to one lung be guaranteed and protected from the ingress of blood or pus from the other side. Under such circumstances, endobronchial tubes may be life-saving; however, insertion and accurate placement, especially in an emergency, may

be extremely difficult and require extensive experience. Furthermore, since these tubes have a double lumen, each lumen is quite small, producing an increased resistance to air flow and moderate to severe difficulty in removing blood and thick secretions. The three main endobronchial tubes used are the Carlen's, White, and Gordon-Green tubes (Fig. 1).

The Carlen's tube is inserted into the left main-stem bronchus, while the White and Gordon-Green tubes are inserted into the right. The White tube has the disadvantage that right upper-lobe atelectasis is apt to occur unless the slit-like opening for ventilating this area is in exact position; fortunately this can usually be readily checked by auscultating over the right upper anterior chest. The Gordon-Green tube obviates this problem, but it has a small carinal hook that has a propensity to become detached. Another instrument, the Machray tube, may be inserted via an intubating (Magill) bronchoscope into the middle or lower bronchial orifices on the right or into the left upper-lobe bronchus. Correct positioning of the bronchoscope within the endotracheal tube is vital to prevent damage to the tracheobronchial tree.

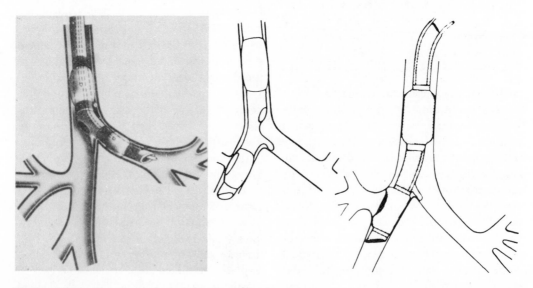

FIG. 1.   Endobronchial tubes. A: Carlen's, B: White, C: Gordon-Green.

In the patient with profuse hemoptysis, the main risk is asphyxiation; exsanguination through the tracheobronchial tree is rare. The first task in management is to localize the site of the bleeding. If the patient has a unilateral penetrating wound, the site of the bleeding is usually obvious; however, if the patient has had blunt trauma, bronchoscopy may be needed. It must be determined whether the bleeding is occurring from the right or left, and if possible the hemorrhage should be localized to a specific lobe or bronchopulmonary segment. The bleeding site should then be blocked off or isolated while the remaining lung tissue is ventilated. If an endobronchial tube or blocker cannot be inserted properly, the Parry-Brown or Overholt prone position and a posterior thoracic surgical approach should be considered.

Respirators

During any anesthesia, but particularly general anesthesia, it is vital to maintain adequate ventilation. Although the "educated hand" squeezing the breathing bag can rapidly detect relatively minor but important changes in lung compliance, it can quickly become the "tired hand" with a resultant decrease in tidal and minute volume. The other advantage of a respirator is that it frees the anesthetist to perform other tasks, including monitoring vital signs and administering blood and fluid, which are especially important if massive blood loss has occurred.

The objectives of ventilation are to prevent atelectasis and to maintain normal blood gases with a Pco_2 of 40 mm Hg or less and a Po_2 of 80 mm Hg or higher. It is, therefore, essential that a respirator of some type be used to help the anesthetist. Volume-cycled respirators are generally preferable to pressure-cycled respirators because they better maintain the desired levels of ventilation.[20] They do, however, have certain disadvantages related to the high ventilatory pressures they may develop, es-

pecially if a portion of the tracheobronchial tree becomes occluded.

High intrapulmonary pressures can reduce venous return and increase the chances of a pneumothorax. The impaired venous return may cause severe hypotension, especially if the patient is hypovolemic. The patient with emphysematous blebs, penetrating lung wounds, or prolonged shock is particularly apt to develop a pneumothorax. These risks are of increased concern if intrathoracic surgery requiring partial collapse of one lung is performed.

Monitoring

Monitoring of the trauma patient during anesthesia is generally much more exacting than during elective procedures. Less time and opportunity are available for preoperative preparation and the patient is affected not only by the anesthetic and surgery but also by the trauma, which may have severe immediate or delayed effects. Continuous monitoring is essential in these patients because the *trend* of the physiologic parameters provides the most important physiologic information.

VENTILATION. In addition to careful and continuous observation of tidal volume, ventilation pressures and the color of the skin, mucous membranes, and blood in the operative wound, facilities for rapid arterial blood gas analysis should be readily available at all times. It may be wise, especially in critically ill or injured patients, to insert an arterial needle or catheter preoperatively to facilitate frequent acid-base and blood gas analysis.

CARDIOVASCULAR. In addition to the routine frequent monitoring of the blood pressure and pulse during any general anesthetic, in the patient requiring emergency surgery for trauma, EKG (cardioscope) and CVP monitoring are extremely important. This is especially true if the patient has cardiac disease or injury, if massive hemorrhage has occurred, or if the surgery is to be difficult or prolonged.

Cardioscope

PITFALL

IF CARDIAC FUNCTION IS MONITORED ONLY BY THE CARDIOSCOPE, DIAGNOSIS OF IMPORTANT REDUCTIONS IN CARDIAC CONTRACTILITY AND OUTPUT MAY BE SERIOUSLY DELAYED.

Although the cardioscope is essential for early warning of arrhythmias and conduction abnormalities, it may provide little or no information on actual mechanical function. Blood pressure and cardiac output may be greatly reduced for some time with no change in the EKG. On occasion, moreover, we have noted normal EKG activity in a situation in which the blood pressure was unobtainable and the cardiac output was negligible.

Central Venous Pressure (CVP). The CVP, especially its response, is an important guide to the rate and volume of fluid administration. In seriously injured patients, especially those requiring massive transfusions, the CVP should be measured almost continuously. This, of course, requires having one or two additional large I.V. lines for administering drugs, blood, or other fluids as needed.

PITFALL

IF THE INFUSION OF BLOOD AND FLUID IN A HYPOTENSIVE PATIENT IS RESTRICTED BECAUSE HE HAS A HIGH CVP, DANGEROUS HYPOVOLEMIA MAY BE ALLOWED TO PERSIST.

Estimation of blood and fluid needs during general anesthesia is notoriously difficult. Positive-pressure ventilation and the cardiodepressant effects of most general anesthetics tend to raise the CVP to much higher levels than might otherwise be present. The pulmonary wedge pressure may be a much better fluid guide. Close measurement of blood loss into the suction bottles and onto the sponges must be correlated with the amount of fluid and blood given and the response of *all* physiologic parameters.

TEMPERATURE. Monitoring of rectal and esophageal temperatures should be routine during most general anesthetics, especially if the patient is critically injured or septic, or is younger than two years. Hypothermia tends to develop if the surgery is prolonged and large incisions are used, especially if large amounts of cold blood or fluid are administered and the patient is hypotensive. On the other hand, severe hyperthermia may occur in small infants who are covered with heavy drapes and in patients who are septic.

In rare instances a syndrome of "hereditary idiopathic hyperthermia" may occur, with sudden development of extremely high temperatures and death. This syndrome is believed to be due to a hereditary idiosyncrasy to some of the anesthetics and succinylcholine causing phosphorylase uncoupling and depletion of muscle cell potassium. Early recognition of a rising temperature may allow the institution of cooling procedures before hypoxia, hypercarbia, and convulsions occur.

THE APPROACH TO SPECIAL PROBLEMS

A number of situations pose special problems for the anesthesiologist, especially when he is required to give anesthesia for emergency surgery on trauma victims. Some of these special problems include: diabetes mellitus, alcoholism, head injuries, eye trauma, chest trauma, blast injuries, smoke inhalation, abdominal distension, obesity, antibiotics, air embolism, pacemakers, and cardiopulmonary bypass.

Diabetes Mellitus (Chap. 4)

PITFALL

IF SPECIAL EFFORTS ARE NOT MADE TO IDENTIFY THE DIABETIC OR PREDIABETIC PATIENT PREOPERATIVELY, DANGEROUS METABOLIC AND ELECTROLYTE PROBLEMS MAY DEVELOP DURING THE ANESTHESIA.

General anesthetics, severe trauma, hypotension and sepsis tend to cause hyperglycemia and ketosis. If the patient is diabetic or prediabetic this tendency is greatly increased, and the resultant metabolic and electrolyte changes may be extremely difficult to treat. Frequent measurements of blood and urine glucose and acetone are essential. Since these patients also tend to develop osmotic diuresis and gastric stasis or vomiting, all fluid deficits must be corrected rapidly before the anesthetic is administered.

PITFALL

IF A MILD TO MODERATE DIABETES MELLITUS IS TREATED TOO AGGRESSIVELY WITH INSULIN, A RELATIVELY HARMLESS HYPERGLYCEMIA MAY BE CONVERTED INTO A DANGEROUS HYPOGLYCEMIA.

A mild amount of glycosuria without acetonuria is usually welcome during the anesthetic and indicates that an adequate amount of glucose is available to meet current metabolic needs. Attempts to reduce the blood glucose levels to normal may result in hypoglycemia, which is dangerous not only because it is apt to cause severe hypotension or death but also because it is difficult to recognize under anesthesia.

Insulin is given primarily to control acetonuria. Long-acting insulins, such as PZI, lente, and NPH, are avoided because their effects may not be seen until much later, when the patient is in the recovery room or on the ward. Multiple small doses (10 to 25 units) of regular insulin intravenously every one to two hours, with or without 10 to 25 units added to each liter of fluid containing 5% glucose, are preferable to larger less frequent doses.

Alcoholism (Chap. 6)

The alcoholic presents many special problems related to acute alcoholic intoxication, cirrhosis, and delirium tremens. These patients are apt to develop sudden cardiovascular collapse, respiratory depression or obstruction, aspiration of gastric contents, and resistance or intolerance to anesthetic agents.[21,22]

If emergency surgery is needed, proper management for even relatively minor procedures includes careful volume replacement, emptying of the stomach with a nasogastric tube, and control of ventilation through an endotracheal tube. If the patient has frank or impending delirium tremens, the risks of anesthesia and surgery are extremely high; all except the most vital emergency operations should be delayed. If surgery cannot be put off, $MgSO_4$ (1 to 2 gm I.M. every 4 to 6 hours) and Valium (diazepam) (5 to 10 mg I.V. every 1 to 4 hours) as needed may help to control many of the neuromuscular problems. The use of I.V. 10% alcohol infusion is controversial, but may be helpful if the patient develops delirium tremens in spite of other measures.

Head Injuries (Chap. 14)

In addition to difficulties in gauging the depth of anesthesia in patients with head injuries, special problems are related to intracranial hematomas, cerebral edema, and the positions required for neurosurgery. Occasionally after the removal of an epidural or subdural hematoma, the previously unconscious patient may become severely restless, disturbed and combative; it is essential, therefore, that the anesthesiologist be made completely aware of each step in the procedure so he can properly anticipate such reactions.

Cerebral edema due to trauma or hypoxia may make control of the respiratory and cardiovascular systems extremely difficult. If an intracranial procedure is performed, severe brain swelling may make the operation extremely difficult and dangerous. Under these circumstances, osmotic diuretics may be needed to shrink the brain; later, however, a rebound effect and increased cerebral edema and hypertension may develop. Since hypocarbia and hyperoxemia cause cerebral vessels to constrict, hyperventilation can also be used to help reduce the cerebral edema.

The positions required for certain neurosurgical procedures can also create a number of problems. The prone position reduces the ventilatory capacity of relatively normal patients by as much as 25%; in obese patients, the reduction is even greater and can be extremely dangerous. If the patient must lie prone, his body must be supported and positioned so that abdominal or thoracic expansion is not limited. All pressure points must be well padded to prevent nerve damage, and the eyes must be well protected. The sitting position, since it tends to cause dependent pooling of blood, may be associated with severe hypotension, especially if the patient is hypovolemic. The erect position also increases the likelihood of air embolus through any open vein in the head or neck.

Eye Disease or Trauma (Chap. 15)

The possibility of frank or incipient glaucoma must be considered in any patient over 35 years of age. Although much has been written about the dangers of causing exacerbation of glaucoma with belladonna derivatives,[23,24] there is relatively little danger when these drugs are given in their usual dosages. Succinylcholine on the other hand is much more dangerous.[25,26] Even at low dosages this agent produces fasciculations of the orbicularis oculi muscle with a resultant constriction or narrowing of the canal of Schlemm. In narrow-angle glaucoma the occlusion may become complete, causing a rapid increase in the intraocular pressure. Even in normal patients succinylcholine can raise intraocular tension by an average of 7.5 to 8.5 mm Hg, and has been implicated in vitreous extrusion in patients with eye injuries. These dangers can be reduced by adding Mylaxen (hexafluorenium), which reduces the probability of orbicularis oculi fasciculation and prolongs the activity of the succinylcholine. An older technique using d-tubocurarine with succinylcholine produces less predictable effects.

AXIOM

IF THE PATIENT HAS A RETINAL INJURY, HE MUST NOT BE ALLOWED TO BEAR DOWN OR STRAIN.

The possibility of a retinal detachment should be considered in any patient with a history of a sudden blow to the head, neck, or thorax, especially if he is hypertensive. This problem is uncommon; however, if a patient with this injury gags, coughs, retches or performs a Valsalva maneuver during the anesthetic, the increased venous pressure can severely aggravate the detachment. Early ophthalmologic consultation is necessary and, at the end of the operation, extubation should be done during the apneic state with full awakening under mask control.

Anesthetic masks must be used with great care in anyone with a possible facial injury, especially if the eyes are involved. The pressure applied by the mask, particularly in the area of the supraorbital notch, can severely aggravate injuries in that area. Prolonged pressure can also interfere with the lymphatic and venous drainage from the periorbital and nasal structures, causing increased swelling and hemorrhage.

Chest Trauma (Chap. 20)

Hemothorax, pneumothorax and pulmonary contusion, especially if large, may reduce vital capacity and interfere with ventilation and venous return; not uncommonly, moreover, the pneumothorax may increase rapidly during the anesthetic because of the positive-pressure ventilation. Even a small pneumothorax should be removed and controlled with a chest tube prior to giving a general anesthetic.

Hemoptysis, as mentioned earlier, is cause for great concern; bleeding into the bronchi can cause bronchial occlusion, atelectasis, and severe postoperative pneumonia. In some instances the hemorrhage may be severe enough to require the use of a Carlen's tube or endobronchial blocker.

Myocardial contusion can be associated with arrhythmias and/or impaired contractility, which are apt to become worse during anesthesia. Pericardial tamponade should be at least partially relieved prior to anesthesia.

If a rupture of the thoracic aorta is suspected, the anesthetist must be especially careful not to allow the patient to cough, retch, buck, or perform a Valsalva maneuver; a partially torn aorta in one recent patient completely ruptured when the patient bucked during insertion of a Levin tube.

Blast Injuries

Blast injuries may damage the lungs directly and indirectly. During the positive phase of the blast, alveoli and emphysematous blebs may rupture creating bilateral tension pneumothoraces. During the negative phase, intrapulmonary hemorrhage and pulmonary edema may develop. Unfortunately, although many of these changes may not be apparent initially, they may cause progressive pulmonary difficulty later during anesthesia. Repeated careful evaluation of the lung, with judicious use of fluids and ventilatory pressure, is essential in such individuals.

Smoke Inhalation

Patients with burns or smoke inhalation in closed spaces may have heat damage to the upper airway and may develop a severe chemical (smoke) pneumonitis. Ciliary action and surfactant may be destroyed, and there may be acute pulmonary edema

with petechial hemorrhages. In some instances bronchoscopy may be necessary to remove tracheobronchial casts. These patients also tend to develop severe bronchospasm, which may require treatment with bronchodilators, nebulizer-humidifiers, helium-oxygen mixtures[20] and positive-pressure volume-controlled ventilator assistance.

AXIOM

PULMONARY CHANGES DUE TO BURNS ARE OFTEN DELAYED.

Not uncommonly there may be little or no clinical evidence of lung damage when the patient is first seen. Pulmonary changes, however, can be rapidly progressive over the next 24 to 48 hours. Under these circumstances the chemical pneumonitis may not be recognized until respiratory failure is well established and extremely difficult to treat. Steroids may be of some help with this problem, especially if given prophylactically, by reducing the inflammatory changes in the lung.

Abdominal Distension

Distension of the abdomen with ascitic fluid, blood or gastrointestinal air or fluid limits diaphragmatic motion and ventilation. If severe ascites is present in a patient with marginal pulmonary function, the ascites should be partly relieved prior to or shortly after the induction of the general anesthetic. The ascitic fluid should be removed slowly to allow the patient to accommodate to the altered hemodynamics. Additional fluid may have to be given later as the ascites reaccumulates at the expense of the intravascular volume.

If there has been massive bleeding into the abdomen, the surgeon and the anesthetist must cooperate closely, recognizing that the release of the abdominal tamponade may be followed by torrential hemorrhage and sudden severe hypotension. Efforts must be made to transfuse such patients rapidly just before and after the abdomen is opened. If the hypotension cannot be corrected preoperatively, some surgeons will open the chest to clamp the descending aorta just above the diaphragm before performing the laparotomy.

Obesity

PITFALL

IF RESPIRATION IN THE OBESE PATIENT IS NOT ASSISTED UNTIL HE HAS COMPLETELY REACTED FROM THE GENERAL ANESTHETIC, VENTILATION MAY BE DANGEROUSLY IMPAIRED.

Obese patients present a number of anesthetic problems related to airway management and ventilation. They frequently have a short bull neck which can make endotracheal intubation or tracheostomy extremely difficult. Because of the great weight of the chest wall and the pressure of the abdominal wall and viscera against the diaphragm, it takes great effort to inflate the lungs of severely obese patients. In these patients, direct inflation of the lungs with a volume-cycled respirator is necessary throughout the procedure and until the patient is almost completely awake and can definitely breathe adequately on his own. Pressure-cycled respirators in such individuals are almost useless.

Other problems with very obese patients include difficulties in positioning the patient and in producing enough relaxation of the abdominal wall to provide the surgeon with adequate exposure. Fortunately, spinal anesthetics (subarachnoid blocks) can usually be accomplished, even in extremely obese patients.

Antibiotics

AXIOM

DURING GENERAL ANESTHESIA ANTIBIOTICS WHICH MAY HAVE NEUROMUSCULAR EFFECTS SHOULD BE AVOIDED.

A number of antibiotics can interfere with neuromuscular ganglionic transmission mechanisms[27,28] and may cause prolonged postoperative apnea or hypopnea, especially if the anesthetist uses ether or any drugs which also have a ganglionic blocking effect (Table 1). Such antibiotics should *not* be given I.V., I.M., or into any body cavities during anesthesia.

TABLE 1. ANTIBIOTICS APT TO CAUSE ANESTHESIA COMPLICATIONS

Streptomycin	Dihydrostreptomycin
Kanamycin (Kantrex)	Paromomycin
Polymyxin A	(Humatin)
Viomycin (Vinactane, Viocin)	Polymyxin B (Aerosporin)
Neomycin B and C	Colistin (Coly-Mycin)

The neuromuscular blockade produced by these antibiotics appears to be similar to that caused by high doses of magnesium. These agents decrease acetycholine liberation at the motor end-plate and, by suppressing calcium activation of adenosine triphosphate in the myosin, also increase the resistance of the end-plate to any acetycholine that is released. This effort is the same whether depolarizing or nondepolarizing agents are used and can be antagonized or reversed by ionic calcium.

All new antibiotics should be viewed with suspicion and should not be used with a general anesthetic until they have been thoroughly investigated and found to be free of neuromuscular effects. At the present time, the tetracyclines, chloramphenicol, penicillins, and erythromycin appear to be safe during anesthesia, except for possible allergic reactions.

Air Embolism

Air embolism is one of the most dreaded complications of anesthesia. This problem is most apt to occur during operations that involve the head or neck, especially if the head is elevated. Large amounts of air in the right heart can cause severe foaming and blockade of the right ventricle or pulmonary artery similar to that seen with multiple or large pulmonary emboli. On the left side of the heart, even a small amount of air, as may develop during cardiac surgery or through congenital or traumatic right-to-left heart shunts, may be pumped without warning into the coronary or cerebral circulation with a resultant myocardial or cerebral infarct.

The diagnosis of air embolism must be suspected any time hypotension or cardiac abnormality develops suddenly, especially if surgery is being performed on the head or neck of a patient whose head is elevated. The characteristic murmur is a loud, churning, so-called mill-wheel murmur. Other diagnostic features include sudden cyanosis, hypotension, enlarged neck veins, tachycardia and respiratory distress. In this situation the esophageal stethoscope can be extremely valuable.

If the diagnosis is suspected, the surgeon must immediately search for and occlude any open vein. Therapy includes placing the patient in the head-down position with the right side up, allowing the air to rise to the apex of the heart and permit the aortic and pulmonary valves to be bathed with blood. A long needle is then inserted into the apex of the right ventricle to aspirate the air and foamy blood.

Pacemakers

Even without a proper preoperative history, chest x-ray or EKG, the presence of an epicardial pacemaker should be suspected by the presence of a scar on the chest and is confirmed by palpation of the battery case under the skin of the chest or abdomen. The endocardial pacemaker, however, may be more difficult to discover.

Trauma may cause intermittent or complete malfunction of a pacemaker. The electrodes may be displaced, or the implantation site or batteries may be damaged. If there is any indication of malfunction, a temporary transvenous pacemaker should be inserted and its proper function confirmed preoperatively. Special care must be taken not to disengage such a transvenous electrode while positioning or moving the patient. Even if the implanted pacemaker is functioning properly, a temporary pacemaker should be available in the operating room. The EKG monitor attached to such patients should have an external pacing attachment in case of failure of the transvenous system. An isoproterenol solution (0.2 mg in 100 ml) should be prepared and hung up so that an infusion can be begun immediately if the need arises.

Once continued proper function of the pacemaker is assured, it must be determined that cardiac filling is adequate. The pulse rate is often either fixed or incapable of adjusting properly if hypovolemia or hypotension develops. Accordingly, changes in cardiac output are determined primarily by venous return and resultant stroke volume.

It is especially important when operating on individuals with pacemakers that all electrical equipment be grounded properly. Electrocautery is also often contraindicated because it can interfere with the electric circuitry of the pacemaker.

Cardiopulmonary Bypass

Anesthetic management for emergency cardiopulmonary bypass requires a high degree of organization, preparation, and checking of drugs and monitoring equipment prior to surgery. The availability and effectiveness of back-up equipment must also be checked. Checklists are valuable, especially for the setting up of the pump. All probable medications should be drawn preoperatively and other agents should be in tabletop readiness. The availability and cross-matching of blood and/or blood components should be personally checked by the anesthesiologist. The proper nursing and laboratory personnel must be present in the operating room or in the hospital. Everything must be checked; nothing can be assumed.

POSTANESTHETIC MANAGEMENT

PITFALL

IF THE PATIENT IS NOT FOLLOWED CLOSELY
IN THE RECOVERY ROOM, ANESTHETIC COM-
PLICATIONS INCREASE MARKEDLY.

The responsibility of the anesthetist does
not stop when the patient leaves the operating room. Not infrequently the serious
complications of the anesthetic occur while
the patient is being removed or after he
has arrived in the recovery room. Reversal
of the effects of any muscle relaxants may
not be as complete as is clinically suggested, particularly if nerve stimulator
monitoring was not utilized throughout the
course of the anesthesia. In addition, removal of the stimulus of the endotracheal
tube may permit the patient to slip into a
greater depth of sleep. With few exceptions, the anesthesiologist should not feel
compelled to remove the endotracheal tube
early in the recovery phase. By leaving the
tube in place, dead space and the consequent energy required for ventilation are
reduced. Indeed, an assistor-ventilator may
be readily attached to the endotracheal
tube with a view to thoroughly and rapidly
washing out the inhalation anesthetic agent
and diminishing the incidence and severity
of postoperative atelectasis.

The patient who can remove his own
endotracheal tube is usually alert and
strong enough to maintain his own airway
even in the event of postoperative nausea
and retching. Exceptions to this policy of
leaving the tube in place, as mentioned
previously, include patients with possible
retinal detachments or intracardiac shunts,
where even the slightest increase in venous
pressure may have significant adverse results.

SUMMARY (Table 2)

Application of the scientific method of
logic plus data interrelation, together with
a complete understanding of the technical
requirements of the proposed procedures
and the pathophysiologic situation presented, serve as the basis for rational anesthesiologic management.

Preoperative evaluation of critically injured patients must be rapid and thorough,
even if only minor surgery is contemplated.

TABLE 2.   MOST FREQUENT ERRORS IN ANESTHETIC MANAGEMENT OF CRITICALLY
INJURED PATIENTS

1. Failing to take time and effort to effectively evaluate the patient's vital status.
2. Delaying surgery for diagnostic studies on parameters either not vital for the *immediate* surgico-
   anesthetic management or impossible to change in the time available.
3. Allowing oneself to be rushed into a method of anesthetic management that, on reflection, one
   would not ordinarily choose.
4. Proceeding without adequate blood products or substitutes, and/or proceeding without adequate
   routes for administration of fluids (colloid and noncolloid) and electrolytes.
5. Giving too much medication to patients scheduled for imminent operation, particularly during the
   induction phase of anesthetic management.
6. Failing to have an emergency drug and equipment setup ready on a 24-hour basis.
7. Failing to communicate with others involved in management of the patient.
8. Failing to anesthetize the patient adequately before endotracheal intubation is begun.
9. Failing to anticipate and be prepared for the possibility of regurgitation and resultant aspiration.
10. Failing (on the part of the entire team) to maintain vigilance and direct personal attention during
    the period immediately after surgery and after transfer to the recovery room or other special-care
    facility.

The choices of drugs, fluids and positioning should be discussed with the surgeon pre-operatively and constant communication must be maintained during and after the surgery. Cardiovascular and pulmonary function must be monitored closely on an almost constant basis, with no letdown in the postoperative period.

REFERENCES

1. Thornton, H. L., and Knight, P. F.: *Emergency Anesthesia*. Baltimore, Williams & Wilkins, 1965.
2. Green, N. M.: *Anesthesia for Emergency Surgery*. Philadelphia, F. A. Davis, 1963.
3. Symposium on Trauma. Brit. J. Anaesth., 38:4, 1966.
4. Norton, M. L.: Pre-operative appraisal of the surgical patient. J. Int. Coll. Surg., 38:308, 1962.
5. Jenkins, M. J.: *Common and Uncommon Problems in Anesthesiology*. Philadelphia, F. A. Davis, 1968.
6. Guyton, Arthur C.: *Functions of the Human Body*, 4th ed. Philadelphia, W. B. Saunders, 1974.
7. Egbert, L. D., et al.: A comparison in man of the effects of promethazine, secobarbital, and meperidine, alone and in combinations, on certain respiratory functions and for use in pre-anesthetic medication. Southern Med. J., 51:1173, 1958.
8. Index X. Acta Scand. Anaesth., 1966.
9. Lerner, A. M.: Primary gram negative pneumonias. Med. Times, 97:118, 1969.
10. Laborit, H.: *Stress and Cellular Function*. Philadelphia, J. B. Lippincott, 1959.
11. Feldman, S. A.: Muscle relaxants. In: *Major Problems in Anesthesia*, Vol. 1. Philadelphia, W. B. Saunders, 1973.
12. Moncreif, J. A.: Complications of burns. Ann. Surg., 147:443, 1958.
13. Belin, R. P., and Karleen, C. I.: Cardiac arrest in the burned patient following succinylcholine administration. Anesthesiology 27:516, 1966.
14. Schaner, P. J., et al.: Succinylcholine-induced hyperkalemia in burned patients. Anesth. Analg., 48:764, 1966.
15. Editorial: Succinylcholine and trauma. JAMA, 210:549, 1969.
16. Dripps, R. D., et al.: *Introduction to Anesthesia*, 4th ed. Philadelphia, W. B. Saunders, 1972.
17. Norton, M. L.: Development of a program in laryngoscopy, therapeutic bronchoscopy and endobronchial blocking techniques. Michigan Med., 68:217, 1969.
18. Sellick, B. A.: Cricoid pressure to control regurgitation of stomach contents during induction of anesthesia. Lancet, 2:404, 1961.
19. Giuffrida, J. G., and Bizzari, D.: Intubation of the esophagus: Its role in preventing aspiration pneumonia and asphyxial death. Amer. J. Surg., 93:329, 1956.
20. Egan, D. F.: *Fundamentals of Inhalation Therapy*. St. Louis, C. V. Mosby, 1969.
21. Harger, R. N., and Hulpieu, H. R.: The pharmacology of alcohol. In: *Alcoholism* (Thompson, G. N., Ed.). Springfield, Charles C Thomas, 1956.
22. Kapant, H.: The pharmacology of alcohol intoxication. Quart. J. Stud. Alcohol, Suppl. 1, 1961.
23. Leopold, I. H., and Comroe, J. H., Jr.: Effect of intramuscular administration of morphine, atropine, scopalomine and neostigmine on the human eye. Arch. Ophthal., 40:285, 1940.
24. Schwartz, H., et al.: Pre-anesthetic use of atropine and scopalomine in patients with glaucoma. JAMA, 165:144, 1957.
25. Lincoff, H., et al.: The effect of succinylcholine on intraocular pressure. Amer. J. Ophthal., 40:54, 1955.
26. Schwartz, H., and deRoetth, A., Jr.: Effect of succinylcholine on intraocular pressure in human beings. Anesthesiology, 19:1, 1958.
27. Symposium on muscle relaxants. Anesthesiology, 20:4, 1959.
28. Emery, E. R. J.: Neuromuscular blocking properties of antibiotics as a cause of postoperative apnoea. Anaesthesia, 18:57, 1963.

Suggested Reading

1. Aviado, D. M.: *Krantz and Carr's Pharmacologic Principles of Medical Practice*, 8th ed. Baltimore, Williams & Wilkins, 1972.
2. Katz, J.: *Experimentation with Human Beings*. New York, Russel Sage Foundation, 1972.
3. Snow, J. C.: *Anesthesia in Otolaryngology and Ophthalmology*. Springfield, Charles C Thomas, 1972.
4. Katz, J., and Kadis, L. B.: *Anesthesia and Uncommon Diseases: Pathophysiologic and Clinical Correlations*. Philadelphia, W. B. Saunders, 1973.
5. Smith, R. B.: Anesthesia in ophthalmology. Int. Ophthal. Clin., 13:2, 1973.
6. Mushin, W. W.: *Major Problems in Anesthesia*, Vol. 2. Philadelphia, W. B. Saunders, 1973.
7. Eckenhoff, J. E., et al.: *Yearbook of Anesthesia*. Chicago, Year Book Medical Publishers, 1973.
8. Oyama, T.: Neuroleptanesthesia. Int. Anesth. Clin., 11:3, 1973.
9. Hewer, C. L.: Recent advances in anaesthesia and analgesia. Int. Anesth. Clin., 11:1, 1973.
10. Ingelfinger, F. J., et al.: *Controversy in Internal Medicine*, Vols I and II. Philadelphia, W. B. Saunders, 1974.

13 RADIOLOGIC CONSIDERATIONS IN TRAUMA

R. KURTZMAN

LOCATION, FACILITIES, AND PERSONNEL

To care for injured patients efficiently and safely, a major diagnostic radiology facility must be immediately available in or near the emergency area. Further facilities to perform angiographic and other sophisticated radiologic procedures must be available either in the same suite or in an easily accessible area elsewhere in the hospital.

The necessary x-ray equipment includes generators and tubes capable of very rapid exposures of at least 1/120 second when not using a Bucky diaphragm to 1/30 second when using a high-speed reciprocating Bucky. The generators should be rated at a minimum of 500 milliamperes at 150 kvp. The x-ray tubes should be heavy-duty, ceiling-hung types. An upright Bucky and tilt-table are necessary, as is a rack for examination of the chest. Each room must be equipped with appropriate restraints for examinations of the skull, chest, abdomen, and extremities. Radiotranslucent stretchers are also desirable, since with them examinations can be performed on seriously injured patients without their having to be moved.

Even more important than the required space and equipment is the need for technologists, nurses, and other personnel trained to the special circumstances of an emergency department. The radiology facility must be staffed on a full 24-hour basis, every day of the year, and a radiologist must be available for consultation at all times. The personnel in the x-ray department routinely should be given the following information on each case:

1. where the patient is
2. how he is to be transported
3. what precautions should be observed
4. what the presumptive diagnoses are
5. what is to be examined.

Films must be taken carefully and processed and interpreted rapidly so that any further or repeat examinations needed can be obtained without moving the patient unnecessarily.

PLANNING FOR X-RAYS

When Should X-rays be Obtained?

CLINICAL INDICATIONS. When it is perfectly clear that an injury is superficial and does not involve bones or viscera, an x-ray examination is wasteful and therefore undesirable. At the other extreme, some patients are so severely injured that roentgenologic examinations may waste time vitally needed for resuscitation and treatment, and may in fact be directly harmful if much movement of the patient is involved.

Between these two poles, there are circumstances where the value of x-rays is unequivocal:

1. All patients for whom general anesthesia is contemplated should have preliminary chest x-rays, except those desperately in need of immediate operation. If a preoperative chest x-ray is not taken and examined, the anesthesiologist should be informed of this deliberate omission so that the possibility of an occult pneumothorax or other thoracic lesion is kept in mind.

2. All overt or suspected fractures should be x-rayed. With the latter, apart from the desirability of establishing a definitive diagnosis, later medicolegal harassment may be avoided.

3. In soft-tissue injuries in which, after exploration, there is even a remote possibility of a residual foreign body such as glass, x-rays must be taken. Certain foreign bodies, particularly wood, plastic, and some types of glass, however, are not radiopaque and are, therefore, invisible radiologically.

4. With injuries which may be serious but cannot be adequately evaluated by physical examination alone, appropriate x-rays may be the only preoperative method of uncovering the lesion. This situation is typified by some cases of rupture of the diaphragm or thoracic aorta and certain renal injuries.

MEDICOLEGAL ASPECTS. In these litigious times, increasing numbers of lawsuits are being filed against physicians. A simplistic view of the nature of x-ray examinations had led to the application of the principle of "res ipsa loquitor" (the thing speaks for itself) in cases of trauma. In other words, it has been considered negligent not to have had x-rays made of an injured area, even if the physician believed such examinations to be unnecessary. From the strictly medical position, if treatment is the same and outcome identical regardless of the x-ray, the importance of radiologic examinations is dubious. Careful clinical notes, with appropriate instruction given to the patient to return if symptoms persist, could eliminate a large percentage of unnecessary x-ray examinations in trauma patients without prejudicing the patient's well-being or jeopardizing the physician. In practice, however, many clinicians because of current social pressures often feel forced, for their own protection, to request unnecessary radiologic examinations. At the same time, physicians are held accountable for the rising costs of medical care. This is a dilemma for which no solution can be offered here.

History and Physical Examination

Important but often neglected prerequisites of an accurate and useful roentgenologic examination are a careful history and physical examination. In dealing with minor fractures, it is helpful to know the site of tenderness when trying to evaluate a shadow which could be a normal variant or the result of an old injury. Clinical histories which say "fell off bus on corner of Woodward and Michigan" or "beat up by boy friend" or "stabbed with hat pin by old lady resisting arrest, please x-ray abdomen," while illuminating, do not illuminate the right things. Statements such as "bruised left shoulder with crepitus," or "marked swelling of face and lids," or "board-like abdomen with no bowel sounds" are much better.

Consultation and Preparation

The radiologist can be of great benefit to the clinician if he is used as a consultant. Once the radiologist knows the information the clinician wants and the most pertinent facts from the clinical examination, he can intelligently direct his technicians to obtain the most rewarding examinations. Limitations of methods, and possible rewards, can be better understood through a dialogue between clinician and radiologist.

Not only does careful planning save time but it also decreases the chances of serious complications developing unnoticed while the patient is being x-rayed. Aspiration, serious bleeding or cardiac arrest may occur in the x-ray department when the patient's stay there is prolonged. Some of the important aspects of planning are:

1. Evaluation of the complete radiologic needs of the whole patient, to avoid a series of trips to the x-ray facility.
2. Communication by the clinician of the urgency of and amount of time available for getting these studies.
3. Assessment of technical considerations— time and number of exposures required, safe positioning of the patient, potential need for special investigations such as arteriography, etc.
4. Assurance that appropriate medical or nursing personnel are at hand to supervise the airway, monitor I.V. fluids and prevent undesirable movement of the patient while he is being x-rayed.

X-RAY REPORTS. It should be understood that a record of the radiologic report and diagnosis, typed if possible, should be made available rapidly and included in the patient's chart. Rapid reporting is important to physicians and nurses for guiding and accelerating therapy and for ensuring completeness of the record.

Wherever possible, the clinician should review the films, especially if there is a dis-

AXIOM

ALWAYS CROSS-CHECK THE X-RAYS WITH THE PATIENT'S IDENTIFICATION AND CLINICAL FEATURES. IN A BUSY EMERGENCY DEPARTMENT, IT IS EASY TO MIX X-RAY REPORTS AND ATTACH THEM TO THE WRONG PATIENTS. SUCH MISTAKES MAY HAVE EMBARRASSING, DISASTROUS, AND EXPENSIVE RESULTS.

crepancy between the clinical picture and the initial radiologic interpretation. Ideally, all x-ray examinations should be reviewed by the radiologist and clinician together.

THE RADIOLOGIC EXAMINATION

Some General Considerations

Negative or normal x-rays do not mean that a fracture is not present. Some fractures are not visible on the initial x-rays even with examinations of the highest quality. Generally this is not important as long as both physician and patient understand

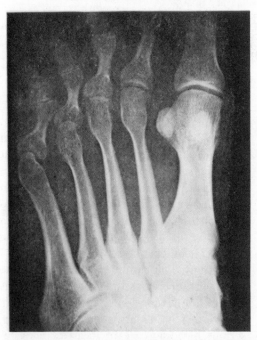 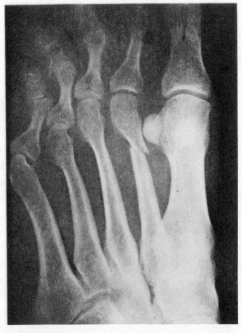

FIG. 1. Fracture not visible on initial examination. These are radiographs of a friendly psychiatrist who hobbled into the x-ray department after having dropped a heavy object on his foot. The initial study was normal (left). Five days later, while he was still hobbling, a reexamination showed a displaced fracture of the second metatarsal (right).

this possibility. However, in the case of a suspected fracture of the femoral neck, this pitfall has special relevance. When the clinical evidence strongly suggests such a possibility, the patient should be kept at bed rest despite the absence of an immediately demonstrable fracture. Patients with suspected fracture of nonweight-bearing bones can be given a splint or sling, and instructions to return if symptoms persist. Occasionally, as little as one day can be sufficient time for resorption of bone to permit visualization of the fracture line on x-ray. In general, if a fracture line is not seen within a week on good films, there is probably no fracture (Fig. 1). Some of the easiest fractures to miss on the original x-rays are those involving the carpal-navicular bones. If such a fracture is suspected but the original films are negative, a cast or splint should be applied to the forearm and hand and the x-rays repeated in a week or two.

Children require x-rays of both the injured and normal extremities. Since the ends of the long bones in children are partially uncalcified cartilage, severe disruptions of the epiphyses can occur with relatively little or no appreciable radiologic change. It is, therefore, important that the injured extremity be compared with the normal; x-rays of the opposite uninjured extremity must be routinely compared in anyone under the age of 12 years. Sometimes it is only in this manner that normal anatomic variations of the growing skeleton can be differentiated from changes due to trauma.

Fractures may be due to underlying disease. It is not uncommon for fractures to occur through preexisting lesions of bone, especially tumors, cysts, or osteoporosis (Fig. 2). These conditions may not be readily apparent radiologically but should be suspected if a fracture occurs after relatively mild trauma.

The Skull

PITFALL

EXCESSIVE ATTENTION IS OFTEN GIVEN TO THE SKULL, WITH INADEQUATE ATTENTION TO THE BRAIN

The linear skull fracture itself is relatively unimportant except as a gross indication of the presence and possible severity of trauma. The patient with a skull fracture and little or no important damage internally is in far better condition than the patient with injury to the brain or meninges and no fracture.

AXIOM

IT IS AN ERROR TO ASSUME THAT NO SKULL FRACTURE IS PRESENT (ESPECIALLY IN THE BASAL AREA) BECAUSE NO FRACTURE LINE IS VISIBLE.

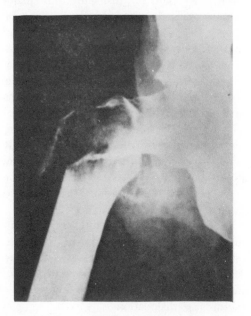

FIG. 2. Fracture through pathologic bone. The patient simply stepped off a curb, fracturing his hip. The fracture extends through a large area of destroyed bone, the result of metastasis from a primary carcinoma in the lung which had previously been occult.

Although fractures of the cranial vault are usually relatively easy to recognize, basal-skull fractures are often impossible to see, even in retrospect.

Facial Bones and Orbits

Fractures of the zygomatic arches, paranasal sinuses, and orbits are frequently difficult to recognize but are of great importance because of the potential consequences of failing to diagnose and treat them. Zygomatic fractures can lead to major cosmetic defects. The arches are best seen in the submental-vertex projection or in the Towne view. All fractures of the paranasal sinuses are compound by definition. Therefore the presence of an air-fluid level in a sinus following injury may be the clue to recognition of this frequently subtle fracture. Laminagraphy is of considerable importance in this area. Orbital fractures, particularly the blowout fracture of the floor of the orbit, may be invisible except for a soft-tissue density, representing orbital contents, projecting into the maxillary

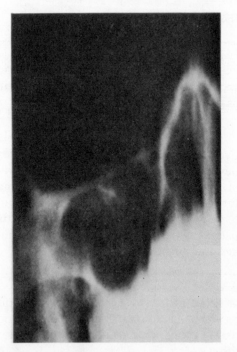

FIG. 3. Laminagram of blowout fracture of the orbit due to blunt trauma (clenched fist). There was marked swelling about the left eye which made physical examination impossible. The x-ray examination shows a soft-tissue mass protruding into the maxillary sinus. The soft-tissue mass represents orbital fat which has herniated through a fracture of the floor of the orbit. The fracture itself cannot be seen otherwise.

sinus from above (Fig. 3). This injury can lead to diplopia if uncorrected. In the acute phase, swelling of the soft tissues is such that the eye may be shut and clinical evaluation impossible (Chap. 15). Again, laminagraphy can be invaluable in demonstrating the soft-tissue density and the defect in the floor of the orbit.

Spine

PITFALL

IF A PATIENT WITH A CERVICAL FRACTURE IS MISHANDLED IN THE COURSE OF X-RAY EXAMINATION, THE SPINAL CORD MAY BE DAMAGED AND PARALYSIS MAY RESULT.

If there is a question of injury to the vertebral column, especially the cervical spine, the patient should be examined with the least possible handling. Cross-table lateral films of the neck, using an upright Bucky or grid cassette, should be obtained first, and only after these are seen and it is determined that no dislocation or major fracture is present should the patient be moved. Because of intervening tissue and because muscle spasm may be present, injuries to the lower cervical and upper thoracic spine are especially hard to visualize. Not uncommonly several x-rays of this area must be taken before the seventh cervical vertebra can be seen clearly. In some patients laminagraphy may be the only method by which fractures of the cervical spine, particularly those involving the lower cervical vertebrae or the odontoid process, may be demonstrated.

As in the case of the skull, serious injuries to the spinal cord can be sustained without evidence of fractures or dislocation of the spine. Patients with the most painful whiplash injuries of the neck seldom have fractures or dislocations.

Neck

X-ray examination of the soft tissues of the neck are of special diagnostic value following penetrating wounds of the pharynx, larynx, or esophagus. Although the initial wound of entry may be relatively small, these injuries can lead to lethal infections in the fascial spaces of the neck or mediastinum unless recognized and treated early (Chap. 19). Penetration or laceration of the upper airway or esophagus may be suspected radiologically by the presence of air in the soft tissues of the neck and mediastinum and particularly in the retropharyngeal space, which is best seen in the lateral view of the neck. If the space between the larynx or esophagus and cervical spine is more than 1.0 cm, an abnormal fluid collection should be suspected. It should be remembered, however, that injuries to the esophagus, pharynx, or trachea can occur with little or no evidence of this on routine chest or neck films. Although abnormal collections of air or fluid in the mediastinum or pleural spaces should suggest this diagnosis, barium or aqueous contrast studies under fluoroscopy may be needed to confirm it. Even these examinations, however, are not absolutely definitive, because the defect in the wall may be occluded by clot, fibrin, or food.

Thorax

RIB CAGE AND STERNUM

AXIOM
DO NOT ASSUME THAT THE THORACIC CAGE IS INTACT BECAUSE NO FRACTURE IS VISIBLE.

It is usually far more important to recognize damage to the intrathoracic organs than it is to diagnose fractures of the rib cage or sternum. Injuries to the anterior noncalcified cartilaginous ends of the ribs are seldom detectable. Indeed, many fractures of the lateral and posterior osseous portions of the rib are also invisible on the initial radiologic examinations, even in retrospect.

In evaluating the sternum and sterno-clavicular joints, laminagraphy is the best method of radiologic examination. Posteroanterior oblique views of these areas are not reliable and are difficult to perform correctly, even in a healthy person who has no pain.

PLEURA

AXIOM
LARGE QUANTITIES OF FLUID MAY NOT BE VISIBLE ON ROUTINE X-RAYS OF THE CHEST.

Although the presence of relatively large amounts of pleural fluid can be suspected on recumbent films, upright and decubitus views are often necessary to establish the diagnosis and to see smaller collections. If even a minimal amount of fluid is demonstrated by slight blunting of the costophrenic angle, it can usually be assumed that at least 300 ml are present. Frequently fairly large quantities of fluid will remain in a subpulmonic position between the diaphragm and the base of the lung and may be undetected except on decubitus films.

Pneumothorax can arise not only from tear of the visceral pleura but also from internal rupture of the lung with extension of the interstitial pulmonary emphysema along the bronchi into the hilum and then into the free pleural space. When a small pneumothorax is suspected or difficult to see on routine chest x-rays, decubitus views and films taken during expiration may be of help.

LUNGS. Contusion of the lung produces a transudation of fluid and blood into and around the bronchioles and alveoli, resulting in increased density of the involved area. These changes may progress rapidly to a superimposed atelectasis and infection. Later, necrosis and infection in some of these contused areas may result in abscess formation with an air-fluid level or a pneumatocele.

Pneumatoceles may develop soon after injury and persist as radiolucent "holes" in the lung. Occasionally, however, they may initially be filled with blood and appear to be solid. These spherical defects can persist and are sometimes removed in later years as "coin lesions" if their etiology is not apparent.

Fracture of a bronchus, although rare, is important to diagnose early. While this injury usually results in massive pneumothorax, the initial x-ray may be normal. Although minimal amounts of subcutaneous emphysema can be expected with any penetrating injury, larger amounts, particularly if they occur after blunt trauma, are suggestive of damage to the trachea or large bronchi. Even if the massive air leak stops spontaneously later, if a bronchial fracture is suspected but not found on bronchoscopy, a bronchogram may outline the defect clearly.

If the patient has a penetrating wound of the chest and/or abdomen, the entrance and exit wounds should be marked with radiopaque markers. These markers help delineate the bullet track and assist considerably in focusing the attention of the radiologist and clinician on the areas likely to be injured.

HEART. The condition of patients with penetrating wounds of the heart is usually so precarious that there often is no time to obtain roentgenologic examinations. Occasionally, however, the nature of the patient's problem is not immediately clear and changes in the size or configuration of the heart may be helpful diagnostically. If the normal pericardial cavity rapidly fills with more than 200 to 300 ml of blood or fluid, tamponade usually occurs with a resultant significant decrease in the filling of the heart during diastole. Although this amount of fluid can cause severe hypotension, the enlargement of the heart shadow which it produces may be so slight that it can be easily overlooked. If it is important to determine how much of the cardiac shadow is due to pericardial blood or fluid, and if pericardicentesis is unsuccessful or inconclusive, CO_2 angiocardiography may be helpful. This technique is safe and can

usually be performed with minimal difficulty. With the patient lying on his left side, cross-table lateral x-rays are taken while 100 ml of CO_2 is rapidly injected through a catheter into the superior vena cava or right atrium or through a needle in a peripheral vein. If the distance between the right heart border and the CO_2 in the right atrium is more than 1 cm, a significant pericardial effusion is probably present.

Contusion of the heart can produce myocardial and pericardial changes with progressive cardiomegaly. Indeed, there is a well-documented entity of chest pain, fever, and pericardial effusion, apparently related to the postpericardiotomy syndromes, which may occur a month to six weeks after blunt trauma to the chest.

GREAT VESSELS. Any of the great vessels in the thorax can be injured by penetrating wounds; this can result in a mediastinal hematoma and extrapleural or intrapleural bleeding, depending on the site of the injury. Blunt trauma can also produce lacerations of the major arteries and veins in the chest. Of particular interest are the tears of the aorta, produced most typically by severe deceleration injuries and resulting in false aneurysms of the aortic isthmus just distal to the left subclavian artery. In such cases, while the diagnosis can be suspected if there is widening of the upper mediastinum on plain roentgenograms, angiography is usually necessary to determine the precise nature of the lesion. It should always be remembered that the mediastinum appears wider on AP views than on standard PA projections.

Aortography can be performed using the forward technique of venous injection; the results of studies with a catheter inserted into the aorta through the axillary or femoral arteries are far more reliable, however.

THE DIAPHRAGM. Both blunt and penetrating wounds can produce disruption of the diaphragm. Tears with blunt trauma are more common on the left than on the right and, because the liver acts as a shield on that side, organs are less likely to pass into the right chest. Diaphragmatic injury must be suspected in anyone who has severe blunt trauma to the abdomen, such as the patient who is crushed or falls from a height. Associated injuries often include a fractured pelvis and upper- and lower-limb damage. Although herniation of abdominal contents into the chest may compromise ventilation, the major complications or dangers related to the hernia itself are strangulation or obstruction of the stomach or intestine by the relatively small diaphragmatic wound. Even though a ruptured diaphragm may cause no immediate difficulty, strangulation of the stomach, colon, or small bowel can occur many years later.

AXIOM

TRAUMATIC DIAPHRAGMATIC HERNIAS MAY BE DIFFICULT TO RECOGNIZE ON THE INITIAL X-RAYS OF THE CHEST.

Although this injury may be difficult or impossible to diagnose initially on plain films of the chest or abdomen, it should always be suspected when the diaphragm is elevated, when it moves abnormally on fluoroscopy, or if unusual gas shadows are seen above the diaphragm, especially on the left.

Not uncommonly, the walls of abdominal viscera which have herniated in the chest have been mistaken for a high diaphragm. The diagnosis is sometimes first made when the end of a radiopaque nasogastric tube is noted to pass from the abdomen into the left chest. Decubitus views and studies with opaque contrast agents may help to confirm the diagnosis. Occasionally, insufflation of 200 to 300 ml of air into the stomach through a nasogastric tube may outline the stomach or intestine in the chest. Herniation of bowel into the chest is often better seen with the patient supine, since intrathoracic abdominal contents may slide back below the diaphragm when the patient is upright.

The Abdomen

ABDOMINAL WALL. The use of contrast media has been advocated to assess peritoneal penetration in cases where, after digital and visual exploration of a stab wound, the indications for laparotomy are questionable. After a Foley catheter is inserted as far as possible into the wound, the balloon is inflated, the outside of the wound is sutured to make it water tight, and 50 ml of a water-soluble contrast material is injected into the wound through the catheter. If the wound is small and the patient has much pain, or if much resistance is encountered, lesser amounts of solution should be used. Sometimes communication with the bowel or free peritoneal cavity is demonstrated by this technique. It is important to remember, however, that there may be false negatives. This is especially true when the wound tract is long and oblique. The examination is not to be trusted except when it is positive, therefore, and has very limited application.

HOLLOW VISCERA. *Penetrating Wounds.* The incidence of free air in the abdomen following penetration of the stomach or colon by a knife or bullet is surprisingly low. The small intestine is generally collapsed or filled with fluid, so that even multiple perforations may not result in visible free air. In the stomach or colon the penetrating wound may be temporarily self-sealing, thereby limiting the quantity of gas released into the peritoneum. Although as little as 5 cc of air may be visualized with good radiographic technique with the patient upright, the diagnosis of free air on films made with the patient recumbent generally is possible only if a large amount of air is present. Therefore, in any proper attempt to recognize free air, films of the abdomen should be taken with the patient in the upright and the left lateral decubitus positions. In addition, upright PA and lateral projections of the chest are desirable, not only to evaluate the chest but also to allow small collections of free air to be demonstrated below the diaphragm. If at all possible, the patient should be kept in the upright or decubitus position for at least 5 to 10 minutes before the x-rays are taken. With a patient too ill for this, a cross-table lateral can supplement the lateral decubitus view. Although it is generally wise to explore the patient surgically if perforation of a hollow viscus is suspected, in some patients contrast studies can confirm the diagnosis preoperatively. In such cases, a water-soluble agent such as Gastrografin should be utilized. Barium should not be used in the evaluation of possible gastrointestinal trauma because it may produce peritoneal adhesions or granulomas if it enters the peritoneum.

Even with an optimal study, only some of the leaks are seen; most of the smaller perforations seem to seal over rapidly, at least temporarily. Since aqueous contrast media are absorbed rapidly from the peritoneum, an indirect sign of a perforation is the rapid appearance of a relatively intense pyelogram during or immediately following the gastrointestinal study. Some of the contrast medium may also be absorbed directly through mucosa of the bowel, but this produces a later and much fainter pyelogram.

Blunt Trauma. Rupture of the descending or retroperitoneal portion of the duodenum following blunt trauma to the abdomen merits special attention. Both the radiologic and clinical pictures may be subtle, and any delay in treatment greatly increases morbidity and mortality. Roentgenologically, this lesion is characterized by obliteration of the right psoas shadow, with bubbles of air in the right upper quadrant, in the right perinephric space, or along the borders of the psoas muscle.

Injury to the duodenum can also produce intramural hematoma involving the retroperitoneal portion of the duodenum. Clinically, patients with this abnormality may show signs of high small bowel obstruction. Radiologically, this entity can be identified by the typical coil-spring appearance of the involved segment as seen following the ingestion of barium.

LIVER AND SPLEEN. Occasionally, when the clinical picture is unclear, radiologic techniques can be employed to determine whether or not the liver or spleen has been injured. Although arteriography is the only precise method of evaluating such injuries, a number of indirect signs can be helpful. Fractures of the lower ribs are often associated with blunt trauma to the liver or spleen, and there may be a visible mass in the region of these organs. The involved organ occasionally is not as sharply defined as it usually is radiographically. Frequently there is a pleural effusion on the involved side; the gastric air bubble is often displaced and the splenic flexure may be depressed. The gastric rugae along the greater curvature tend to be thicker than normal because the adjacent blood acts as an irritant, producing submucosal edema. Occasionally the use of radioactive materials can demonstrate hematobilia, subcapsular hematoma, or abscess of the spleen or liver.

URINARY TRACT. The roentgenologic evaluation of trauma to the urinary tract requires opacification procedures of one sort or another. Although excretory urography is relatively convenient and an important aid in the study of renal trauma, selective renal arteriography is the most reliable method of determining the extent of renal parenchymal or vascular injury. In the patient with post-traumatic hematuria, the excretory urogram can be performed immediately, without prior preparation, by infusing a relatively high dose of contrast medium, usually 50 to 100 cc, to obtain a "drip pyelogram." Damage to the renal artery is suggested when one kidney is not visualized. Renal-vein injuries can produce a swollen kidney. Parenchymal injuries can be manifested by distortion of the collecting systems or by recognition of extravasated contrast material. Tears of the renal pelvis or ureter are best evaluated by retrograde pyelography, and injuries to the bladder by opaque cystography. The problems of diagnosis of urinary tract injuries are discussed in more detail in Chapter 24.

ARTERIOGRAPHY

In recent years there has been considerable interest in the use of arteriography to evaluate the injured patient. Many severe arterial injuries may not show clinical evidence of distal ischemia or an expanding hematoma until the chances of successful treatment are greatly reduced. Any suspected vascular injury to an extremity should be explored surgically or angiographically to be sure that an important lesion is not missed. In some instances a good distal pulse can be felt readily, even with complete obstruction of the proximal main vessel. Other lesions that can be demonstrated on angiography include lacerations, false aneurysms and arteriovenous fistulae. Although arterial spasm occasionally occurs following trauma, narrowing of a vessel, even if only mild, should not be dismissed casually since this may be a sign of an important vascular injury. If there is any question of the integrity of the popliteal artery, arteriography is especially important; the amputation rate following any delay in treatment of an injury to this artery is alarmingly high. Study of the vascular supply to the lower extremities is simple and can be accomplished in any emergency room. The procedure involves insertion of a needle into the femoral artery, hand injection of radiopaque contrast agents, and radiography. Although serial rapid filming is preferable, adequate examinations can be obtained by using a single film with the understanding that repeat injections may be necessary to demonstrate the anatomy.

Examination of the thoracic, abdominal, and pelvic arteries is substantially more complex than peripheral arteriography and requires insertion of an intra-arterial catheter, fluoroscopic control and serial filming. An intra-arterial catheter can be placed either by arteriotomy or by using the familiar percutaneous needle-replacement Seld-inger technique in which an artery is entered with a needle, a guidewire is inserted through the needle, the needle is withdrawn, leaving the guide, and an appropriate catheter is passed into the artery over the guide. Generally arteriotomy is preferred for entering the brachial artery, but for approaches via the femoral, axillary, or subclavian arteries the Seldinger technique is routine.

These studies are time-consuming and require refined and costly equipment and highly skilled personnel. In addition, they carry certain inherent risks and definite morbidity and mortality of their own. Complications of the catheterization procedure include laceration or thrombosis of the vessel used for the study, hematomas at the puncture site, and vascular damage internally by the tip of the catheter as it is manipulated in the dark recesses of the body cavities. Intramural injection of contrast materials can cause arterial dissection with or without occlusion. "Reactions" to the opaque materials are well known although not fully understood, and can cause paralysis, shock, or death.

In spite of the potential problems with the procedure, catheter arteriography can provide information on the status of the thoracic and abdominal aorta and their major branches that may be unobtainable in any other way. The technique is especially valuable for diagnosing tears of the aortic isthmus due to deceleration trauma. In the abdomen, selective catheterization of the renal, hepatic, and splenic arteries can provide specific information of the status of these vessels and the organs they supply.

Recently, a number of efforts have been made to provide therapy as well as diagnose through selective arterial catheterization. Gastrointestinal bleeding can occasionally be controlled by arterial infusions of vasopressor drugs, and pelvic bleeding can be controlled in some cases by the infusion of autologous clot. These approaches are extremely interesting and provide a hope of alternative therapeutic approaches for patients who are either unacceptable surgical risks or whose injuries are so complex and multiple that it is difficult to know the problem to attack first.

These studies (as all elective procedures) should be performed only when the rewards are likely to exceed the risks incurred. The overriding consideration in dealing with major injuries is the condition of the patient. Frequently, the information which could be obtained from arteriography would be helpful but the time spent in doing the studies would delay treatment unjustifiably. When the "need to know" is exceeded by practical considerations, studies should be delayed until circumstances make the risk significantly less than the potential rewards.

NUCLEAR MEDICINE TECHNIQUES

Thus far radioactive isotopes have only limited application in the early study of the injured patient. With the increasing availability of short-life isotopes the injection of substantially greater quantities of radioactive materials is possible, providing more "counts" with less total radioactive dose to the patient. Devices such as the gamma camera not only allow rapid organ scanning but can also be used in a number of areas to determine regional blood flow and perfusion ratios.

Blood volume determinations with radioisotopes can be useful, especially if they are done serially to follow relative changes rather than absolute values. Scanning of the lungs can be helpful in the diagnosis of pulmonary embolism or other causes of reduced circulation to the lung. Spleen scans may confirm a diagnosis of subcapsular hemorrhage. Liver scans are seldom indicated in the initial study of hepatic injury, but can be helpful later when evaluating the patient for a possible hepatic hematoma or abscess or subphrenic collection. Hematobilia can also be evaluated using radioactive materials. With continued tech-

nologic progress in this field, further applications no doubt will be forthcoming.

ULTRASOUND

Using sonar, a number of applications of ultrasound to the problems of the acutely injured patient are available. In the brain, a midline shift can be determined rapidly and simply. Collections of fluid, notably in the pericardium but also in the abdomen and retroperitoneum, may be studied noninvasively. Even when pulses are absent, blood flow to an extremity can be evaluated in a semiquantitative fashion. Ultrasound is a relatively recent technologic aid to modern medicine, and many more applications can be expected in the future.

SUMMARY (Table 1)

The use of roentgenologic techniques in the evaluation of trauma involves all clinical disciplines. Some of these examinations are relatively simple, others extremely complex. High-quality studies are absolutely necessary if results are to be relied upon. Appropriate equipment, space, and well-trained people used to dealing with injured patients are required for proper examinations. A careful and complete history and physical examination and close communication between the clinician and radiologist are essential if the radiology of

TABLE 1. COMMON PLATITUDINOUS DO'S AND DON'T'S

1. DO have proper organization, people, and equipment.
2. DO be certain to provide appropriate clinical information.
3. DO *NOT* be satisfied with inferior radiologic examinations.
4. DO remember that not all injuries or illnesses can be recognized radiologically, particularly at the time of initial examination.
5. DO remember that soft-tissue abnormalities can be at least as important as skeletal abnormalities.
6. DO remember that clinical considerations must override apparently normal x-ray studies.

trauma is to be as rewarding as it can be, for both the patient and the physicians charged with his care.

Suggested Reading

1. Compere, C. L., and Banks, S. W.: *Pictorial Handbook of Fracture Treatment*, 5th ed. Chicago, Year Book Medical Publishers, 1963.
2. Evans, G. W., et al.: Scintigraphy in traumatic lesions of liver and spleen. JAMA, 222:6, 1972.
3. Felson, B.: *The Acute Abdomen*. New York, Grune & Stratton, 1973.
4. Finley, J. W., et al.: Selective arteriography and infusion in diagnosis and treatment of acute gastrointestinal bleeding. Amer. Surg., 39:448, 1973.
5. Fontan, F., et al.: Aneurysm caused by traumatic rupture of aortic isthmus—interest of repair by direct suture. Ann. Chir., 26:29, 1972.
6. Frimann-Dahl, J. C.: *Roentgen Examinations in Acute Abdominal Disease*, 2nd ed. Spring-field, Charles C Thomas, 1960. (Third edition due in 1974.)
7. Linn, R. C. Jr., et al.: Angiography in patients with blunt trauma to the chest and abdomen. Surg. Clin. N. Amer., 52:551, 1972.
8. Margolies, M. N., et al.: Arteriography in the management of hemorrhage from pelvic fractures. New Eng. J. Med., 287:317, 1972.
9. McGee, E. M., et al.: Pulmonary contusion: pathogenesis and current management. Rev. Surg., 29:224, 1972.
10. Sadler, R. B., and Chinn, J.: JAMA, 221:7, 1972.
11. Shopfner, R. F.: Plain skull roentgenograms in children with head trauma. Radiology, 114:230, 1972.
12. Stanley, R. J., et al.: Arteriography in diagnosis of acute gastrointestinal tract bleeding. Arch. Surg., 107:138, 1973.
13. Tippens, J. K., et al.: How sinograms can help you evaluate wounds. Med. Times, 101:124, 1973.
14. Westfall, R. H., Nelson, R. H., and Musselman, M. M.: Barium peritonitis. Amer. J. Surg., 112:760, 1966.

Part 4

SPECIFIC INJURIES AND
THEIR MANAGEMENT

14 SOME CONSIDERATIONS IN THE INITIAL MANAGEMENT OF INJURIES TO THE HEAD AND SPINE

L. M. THOMAS
E. S. GURDJIAN

INJURIES TO THE HEAD

In these days of high-speed transportation, motorcycle enthusiasts, and civil disturbances, few accident rooms will escape their share of head and spine injuries. All concerned, physicians and laity alike, recognize and fear head injury, often to the point of neglecting to pursue an orderly course of management.

AXIOM

THE SINE QUA NON OF HEAD-INJURY MANAGEMENT IS CAREFUL AND REPETITIVE OBSERVATION AND TIMELY INTERVENTION.

Unfortunately, no magic cures or shortcuts to diagnosis and management are available either to the emergency-room physician or to the neurosurgeon. All patients with injury to the head do not require neurosurgical consultation but all do require careful and accurate assessment.

In an average year the neurosurgical department of Detroit General Hospital will be called upon to see approximately 900 patients with head injuries. About three fourths of these injuries are accidental and one fourth the result of intentional trauma[1] (Table 1). The role of alcohol is important in these injuries not only as an etiologic factor (about one in five patients had been drinking prior to trauma) but also as a factor which often makes examination and evaluation extremely difficult.

PITFALL

FAILURE TO LOOK BEYOND THE OBVIOUS HEAD INJURY IN ASSESSMENT OF A PATIENT PRECLUDES THE RECOGNITION OF ASSOCIATED TRAUMA.

TABLE 1. ETIOLOGY OF HEAD INJURIES AND THEIR ASSOCIATION WITH ALCOHOL, 1961

Etiology	TOTAL		ASSOCIATED WITH ALCOHOL	
	Number	%	Number	%
Falls	301	33.4	67	22.3
Direct blows	205	22.8	55	26.8
Auto accident	159	17.7	37	23.3
Pedestrian accident	107	11.9	13	12.1
Gunshot wounds	22	2.4	2	9.1
Other	63	7.0	16	25.4
Unknown	43	4.8	—	—
Total	900	100.0	190	21.1

An important complicating factor in patients with head injuries is the high incidence of associated injuries. Almost one in four of our patients has had significant damage to the other parts of the body, with the greatest number of problems involving the extremities, face, and chest (Table 2). A team leader must be agreed upon early in the management of such patients; although the neurosurgeon may be called on for such duty, more frequently this responsibility will fall upon the general surgeon.[2]

TABLE 2.   ASSOCIATED INJURIES IN PATIENTS WITH HEAD INJURIES, 1961

Associated Injury	%
Pelvis and extremity fractures	7.0
Chest injuries	6.1
Facial fractures	5.9
Spinal-cord injuries	5.6
Thoracic or lumbar-spine injuries	4.4
Cervical-spine injuries	2.2
Shoulder injuries	1.8
Abdominal injuries	1.4
Other	9.4

Initial General Management of Extracranial Problems

Circulation and oxygenation are of prime importance to the central nervous system. Immediate attention must be directed toward establishment of an adequate airway and ventilation, control of hemorrhage and treatment of shock.[3]

If there is any question about the adequacy of the airway or ventilation, endotracheal intubation or tracheostomy may be required; it is poor judgment to err on the side of conservatism in this regard. While manipulating the neck to perform these procedures, extreme caution is necessary unless cervical fracture has been ruled out by appropriate x-rays; however, establishment of an adequate airway *must not* be delayed.

A careful and complete search must be made for the etiology of hypotension in any

AXIOM

SHOCK IS NEVER TO BE CONSIDERED THE RESULT OF HEAD INJURY ALONE.

trauma victim. It is extremely rare to find shock resulting from head injury alone unless massive external bleeding from the scalp is present.[4] The rare exceptions to this are tiny infants, who can lose relatively large amounts of blood into the subgaleal space.

Pathophysiology of Head Injuries

An understanding of the pathophysiology of craniocerebral trauma is essential for proper management. Damage from penetrating wounds is largely related to direct tissue damage but may also involve some of the problems seen in nonpenetrating (closed) injuries. A closed head injury may result in cerebral concussion, due to depression of the reticular formation of the brain stem, with a period of unconsciousness and some amnesia. This type of injury is usually reversible without residual effects, but in rare cases it may be fatal.

Contusion and lacerations of the cortex after nonpenetrating trauma are caused by movements of the brain relative to its bony dural coverings, direct and contrecoup impacts and the effects of acceleration-induced pressure gradients. Such injuries cause focal neurologic deficits from the time of injury, but increases in neurologic loss may result from local bleeding and swelling.

In many instances brain swelling may cause increased intracranial pressure.[5] Cerebral edema is aggravated by hypoxia, hypercarbia, and acidosis, all of which dilate cerebral vessels.

Intracranial hematomas may further complicate the picture. The epidural clot is most frequently associated with a skull fracture crossing and lacerating one of the dural vessels, commonly the middle meningeal artery or vein. Subdural clots result from tears of small connecting veins and/or cortical vessels, presumably due to movements of the brain relative to its dural covering. Traumatic intracerebral clots result from brain deformation and distortion, with resulting tissue necrosis and hemorrhage.

Assessment of the Head Injuries

The treatment of the head injury in an individual patient may be conservative or operative, depending upon the type and severity of craniocerebral damage. Approximately 12% of patients with an acute severe head injury causing unconsciousness require surgical intervention. The interpretation of signs and symptoms must be cautious and the dynamic state of the injury must always be kept in mind. Treatment plans must be modified if changes in the clinical picture develop.

HISTORY. An adequate history may provide information about changes of consciousness and neurologic function occurring before the initial examination. Further observation will permit an accurate assessment of any neurologic changes and indicate the need for changes in management.

The details of the accident should be sought for meticulously. If the patient is unable to delineate the events clearly, other witnesses should be questioned. An awareness of the mechanism of injury and of the magnitude of the energy involved will aid in decisions regarding management.

It is particularly important to determine the presence or absence of a period of unconsciousness. Occasionally it is difficult to differentiate between a dazed state and true unconsciousness. The presence of amnesia is of great value in this regard. The more serious and prolonged the initial unconsciousness, the more marked will be the retrograde amnesia. If the period of unconsciousness is short, less than five minutes, the patient should be carefully observed for 6 to 12 hours. Frequently this can be done in the emergency room and does not require hospitalization. Patients with periods of unconsciousness lasting more than five minutes should be hospitalized overnight. An equally careful inquiry must be made regarding changes in consciousness since the accident, for even minor changes may herald the beginning of brain decompensation.

MININEUROLOGIC EXAMINATION. The minineurologic examination is named advisedly; it is long enough to cover the essentials but short enough to maintain the interest of the observing physician. An assessment of the conscious state and orientation of the patient serves as the foundation. Inasmuch as most patients will be seen on admission to the emergency room and again some time later after their x-rays have been completed, it is possible to make a determination of changes in the conscious state based on this interval in time. The patient's alertness, awareness, and ability to comprehend and abstract should be noted. Deterioration in these functions is an indication for further continued careful observation.

Examination of pupillary function is of particular importance. Frequently a unilateral dilating pupil, still reactive to light, may be the first sign of an expanding mass in the temporal lobe or an epidural hematoma of the middle fossa. The reaction of the pupils, both to light and to accommodation, should therefore be observed. Extraocular movements and visual fields should also be carefully checked.

In examining the cranial nerves following trauma, it is advisable to pay some attention to the function of the first cranial nerve. Simple solutions (methylsalicylate, rose water, tincture of benzoin) can be utilized to determine the presence or absence of the function of smell. Gross examination of hearing should be carried out and the external ear canals carefully examined for CSF drainage and for bleeding through or behind the tympanic membranes.

The sensory functions of the fifth cranial nerve and the motor functions of the seventh cranial nerve should be examined together; this should include a careful check of the corneal reflexes. The functions of the lower cranial nerves 10, 11, and 12 should not be overlooked, and may be easily evaluated by observing the patient's ability to swallow and the functions of the palate, trapezius muscle and tongue.

The ability of the patient to perform rapid alternating movements, finger-to-nose and finger-to-finger pursuits, and movement of the heel down the shin will screen for slight degrees of weakness and for cerebellar dysfunction. Station and gait should be carefully observed and the deep tendon reflexes, superficial reflexes and Babinski phenomenon should be examined and recorded.

OBSERVATION

AXIOM

OBSERVATION MEANS REPEATED CAREFUL EXAMINATION OF THE PATIENT BY A PHYSICIAN.

Continued and repeated observation is the keynote to the evaluation and management of neurosurgical problems. The state of consciousness and other neurologic functions in patients who may require neurosurgical intervention are seldom constant except in the terminal irreversible stages. Merely keeping the patient in a hospital bed or in the emergency room does not imply that he is being adequately observed. All too often, patients languish in these areas without being seen by a physician at all.

Treatment

NONSURGICAL MANAGEMENT. *Position.* The unconscious patient is best nursed in a slightly head-up (10°) position. A patient in coma breathes poorly in the supine position but may do very nicely on his side. Such positioning may obviate the need for a tracheostomy. Although careful physical examination of the patient's breathing is important, serial arterial blood gas determinations are more accurate.

Fluids. Although excessive administration of water and salt may contribute to the formation of cerebral edema, dehydra-

tion is also to be deplored; certainly the danger of slight overhydration is much less than that of persistent hypotension and poor tissue perfusion. In the unconscious patient with no other serious injuries 1500 to 2000 ml 5% glucose in water per day will usually be adequate for the first two to three days. Following this, feedings through a small nasogastric tube are usually efficacious.

Hypothermia. Body temperature should be monitored frequently and kept within normal limits by sponging and/or the use of special hypothermia blankets. Certainly high fever should be prevented because of its possible adverse effect on brain swelling. Hypothermia, on the other hand, does not have a place in the management of head trauma. In a long careful study at Detroit General Hospital, it was found that hypothermia did not improve the survival rates of patients with head trauma.

Steroids. Steroids are of value in combating cerebral edema, perhaps by reducing the local inflammatory reaction to injury. The dosage of steroids currently used is 10 mg of dexamethasone (Decadron) I.V. followed by 4 to 6 mg I.M. every four hours for two to three days with a gradual reduction in dosage thereafter, depending upon the patient's response.

Osmotic Diuretics. Osmotic diuretics such as mannitol and urea may reduce brain swelling dramatically. The effect is to decrease intracranial pressure and by this mechanism reduce or delay the phenomenon of brain-stem herniation. The benefit lasts only a few hours; a rebound phenomenon follows and the intracranial pressure again rises.

SURGICAL MANAGEMENT. *Open Wounds.* Although patients with open wounds of the head with depressed, perforating or penetrating fractures may not lose consciousness, they clearly require neurosurgical aid.[7] Sterile dressings, routine measures for shock, and antibiotic administration will usually suffice until the neurosurgeon can be summoned to elevate any depressed fragments and remove any intracranial foreign bodies, necrotic tissue, or collections of blood. Such injuries are usually well managed by all concerned; it is the closed head injury with its complications of brain swelling and intracranial hematomas that causes the most problems.

Skull Fractures. Fractures of the cranial vault may be divided into linear and depressed fractures.[8] The linear fracture rarely needs treatment and causes difficulty only when it tears an underlying vessel or causes a cerebrospinal leak. A depressed fracture on the other hand may cause damage to the underlying brain and requires elevation unless the depression is minimal. Elevation of a closed depressed skull fracture is rarely an emergency.

An open fracture requires debridement. Linear fractures rarely require more than soft-tissue debridement and irrigation, but open depressed fractures may require extensive bony debridement as well. With modern antibiotics the "golden period" for primary repair may be extended to 12 to 24 hours, and patients can be transferred to a neurosurgical facility for debridement.

Closed Head Injuries. NATURAL HISTORY OF EXPANDING INTRACRANIAL HEMATOMAS. The evacuation of an expanding intracranial mass constitutes the main indication for surgical intervention in patients with closed head injuries. Continued intracranial bleeding following a head injury produces a characteristic dynamic pattern which may ·be illustrated by the following case report.

A 24-year-old motorcyclist was brought to the accident room by his friends. Although the patient was awake and alert, he remembered little of the accident. A history taken from his friends revealed that this young man fell from his bike when the front wheel struck a stone and skidded. He was not wearing a helmet, and his head struck the pavement. He was immediately unconscious and at first did not breathe. Within five minutes, however, he was aware of his surroundings, and shortly thereafter seemed fully conscious. He complained of a severe generalized headache.

It was observed by the accident-room physician that the patient would tend to "drowse off" while his friends were being questioned, although he seemed alert when attention was directed to him. Except for this, the neurologic examination was negative.

If the events are reconstructed, the mechanics of the injury can be demonstrated. At the time of the fall, the impact was first directed against the skull and its overlying padding, the scalp. The head was decelerated rapidly by the unyielding ground and the skull was deformed. Both events cause an increase in pressure within the cranial cavity. The result of the increase in pressure is a movement of the intracranial contents toward and through the incisural notch of the cerebellar tentorium and through the foramen magnum at the base of the skull. Since the skull is nonexpansile, this is the only direction in which such movement or extrusion can occur. The shear stress developed by this movement paralyzes cells in the reticular activating system of the midbrain and loss of consciousness, or cerebral concussion, results. Ordinarily, this depression of the reticular activating system is short lived and consciousness soon returns. In some patients, however, this mechanism can cause severe damage and may result in death.

Upon examining the patient again, it was observed that the right pupil, which was the same size as the other pupil on initial examination, was now slightly larger than the left. An x-ray of the skull was taken and revealed a fracture line across the temporal bone on the right. By this time the patient was stuporous and obeyed commands only sluggishly. The pupillary dilatation on the right was much greater, and the pupil no longer reacted to light.

PITFALL

IF THE CONSCIOUS STATE AND PUPILLARY SIGNS ARE NOT ADEQUATELY OBSERVED ON ADMISSION AND AT FREQUENT INTERVALS THEREAFTER, THE EARLY SIGNS OF BRAIN-STEM FAILURE WILL BE MISSED.

The period of consciousness lasting from the concussion until the lapse into stupor is called the "lucid interval" and is diagnostic of an expanding intracranial mass.

AXIOM

PROGRESSIVE DETERIORATION IN CONSCIOUSNESS IS THE GUIDON BEARER OF INCREASING INTRACRANIAL PRESSURE.

As the contents of the supratentorial compartment enlarge, the brain stem and diencephalon are forced through the incisura, leading to progressive loss of consciousness and followed in order by impaired brain-stem function with changes in respiration and vasomotor control. The increase in supratentorial bulk may result from an expanding hematoma, from brain swelling, or from a combination of causes.

The case described above typifies an epidural hematoma. Since this lesion is usually temporal in location, the early detection of a unilateral pupillary dilation (due to uncal herniation involving the third cranial nerve) is of great importance. A similar story, as exemplified by the following case report, can develop either with a subdural or intracerebral mass or from brain swelling alone.

A 45-year-old male was brought to the emergency room by the police. He had driven his car into an expressway embankment and was found unconscious in the car. When seen in the emergency room, he was deeply stuporous, responding only to painful stimulation. The response to pain was purposeful, however, and the pupils reacted to light. Both sides appeared to move equally well and deep tendon reflexes were present and symmetrically equal. An equivocally positive Babinski sign was present on the right side. X-rays of the skull showed no evidence of fracture. When the patient was examined again later, he was noted to have a dilated left pupil which was not reactive to light and an irregular respiratory pattern of the Cheyne-Stokes variety. Painful stimuli at this time caused stiffening and extension of all four extremities with associated internal rotation of the arms and legs.

This decerebrate state is the result of upper brain-stem depression and represents a severe, often irreversible, deterioration in neurologic status.

PITFALL

FAILURE TO APPRECIATE DETERIORATION IN THE STUPOROUS OR COMATOSE PATIENT RESULTS FROM INSUFFICIENT AND INFREQUENT PATIENT OBSERVATION. EVEN PATIENTS IN AN ALCOHOLIC STUPOR CAN BE FOLLOWED ADEQUATELY BY THEIR REACTION TO PAINFUL STIMULI.

THE NEED FOR ACCURATE DIAGNOSIS. Proper management of patients with closed head injuries depends on an accurate diagnosis. At present the neurosurgeon frequently is able to evacuate a clot, thus removing part of the damage-producing mechanism. Little surgical treatment, in fact little treatment of any variety, however, benefits the patient with brain contusions, lacerations, and edema.

AXIOM

IN PATIENTS WITH HEAD TRAUMA, ATTENTION MUST BE DIRECTED TOWARD THE EARLY DISCOVERY OF INCIPIENT INTRACRANIAL HEMATOMAS.

Cerebral angiograms will permit the identification and location of subdural hematomas as well as intracerebral masses, singly or in combination. It can also exclude the presence of a mass lesion when brain swelling is the principal culprit and prevent an unnecessary exploration. Angiography should not be undertaken by the inexperienced or without adequate facilities. Although echoencephalography may be of value in the hands of personnel experienced in its use, it is not generally available.

The detection and removal of an intracranial clot is so important that, if angiography is not available or if rapid deterioration does not permit delay for x-ray studies, emergency "diagnostic" trephination may be required. An epidural hematoma is the classic example of a curable lesion in which a few minutes' delay may be fatal.

Because of the associated brain contusion and laceration resulting from the impact, the mortality rate in patients with acute subdural hematomas requiring operation within the first 12 to 24 hours is extremely high, even in alert and sophisticated head-injury centers.[9] The patient's only hope lies in early recognition and clot evacuation before the brain damage has become irreversible.

TREPHINATION. General surgeons practicing in areas where immediate neurosurgical aid is not available should have the ability to make cranial trephine openings (burr holes). Endotracheal intubation obviates worry about the airway during the procedure. The entire scalp should be shaved; draping, however, can be minimal.

If preoperative angiography has not been performed the trephine openings should be made bilaterally. The following locations for trephine openings are suggested:

1. Frontocoronal: 3 cm lateral to the midline at the coronal suture.
2. Temporal: 2 cm anterior to the ear and 2 cm superior to the zygoma.
3. Parietal: 2 cm above and 2 cm posterior to the ear.

INJURIES TO THE SPINE AND SPINAL CORD

Trauma to the spine and spinal cord may produce devastating neurologic deficits. Injuries of this sort are relatively uncommon and are, therefore, frequently overlooked. If injury to the spine and the spinal cord is borne in mind as a possibility, the physician can evaluate the picture in the conscious patient by the presence of pain or tenderness around the spine and paralysis or anesthesia in the extremities. The testing of the patient's response to pinprick at various levels, his reactions to the pain and the movement of the extremities, will ascertain the degree and extent of any sensory and motor loss. Such observations are

difficult when the patient is stuporous or unconscious, and x-rays must be relied upon under such circumstances.

X-rays of the cervical spine should be obtained in patients who have sustained a head injury, particularly if the energies involved in the accident were great. Such x-rays must not, however, delay treatment of airway obstruction, shock or a rapidly expanding intracranial mass. If there is any suspicion that the cervical spine may be fractured, the neck must be handled with great care during these procedures. In some instances, it may be wise to apply a neck brace to prevent inadvertent excessive motion.

AXIOM

AN INADEQUATE INITIAL EXAMINATION OF THE MOTOR FUNCTION OF THE EXTREMITIES AND A FAILURE TO SEARCH FOR A SENSORY LEVEL MAY RESULT IN FAILURE TO DETECT A SERIOUS SPINAL-CORD INJURY AND SERVE TO CONFUSE THE PICTURE IN SUBSEQUENT FOLLOW-UP EVALUATIONS.

Patients who sustain immediate motor and sensory loss below the level of injury, with absent reflexes, have little chance for recovery by surgical decompression, and in fact may suffer additional loss as a result of surgical intervention. If the motor and/or sensory loss is incomplete or progressive, a more aggressive approach is indicated. Under such circumstances a decompressive laminectomy may provide the margin necessary to allow significant recovery. Unstable fractures and fracture dislocations of the cervical spine should be treated by skeletal tong traction, followed later by

---

PITFALL

IF THE SEVENTH CERVICAL VERTEBRA IS NOT SEEN CLEARLY ON X-RAY, ONE OF THE MOST COMMON SITES FOR FRACTURE DISLOCATION OF THE SPINE WILL BE INADEQUATELY EXAMINED.

---

definitive treatment if indicated. Adequate x-ray examination is mandatory in all cases of suspected spine injury.

SUMMARY

The greatest failing in emergency-room management of injury to the central nervous system is inadequate observation of the patient. A careful recording of the initial examination followed by pertinent and frequent reevaluation will permit the early recognition of expanding intracranial masses. Inadequate or careless observation may permit the patient to deteriorate beyond the point of useful salvage.

In addition to observation, the patient with severe head injury requires careful evaluation and management of respiratory function, including blood gas studies and respiratory assistance. Corticosteroids in large doses may be of value. If intracranial clots are excluded, the use of the osmotic dehydrating agents such as mannitol may also be of benefit in combating brain swelling.

Injuries to the spine and spinal cord are frequently overlooked at the initial examination because the pertinent functions are not tested. This negligence may result in failure to immobilize a fractured spine and/or recognize a progressive and possibly curable lesion. It may also result in the improper assumption by later observers that the paralysis resulted from movement or manipulation after the accident.

REFERENCES

1. Gurdjian, E. S., Hodgson, V. R., Thomas, L. M., and Patrick, L. M.: Impact head injury—mechanisms and prevention. Gen. Pract., 37:78, 1968.
2. Gurdjian, E. S., and Thomas, L. M.: Survey shows importance of team care. Mod. Hosp., 106:90, 1966.
3. Thomas, L. M., and Gurdjian, E. S.: Head injury. In: *The Craft of Surgery*, 2nd ed. (Cooper, Phillip, Ed.). Boston, Little, Brown and Company, 1971.
4. Youmans, J.: Causes of shock with head injury. J. Trauma, 4:204, 1964.
5. Thomas, L. M., and Gurdjian, E. S.: Cerebral edema. In: *Surgery Annual, 1969.* New York, Appleton-Century-Crofts, 1969.
6. Gurdjian, E. S., and Thomas, L. M.: Surgical management of the patient with head injury. Clin. Neurosurg., 12:54, 1965.
7. Jackson, F. E.: Neurosurgical advances in the treatment of missile wounds of the brain. Far East Med. J., 4:57, 1968.
8. Miller, J. D., and Jennett, W. B.: Complications of depressed skull fracture. Lancet, 2:991, 1968.
9. Gutterman, P., and Shenkin, H. A.: Prognostic features in recovery from traumatic decerebration. J. Neurosurg., 32:330, 1970.

Suggested Reading

1. Thomas, L. M., and Gurdjian, E. S.: Intracranial hematomas of traumatic origin. Neurol. Surg., in press.
2. Thomas, L. M., and Gurdjian, E. S.: Cerebral contusion and closed head injury—the nonsurgical management of head injury. Neurol. Surg. in press.
3. Gurdjian, E. S., and Thomas, M. D.: *Operative Neurosurgery*, 3rd ed. Baltimore, Williams and Wilkins, 1969.
4. Kahn, E. A., Crosby, E., Schneider, R. C., and Taren, J. A.: *Correlative Neurosurgery.* Springfield, Charles C Thomas, 1969.
5. Gurdjian, E. S., and Thomas, L. M.: The diseases and injuries of the scalp and skull. In: *Christopher's Textbook of Surgery* (Loyal, David, M. D., Ed.). Philadelphia, W. B. Saunders, 1969.
6. Gurdjian, E. S., and Thomas, L. M.: Management of head injury in the United States. In: *Head Injury Conference Proceedings* (Caveness, Wm. F., and Walker, A. E., Eds.). Philadelphia, J. B. Lippincott, 1966.
7. Richards, D. E., et al.: Inappropriate release of ADH in subdural hematoma. J. Trauma, 11:758, 1971.
8. Talalla, A., and Morin, M. A.: Acute traumatic subdural hematoma: A review of one hundred consecutive cases. J. Trauma, 11:771, 1971.
9. Mathews, W. E.: The early treatment of craniocerebral missile injuries: Experience with 92 cases. J. Trauma, 12:939, 1972.
10. Hoff, J., et al.: Traumatic subdural hygroma. J. Trauma, 13:870, 1973.
11. Gonzalez, N. C., and Overman, J.: Cardiopulmonary responses to uniformly elevated CSF pressure. J. Trauma, 13:727, 1973.
12. Gurdjian, E. S.: Prevention and mitigation of head injury from antiquity to the present. J. Trauma, 13:931, 1973.

15 TRAUMA TO THE EYE

O. BROWN°

"Truly the light is sweet, and a pleasant thing it is for the eyes to behold the sun."

ECCLESIASTES 11:7

EVALUATION OF TRAUMA TO THE EYE

Three cardinal rules for the initial evaluation of trauma to the eye are: listen, question, examine carefully. This means *listen* to the patient as he describes his difficulty, *ask* specific and pertinent questions to complete a good history, and *examine* carefully the injured *and* the uninjured eye.

History Taking

As in any good history, the patient must be given an opportunity to describe, in his own words, the nature of the injury and any symptoms or changes which occurred following the injury. Special attention must be given to a history of pain or any diminution of vision.

After listening carefully to the patient's description of the injury, the examiner should be sure that he has answers to all of the following questions:

1. How and when was the trauma sustained?
2. Was there pain at the moment of injury and/or did pain develop later?
3. Was there any change in vision? If so, was the change sudden or gradual?

°The artwork in this chapter was done by Hedwig Murphy, to whom the author expresses gratitude.

4. In the case of a possible penetrating foreign body, does the patient have a sample of the foreign body or the object from which the foreign body came? This is particularly helpful if the intraocular foreign body is metallic.

PITFALL

IF THE PHYSICIAN ATTEMPTS TO REMOVE A NONMAGNETIC FOREIGN BODY FROM INSIDE THE GLOBE WITH A MAGNET, HE WILL ONLY INCREASE THE TRAUMA.

---

5. Has the patient ever been treated for iritis or glaucoma?
6. Has he any known sensitivity or allergy to topical or systemic medications?

Examination of the Eye

In most cases the examination of the eye may be easily done by any physician, provided a systematic approach is adopted.

VISUAL ACUITY. The visual acuity should be determined early in the examination. If a Snellen chart is available, this should be used at a stated distance, preferably 20 feet. Patients with corrective lenses should wear these while being tested. Near vision should also be tested, again with a standard eye chart if possible, and the results recorded. If standard eye charts are not available or if the patient is unable to read any of the Snellen chart, then some record of visual acuity should be noted (counts of fingers at 1, 2, 6 feet, etc.). For near vision, the patient's ability to read newspaper print at various distances can be recorded.

EXTERNAL INSPECTION. After visual acuity has been determined, the following features are noted: What is the appearance of the lids? Are they open? Is there swelling? Is there spasm due to sensitivity to light or to pain? Is there a laceration, abrasion or ecchymosis? Is there ptosis of one lid while the contralateral lid is normal?

LID RETRACTION. If the lids are so swollen that the patient cannot voluntarily open his eyelids enough to allow the physician to inspect the eye directly, they will have to be retracted with the fingers or special small lid retractors. In opening the lids with the fingers, care must be taken not to apply pressure on the globe. The proper technique for opening the lids to examine the eye or to instill medication is: For the lower lid, the tip of the thumb should be placed almost up to the lid margin after which, with the ball of the thumb resting lightly against the infraorbital rim, the lid is retracted downward so that the end of the thumb now holds the lid margin fairly firmly against the orbital rim. A similar procedure is carried out to elevate the upper lid, but with the ball of the thumb on the supraorbital rim.

PITFALL

IF THE EYELIDS OF AN UNCOOPERATIVE PATIENT WHO HAS LACERATION OF THE CORNEA OR SCLERA ARE RETRACTED, THE INTRAOCULAR CONTENTS MAY EXTRUDE FROM THE GLOBE.

ANESTHESIA. If the eye of a child or uncooperative adult has been lacerated or ruptured, the patient should be anesthetized for the examination. The restless or struggling patient, by increasing intraocular pressure, may cause ocular contents to be extruded through any defect in the surface of the eye once the protection of the lids is lost. When such an injury is suspected or found, the eye should be carefully patched and covered with a metal shield until the patient can be seen by an ophthalmologist who is prepared to repair any damage at the time of examination. It is the strong opinion of the author that whenever repair of a lacerated cornea, globe or ruptured eyeball is required, general anesthesia is the anesthetic of choice, even in adults. Not only can examination and treatment be performed more completely under general anesthesia, but local anesthesia entails a risk of retrobulbar hemorrhage.

EQUIPMENT. The equipment which should be available for examining the patient with a suspected eye injury includes:

1. disposable flashlights with white (clear) and blue bulbs
2. fluorescein strips
3. ophthalmic irrigating solutions
4. small lid retractors
5. magnifying loupe
6. topical ophthalmic solutions including Ophthaine, 10% Neo-Synephrine, 1% pilocarpine
7. small disposable syringes with 22-gauge needles
8. Schiotz tonometer
9. slit lamp.

SCLERA AND CORNEA. The initial inspection of the eyeball or globe itself should begin with an examination of the sclera for any defect (laceration or perforation) in its surface and the presence or absence of increased redness or vascularity (injection). The cornea should next be examined to ascertain that it is clear, shiny, and intact.

If the apparently intact eyeball seems soft when it is pressed lightly, or if there is wrinkling of the cornea or sclera, this suggests a posterior laceration or rupture of the globe. If there is any limitation of motion of the eye, usually checked by asking the patient to follow an object or finger, this suggests a fracture of the orbital floor or wall.

Whenever the history suggests abrasion, laceration, or damage by a foreign body, the cornea should be stained with fluorescein, which produces a greenish fluorescence in any surface defect when observed under a blue light from a Woods lamp or special disposable flashlight. The eye is best examined with a flashlight which provides a small direct spot of light, using both clear and blue bulbs. In many instances, however, reflected light may provide better visualization of corneal foreign bodies, ulcerations, abrasions, and other distortions. If available, a magnifying loupe and a slit lamp should also be used to examine the eye. Even if the examiner has perfect eyesight himself, the visibility with a magnifying loupe is considerably better. A slit lamp provides even greater detail and, unless an ophthalmologist is immediately available, the emergency physician should be familar with its use.

Fluorostrips, rather than fluorescein drops, are recommended because the solution may contain microorganisms, especially Pseudomonas. The exposed strip of fluorescein paper is moistened with a drop of an ophthalmic irrigating fluid, and a drop of the resultant solution is then placed either in the lower cul-de-sac or, with the patient looking down and the upper lid lifted by the examiner, on the exposed portion of the sclera above the cornea. After one or two blinks, the dye is usually well distributed over the outer portion of the eye. The fluorescein will not stain an intact healthy epithelium but will stain an abnormal area, often in a characteristic fashion (Fig. 1).

PUPIL. When examining the pupil its size and shape should be noted, as should its reaction to both direct and consensual stimulation with a light. This light source should be as small as possible. Any photophobia should also be noted. Except to determine the reaction of the pupil, the light should not be shone directly into the patient's eye; light which enters from the side is less uncomfortable.

ANTERIOR CHAMBER. In examining the anterior chamber, the physician should

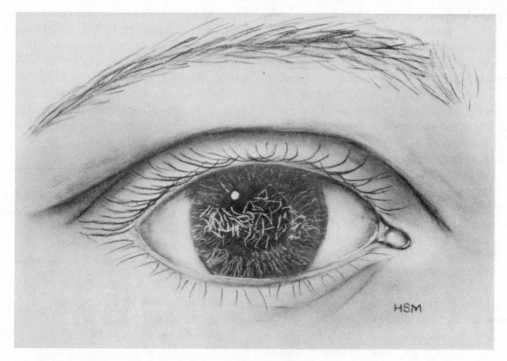

FIG. 1. Corneal abrasion which may occur with a fingernail, hairbrush, piece of paper, or branch from a tree.

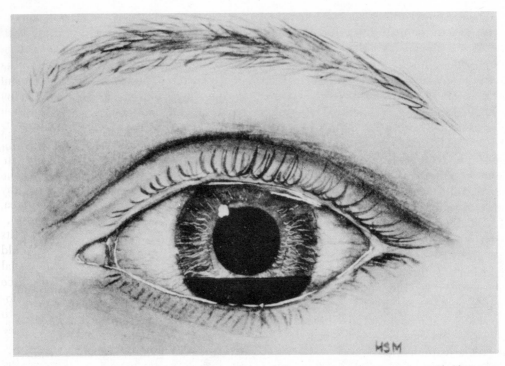

FIG. 2. Hyphema or pooling of blood in the lower portion of the anterior chamber may occur with blunt trauma of the eye.

note its depth and the presence of any blood (hyphema) (Fig. 2) or foreign bodies. With penetrating injury the anterior chamber may be absent, with no space between the cornea and iris. With posterior rupture of the eyeball the anterior chamber may be deeper than normal. At this same time the iris should be examined carefully for any abnormal position or motion; one of the earliest signs of a dislocated lens is "shaking" of the iris with slight movements of the eye.

FUNDUS. After the cornea, the iris and the anterior chamber have been examined, the fundus is observed. Serious limitations are imposed on the examiner if the pupil is not dilated; all he can determine under such circumstances is whether the vitreous is clear, whether there is a good red reflex from the posterior portion of the eye, and whether the optic nerve and the vessels near it are within normal limits. Peripheral holes, hemorrhages, tears, disinsertions can all be missed unless the fundus is examined with the pupil dilated. In any type of injury to an eye, therefore, the examination must be considered to be incomplete until the fundus is properly examined. At this point, unless there are other injuries which contraindicate dilatation of the pupils, 10% Neo-Synephrine eye drops are instilled every 10 minutes for two to three instillations; 20 minutes are then allowed for optimal dilatation of the pupil.

PITFALL

IF A PATIENT IS SENT AWAY FROM THE EMERGENCY ROOM WITH A WIDELY DILATED PUPIL, AN EPISODE OF ACUTE ANGLE-CLOSURE GLAUCOMA MAY BE PRECIPITATED.

The effects of the Neo-Synephrine can usually be overcome with one or two drops of 1% pilocarpine.

When instilling drops or ointment into an eye, the lower lid should be retracted downward and the patient asked to look upward. This technique reduces the possibility of irritating the cornea with the tip of the dropper. The solution should not be allowed to fall directly onto the cornea from a distance of several inches.

TONOMETER. When using a Schiotz tonometer, the cornea must be well anesthetized and care must be taken that the patient does not "squeeze" or move the eye while the tonometer is in contact with the cornea; otherwise, corneal abrasions may occur. All emergency physicians should be familiar with the use of this instrument.

TREATMENT

Foreign Bodies

SUPERFICIAL FOREIGN BODIES. Loosely adherent foreign bodies are usually located in the lower cul-de-sac, under the upper lid and occasionally on the cornea. This type of foreign body can generally be removed

easily by irrigation with a sterile isotonic solution or with a moistened cotton-tip applicator. If these techniques fail, the foreign body is probably embedded in the surface, often involving the cornea. Under these circumstances, it can generally be removed using a 22-gauge sterile disposable needle and a magnifying loupe after the surface of the eye has been anesthetized with a drop of topical anesthesia.

PITFALL

IF VIGOROUS ATTEMPTS ARE MADE TO DIG OUT AN EMBEDDED CORNEAL FOREIGN BODY, THEY MAY PRODUCE A CORNEAL WOUND WHICH WILL SCAR AND CAUSE DISTORTED VISION.

If there is no history of or suggestion of glaucoma, after the adherent or embedded foreign body has been removed antibiotic

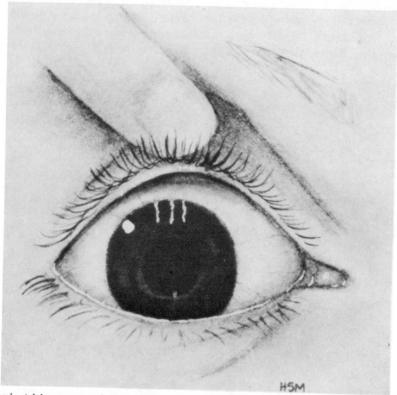

HSM

FIG. 3. Fluorescein staining may reveal small scratch marks on the upper cornea if there is an embedded foreign body under the upper lid.

or sulfa eye drops and a short-acting mydri-atic, such as 2% homatropine, should be instilled and the eye patched. The patch should be removed four times a day and 1 or 2 fresh antibacterial and mydriatic eye drops instilled. The patient should be seen again in 24 hours. As part of the repeat examination, the cornea should be stained with fluorescein. If a corneal stain is present, the patching should be continued with the drops for another 48 hours. If a rust ring remains it should be removed very carefully, using topical anesthesia and the edge, rather than the point, of a 22-gauge needle; this should be done, if at all possible, by an ophthalmologist. After the first 48 hours, the mydriatic drops may be stopped if there is no pain or redness. The patient must be warned that the drops will cause some sensitivity to light and will temporarily impair his ability to focus on close objects or print.

Occasionally, the sole clue to the presence of a foreign body embedded in the underside of the upper lid may be small scratch marks on the upper portion of the cornea, visible only with the fluorescein staining (Fig. 3).

CONTACT LENSES. The patient who has trouble with contact lenses gives a rather typical history of having worn them a bit longer than usual and then awakening with severe pain within one to two hours after removing them. Examination reveals a diffuse corneal edema (Fig. 4).

Other problems for the emergency-room surgeon include the "lost" contact lens or the contact lens which cannot be removed from the eye. Patients are usually upset not only because the lens is lost or because they are unable to remove it but because, in attempting to remove the lens, they have also managed to scratch the cornea. Careful examination will usually reveal the position of the contact lens. If irrigation of the eye does not wash it out, a small suction cup may be used or the lens may be carefully "lifted" out with the cotton tip of a moistened applicator after a drop of topical anesthetic has been placed in the eye. After removal of the lens, the cornea should be carefully examined for abrasion. If such

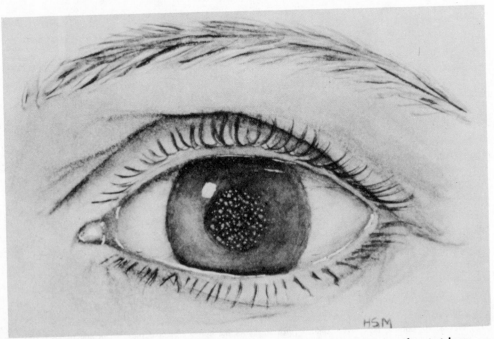

FIG. 4. Fluorescein staining of the cornea revealing corneal edema after prolonged wearing of contact lenses.

a lesion is found, it should be treated with eye drops and patching. At present there is an increased use of the "soft" contact lenses and a word of precaution concerning these lenses is important.

PITFALL

IF FLUORESCEIN IS PLACED IN AN EYE WITH A SOFT CONTACT LENS IN PLACE, THE CONTACT LENS WILL BECOME STAINED.

Because these lenses tend to soak up fluids and stain easily, no medications should be placed in an eye which has a soft contact lens in place. Since they are so fragile, an inexperienced examiner can easily cause damage or distortion in the course of removing and handling them. If it is necessary to remove such a lens, sharp fingernails or metallic instruments should not be used. The lens should not be replaced in the emergency room other than at the direction of the ophthalmologist. The soft contact lens must be sterilized before putting it back in the eye.

AXIOM

A PATIENT WITH A CORNEAL ABRASION SHOULD NEVER BE GIVEN A TOPICAL ANESTHETIC TO INSTILL IN THE EYE AT HOME.

Use of a local anesthetic by the patient at home to obtain relief of pain from a corneal abrasion, ulcer, or edema can mask progression of the condition to penetration of the cornea. Pain in the eye is a protective mechanism, and to relieve the pain without adequate treatment of the basic problem can only produce more trauma.

PARTIALLY PENETRATING FOREIGN BODIES. Occasionally a partially penetrating foreign body, or a foreign body which has completely penetrated the eye but still has a portion remaining outside the eye, may be encountered. In these circumstances, the question arises as to whether or not the foreign body should be removed in the

emergency room. This decision is best left to the judgment of an eye surgeon, who can carefully examine the eye under a slit lamp and who is prepared to suture the eye after removal of the foreign body if this is necessary. The necessity for suturing exists whenever the penetration occurs in the cornea and if the anterior chamber collapses after removal of the foreign body and fails to reform in one or two hours after patching. The danger in trying to remove a penetrating but partially protruding corneal foreign body is that, in addition to the risk of loss of the anterior chamber, the protruding portion may break, leaving the remaining portion buried in the cornea and protruding through the posterior portion of the cornea into the anterior chamber. This situation increases the possibility of significantly greater trauma to the cornea in the course of the surgical intervention necessary to remove the foreign body.

In the case of the penetrating but partially protruding corneal foreign body, antibiotics and drops to constrict the pupil should be instilled. Miotic drops, such as 1% or 2% pilocarpine, are instilled every five minutes for three doses to ensure a miotic pupil to protect the lens.

PENETRATING FOREIGN BODIES. Whenever the history suggests foreign-body penetration into the eye, and especially if the entrance is anteriorly through the cornea, not only should the point of entrance on the cornea be identified but the iris should also be carefully examined for any tear or hole indicating that the foreign body passed into or through it. It is possible for a small metallic foreign body of high velocity to enter the eye and cause only a minimal amount of discomfort, producing no immediate visual changes. Such an object may be ignored for several days. The author has seen instances where a child playing around a garage or machine shop complained of a foreign-body sensation in the eye at the time someone on the other side of the shop was pounding metal against metal. When nothing was found under the lids or on the cornea nothing was done until, because the eye remained red and became painful, x-rays were taken and revealed the presence of a foreign body. In such a case, a careful history, awareness of the possibility that a foreign body might be present and the taking of x-rays in the emergency room may help to make a diagnosis earlier and enhance the possibilities of saving the eye.

Foreign bodies that penetrate the eye and remain in the anterior chamber tend to lie on or embed in the iris or float loosely in the lower portion of the anterior chamber toward the angle. If the foreign body is loose but inferior and anterior to the iris, the patient should be kept in the sitting position and the pupil constricted with miotic eye drops such as 1% or 2% pilocarpine. This reduces the possibility of migration through the pupil onto the lens or into the posterior chamber behind the iris. A foreign body which has completely penetrated into the eye and lies in the deeper structures should obviously not be removed in the emergency room. After it has been ascertained that a foreign body is present, either by visualization with an ophthalmoscope or by appropriate x-ray studies, antibiotic drops should be instilled and the eye covered with a protective patch until an ophthalmologist assumes care of the patient.

Nonforeign Bodies With Foreign-body Symptoms

A number of conditions exist which cause patients to come to the emergency room complaining of a foreign body in the eye but with no apparent foreign body even on careful examination. The symptoms may be associated with trauma of a mild degree (hair spray entering the eye) (Fig. 5), corneal ulcers (Fig. 6), iritis, corneal edema secondary to other conditions such as glaucoma, corneal abrasions, flash burns, chemical irritants and overlong wearing of con-

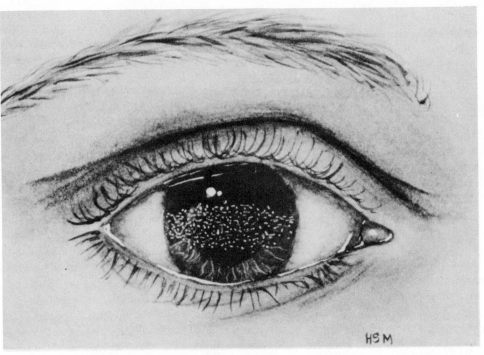

FIG. 5. Fluorescein staining of the cornea which may appear after hair spray enters the eye. Note the lack of staining superiorly and inferiorly where the cornea is often protected by the lids.

tact lens. Most of these conditions are accompanied by a certain degree of photosensitivity and protective blepharospasm of the affected eye. It is therefore important to stain the cornea with fluorescein whenever the symptoms suggest the possibility of a foreign body.

The corneal abrasion and corneal edema associated with the wearing of contact lenses, and the edema due to hair sprays and similar irritants, are best treated with antibiotic and cortisone drops every four hours, mydriatic drops such as 2% homatropine every six hours, and patching of the eye for 24 hours. The patch is removed every four to six hours to instill the medication, then replaced. Eyes should be reexamined within 24 hours by an ophthalmologist, especially if there is no improvement after 24 hours.

If a foreign-body sensation is present, but the corneal surface is normal even when examined after fluorescein staining, iritis should be suspected, especially if vision is impaired, the pupil is small and does not react well to light, and the anterior chamber appears cloudy or muddy. Iritis is usually treated symptomatically at first, using cortisone drops topically every 2 to 3 hours when the patient is awake and mydriatic drops (2% homatropine) every 6 hours. Analgesics may also be needed. Follow-up by an ophthalmologist is essential.

PITFALL

IF AN EYE WITH A BACTERIAL OR VIRAL ULCER IS PATCHED AND KEPT CLOSED, THE ULCER BECOMES RAPIDLY WORSE.

It is important to recognize the typical corneal lesion of herpes (Fig. 7), because such a lesion should not be treated with antibiotics, cortisone drops, or patching of the eye. Ulcers of the eye are usually due to viral or bacterial etiology and eye patching tends to cause the eye to act as an incubator, enhancing the growth of the microorganisms. A viral ulcer usually has reduced corneal sensitivity.

Blunt Injuries

It must be remembered that injury to the visual system can occur in head injuries.

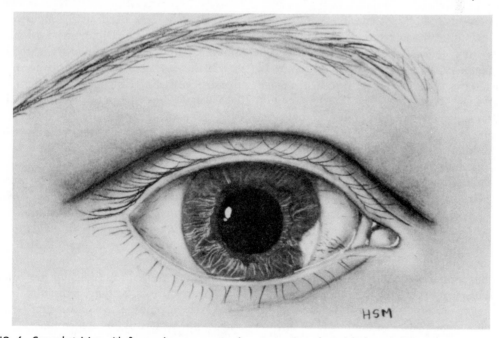

FIG. 6. Corneal staining with fluorescein as may occur in a traumatic or bacterial ulcer of the cornea.

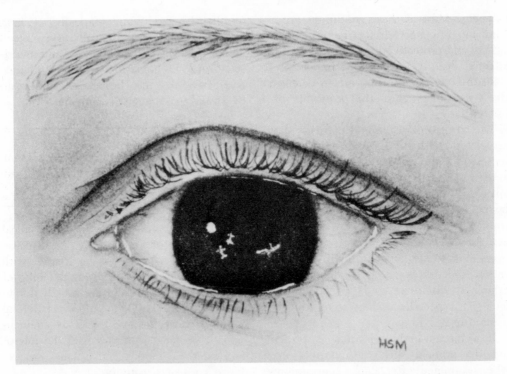

FIG. 7. Typical appearance, after fluorescein staining of cornea, of a dendritic (herpetic) ulcer of the cornea.

The clinical picture may be extremely confusing; vision may be impaired but there may be no observable injury to the eye and no associated skull fractures. Careful follow-up in the hospital by an ophthalmologist and neurologist is essential.

PERIORBITAL HEMATOMAS. Contusions of the periorbital area with resultant hematoma or "black eye" are fairly common after any facial trauma. Most of these injuries are uncomplicated and require only symptomatic therapy with analgesics. Ice packs and enzymes (such as Chymoral or Ananase) may help to reduce the swelling. Nevertheless, when such an injury is seen in the emergency room, the possibility of a more serious injury (fracture of the orbit, retrobulbar hemorrhage, hyphema [blood in the anterior chamber], rupture of the globe, retinal detachments, traumatic iritis, macular contusions, choroidal tears, or subluxation of the lens) must be considered. Unless a complete eye examination, including visual acuity, motility, and fundus-

copy, is performed, these injuries will be missed.

ORBITAL FRACTURES. A fracture of the orbit must be suspected with any severe trauma near the eye. Diplopia and limitation of motion of the eye due to incarceration of the extraocular muscles in the fracture are virtually pathognomonic. Both of these signs, however, may be absent initially even with a large defect in the orbital floor. If severe edema prevents prolapse of the eye into the maxillary antrum, or if visual acuity is markedly reduced, diplopia may not be noted for a period of time. Routine x-ray views of the orbits and facial bones may not demonstrate a fracture, but clouding of the antrum may be seen on the involved side. The exact location and extent of the fracture are best demonstrated with laminagrams. Fractures of the orbit do not require immediate reduction, but whenever diagnosed or suspected they should be treated by an eye surgeon.

BLUNT INJURIES OF THE GLOBE. Damage

to the globe itself following blunt trauma can range from a mild traumatic iritis to posterior bilateral rupture. If there is any decrease in visual acuity, macular edema, vitreous hemorrhage or retinal detachment must be suspected. Certain complications such as retinal holes or hemorrhages, iritis, traumatic cataract, and secondary glaucoma may not appear until later, and for this reason the emergency-room examination must be followed in 24 hours by a complete eye examination. A luxated or subluxated lens may be difficult for the emergency-room physician to diagnose, but should be sought for carefully.

Ruptures of the Globe. Ruptures of the globe following blunt trauma to the eye occur because the high intraocular pressure disrupts the outer layers of the eye and the inner contents extrude. An anterior rupture is not likely to be missed, as there will be absence of the anterior chamber and loss of corneal contour and wrinkling of the eye if the lid is pressed against the globe. If posterior rupture of the globe occurs, the anterior chamber will remain full or will be deeper than normal. The eye will be soft and the cornea will wrinkle when the lid presses against it.

When the rupture of the globe is diagnosed or suspected, great care must be taken not to damage the eye further. Complete examination should be reserved until the patient can be properly anesthetized and a complete repair can be carried out at the time of evaluation. Antibiotic drops should be placed in the cul-de-sac and the eye patched carefully so that there is no movement of the lid. In some instances the contralateral eye must also be patched to prevent lid movement over the eye.

Contusions of the Globe without Rupture. This type of injury may occur in a variety of ways and can be caused by a number of instruments such as suction-tipped arrows, projectile type toys, rubber bands, BB pellets, air gun pellets, poking fingers, baseballs, handballs, fists, and tennis balls. All may cause corneal abrasions,

hyphemas, iridocyclitis, subluxated lens, traumatic cataract, intravitreal hemorrhage, retinal hemorrhage, retinal holes, retinal dialysis, macular hemorrhage, macular edema or choroidal tear. If any of these lesions is suspected or diagnosed, the patient should be admitted to the hospital, sedated and kept at strict bed rest with the eye patched. Consultation with an ophthalmologist should be obtained without delay.

LACERATIONS OF THE LIDS. To avoid notching of the lid margins after a laceration, the repair must be meticulous. Notching of an upper lid, especially in its center, may cause exposure of the cornea during sleep. Notching of the lower lid can cause bothersome epiphora due to leakage of the tears through the notch before they reach the punctum.

PITFALL

IF THE PUNCTA ARE NOT CAREFULLY IDENTIFIED AND THE TEAR DUCTS PROBED BEFORE REPAIR OF LACERATIONS OF THE INNER THIRD OF THE EYELIDS, SERIOUS DAMAGE TO THE TEAR DUCTS MAY OCCUR.

The most opportune and effective time to repair lacerations of the tear ducts is at the time of original surgery. Supports such as sutures, silicone tubes or probes should be inserted in the tear ducts to maintain patency during the repair and the period of healing.

LACERATIONS OF THE GLOBE. Lacerations of the globe, including those of the cornea, are usually not difficult to diagnose if a proper examination is performed. The most dangerous lacerations, because they are easily missed, are those associated with a small laceration of an eyelid.

PITFALL

IF THE EYE OPPOSITE A LID INJURY IS NOT EXAMINED, AN UNDERLYING LACERATION OF THE GLOBE IS LIKELY TO BE MISSED.

Every ophthalmologist has had the experience of having a patient enter his office with a laceration of the cornea or globe, with subsequent prolapse of intraocular contents or iris, two or three days after a minor lid laceration was sutured in an emergency room. In examining and evaluating lid lacerations, it must be remembered that when the lids close the globes rotate upward. Consequently, a laceration which has penetrated the upper lid may involve the cornea or the sclera inferior to the cornea. Similarly, a penetration of the lower lid may result in a laceration of the globe which can be seen only when the eye is rotated upward.

Chemical Burns

Depending upon the type and amount of material contacting the eye, the severity of a chemical burn may range from simple irritation requiring only irrigation to eventual extensive necrosis. With the classic exception of mustard gas, any eye that is exposed to a chemical substance should be copiously irrigated with saline, distilled water, or special ophthalmic irrigating solutions such as Dacriose.

ALKALI BURNS. The most destructive chemicals to enter the eye are alkaline substances such as lye, ammonia, and plaster. With such substances, there must be no delay in instituting irrigation, and it is doubtful whether there can ever be too much irrigation. Special tubes are available which can be inserted through the upper lid so that continuous irrigation from an intravenous type of bottle is possible. The eye must be examined carefully after irrigation, especially if the chemical was in a powder or granular form, to be sure that all of the chemical material is removed; otherwise the chemical substance will continue to react with the ocular tissues, producing progressively more severe damage. After copious irrigation and careful removal of any particles, antibiotic and mydriatic drops should be instilled into the eye and the patient immediately referred

to the nearest ophthalmologist. There should be no delay whatever in the continuing treatment of the eye; if a consultant is not available, the patient should be transferred as soon as possible.

ACID BURNS. Acid burns are usually not as devastating to the eye as those due to alkali. Similar principles of management apply: early complete irrigation followed by antibiotic, mydriatic, and steroid eye drops to prevent secondary infection and to reduce local pain and inflammation.

OTHER INJURIES. Other chemicals and instruments which may injure the eye include misdirected hair spray, deodorants, perfumes, mascara brushes, eyelash curlers, and eyelash glues. These injuries usually involve the portion of the cornea not protected by the eyelids and usually show up well with fluorescein staining. Treatment in each case will vary with the extent and type of the damage. Follow-up examination by an ophthalmologist is important even with what initially appear to be mild injuries.

CONCLUSIONS

Careful complete examination of the eye is essential even with what may appear to be a mild ocular injury. Consultation with an ophthalmologist should be obtained if there is any question at all about the seriousness of the problem or its treatment. Follow-up examination in 24 hours is essential and may prevent considerable eye damage. The margin of safety with any eye injury is extremely narrow. The thickness of the cornea is less than a millimeter, and one diopter of induced astigmation can reduce visual acuity by 10%. Further, appearance of the eyes can have an important influence on the patient's personality and social acceptability.

REFERENCES

1. Kelman, C., and Brooks, D.: Ultrasonic emulsification and aspiration of traumatic hyphema. A preliminary report. Amer. J. Ophthal., 71:1289, 1971.

2. Dodick, J., Galin, M., and Kwitke, M.: Concomitant blowout fracture of the orbit and rupture of the globe. Arch. Ophthal., 84:707, 1970.

3. Smith, R., and Blount, R.: Blowout fracture of the orbital roof with pulsating exophthalmos, blepharoptosis and superior gaze paresis. Amer. J. Ophthal., 71:1052, 1971.

4. Frueh, B.: Transient blindness following blunt trauma to the eye. Amer. J. Ophthal., 71:1034, 1971.

5. Ide, C., and Webb, R.: Penetrating transorbital injury with cerebrospinal orbitorrhea. Amer. J. Ophthal., 71:1037, 1971.

6. Bleeker, G., and Keith, L.: *Fractures of the Orbit.* Baltimore, Williams & Wilkins, 1970.

7. Ferguson, C.: Deep, wooden foreign bodies of the orbit. Trans. Amer. Acad. Ophthal. Otolaryng., 74:778, 1970.

8. Girard, L., Alford, W., Feldman, G., and Williams, B.: Severe alkali burns. Trans. Amer. Acad. Ophthal. Otolaryng., 74:788, 1970.

9. Laibson, P., and Oconor, J.: Explosive tear gas injuries of the eye. Trans. Amer. Acad. Ophthal. Otolaryng., 74:811, 1970.

10. Snow, J.: The management of orbital wall fractures. Trans. Amer. Acad. Ophthal. Otolaryng., 74:1045, 1970.

11. Thompson, E.: Orbital rim and arch fractures. Trans. Amer. Acad. Ophthal. Otolaryng., 74:1052, 1970.

12. Treister, G.: Review of ocular injuries in the six day war. Amer. J. Ophthal., 68:675, 1969.

13. Krolman, G., and Pidibe, W.: Early ethanol therapy for acute methyl alcohol poisoning. Canad. J. Ophthal., 3:270, 1968.

14. Griffith, J. D.: Transient blindness following seemingly trivial head injury in children. New Eng. J. Med., 278:648, 1968.

Suggested Reading

1. Goldman, R. J., and Hessbury, P. C.: Appraisal of surgical correction in 130 cases of orbital floor fracture. Amer. J. Ophthal., 76:152, 1973.

2. Edwards, W. C., and Layden, W. E.: Monocular versus binocular patching in traumatic hyphema. Amer. J. Ophthal., 76:359, 1973.

3. Fryer, M. P., et al.: Repair of trauma about the orbit. J. Trauma, 12:290, 1972.

4. Asch, M. J., et al.: Ocular complications associated with burns: Review of a five-year experience including 104 patients. J. Trauma, 11:857, 1971.

16 TRAUMA TO THE FACE

R. F. WILSON
P. ZAMICK

Severe facial trauma is becoming increasingly common, and up to three quarters of the automobile accident victims seen in the emergency room sustain soft-tissue or bony injury to the head or neck.[1] These injuries may compromise the upper airway, can cause sensory damage to the eyes and ears, and can result in severe functional and cosmetic deformities. Although the exposed nature of the face makes most of these injuries fairly obvious, intra-oral, intranasal, and intra-aural damage may not be detected unless special efforts are made to examine for them.

INITIAL MANAGEMENT

The most important objectives in the initial or emergency treatment of severe injuries to the face are: (1) provision or maintenance of an adequate airway, and (2) control of bleeding.

Maintenance of an Airway

The mouth must be opened and examined visually and directly with the gloved finger for blood, vomitus, broken dentures, loose teeth, or foreign bodies. A bite-block, oral airway, or several tongue blades should be held between the patient's teeth so that he cannot, voluntarily or involuntarily, bite the examiner. Blood and vomitus should be aspirated from the pharynx, mouth, and nose; a large-bore suction apparatus such as the "tonsil-sucker" is ideal for this purpose.

If the tongue is falling back into the pharynx because the jaw is fractured or because the patient is severely depressed from a head injury, alcohol, or drugs, the mandible should be held forward until an oral airway can be inserted. If it is absolutely certain that there are no injuries except to the face, the tongue and jaw can be maintained in a forward position by turning the patient on his side. If there is massive intra-oral hemorrhage, insertion of an endotracheal tube may be extremely difficult, and a coniotomy or tracheostomy may be required to maintain the airway.

Control of Hemorrhage

PITFALL

IF BLEEDING VESSELS ON THE SIDE OF THE FACE ARE CLAMPED WITHOUT CAREFULLY DISSECTING THEM FROM THE SURROUNDING TISSUE, BRANCHES OF THE FACIAL NERVE ARE LIABLE TO BE DAMAGED.

Whenever possible, hemorrhage from the face should be controlled by direct pressure. If a vessel must be clamped, care must be taken not to include branches of the facial nerve which may run alongside the vessel.

Intra-oral bleeding can be especially hazardous because, if the patient has lost his gag or cough reflexes through brain damage, drugs, or alcohol, he is apt to aspirate the blood. In some instances massive bleeding from the nose or pharynx may go unnoticed until the patient vomits up a large quantity of blood.

In instances of severe intra-oral or pharyngeal bleeding which are difficult to control directly, some physicians have attempted indirect control by unilateral or bilateral ligation of branches of the external carotid artery in the neck. These efforts are generally ineffective because of the rich collateral blood supply; such endeavors should be discouraged except as a last resort, to be combined with packing of the area, when all other methods have failed.

Although the face and scalp can bleed massively, especially from long deep lacerations, and may occasionally cause severe shock, the physician should be reluctant to ascribe any persistent hypotension to a facial or head injury alone; in such circumstances, special efforts must be made to rule out the abdomen or thorax as a site of continued hemorrhage.

EXAMINATION OF THE PATIENT

Physical Examination

PITFALL

IF THE PHYSICIAN ALLOWS A SEVERE FACIAL INJURY TO DIVERT HIM FROM A COMPLETE EXAMINATION OF THE PATIENT, SUBTLE BUT MORE LIFE-THREATENING INJURIES MAY GO UNNOTICED.

All patients with facial injuries must be examined completely before definitive repair is attempted. Special attention in such individuals should be directed to the brain, cervical spine, abdomen, and chest.

PITFALL

IF X-RAYS ALONE ARE RELIED ON TO DIAGNOSE FACIAL FRACTURES, MANY IMPORTANT INJURIES WILL BE MISSED.

Although there seems to be increasing reliance placed on the x-ray to diagnose all bony injuries, especially in medicolegal proceedings, a complete early physical examination of the face is often far more revealing and accurate. During the initial external inspection, any unusual swelling or loss of facial symmetry and any impaired movement of the facial muscles or jaw should be sought. The face should be carefully palpated bilaterally before the severe edema and hematoma formation accompanying most facial injuries obscures the bony landmarks. All bony prominences, especially the nasal bones, zygomatic arch, the alveolar ridge, teeth, and orbital rim should be checked for any unusual mobility. Loss of sensation to pinprick over the lower or upper lips may be an indication of a fracture of the mandible or maxilla.

X-rays

With any severe facial injury, x-rays should be taken of the skull and cervical spine as well as of any site of suspected facial fracture. X-rays of the facial bones are often misleading and difficult to interpret. Special views are frequently necessary, and careful early review of the films with a radiologist is essential.

Because of the special problems and pitfalls involved in the treatment of trauma to various portions of the face, the discussion of this area has been divided into four sections: 1. Soft-tissue injuries of the face. 2. Maxillofacial trauma. 3. Trauma to the midportion of the face. 4. Trauma to the ears and facial nerves.

Section 1

SOFT-TISSUE INJURIES OF THE FACE

The common soft-tissue injuries of the face, such as abrasions, contusions, and simple lacerations without loss of tissue, can be managed quite adequately by most E.D. physicians. More complex trauma involving loss of tissue or avulsion flaps should be referred to a surgeon specializing in the management of these problems. Since a facial scar is often a lifetime reminder of the primary repair, proper initial treatment is vital (Table 1).

After the patient's condition has been stabilized with proper control of the airway and any hemorrhage, complete examination of the patient performed, and appropriate x-rays obtained, attention can be directed to definitive repair of the facial injuries. In general this can follow a logical series of steps: (1) anesthesia, (2) cleansing and debridement of the wounds, (3) reduction and stabilization of fractures, (4) repair of special structures, and (5) repair of the muscle, subcutaneous tissue, and skin.

The optimal time to repair most facial injuries is as soon as the patient's condition permits. Shock, severe burn injury, unstable cervical spine fractures, and severe alcohol intoxication, however, are contraindications to early repair. Nevertheless, if repair of facial injuries is delayed for more than seven days, the bony fragments may begin to heal with fibrous union, and proper reduction may require refracture of the fragments.

ANESTHESIA

Small- or moderate-sized lacerations in cooperative adults may be treated under direct local infiltration anesthesia or by regional blockade of the infraorbital, supraorbital, or mental nerves. The ideal local

---

TABLE 1. FREQUENT ERRORS IN TREATING FACIAL TRAUMA

1. Unnecessary trauma in the handling of skin wounds.
2. Failure to remove foreign bodies, resulting in dirt-engrained tattoo wound scars.
3. Failure to align key anatomic points (for example, in the margin of eyelids, eyebrow, ear and lip wounds).
4. Use of inappropriate instruments, needles, and suture material.
5. Failure to examine the eyes for possible injury.
6. Failure to diagnose injury to the facial nerve or parotid duct or canaliculi.
7. Failure to retain cartilage or bone essential for secondary reconstructive procedures.
8. Excessive debridement of traumatized facial wound margins.
9. Use of intricate flaps for primary repair of traumatized wounds.
10. Use of strong detergents in cleansing of facial wounds.
11. Failure to keep a proper record and photographs of the initial injury which may be required for medicolegal problems.
12. Failure to protect the cornea when repairing wounds near the eyes.
13. Failure to suture mucosa to skin in full-thickness cheek loss.
14. Improper removal of sutures and delay in removal of sutures.
15. Failure to follow up the patient after primary repair of a facial wound.

PITFALL

anesthetic is usually 0.5% Xylocaine with
1:100,000 epinephrine. The vasoconstriction produced by the epinephrine helps to
reduce bleeding in the area but this vasoconstrictor should not be used in the external ear or in the tip of the nose.

Facial injuries in infants and children
and in uncooperative adults, except for the
smallest clean lacerations, should be repaired under general anesthesia; repair of
lacerations in such individuals is especially
hazardous if the injury is anywhere near
the eyes. Obviously, if the patient has an
injury to the brain or if his general condition is unstable, it is safer to delay definitive repair and merely cover the injured
areas with sterile dressings.

CLEANSING AND DEBRIDEMENT

Except for the eyebrows, all hair should
be shaved for at least an inch around any
wound. A doughnut compression dressing
around the scalp wound may help control
bleeding while the area is shaved and
cleaned. As mentioned in Chapter 15, it is
extremely important to preserve the eyebrow as a landmark for proper repair. The
skin for several inches around the wound
should then be cleaned with a nonirritating
solution, taking special care not to allow
any solution to get into the eyes. As an
extra precaution, it is wise to put a protective ointment into the eyes while the
surrounding skin is being cleansed. If there
is grease in or around the wound, benzene,
acetone, or 70% alcohol may be used as a
solvent.

The usual routine for cleaning is to cover
the wound with moist sterile gauze while
washing the surrounding skin radially away
from the wound. One can then concentrate
on cleaning the wound itself. All foreign
material and necrotic tissue are removed,
and then the wound is copiously irrigated
with sterile saline. Since any dirt or carbon
particles left behind can cause permanent
tattooing of the skin, the tissue with
ground-in foreign material may have to be
either excised or scrubbed vigorously with
a brush. Nonviable and badly traumatized
flap edges should be trimmed back to
bleeding margins; however, as a general
rule, irregular wound edges in facial lacerations require minimal debridement because of the excellent blood supply.
Healthy, small slicing trapdoor flaps should
be replaced in the defect and held with a
few tacking 6–0 interrupted nylon sutures.

Composite tissue from the ear, nose, or
eyelid containing either bone or cartilage
should never be discarded. Such tissue
should be placed in a sterile solution of
normal saline and penicillin and put into a
refrigerator for possible future use in reconstruction of the involved area.

Dirty lacerations and animal (especially
human) bites require thorough irrigation
and debridement of the heavily contaminated or necrotic tissue. Although some of
these injuries will heal if cleaned and
closed carefully with appropriate antibiotic
coverage, it is usually safer to close them
several days later after healthy granulation
tissue has developed in the base of the
wound.

REDUCTION AND STABILIZATION OF FRACTURES

The actual techniques of reducing and
stabilizing facial fractures are similar to
those used in reducing long bone fractures,
namely, disimpaction, realignment, and
then immobilization using wire splints or
denture fixation. These are discussed in detail in many texts and will consequently
not be presented here. It should be noted
that initial attempts at reduction and healing are much more apt to be successful
than later attempts at reconstruction.

REPAIR OF SPECIAL STRUCTURES

Parotid Gland and Duct

Any deep laceration involving the cheek from the anterior border of masseter muscle back toward the ear should arouse suspicion of an injury to the parotid gland, parotid duct, or facial nerve (Fig. 1). Intraoral catheterization of the parotid duct through its opening opposite the second upper molar tooth with or without a sialogram may be very helpful in diagnosing parotid injuries which later can be repaired (Fig. 2). If the gland is injured, the cap-sule should be carefully approximated. Since there is usually some drainage of saliva from the injury for at least a few days, a Penrose drain should be inserted near the site of repair.

Facial Nerve

The diagnosis and management of facial nerve injuries are discussed in Section 4 of this chapter.

Repair of Complex Lacerations

Lacerations which are stellate or which have one or more angular flaps require a special suturing technique to prevent loss of the tips of the angles (Fig. 3). The sutures for such lacerations should pass through one side of the triangular defect, through the subdermal angular flap tip, and out the opposite side of the triangle equidistant from the tip. This angle suture can be used for several types of flap lacerations including those shaped like a T, V, Z, W, Y, X, L, and H.

With lacerations in which there is loss of tissue greater than 1.0 cm in diameter, the skin on either side should be undermined subdermally for a distance equal to the diameter of the defect (Fig. 4). This produces sufficient laxity of the skin to allow bilateral advancement of the wound edge in the longitudinal axis of the defect.

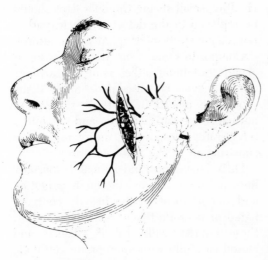

FIG. 1. Divided parotid duct and branches of the facial nerve.

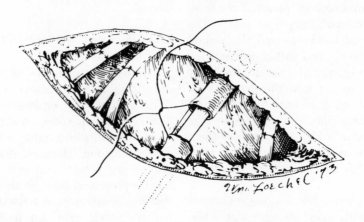

FIG. 2. Catheterization of the parotid duct and suture of its divided ends. Suture of branches of the facial nerve.

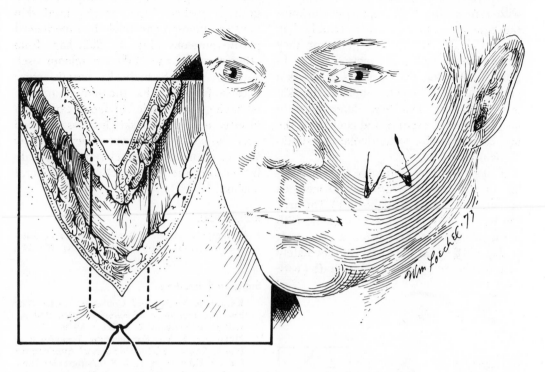

FIG. 3. The angle suture technique for repair of triangular flap defects.

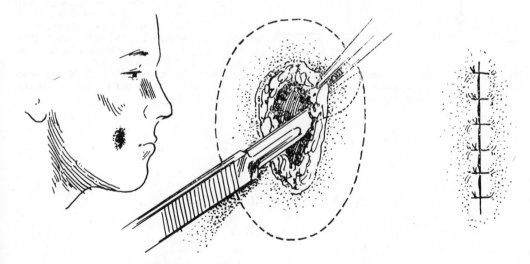

FIG. 4. Repair of a laceration with loss of tissue, illustrating the undermining technique, bilateral advancement of the wound edges and primary closure without tension.

Superficial loss of skin is best replaced with skin grafts. Very thin split-thickness skin grafts tend to "take" more readily than thicker grafts, but thicker grafts, if they remain viable, look and function better. In general, however, the thickness of the skin graft should be about the same as the skin it is replacing. The best donor sites to match the color, texture, and contour of the face come from the postauricular and supraclavicular regions.

If there has been extensive full-thickness loss of skin from the face several methods of management are available: (1) The area can be left open to granulate initially, with secondary closure later using a skin graft or flap, (2) it can be covered immediately with a thin split-thickness skin graft (with

later coverage using a full-thickness skin graft or pedicle flap), or (3) local skin flaps can be used effectively by experienced plastic surgeons (Fig. 5). Skin flaps from other areas of the body are seldom used and are often cosmetically unsatisfactory because facial skin has the unique property of having the muscles of facial expression inserted into it. If the skin loss has occurred over the cheek and is very deep, the raw area can sometimes be closed temporarily by suturing the skin directly to the buccal mucosa.

REFERENCES

1. Braunstein, P. W.: Medical aspects of automotive crash injury reach. JAMA, 163:249, 1957.

Suggested Reading

1. Kazanjian, V. H., and Converse, J. M.: *The Surgical Treatment of Facial Injuries,* 2nd ed. Baltimore, Williams & Wilkins, 1959.
2. McGregor, I. A.: *Fundamental Techniques of Plastic Surgery and their Surgical Applications,* 3rd ed. Edinburgh, E. & S. Livingstone, 1962.
3. Grabb, W. C., and Smith, J. W.: *Plastic Surgery, a Concise Guide to Clinical Practice.* Boston, Little, Brown and Company, 1968.
4. Dingman, R. O.: The management of facial injuries and fractures of the facial bones. In: *Reconstructive Plastic Surgery* (Converse, J. M., Ed.). Philadelphia, W. B. Saunders, 1964.
5. Schultz, R. C.: *Facial Injuries.* Chicago, Year Book Medical Publishers, 1970.
6. Broadbent, T. R., and Wolff, R. M.: Gunshot wounds of the face: initial care. J. Trauma, 12:229, 1972.

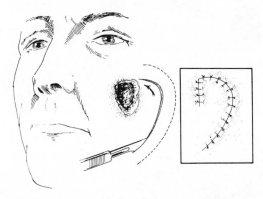

FIG. 5. Laceration with loss of tissue managed by outlining a local flap which is advanced medially following undermining of the wound edges.

Section 2

MAXILLOFACIAL TRAUMA

F. MONACO

Proper management of maxillofacial trauma requires a complete understanding of the complex architecture and function of the face, teeth, and jaws. Unfortunately, many surgeons attempt repair of severe injuries in this area without first acquiring a

sound fundamental background in the anatomy and physiology of the dental apparatus.

There are many excellent texts which describe in detail the various procedures used to manage maxillofacial trauma. Our primary interest here, however, will be to out-line briefly the principles of management of these injuries and to identify some of the pitfalls that await physicians and dentists who may be called on to treat these problems.

DIAGNOSIS

Fractures of the Mandible

The usual signs and symptoms of a fractured mandible include pain, swelling, ecchymosis, loss of function, and deformity. Paresthesias or anesthesia of the lower lip and chin due to damage to the inferior alveolar nerve in its mandibular canal or at the mental foramen should also cause one to suspect this injury.

AXIOM

MALOCCLUSION FOLLOWING TRAUMA INDICATES MANDIBULAR OR MAXILLARY FRACTURE UNTIL PROVEN OTHERWISE.

With the less obvious injuries, the most important clue to the presence of a frac-tured mandible or maxilla is malocclusion, that is, the cusps of the teeth do not fit together properly. Anyone who has had dental caries restored realizes how obvious even a mild protrusion of a filling can be.

When examining the mandible, the condyloid and coronoid processes, the horizontal and vertical rami, and the symphysis should be systematically evaluated for deformity, point tenderness, and abnormal mobility.

With a unilateral fracture dislocation of the condyle of the mandible, the jaw will deviate to the fractured side, and palpation will elicit preauricular pain. Displaced bilateral fractures of the condylar region tend to produce a retruded position of the mandible and an open-bite deformity (Fig. 6).

Certain mandibular injuries tend to be associated with damage to other structures. If the horizontal ramus is fractured on one side of the mandible, for example, there is often a corresponding fracture of the neck of the condyle on the opposite side (Fig. 7). Fractures of the symphysis of the mandible or severe contusions of the chin may

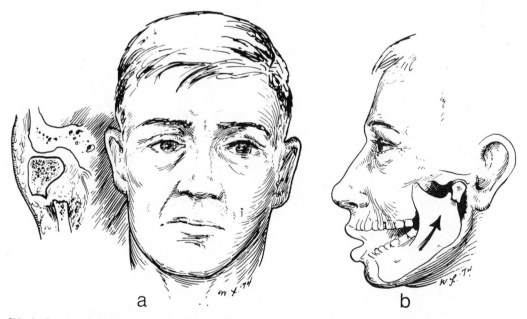

FIG. 6. Fracture of the condyle of the right mandible. a: Note the deviation of the jaw to the right and the lateral displacement of the condylar head. b: Profile view of the bilateral condylar fracture with resultant open bite deformity and retrusion of the mandible.

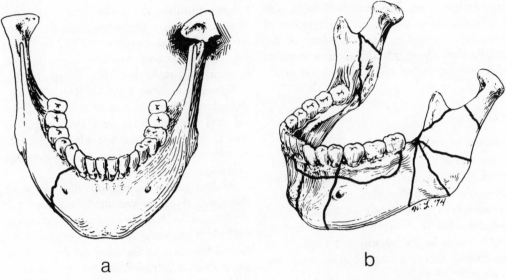

a   b

FIG. 7. *a:* Fracture of the right mandible between the canine and premolar teeth with associate fracture of the left condyle. *b:* Fractures of the jaw may involve the mandible in a wide variety of anatomic areas.

also be associated with bilateral subcondylar fractures.

Fractures of the coronoid process are not common, but when they do occur they are often associated with fractures of the malar bone and the zygomatic process of the temporal bone. Such a fracture can often be suspected if pain is elicited while examining the ascending (vertical) ramus intraorally. In some patients opening and closing the mouth may also cause pain in this area.

Fractures of the Maxilla (Midface)

CLASSIFICATION. Fractures of the maxilla should not be considered as isolated entities because they are often associated with fractures of the nasal and orbital complex. Today's literature contains many references to LeFort's classification of maxillary or midface skeletal fractures. His class I, II, and III designation, in our opinion, however, is overused and often confuses individuals attempting to understand the structures involved in an injury to the midface. We prefer to classify these maxillary fractures as lower third, middle third and orbital complex (Figs. 8, 9, 10).

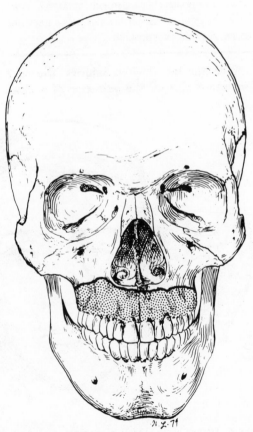

FIG. 8. Fracture of the lower third of the maxilla (LeFort I).

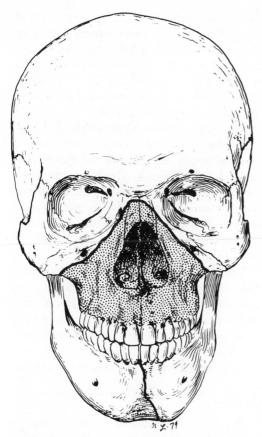

FIG. 9. Fracture of the middle third of the maxilla (LeFort II).

Horizontal fractures of the maxilla at the level of the pyriform apertures involving teeth-bearing bone are referred to as lower-third maxillary fractures. Middle-third fractures involve the nose and that part of the maxilla from the pyriform aperture superiorly to the inferior border of the orbits; this portion of the face is in the shape of a tripod with its apex at the nose (Fig. 9). The orbital complex fractures may be relatively simple and undisplaced or they may involve the frontal, nasal, and sphenoid bones, the zygomas, the zygomatic process of the temporal bone and the lacrimal and ethmoid bones unilaterally or bilaterally with severe facial deformities.

EVALUATION. The signs and symptoms of maxillary fractures are similar to those involving the mandible and include (1) deformity or asymmetry, (2) pain, edema or ecchymosis, (3) infraorbital paresthesias, and (4) malocclusion. Any mobility of the maxilla when pushing or pulling on any of its processes, especially the alveolar process of the upper teeth, confirms the diagnosis.

Fractures of the zygomatic arch are characterized by depression of the cheekbone and, in some cases, by limitation of jaw motion due to impingement on the coronoid process. Although this lesion is usually recognized rather easily, the extensive edema over the site of fracture often makes it extremely difficult to determine if it is an isolated injury or part of a complex problem involving the orbit.

Special x-ray views are often needed to help diagnose fractures of the maxilla.

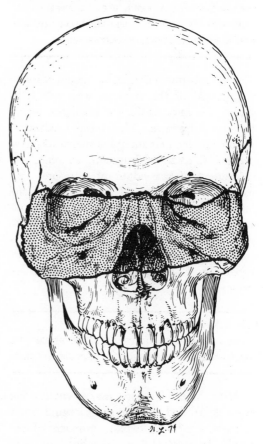

FIG. 10. Orbital complex fracture of the maxilla (LeFort III).

These may include Stereo-Waters views with horizontal shift, submento-occipital views to clarify superimposed bony shadows, and tomography to visualize the orbital floor and condyles. The main points to look for on the x-rays include: comparative size of the antra, discontinuity of the antral wall, clouding of the antra, irregularity of the floor of the orbital rim, difference in the distance between the coronoid and malar bones, separation of the fronto-malar suture line, and fracture of the zygomatic arch.

INITIAL MANAGEMENT

PITFALL

IF TREATMENT OF MAXILLOFACIAL INJURIES IS BEGUN BEFORE A COMPLETE PLAN OF MANAGEMENT HAS BEEN FORMULATED BY AN EXPERIENCED SURGEON, TEETH, BONE, OR TISSUE MAY BE REMOVED UNNECESSARILY.

Some treatment is usually begun prior to the arrival of the surgeon who will ultimately be responsible for management of the facial fractures. This initial treatment, unfortunately, may include removal of loose teeth with attached fragments of bone, debridement of the edges of intra-oral and extra-oral wounds, and suturing of facial lacerations. These well-intentioned attempts unfortunately often work to the detriment of the patient and can greatly complicate the task facing the oral surgeon, especially if soft tissue, teeth, or bone are removed.

AXIOM

NEVER REMOVE TEETH OR BONE FROM THE MANDIBLE OR MAXILLA IF IT CAN BE AVOIDED.

After bleeding from major vessels has been controlled and the open wounds have been lavaged with copious amounts of lactated Ringer's solution or saline and 3.5% hydrogen peroxide, a very careful, meticulous examination of the bony injury should be performed and then appropriate x-rays taken. While waiting for diagnostic studies and repair of the injuries, large soft-tissue flaps should be bathed in body-temperature gauze packs saturated with lactated Ringer's solution or normal saline.

Once an accurate diagnosis of all the injuries has been made and a comprehensive plan of action formulated, definitive treatment may be begun. The bony fragments are now reduced and stabilized with transosseous wire sutures and/or metal splints if indicated. The teeth are replaced in proper occlusion, the jaws immobilized, and, finally, the soft tissue is repaired.

The lacerations are not closed until the bony injuries have been corrected. In general it is simpler to work through an existing wound which exposes the underlying bony injury than it is to wait several days for the laceration to heal and then create a new wound to perform the open reduction.

PITFALL

IF AN AVULSED TOOTH IS NOT REPLACED SOON AFTER THE INJURY, SEVERE COSMETIC DEFECTS AND IMPAIRED DENTAL FUNCTION MAY RESULT.

An avulsed tooth or a loose tooth that must be removed, because it might fall into the larynx or tracheobronchial tree, should be placed in Ringer's solution. When the oral surgeon arrives, he can decide whether or not to immediately replace it by splinting or wiring it into position. If teeth with attached bone and soft tissue were torn free at the time of the injury, they should be retrieved from the scene of the accident and, if less than six hours has elapsed, an attempt can be made to replace them as soon as possible. Even if the replaced bone and tissue do not heal, the temporary splinting can be very helpful. Removal of loose or questionably viable teeth and bone may be permanently disruptive, especially in children and adolescents.

DEFINITIVE MANAGEMENT

Fractures of the Mandible

The main objectives in the reduction of fractures of the mandible are the restoration of proper dental relationships and maximal contact of the bone fragments to provide good immobilization and optimal healing. Inadequate fixation and immobilization of jaw fractures account for the vast majority of failures resulting in malunions, nonunions, fibrous unions and infections. In addition, despite the availability of a large number of readily available antibiotics, osteomyelitis of the mandible is not at all uncommon.

Most jaw fractures can be treated adequately by closed techniques using arch bars secured to the teeth of the maxilla and mandible by wire ligatures. The maxilla can then be used as a splint for the mandible by securing the maxillary and mandibular arch bars to each other with rubber bands or wires. If the fragments cannot be reduced or stabilized adequately by closed techniques alone, an open reduction should be performed orally or extra-orally depending upon the requirements of the case. The jaws are then immobilized by intermaxillary fixation with the use of arch bars.

ALVEOLAR FRACTURES. Some of the most difficult fractures to manage are those which involve only the teeth and their attached alveolar process. Even if these fractures are reduced and immobilized with great care, the teeth often become nonviable later and are lost.

RAMUS FRACTURES

PITFALL

IF GREAT CARE IS NOT TAKEN IN PLACING INTEROSSEOUS WIRES TO REDUCE MANDIBULAR FRACTURES, THE INFERIOR ALVEOLAR NERVE AND DENTAL ROOTS MAY BE DAMAGED.

Inadvertent placement of transosseous holes in the horizontal ramus of the mandible so that they penetrate the inferior alveolar canal may injure the inferior alveolar nerve and cause paresthesias, hyperesthesia, and neuritic pain over the lower lip and jaw. If the roots of the teeth are perforated by the drill, the teeth may die with formation of periapical abscesses. The heat from the high-speed drill can occasionally cause delayed sequestration of bone and, in some cases, extensive bone loss.

CONDYLE FRACTURES. Fractures of the condyles of the mandible can be treated by closed reduction in most cases. Even when the reduction appears to be poor, the fragments will usually eventually unite and mold to provide good function. Early use of the mandible following condylar fractures seems to produce the best results when no other area of the mandible is involved. Open reduction, which will tend to delay use of the mandible, should be used only if, in the judgment of the surgeon, the closed technique will fail to provide good function.

FRACTURES OF THE EDENTULOUS MANDIBLE

PITFALL

IF FRACTURES OF THE EDENTULOUS ATROPHIC MANDIBLE ARE TREATED WITH HEAVY BONE PLATES, THE BRITTLE OSTEOPOROTIC CORTICAL BONE MAY COLLAPSE.

Since the edentulous mandible of long standing and in the aged is usually atrophic and easy to crush or fracture, the usual forms of postreduction splinting with stan-

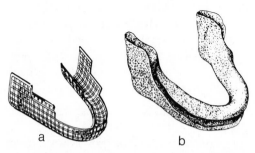

a   b

FIG. 11. Splints used to treat fractures of the edentulous mandible. a: Metal tray (Sampson titanium mesh system). b: Leake mandible (Dacron mesh with polyether urethane). (After Leake, D. L.: Mandible reconstruction with a new type of alloplastic tray: a preliminary report. J. Oral Surg., 32:23, 1974.)

dard bone plates may be difficult to apply and may cause further bony damage. On the other hand, if the mandible is inadequately splinted, the fracture site will not heal. This problem has stimulated many oral surgeons to use custom-made splints of thin but rigid metal or other materials preformed on a cast made from an impression of the jaw (Fig. 11). The splint is then attached to the jaw by wire fixation rather than by self-tapping screws. Additional support can be obtained from a properly prepared intra-oral dental splint which is attached to the mandible with circummandibular wires.

Fractures of the Maxilla

SIMPLE FRACTURES. Most fractures of the maxilla do not require open reduction; however, intermaxillary wiring is necessary to restore proper dental relationships and occlusion. If the patient is edentulous, a denture or acrylic splint should be wired to the maxillary fragments to hold them securely and to maintain adequate jaw space.

COMPLEX FRACTURES. In the most severe maxillary fractures it is usually necessary to suspend the maxillary complex from the zygomatic processes of the temporal bones to prevent elongation of the face. This can be accomplished by placing wires around the zygomatic arch and attaching them to maxillary arch bars between the second bicuspid and first molar teeth (Fig. 12). The zygomatic process of the frontal bone and the infraorbital rim can also be used as suspension points. These wires may have to be left in place for six weeks or longer until proper healing is obtained; after six weeks, however, these suspension wires become less effective.

PITFALL

IF COMPLEX COMMINUTED FRACTURES OF THE MAXILLA ARE TREATED WITH OPEN REDUCTION AND WIRE FIXATION, THE SURGICAL MANIPULATION MAY DESTROY THE BLOOD SUPPLY OF THE MULTIPLE SMALL FRAGMENTS.

The extensive dissection required accurately to reduce and to stabilize multiple small fragments of fractured maxilla will tend to disrupt their mucoperiosteal blood supply with resultant necrosis of the fragments. Such fractures, especially if due to gunshot wounds, should be treated conservatively until osteoid formation has begun. In the initial treatment of such injuries, however, when the orbits are involved one should attempt to keep the medial canthal ligament in its proper position; if it has been displaced, it occasionally can be secured to the contralateral ligament by a wire suture passed transnasally.

Orbital Fractures

AXIOM

ALL FRACTURES OF THE MALAR BONE WITH OR WITHOUT DISPLACEMENT ARE ASSOCIATED WITH CONCOMITANT FRACTURES OF THE ORBITAL FLOOR.

Orbital complex fractures associated with displaced malar fractures are not blowout fractures of the orbit and do not generally require a stent to the orbital floor. Attempts to correct enophthalmos due to periorbital fat atrophy rather than to loss of the orbital floor are unnecessary unless there is persistent diplopia. Simple elevation and reduction of the malar bone and zygomatic process usually restore the infraorbital rim and orbital floor to an acceptable functional position without further intervention. Sometimes it is necessary to stabilize the malar bone at the frontomalar suture with a transosseous wire, but an infraorbital wire suture at the lower border of the orbit is only occasionally indicated.

Fractures of the Zygoma

Fractures of the malar bone or zygoma are frequently found after direct blows to the upper lateral face. These often also involve the zygomatic arch, the infraorbital rim, and lateral orbital rim. Depressed seg-

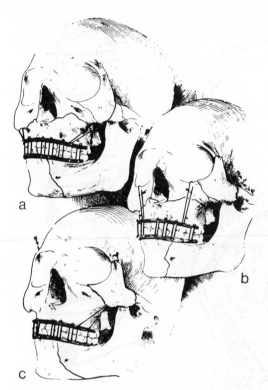

FIG. 12. Methods for suspending the maxillary complex after severe fractures: a: Circumzygomatic wire attached to arch bar, b: intraorbital wire suspension to arch bar, c: frontal bone wire suspension to arch bar.

Centric Occlusion (Fig. 13)

PITFALL

IF A FRACTURED JAW IS WIRED WITHOUT PROVIDING CENTRIC OCCLUSION OF THE TEETH, THE PATIENT WILL DEVELOP FACIAL ASYMMETRY, PAIN, LIMITED MASTICATORY FUNCTION AND EVENTUAL LOSS OF TEETH AND BONE.

When the jaw is closed, the teeth in the maxilla should occlude directly and symmetrically with the teeth in the mandible. Unless this centric occlusion is obtained, the jaws and teeth cannot function properly. Some of the worst complications occurring after maxillofacial trauma are due to unsatisfactory reductions with improper centric occlusion.

VERTICAL-OCCLUSAL DISTANCE

Vertical-occlusal distance (VOD) is the space between the maxilla and mandible when the jaws are in centric relation. When attempting to reduce fractures of the maxilla or mandible coexisting in the same patient, it can be extremely difficult to estimate the proper VOD and centric occlusal relation; however, the proper VOD will usually be attained if the jaws appear symmetrical and unstrained.

DELAYED INTERVENTION

PITFALL

IF MAXILLARY, ZYGOMATIC, OR ORBITAL FRACTURES ARE NOT PROPERLY REDUCED IN TWO TO THREE WEEKS, REFRACTURE MAY BE NECESSARY.

In patients with severe multiple injuries and unstable hemodynamic function, it may be wise to delay any attempts at reduction and fixation of the maxillofacial fractures. Every effort should be made, however, to reduce maxillary, zygomatic process, and orbital complex fractures within seven days. Reduction of mandibular fractures,

ments of the zygomatic arch usually can be reduced quite simply by an intra-oral approach; however, stabilization of fractures of the lateral orbital rim may require support with wiring or bone grafts. Blowout fractures of the orbit are discussed in Chapter 15.

DENTAL OCCLUSION

Realigning mandibular and maxillary fracture segments so that all teeth meet properly can be difficult even for the most experienced oral surgeon, especially if the fractures are extensive or many teeth are missing. It is extremely important, however, that every effort be made to achieve this. Even mild malocclusion can cause severe deformity, pain, and loss of function.

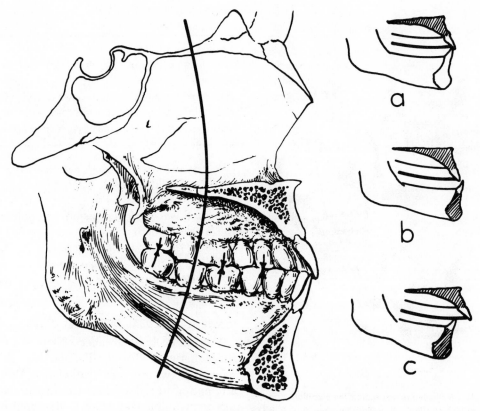

FIG. 13. The large figure represents the ideal centric relation of the jaws and teeth when in contact (centric occlusion). *a:* Centric relation of jaws, *b:* prognathic relation of jaws, *c:* retrognathic relation of jaws.

on the other hand, can often be postponed for as long as six weeks.

Sometimes delay in the treatment of maxillary, zygomatic and orbital fractures cannot be avoided. However, if another surgical procedure is planned during the immediate postinjury period, the fracture fragments can be brought into as near centric relation as possible, and immobilized with simple Ivy loops or splints in the operating room while the other surgery is being performed. It is also frequently possible to stabilize the jaws at the bedside with minimal discomfort to the patient using local anesthesia and some method of fixation. With this initial reduction and stabilization, a more definitive procedure can be accomplished later with greater potential for success functionally and cosmetically.

SUMMARY (Table 2)

Careful evaluation and planning are essential if the treatment of severe maxillofacial fractures of the dentoskeletal masticatory apparatus is to be preserved properly. The cosmetic aspect of facial trauma is taken for granted; however all surgeons, medical or dental, should have as a goal the most precise closure possible for all skin wounds. It must be emphasized that no tissue, teeth, or bone should be discarded or removed unless absolutely necessary. Reconstruction is always best accomplished with the patient's own tissues.

The essentials outlined here serve only to acquaint the reader with the fundamentals of the initial management of these problems. Further reading, particularly from the suggested reading list, is essential for anyone concerned with more definitive care.

TABLE 2. TEN OF THE MOST FREQUENT ERRORS IN THE MANAGEMENT OF MAXILLO-FACIAL FRACTURES

---

1. Unnecessary removal of teeth, bone and/or soft tissue.
2. Inadequate restoration of occlusal relationships.
3. Overzealous debridement of soft tissue.
4. Insufficient wound lavage.
5. Attempts to wire multiple small bone fragments.
6. Inadequate immobilization of the teeth and both jaws.
7. Careless skin closure.
8. Poor or careless aseptic technique.
9. Inadequate dosage and duration of antibiotic therapy.
10. Inadequate planning before treatment is begun.

SUGGESTED READING

1. LeFort, Reni: Experimental studies upon fractures of the upper part of the face. Brit. Dent. J., 71:1, 1941.
2. Rowe, N. L., and Killey, H. C.: *Fractures of the Facial Skeleton*. Baltimore, Williams & Wilkins, 1955.
3. Archer, H. W.: *Oral Surgery*. Philadelphia, W. B. Saunders, 1961.
4. Shires, G. T.: *Care of the Trauma Patient*. New York, McGraw-Hill, 1966.
5. Kruger, G. O.: *Textbook of Oral Surgery*. St. Louis, C. V. Mosby, 1968.
6. Thoma, K. H.: *Oral Surgery*. St. Louis, C. V. Mosby, 1969.
7. Hatti, H.: *Orbital Fractures*. Springfield, Charles C Thomas, 1970.
8. Schultz, R. C.: *Facial Injuries*. Chicago, Year Book Medical Publishers, 1970.
9. Costich, E. R., and White, R. P.: *Fundamentals of Oral Surgery*. Philadelphia, W. B. Saunders, 1971.
10. Waite, D. E.: *Textbook of Practical Oral Surgery*. Philadelphia, Lea & Febiger, 1972.
11. Ferraro, J. W., and Berggren, R. B.: Treatment of complex facial fractures. J. Trauma, 13:783, 1973.
12. Kenepp, N., et al.: Evaluation of maxillary antrostomy in the treatment of fractures of the middle third of the face. J. Trauma, 13:884, 1973.
13. Russell, D., et al.: Treatment of fractures of the mandibular condyle. J. Trauma, 12:704, 1972.
14. Jurkiewicz, M. J., and Nickell, W. B.: Fractures of the skeleton of the face. J. Trauma, 11:947, 1971.

Section 3

TRAUMA TO THE NOSE, NASO-ETHMOID AND FRONTAL REGIONS

G. J. BEEKHUIS

The nose is frequently involved with other facial injuries, and is damaged in about half of all facial fractures. Unfortunately, many of these nasal injuries are overlooked or misdiagnosed, leading to later external nasal deformities or airway obstruction. Since the blood supply to the external nose is so rich, any trauma to it is likely to result in considerable extravasation of blood with hematoma formation and severe swelling. Because of the looseness of the adjoining skin, the blood rapidly moves into the eyelids and cheeks, frequently causing a "black eye." This edema and ecchymosis quickly obscure the normal landmarks and make it difficult to evaluate the extent of the injury.

PITFALL

IF THE PATIENT WITH NASAL TRAUMA IS NOT SEEN SOON AFTER INJURY, ACCURATE EXAMINATION MAY BE EXTREMELY DIFFICULT.

The skin of the nose over the upper bony framework is relatively thin and movable but distally over the cartilaginous support framework it becomes thicker, contains a large number of sebaceous glands, is more firmly adherent to the underlying structures. Because of the rich blood supply, most lacerations, wounds, and incisions to the skin of the nose heal very rapidly and serious infections are quite rare. Lacerations of the skin over the lower part of the nose extending into the mucous membrane of the nares, however, may be difficult to handle. As the configuration of the nostril margin is largely determined by the underlying cartilage, the surgeon repairing lacerations in this region must be careful to approximate the perichondrium of the cartilage before closing the external skin wound. If this is not done, retraction and notching are apt to occur in all through-and-through lacerations. The closure should be started on the inside; the mucous membranes should be reapproximated first, followed by

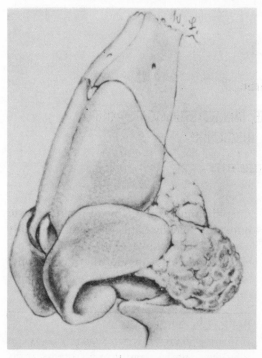

FIG. 14. Framework of external nose showing nasal bones, upper lateral cartilages, and lower lateral cartilages.

the perichondrium of the cartilage, then the subcutaneous tissue, and finally the skin.

The upper and lower lateral cartilages (alar cartilages) provide the cartilaginous support for the lower third of the external nose, and the medial crura provide the support and framework for the columella (Fig. 14). Jointly, they determine the contour and shape of the external nares and nostrils. Because of their resilience, they will usually not be damaged or displaced by blunt injuries unless the nasal bones are fractured. When the bony fracture is adequately reduced, the displaced cartilaginous structures will usually also fall into position and will not require further attention.

The upper bony nasal pyramid is thick and heavy and, therefore, very resistant to trauma; however, in the lower part where it approaches the pyriform aperture, the bones are thin and chip fractures of the lower border are rather frequent. The more severe nasal fractures, especially those originating from lateral blows and involving the nasal process of the maxilla and the frontal bone, are much less common.

The main support of the nose is the nasal septum (Fig. 15) which acts as a tentpole for the rest of the nose and is composed of the septal cartilage, the perpendicular plate of the ethmoid, and the vomer. The septal cartilage has a free border anteriorly where it blends with the membranous septum. Posteriorly it articulates with the ethmoid and vomer, and inferiorly it sits in the crest of the maxilla.

Even minimal nasal trauma may lacerate the very vascular mucous membrane of the septum, causing nasal bleeding which not infrequently requires packing before it is controlled.

Nasal trauma also may disrupt the semimobile septal cartilage rather easily, causing obstruction of side of the nose because of septal deviation, spurs along the floor of the nose because of dislocation from the maxilla, or asymmetry of the nasal tip because of dislocation from the membranous septum. These septal fractures and disloca-

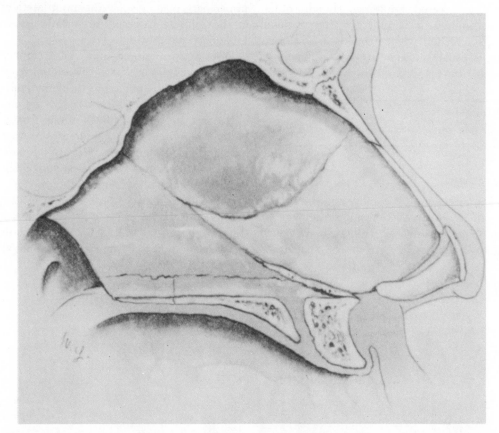

FIG. 15. Framework of nasal septum showing importance of the large quadrilateral septal cartilage in supporting the external nose.

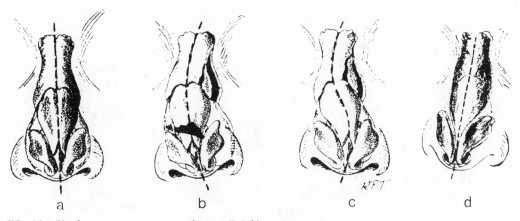

FIG. 16. "As the septum goes—so goes the nose." Goldman.

tions are frequently overlooked, but if they are not corrected simultaneously with other nasal injuries it is unlikely that a good nasal reduction will be obtained. The septum is usually the key to proper diagnosis and treatment of nasal fractures (Fig. 16).

AXIOM

AS THE SEPTUM GOES, SO GOES THE NOSE.

FRACTURES

The direction of the blow and the intensity of its force will determine the type of nasal fracture. Direct frontal blows may fracture the lower portion of the nasal bones separating them from the heavier upper part, or may splay them out laterally at the midline to result in a flattened or broadened nasal bridge.

More severe trauma may cause comminuted nasal fractures with dislocation from the frontal bone and fractures of the lacrimal bones, the ethmoid labyrinth, and the cribriform and orbital plates of the frontal bone. There may also be injuries to the nasolacrimal system and the orbital contents. If the dura is torn, cerebrospinal fluid may leak out through the nose.

The intercanthal distance between the medial ends of the palpebral fissures in the Caucasian varies from 24 to 39 mm, with an average of 33 to 34 mm in males and 32

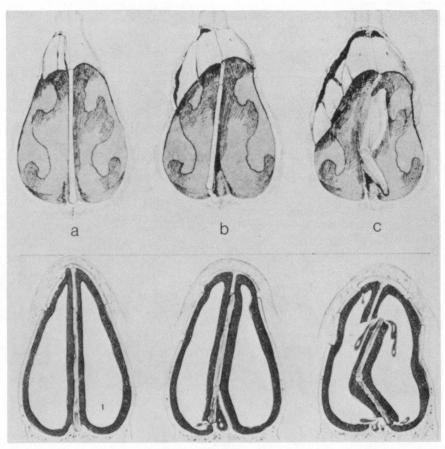

FIG. 17. Progressive degrees of nasal trauma. *a:* Only one nasal bone is involved and there is no septal displacement. *b:* The entire nasal pyramid has been shifted over; the septum follows and is dislocated from the crest of the maxilla. *c:* There is a comminuted fracture of the nasal bones and adjoining maxilla with dislocation of the nasal septum, and tears of the septal cartilage and overlying mucous membrane.

to 35 mm in females; if this distance is widened, we must strongly suspect that there has been a comminuted naso-ethmoid fracture which will require open reduction.

Blows from the side, especially those caused by small objects, can result in fractures in which only one lateral nasal bone is displaced into the nasal cavity (Fig. 17). With more severe blows, however, the entire nasal pyramid may be displaced laterally with the nasal bone and the nasal process of the maxilla pushed inward on the side of the trauma and outward on the other side. The supporting septum will also be moved out of its proper position. The septal cartilage may become dislocated from the crest of the maxilla and may tear or buckle in a horizontal or vertical direction. Unless the septal injury is diagnosed and corrected at the time of the reduction of the nasal bones, the result will be unsatisfactory.

PITFALL

IF THE NOSE IS NOT EXAMINED INTERNALLY AFTER TRAUMA TO THE MIDFACE BECAUSE IT LOOKS NORMAL EXTERNALLY, SERIOUS SEPTAL DAMAGE MAY BE MISSED.

Fractures and dislocations of the septal cartilage without obvious fractures of the nasal bones are usually due to trauma directed at the lower half of the external nose. If the cartilage is torn, the fragments of cartilage may telescope backward, causing duplication and thickening of the septum, shortening of the nose, and retraction of the nasal columella. If these are allowed to heal in this abnormal position, the nasal deformity will be severe and extremely difficult to correct at a later time.

Diagnosis

An accurate diagnosis of any nasal injury due to trauma is made on the basis of a complete history and a careful examination of the external nose, nasal passages, and nasal septum. If the physical examination is difficult because of considerable edema and ecchymosis, there is no harm in waiting several days to make an accurate diagnosis and to perform a definitive correction.

The history should provide detailed information on the cause of injury, the direction of the blow, the extent of any nasal hemorrhage and drainage of any clear fluid which may indicate a cerebrospinal fluid leak. The patient, family or friends should be asked whether there is any significant change in the shape or appearance. It is not uncommon to find that these patients have had a crooked nose for some time because of previous nasal fractures. Under these circumstances it is impossible to achieve a perfect result unless a complete rhinoplasty is performed.

External inspection may reveal that the nose is deviated laterally or considerably flattened and broadened (Fig. 18). The distance between the inner canthi should be measured and the patency of the nasolacrimal system should be noted. Careful,

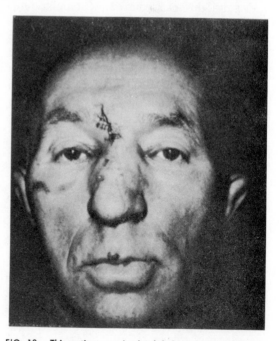

FIG. 18. This patient sustained a left frontal lateral blow to the nose with obvious displacement of the nasal pyramid. The laceration was previously sutured in an emergency room. The patient also had a dislocated septum which required simultaneous correction.

gentle palpation will usually confirm any asymmetry and may also reveal crepitation which is indicative of fracture or dislocation. The root of the nose should be evaluated carefully to see if this has been pressed below the frontal bone. The internal nose should then be examined for the presence of mucosal tears, ecchymosis, septal hematoma, or septal deviation. To perform this examination adequately, proper lighting, suction, and vasoconstricting drugs should be available.

PITFALL

IF A PATIENT WITH SEVERE INJURY TO HIS NOSE IS ALLOWED TO BLOW HIS NOSE, AIR MAY BE FORCED INTO THE SURROUNDING TISSUE OR INTRACRANIAL CAVITY.

If there has been disruption of the nasal mucous membrane or the nasolacrimal system, or if there is a suspected fracture through the cribriform plate, the patient should be cautioned not to blow his nose because this can cause subcutaneous emphysema or intracranial air, with resultant severe local infection or meningitis.

The presence or absence of concomitant orbital injury must be determined. If the eyelids are too swollen, they should be gently opened with special lid retractors to determine whether the globe is intact and whether vision and ocular mobility are normal.

AXIOM

CLINICAL EXAMINATION OF THE NOSE AND FACE IS GENERALLY MORE RELIABLE THAN A RADIOGRAPH.

Radiographs of the skull or facial or nasal bones should be used only to confirm the clinical findings. X-rays by themselves may be misleading and are easily misinterpreted. If there is an obvious displacement of the nose, the surgeon should not be deterred by an x-ray report that is negative for fracture. Conversely, normal suture lines may be misinterpreted as being fracture lines. If the nose and septum appear to be in perfectly normal position, and the patient has noticed no change in his appearance since the trauma, any report indicating the presence of a fracture should be taken skeptically. If a nasal fracture is suspected but the routine skull and facial radiographs are considered negative for fracture, special views of the nasal bones should be obtained.

Treatment

The desired objectives in treating nasal fractures are: (1) to reestablish cosmetic appearance, (2) to reestablish proper function with an adequate airway on both sides. Since the nose is so important, the correction should be based on accurate preoperative diagnosis and should be done under optimal circumstances using the principles of rhinoplastic surgery with careful attention to the condition of the nasal septum and the adequacy of the nasal airway.

Most simple nasal fractures can be managed on an outpatient basis in the emergency room. All too frequently, however, the physician may attempt reduction in the emergency room by inserting an instrument in the nostril and trying to elevate the depressed nasal bones without performing a complete examination. Since this is often done without adequate anesthesia and frequently results in a prompt gush of blood, the patient will usually allow only one attempt at this type of correction. Furthermore, because of the ecchymosis, edema, and bleeding that are present, the surgeon cannot accurately determine whether he has performed a complete reduction. For these reasons we advise that most nasal fractures be reduced in the operating room under optimal circumstances at a properly scheduled time.

PITFALL

IF ALL NASAL FRACTURES ARE TREATED IN THE EMERGENCY ROOM, EXAMINATION, DIAGNOSIS, AND TREATMENT ARE APT TO BE INADEQUATE.

If considerable edema and ecchymosis are found, it is better to wait several days until these have subsided so that a more accurate appraisal and reduction can be performed. Good overhead lighting and a proper headlight should be used, and suction should be available to remove clots or hematomas. Instruments on the surgical tray should include all those needed for open reduction and instruments necessary for performing septal reconstructive surgery should also be immediately available. Proper anesthesia is extremely important. Children usually require a general anesthetic supplemented by local infiltration of a dilute epinephrine solution. In adults, adequate premedication and wide local anesthesia of the type used in rhinoplasty are necessary.

A closed reduction may be attempted first, but if this is not completely satisfactory the surgeon should not hesitate to perform an open reduction. As stated previously, most nasal fractures are accompanied by septal deformities, and these will almost invariably require an open reduction. Unless this is done so as to preserve most of the cartilaginous support of the nasal septum, later nasal deformities, saddling, or retraction of the columella may develop (Fig. 19).

If the septal deformity is corrected but the external nasal appearance is still not satisfactory, open reduction of the nasal pyramid can be attempted using direct approximation of fragments and osteotomies. Following reduction, the position must be maintained by the appropriate use of nasal packing for a few days to act as an internal splint. This packing is merely to give support to the dorsum of the nose and, if too voluminous, may distort the external appearance.

An external nasal splint should also be applied for about a week to help prevent the formation of a hematoma over the nasal dorsum, to reduce the amount of swelling, and to stabilize the fragments.

PITFALL

IF THE SURGEON HAS TO RELY ON PACKING OR SPLINTS, THE REDUCTION WAS NOT ADEQUATE.

The purpose of the packing and splinting is only to help maintain position and prevent postoperative edema, bleeding, or further injury. If the reduction has been properly performed, the structure should be virtually self-supporting.

Accurate diagnosis of nasal fractures in small children can be extremely difficult. The external nose and nasal bones are quite small and any trauma is apt to be accompanied by excessive hematoma, ecchymosis and edema. Minor displacements are difficult to find on x-rays and yet may lead to nasal and septal deformities later in life. Undisplaced fractures or hematomas may also lead to disturbance of the growth centers, causing improper development of the external nose. Very accurate reduction and thorough evacuation of hematomas may help prevent many of these future problems.

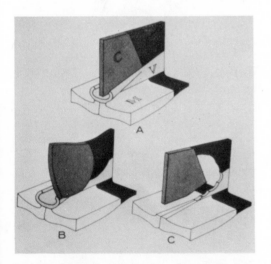

FIG. 19. Schematic representation of anatomic components. A: Normal septum. B: Commonest type of septal deformity; dislocation of septal cartilage from maxilla and columella with maximum deviation at junction with ethmoid and vomer. C: Usual type of surgical correction needed to restore septum to midline position.

COMPLEX FRACTURES

Many severe nose injuries result in a comminuted fracture of the nasal bones and associated fractures of the ethmoid labyrinth, lacrimal bones, and frontal bones (Fig. 20). In many of these severe naso-ethmoid or middle-third facial injuries, the airway may be in jeopardy, especially if excess swelling or bleeding is present. Such patients may require a tracheotomy at an early stage.

Dural Tears

These complex fractures may be associated with a tear in the dura and leakage of cerebrospinal fluid through the anterior or the posterior nares. The patient should be instructed not to blow his nose, and should be placed on systemic antibiotics to prevent meningitis. The cerebrospinal fluid rhinorrhea will usually clear up spontaneously within a week or two; however, if there has been a massive injury with severe

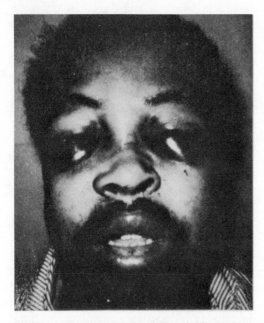

FIG. 20. Patient sustained direct frontal blow with resultant comminuted fracture of nasal bones, septum, and ethmoid labyrinth. Note the depressed nasal bridge, bilateral orbital ecchymosis and widening of the intercanthal distance. This injury will require an open reduction.

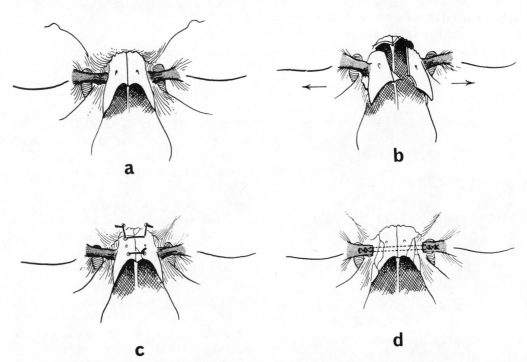

FIG. 21. a: Normal medial canthal ligament. b: Naso-ethmoid fracture with displacement of bony fragments but ligament still attached to the fragment. c: Reduction and immobilization of the fragments will restore the normal medial canthal ligament to its proper position. d: When the ligament is avulsed from its bony attachments, it will require through-and-through suture to reestablish the proper intercanthal distance.

rhinorrhea, it must be assumed either that there is a very large defect in the dura or that bony fragments have been pushed up into the dural tear. The dural tear may be along the cribriform plate, in the posterior wall of the frontal sinus, or in the roof of the orbit leaking out through the ethmoid sinuses. Laminagrams will be helpful in determining the exact site of leakage. Such injuries almost invariably require an open surgical correction with removal or reduction of the bony fragments and direct approximation of the dural tears or the use of fascial grafts to close the defects.

Disruption of the Medial Canthal Ligament

Gross bony injuries of the naso-ethmoid region will almost invariably be accompanied by disruption of the medial canthal ligament. This ligament acts as a tendinous insertion for the orbicularis oculi muscle and extends from the medial border of the eyelid to the bones of the medial orbital wall, the lacrimal bone and the frontal process of the maxilla (Fig. 21). The medial canthal ligament and its insertion determine the appearance and extent of the intercanthal distance. Although the ligament itself may become separated from its

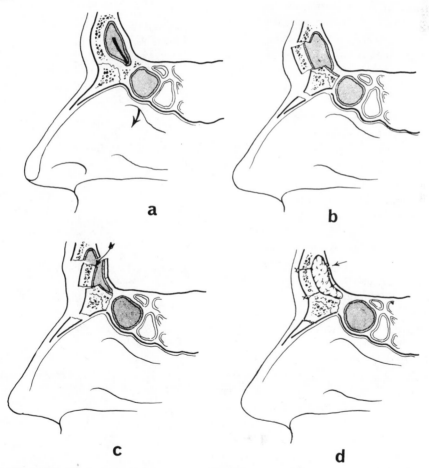

FIG. 22. a: Normal frontal sinus with adequate drainage through nasofrontal duct. b: Fracture through the anterior plate of the frontal sinus readily causes obstruction of nasofrontal duct, and resultant complications. c: Fragments from the anterior plate may fracture posterior plate with dural tears and cerebrospinal rhinorrhea. d: Repair by removal of protruding bony spicules, removal of all mucous membrane from the sinus cavity, obliteration of the sinus with a free fat graft, repositioning of fragments of the anterior plate, and suturing of the periosteum.

bony attachments, it is more usual to find that several large bony fragments at the root of the nose have been displaced, resulting in a widening of the intercanthal distance beyond the average normal of 32 to 34 mm.

Open reduction with restoration of the normal intercanthal distance by direct wiring of the fragments is essential to a proper cosmetic and functional result. If necessary, the ligament may be wired through and through to the opposite ligament or bony attachment. The lacrimal pathways are seldom torn and, if the bony fragments are properly repositioned, the nasolacrimal system will usually function normally without epiphora. However, if the fragments are allowed to heal in their abnormal position with the formation of much scar tissue, disturbances of the nasolacrimal apparatus will frequently result.

Frontal Sinus Fractures

Fractures of the frontal sinus through the anterior table alone, or through both the anterior and posterior table, may result in cerebrospinal fluid rhinorrhea (Fig. 22). If not treated adequately with open reduction, these fractures may result in persistent rhinorrhea and/or depressions over the frontal region; eventually, sometimes years later, these patients may develop recurrent frontal sinusitis, osteomyelitis, or mucocele because of obstruction to the nasofrontal duct.

At the time of surgical correction it is extremely important to evaluate this area carefully. If there is obstruction or laceration in the area of the nasofrontal duct, correction is most difficult; it has been found better to obliterate the entire sinus by removing all of the mucous membrane from the sinus cavity and then filling the entire cavity with a free fat graft taken from the abdominal wall. The bony frag-

ments of the external table are then replaced into their proper position on top of this fat. The free fat graft not only obliterates the sinus cavity, thereby preventing later complications, but also helps stabilize the bony fragments of the external frontal plate. These may then be held in position by suturing the periosteum. If performed through a hairline suprabrow incision, this leads to good cosmetic and functional results.

SUGGESTED READING

1. Converse, J. M.: *Reconstructive Plastic Surgery*, Vol. 2: The Head and Neck. Philadelphia, W. B. Saunders, 1964.
2. Shapiro, H. H.: *Maxillofacial Anatomy with Practical Applications*. Philadelphia, J. B. Lippincott, 1964.
3. Dingman, R. O., and Natvig, P.: *Surgery of Facial Fractures*. Philadelphia, W. B. Saunders, 1964.
4. Denecke, H. J., and Meyer, R.: *Plastic Surgery of the Head and Neck*, Vol. I: Rhinoplasty. Berlin, Springer Verlag, 1934.
5. Shumrick, D., and Paparella, M.: *Textbook of Otolaryngology*. Chapter on nasal fractures by J. Beekhuis. In press.
6. Conley, J.: *Proceedings of the First International Symposium on Plastic Surgery of the Face and Neck*, 1970. In press.
7. May, M., Ogura, J. H., and Schramm, V.: Naso-frontal duct in frontal sinus fractures. Arch. Otolaryng., 92:534, 1970.
8. Stranc, M. F.: The pattern of lacrimal injuries in naso-ethmoid fractures. Brit. J. Plast. Surg., 23:339, 1970.
9. Dingman, R. O., Grabb, W. C., and O'Neal, R. M.: Management of the injuries of the naso-orbital complex. Arch. Surg., 98:566, 1969.
10. Beekhuis, G. J.: Traumatic deformities of the nose. Mich. Med., 63:853, 1964.
11. Beekhuis, G. J.: Use of silicone rubber in nasal reconstructive surgery. Arch. Otolaryng., 86:88, 1967.
12. Beekhuis, G. J.: Nasal fractures. Symposium: Maxillofacial Trauma. Trans. Amer. Acad. Ophthal. Otolaryng., 74:1058, 1970.
13. Robinson, T. J., and Stranc, M. F.: The anatomy of the medial canthal ligament. Brit. J. Plast. Surg., 23:1, 1970.
14. Stranc, M. F.: Primary treatment of naso-ethmoid injuries with increased intercanthal distance. Brit. J. Plast. Surg., 23:8, 1970.

Section 4

INJURIES TO THE EARS AND FACIAL NERVE

P. M. BINNS

Except for the brain, the ear is the sensory organ most frequently damaged during severe head trauma. Injuries to the ear and facial nerve are being recognized with increasing frequency, not only because of the rising incidence of violence in our society but also because of greater awareness of the complications of this trauma and the improved techniques for investigating these problems (Table 3). The importance of these injuries is reflected by the economic and social consequences of the impaired hearing, the vertigo, and the cosmetic changes that may result.

EXTERNAL EAR INJURIES

Foreign Bodies

Most foreign bodies in the external ear canal can be readily identified and removed. Objects such as pieces of paper may be extracted easily using forceps or suction. For more difficult objects such as beads, a blunt right-angled hook is probably the best instrument.

PITFALL

IF THE PHYSICIAN ATTEMPTS TO REMOVE A FOREIGN BODY FROM THE EAR OF A STRUGGLING PATIENT, HE MAY CAUSE SERIOUS INJURY TO THE EAR.

It is imperative that patients hold still or be held motionless during any manipulation in the ear. If the foreign body cannot be easily removed because the patient is struggling, as frequently occurs with frightened children, it is preferable to administer a general anesthetic.

Iatrogenic injuries to the middle ear in an uncooperative patient may include perforation of the eardrum and injury to the ossicles. Dislocation or extraction of the malleus or incus can easily occur during probing in a moving patient, especially if the ear is bleeding; the author has seen the malleus extracted or avulsed by inexperienced doctors on two such occasions. If there is any bleeding, good suction and a good light are mandatory; a general anesthetic and an operating microscope may also be required.

TABLE 3. TEN FREQUENT ERRORS WITH EAR AND NERVE INJURIES

1. Improper removal of foreign bodies from ear canal.
2. Improper care of lacerations of the pinna.
3. Improper care of hematomas of the pinna.
4. Inadequate treatment of perichondritis.
5. Difficulty in differentiating between lacerations of the ear canal and perforation of the eardrum in patients with temporal bone fractures.
6. Missed fractures of the temporal bone.
7. Missed damage to the ossicles.
8. Missed labyrinthitis following head injury.
9. Missed or inadequate appreciation of benign positional vertigo following severe head injury.
10. Missed facial nerve paralysis in seriously injured patients or inadequate appreciation of the degree of facial nerve injury.

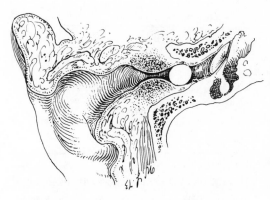

FIG. 23. Foreign body—external auditory meatus.

PITFALL

IF ONE PERSISTS IN EFFORTS TO EXTRACT
AN IMPACTED FOREIGN BODY IN THE EAR, ONE
MAY SEVERELY DAMAGE THE EAR CANAL,
DRUM, OSSICLES, AND FACIAL NERVE.

The great majority of foreign bodies can
be removed from the ear canal through the
endaural route. When this is impossible,
swelling of the skin and submucosa in the
cartilaginous portion of the external auditory meatus external to the foreign body is
the usual cause of the impaction. Under
these circumstances, the foreign body can
be extracted easily through a postauricular
incision at the junction of the cartilaginous
and bony portions of the external auditory
meatus (Fig. 23).

Lacerations and Avulsions

Lacerations of the external ear are usually relatively easy to repair. Careful debridement of the skin and underlying cartilage using sterile technique is extremely
important because of the severe problems
that can result if infection develops. If
a portion of the pinna has been avulsed,
it should be thoroughly cleaned and sutured back into its original position with
antibiotic coverage. Ice packs should be
applied over the ear during the first day or
two postoperatively to reduce the edema
which almost invariably accompanies these
injuries.

Hematoma

Hematoma of the pinna following blunt
trauma should be aspirated under sterile
conditions to prevent the development of an
unsightly cauliflower ear. If a large hematoma is present, surgical evacuation and external packing may be necessary.

Perichondritis

If infection occurs following a hematoma
or laceration of the pinna, a perichondritis
is likely to ensue, causing recurrent abscess
formation and sequestration of cartilage
and eventually resulting in a grossly deformed, shriveled external ear. The initial
treatment of any ear cartilage infection is
wide-spectrum antibiotic coverage. If an
abscess develops, incision under sterile conditions at the site of fluctuation should be
performed promptly.

Fractures of the Ear Canal

PITFALL

IF THE CLEANSING OF AN INJURED EAR IN A
PATIENT WITH A SKULL FRACTURE IS NOT PER-
FORMED UNDER STERILE CONDITIONS, THE RISK
OF MENINGITIS IS GREATLY INCREASED.

Fractures of the bones surrounding the
ear are always potentially dangerous because of the great risk of introducing infection into the middle ear, inner ear, or
brain itself. Any extensive inspection, cleaning, probing or manipulation in this area
should be performed under absolutely
sterile conditions. If the fracture extends
through the dura, there is always a risk of
meningitis and death. In the initial stages of
treatment, it may be wise to insufflate the
ear gently with antibiotic powder and to
administer ampicillin. If there is profuse
bleeding, insertion of a sterile iodoform wick
into the ear canal and then coverage with a
sterile pad may suffice to control the bleeding.

Cerebrospinal Fluid Leaks

A cerebrospinal fluid leak into the ear is
not at all infrequent following fractures of

the temporal bone and is extremely dangerous because of the meningitis which can develop through the fracture site. Fortunately, most of these CSF leaks stop spontaneously. If a CSF leak is suspected, the ear should be covered with a sterile pad, and systemic penicillin and oral sulfonamides should be administered. Nursing in the erect position, fluid restriction, and repeated lumbar punctures may help reduce or stop persistent leakage. If the CSF leak persists after all these measures and if the exact site of the CSF leak can be localized with fluorescent dyes or other techniques, surgical correction of the defect should be attempted.

Meatal Stenosis

PITFALL

IF THE LUMEN OF A LACERATED EAR CANAL IS NOT MAINTAINED BY CAREFUL APPOSITION OF THE WOUND EDGES AND PROLONGED PACKING, MEATAL STENOSIS MAY OCCUR.

Meatal stenosis is most likely to occur following severe lacerations or fractures of the ear canal, particularly if these become infected. Every attempt must be made to prevent meatal stenosis, because once it occurs it is extremely difficult to correct.

Fracture of the tympanic plate following fracture-dislocation of the temporomandibular joint is rare but may also cause meatal stenosis. If lateral laminagrams reveal a displaced fracture of the tympanic plate, the fracture should be reduced promptly.

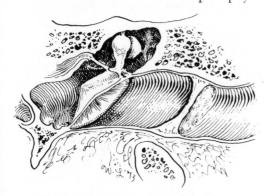

FIG. 24. Secondary tympanic membrane.

Secondary Tympanic Membrane

Secondary tympanic membrane, an extreme form of meatal stenosis, is a rare sequela after injury. It develops as scarring and narrowing of the ear canal and causes a complete membrane to form external to the eardrum (Fig. 24). Initially, the patient will have a loss of hearing and a feeling of fullness in the ear. A cholesteatoma developing from the squamous cell epithelium which is entrapped between the true and secondary tympanic membranes may extend into and damage the middle ear structures. Treatment for this condition is surgical removal of the membrane and correction of the defect with or without skin grafts.

MIDDLE EAR INJURIES

Perforation of the Tympanic Membrane

Perforation of the tympanic membrane very commonly occurs with head injuries or with insertion of pointed instruments into the ear canal. The extent of the perforation and hearing loss depends on the nature of the injury and may include anything from a pinpoint perforation to a subtotal loss of the eardrum. This type of injury may also be associated with injuries to the ossicular transmission mechanism, causing conductive deafness, or with injuries to the inner ear resulting in nerve deafness and vertigo with nystagmus. After any ear injury, the Rinne (Fig. 25a), Weber (Fig. 25b), and absolute bone conduction tests should be performed and the patient should be examined for nystagmus. Voluntary facial movements should also be checked immediately to rule out damage to the facial nerve.

Immediate treatment of traumatic perforation includes blowing of antibiotic powder into the ear to help prevent infection. This insufflation must be done very gently; otherwise marked vertigo, nausea and nystagmus may result from labyrinthine irritation. Oral or parenteral antibiotics may also be indicated with the more se-

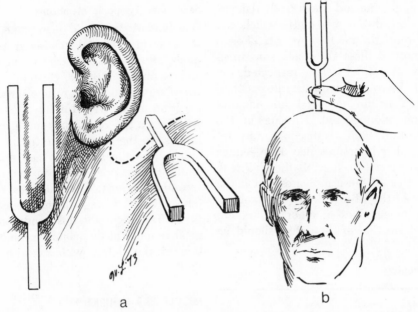

FIG. 25. Rinne test (a) shows bone conduction persisting twice as long as air conduction. In Weber test (b) tuning fork is heard best on the side with middle ear disorder.

vere injuries until the eardrum has healed completely.

PITFALL

IF THE EDGES OF A PERFORATED EARDRUM ARE ALLOWED TO REMAIN INVERTED, INGROWTH OF SQUAMOUS EPITHELIUM INTO THE MIDDLE EAR SPACE CAN CAUSE MULTIPLE COMPLICATIONS AND HEARING LOSS.

The perforation should be inspected carefully as soon as possible to be sure that the edges of the perforation are not turned inward with squamous epithelium facing toward the promontory of the middle ear (Fig. 26). This is unusual, but is very serious because it may lead to the formation of cholesteatoma and serious otologic problems. The author has seen this occur in a few patients, one of whom was a young physician who had a very serious hearing loss and had five or six operations before he was finally cured by a radical mastoid operation.

Repair of the eardrum may be performed under local anesthesia in a cooperative adult, but in children and uncooperative

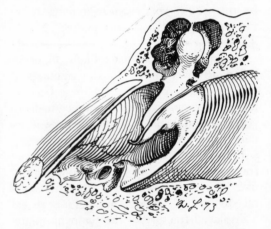

FIG. 26. Perforation of left eardrum with edges of perforation turned inward toward the promontory.

adults general anesthesia is preferred. After the edges of the perforation are everted by gentle suction, Gelfoam is placed in the middle ear behind the perforation and the edges of the perforation are approximated as near normal position as possible. The patient should be instructed not to blow his nose vigorously and not to allow any water to enter the external ear canal until the eardrum has healed. The ultimate hearing result should be assessed audiologically.

Serous Effusions

Serous effusions into the middle ear are common following physical or barotrauma to the ear. This problem is particularly frequent in airline staff and patients who fly a great deal. Pain and impaired hearing are the usual presenting symptoms. Administration of analgesics, ephedrine nasal drops, and antihistaminics will frequently aid the spontaneous resolution of this situation; however, if the problem persists, a myringotomy may be indicated.

Bleeding

Hematomas of the middle ear may arise from a blow to the ear canal or after barotrauma. These will usually resolve following treatment with nasal decongestants, but on occasion a myringotomy may be needed.

Excessive bleeding from the middle ear usually denotes a serious temporal bone fracture and may be due, though rarely, to a rupture of the internal carotid artery or the internal jugular vein into the middle ear. After sterile packing of the ear canal, bleeding into the eustachian tube may continue, but this will almost always subside gradually. If the bleeding is heavy after a minor injury, one should check to be sure that the patient does not have a bleeding tendency and is not receiving anticoagulant therapy.

Fractures

TEMPORAL BONE. The skull fractures most apt to result in damage to the ear are those involving the temporal bone. Of the fractures of the temporal bone, 80% are longitudinal and 20% transverse or mixed in type.[1] The longitudinal fractures may extend from the region of the mastoid antrum across the tegmen tympani, involving the roof of the middle ear, the eardrum or ear canal, and may pass forward along the eustachian tube or into the region of the foramen ovale (Fig. 27). Transverse fractures of the temporal bone stemming from the region of the internal auditory meatus may run along the internal auditory canal to

the lamina cribrosa and may pass into the middle ear with injury to the facial nerve, to the cochlea in front and to the vestibular structures behind (Fig. 28).

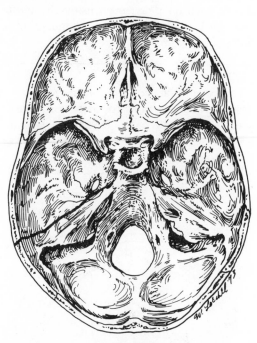

FIG. 27. Longitudinal fracture of temporal bone.

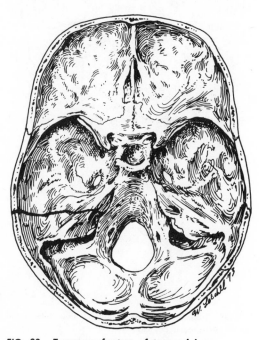

FIG. 28. Transverse fracture of temporal bone.

In addition to these obvious fractures, it is becoming increasingly apparent that there are many more small, previously undetected fractures. It is now thought that about 50% of temporal bone fractures cannot be seen on x-ray, even using the most advanced methods such as laminagrams and polytomography.[2]

PITFALL

IF NASAL CEREBROSPINAL RHINORRHEA IS ASSUMED TO BE DUE TO ANTERIOR FOSSA SKULL FRACTURES ONLY, SEVERE TEMPORAL BONE FRACTURES AND EAR INJURIES MAY BE OVERLOOKED.

Involvement of the dura, meninges, or brain itself may be manifested in several

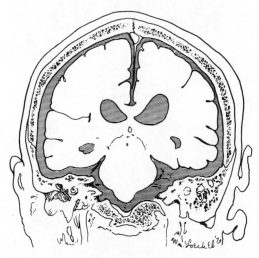

FIG. 29. Mechanism of formation of air encephalocele.

ways. Cerebrospinal fluid may leak externally through the external auditory canal or through the eustachian tube into the nose or pharynx. As mentioned previously, the main efforts in management are designed to prevent infection by use of sterile dressings and antibiotics.

An air encephalocele is occasionally seen with severe head injury if the skull fracture is associated with a dural tear and injury to the eustachian tube, middle ear, mastoid or mastoid air cells (Fig. 29). In rare instances the brain and dura may herniate into the middle ear or mastoid. Treatment includes intensive antibiotic coverage and neurosurgical consultation.

OSSICULAR CHAIN DERANGEMENT. Postinjury conductive deafness due to ossicular chain derangement or disruption was not recorded prior to 1956, and up to 1968 only 45 cases had appeared in the world literature. Once this problem began to be recognized, however, it became apparent that this was not a rare condition. In 1969, Hough reported 33 patients with ossicular chain disruption[3] and this author has seen 15 cases in the past few years.

PITFALL

IF HEARING IS NOT CHECKED IMMEDIATELY IN ALL PATIENTS WITH HEAD INJURIES, CORRECTABLE DEFECTS MAY BE OVERLOOKED.

The most frequent injuries to the ossicles are dislocation of the incus, fracture of the

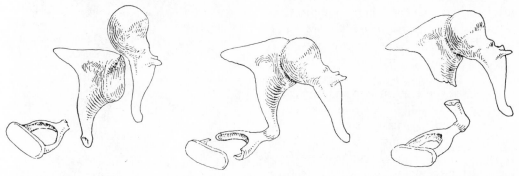

FIG. 30. Traumatic ossicular disruption. From left to right: dislocation of the incus, fracture of crura of stapes, fracture of long process of incus.

crura of the stapes and fracture of the long process of the incus in that order (Fig. 30). Fixation of the incus and malleus may also ultimately develop from adhesions. The absence of a fracture on x-ray does not exclude ossicle chain derangement and the emergency room testing with tuning forks of any patient with a head or ear injury is recommended.

If subsequent clinical examinations and audiology confirm a conductive deafness, laminagrams and polytomography may define ossicular damage which should be treated by a tympanotomy and reestablishment of the ossicular chain. Depending on the injury present, this may involve repositioning of the dislocated bones, or interposition of a part of the incus or a bone graft between the malleus and the stapes. In some injuries a partial stapedectomy, with use of a prosthesis, may be required. Recently, homograft ossicles have been used with increasing frequency.

EUSTACHIAN TUBE DAMAGE. If the eustachian tube becomes occluded and the middle ear, mastoid and mastoid air cells cannot be aerated, the middle ear may fill with a serous effusion resulting in conductive deafness. If the problem is recognized early, a myringotomy and drainage of the middle ear with a small polyethylene tube are indicated.

INNER EAR DAMAGE

Noise Deafness

Noise is a common and important cause of irreversible deafness, occurring most frequently in individuals who work or live in an almost constantly noisy environment. Although this was previously found predominantly in older adults, excessive exposure to loud music produced by high-intensity amplification is causing an epidemic of noise deafness in young adults. The initial hearing loss is usually at 4000 cps, and a marked deafness at this frequency is usually the earliest indication that noise damage is occurring. Occasionally, a complete sudden loss of hearing may occur following a loud noise and this may be associated with vestibular symptoms and signs. There is no treatment for established noise deafness; management must rely on prevention or reduction in exposure to loud noises and use of a hearing aid.

Benign Positional Nystagmus

Benign positional nystagmus is a very common condition following injury in which the patient complains of unsteadiness or vertigo on certain movements, such as suddenly extending or turning the head or lying down in certain positions. This condition has been neglected in the past but may be responsible for considerable lost time before the patient can return to work. One theory on the cause of this symptom complex is that the calcium calcite bodies of the otolith organs are shaken free at the time of the head injury and lie floating in the endolymph; certain movements then cause these particles to move, thereby stimulating the crista of the semicircular canals so that the sensation of vertigo is produced.[4] If the patient is placed in the position which produces the vertigo, there is usually a latent or lag period of a few seconds before he exhibits nystagmus combined with a sense of rotation. Fortunately, this condition is usually self-limiting and the symptoms generally disappear in three to six months.

Vestibular Neuronitis

Vestibular neuronitis due to head injury may cause sudden onset of vertigo and ataxia without hearing loss. The diagnosis may be confirmed by finding a reduced response to caloric testing on the afflicted side.

Labyrinthitis

Bleeding into the endolymph may cause a reactive labyrinthitis with vomiting, vertigo and nystagmus. If the injury is sufficiently severe, the labyrinth may be completely destroyed, resulting in severe vomiting, vertigo, nystagmus, and difficulty with locomotion. This type of inner ear damage is difficult to diagnose in its early stages because the associated head injury is usually very severe and the labyrinthitis may be associated with unconsciousness or with a combination of other ear injuries.

FACIAL NERVE INJURIES

A wide variety of facial nerve injuries are being seen with increasing frequency. Damage to the cerebral cortex or corticobulbar fibers can result in upper motor neuron lesions with loss of movement on the lower part of the face on the opposite side. Lower motor neuron damage to the facial nerve may occur intracranially, in the middle ear, in the mastoid, in the stylomastoid foramen, or on the face. The facial nerve divides into two major divisions within the parotid gland and forms the pes anserinus. Individual branches develop beyond the parotid gland.

PITFALL

IF THE FUNCTION OF ALL PORTIONS OF THE FACIAL NERVE ARE NOT TESTED SOON AFTER TRAUMA, THE EXTENT AND SITE OF THE INJURY MAY BE MISSED.

It is essential to test facial nerve function in any facial or head injury, especially if it involves the region of the mastoid. If voluntary facial nerve function is present immediately after the accident but disappears subsequently, the nerve is probably intact but bruised.

The site of any injury to the facial nerve may be determined rather exactly by checking the function of its various branches. The greater superficial petrosal nerve which supplies the sphenopalatine ganglion arises from the interosseous portion of the facial nerve. This ganglion innervates tear production from the lacrimal gland. Its function can be tested by the Schirmer test, using thin strips of filter paper under the lower eyelids and comparing function on the involved side with that of the normal eye.

The nerve to the stapedius muscle, arising from the vertical portion of the facial nerve, is responsible for the damping of sound. Loss of stapedius muscle function results in undue sensitivity to loud noises and may be detected by measurements using an acoustic impedance bridge. The chorda tympani, also arising from the vertical portion of the facial nerve, supplies taste to the anterior two thirds of the tongue and innervates the submandibular salivary gland. This nerve is easy to check by evaluating taste and saliva production.

The peripheral muscular function of the facial nerve can also be assessed to determine the site of injury. For example, if the facial nerve were completely cut at the stylomastoid foramen, no voluntary facial movement would be present on the involved side. However, if the nerve were only bruised by passage of a bullet close to the nerve, there may be partial loss of muscular movement of the whole face on that side. The degree of recovery will depend on whether the nerve degenerates or not.

Electrical testing of the main trunk of the facial nerve and its branches can also help determine where the lesion is located, if the injury is complete, and if degeneration has occurred. In humans, the distal nerve will still respond to electrical stimulation for about three days after transection.

REFERENCES
1. Kettel, K.: *Peripheral Facial Palsy: Pathology and Surgery.* Springfield, Charles C Thomas, 1959.
2. Binns, P. M.: *Facial Nerve Disease.* To be published.
3. Hough, J. V. D.: Restoration of hearing loss after head trauma. Ann. Otol., 78:210, 1969.
4. Schuknecht, H. F.: Mechanism of inner ear injury from blows to the head. Ann Otol., 78:253, 1969.

Suggested Reading
1. DeWeese, D. D., and Saunders, W. H.: *Textbook of Otolaryngology.* St. Louis, C. V. Mosby, 1968.
2. Scott-Brown, W. G., et al.: *Diseases of the Ear, Nose and Throat,* 2nd ed. New York, Appleton-Century-Crofts, 1965.
3. Shambaugh, G., Jr.: *Surgery of the Ear,* 2nd ed. Philadelphia, W. B. Saunders, 1967.

17 MUSCULOSKELETAL TRAUMA

J. RYAN

". . . that they may mend mankind and, while they captivate, inform the mind."

WILLIAM COWPER

Rather than present the specific details of management of fractures and dislocations, which can be found in many orthopedic texts, this chapter will attempt to delineate briefly the more common injuries encountered in the emergency department and to draw attention to common pitfalls which may lead to serious functional problems for the patient and medicolegal difficulties for the physician (Table 1).

PRIORITIES

AXIOM

THE LEAST OBVIOUS INJURIES ARE OFTEN THE MOST IMPORTANT.

It is important to recognize that in the patient with multiple injuries the osseous component is seldom the most urgent. Unfortunately, severe deformities of the extremity are often so striking that they tend to receive much of the initial attention, with consequent neglect of other, often more serious, injuries. Maintenance of an adequate airway, control of hemorrhage, and correction of hypovolemia and shock take priority over injured bones.

HISTORY. After the initial resuscitative measures have been accomplished, a more thorough evaluation of the patient can be made (Chap. 7). In relation to the musculoskeletal injuries themselves, special attention should be given to the mechanism of injury, location of pain, limitation of motion, and neurovascular function.

TABLE 1. COMMON PITFALLS LEADING TO SERIOUS PROBLEMS

1. Missing injuries because of failure to examine the entire unclothed patient.
2. Treating fractures before other more life-threatening problems are corrected.
3. Underestimating the amount of blood that can be lost from a fractured bone.
4. Incompletely evaluating the neurovascular status of the fractured extremity both before and after treatment.
5. Failing to splint a fracture adequately before the patient is sent to the radiology department.
6. Not handling every spine injury as though it were an unstable fracture until proper evaluation and immobilization can be obtained.
7. Forgetting to x-ray the entire broken bone, including the joints above and below the fracture.
8. Failing to realize that most ligamentous joint injuries will have normal x-rays and that diagnosis depends primarily on physical examination.
9. Not warning the parents of the possible complications of epiphyseal fractures.
10. Failing to debride and copiously irrigate open fractures.

251

PHYSICAL EXAMINATION. The physical examination should be thorough and must include a careful evaluation of the central and peripheral nervous systems and distal blood flow.

AXIOM

AN EXTREMITY CANNOT BE ADEQUATELY EVALUATED IF IT IS COVERED OR CLOTHED.

Any obvious deformities of the extremities should be recorded, as should the location and size of any contusions, abrasions, swellings, or lacerations. All extremities should be gently palpated, noting the location of any tenderness and its severity; in the comatose patient areas of crepitation must be sought for and may be the only objective evidence of a fracture. The joints should be evaluated for range of motion, tenderness or effusion.

SPLINTING. All fractures should be splinted to reduce pain and associated tissue damage. Because no single splint fits all people, a metal splint should not be applied for any extended period, especially to the lower extremity. Since the foot often rides up out of the bottom of such a splint, pressure sores may rapidly develop on the heel (Fig. 1). Nothing makes a better splint than plaster of Paris, either as a cast or as a mold. For femoral-shaft fractures, a Thomas splint utilizing skin traction provides excellent temporary immobilization.

X-RAYS. After any immediate life-threatening problems have been treated or controlled and appropriate dressings and splints have been applied, the patient may be taken to the x-ray department. The x-ray request should contain as much pertinent information about the injury as possible, and should list all areas that might conceivably require an x-ray. It is important to remember that pain from fractures is occasionally referred to more distal portions of the extremity; hip fractures, for example, not uncommonly cause pain in the knee.

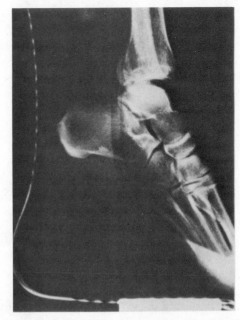

FIG. 1. The foot in this patient with a fractured ankle is riding up in the metal splint and an ulcer on the heel will result.

AXIOM

POOR-QUALITY X-RAYS ARE NOT ACCEPTABLE.

Poor x-rays must not be accepted regardless of time, effort and expense (Chap. 13). The x-rays should be reviewed by the radiologist and also by the physician who has examined the patient and will treat him. Most fractures are missed either because the patient was examined improperly or because the x-rays were of poor quality.

GENERAL CONSIDERATIONS
Open Fractures

All open wounds associated with an underlying fracture should be covered with a sterile dressing and a splint applied until the evaluation of the patient is completed and he is ready to be taken to the operating room. The primary treatment of open fractures is debridement and copious irrigation. Although most open wounds can now be closed primarily after proper care in the operating room, it is dangerous to close a severely contaminated wound. If there is any problem, the skin and subcutaneous tissue can usually be left open; however, cartilage, bone, and tendon should be covered whenever possible.[1,2]

Associated Nerve Injuries

It is important to emphasize that the neurovascular status of an injured extremity should be evaluated both before and after any manipulation. Neurologic deficits following fractures and dislocations are not uncommon; however, nerve injuries may also be caused by manipulation of a fracture or dislocation or by improper application of a cast. If the extremity is not examined carefully initially and if neurologic damage is not detected until after treatment, it will generally be assumed that the physician was responsible.

UPPER EXTREMITIES. The neurologic lesions most frequently seen in the upper extremities include: (1) laceration, contusion, or stretching of the axillary nerve or brachial plexus in dislocations of the shoulder, (2) injury to the radial nerve in humeral-shaft fractures, especially at the junction of the middle and distal third where the radial nerve is relatively fixed in the lateral intermuscular septum, (3) injuries to the radial nerve or median nerve in supracondylar fractures and posterior dislocations of the elbow, and (4) injuries to the median nerve in fractures about the wrist.

LOWER EXTREMITIES. In the lower extremity, injury to the sciatic nerve, especially the peroneal portion, is occasionally seen in posterior dislocations of the hip. The peroneal nerve itself may be involved distally in injuries about the knee joint, especially when there are tears of the lateral collateral ligament or fractures of the proximal fibula. Such nerve injuries, if not detected initially, may be difficult to differentiate from those caused by improper

padding over the head of the fibula when a long-leg cast is applied.

TREATMENT. In general, closed fractures and dislocations seldom completely disrupt the nerve, and contusion or stretching is the usual cause of any neurologic deficit. The fracture should be treated and the extremity splinted in the position of function until the fracture is healed. Nerve function can then be evaluated both clinically and by electromyographic and conduction studies; if there is no evidence of renervation, the nerve should be explored. In nerve injuries with open fractures where there is much contamination, or if the surgeon does not feel capable of performing an accurate anastomosis, the wound should be debrided and irrigated and nerve repair should be delayed until the wound has healed. Some physicians feel that all open nerve injuries should be repaired secondarily.

SPECIFIC FRACTURES AND DISLOCATIONS

Spine

CERVICAL SPINE

PITFALL

IF ALL PATIENTS WITH HEAD AND NECK INJURIES ARE NOT INITIALLY MANAGED AS IF AN UNSTABLE CERVICAL-SPINE FRACTURE WERE PRESENT, UNNECESSARY PARALYSIS MAY RESULT.

Every patient with a suspected cervical-spine injury should be handled with great care until full evaluation can be obtained. He should be put in head-halter traction or placed on a flat stretcher with sandbags on either side of the head (to prevent any motion from side to side). After a thorough neurologic evaluation is performed, AP and lateral scout x-rays should be taken, moving the patient as little as possible. If these initial views do not reveal any abnormality, more detailed studies, including oblique and flexion-extension views, can be ordered. All cervical-spine films should also include the odontoid process and the seventh cervical vertebra. Unfortunately, it is often difficult in the obese or muscular patient to get good views of C-7, and several attempts may be needed before an adequate examination can be obtained; not infrequently, it is necessary for the physician to help position the patient for the x-rays.

If a fracture is demonstrated, it should be determined whether it is stable or unstable and whether a neurologic deficit is present. If there is a fracture of the posterior facets, a fracture dislocation, or evidence of a neurologic deficit, the patient should be placed in skeletal traction using either Vinke or Crutchfield tongs. If there is any question about the extent of the injury after the initial studies, the patient should be placed in head-halter traction pending more sophisticated evaluation.[3]

THORACIC SPINE. The thoracic spine is injured relatively rarely by blunt trauma. Although these injuries are usually less dangerous than those involving the cervical spine, the principles of management are similar.

LUMBAR SPINE. If there is question of a lumbar-spine injury, the patient should be placed on his back on a flat firm cart or stretcher. A careful history and physical examination will usually reveal a neurologic deficit if it is present. If possible, AP and lateral scout films of the lumbar spine should be taken without transferring the patient to the x-ray table.

Minimal compression fractures of the lumbar spine may be treated conservatively by keeping the patient at bed rest until his acute pain subsides. Following this, he can be fitted with a back brace and allowed to ambulate. Patients with unstable fractures, fracture dislocations, and injuries with neurologic deficits may require prolonged treatment on a flat surface which can be turned, such as a Stryker frame. Each of these patients should be evaluated by an orthopedic surgeon to decide whether surgical intervention with decompression or

with fusion of the fracture or fracture dislocation will be necessary.[4,5]

Shoulder Girdle

SCAPULA. Fractures of the body of the scapula may be due to either direct or indirect violence. The displacement is usually minimal because the powerful muscles attached to the scapula tend to hold the fragments in place. If the injury is due to direct violence, the scapular fracture is of relatively little significance compared to the damage to the underlying ribs and viscera, which may be severe but is easily overlooked (Fig. 2).

Fractures of the spine of the scapula are almost always due to direct violence, and the patient should be examined for other injuries. The fractures themselves can usually be treated symptomatically with a "sling-and-swath" for a few days, followed by early motion of the arm so that a frozen shoulder does not result. Fractures of the neck of the scapula and fractures extending into the glenoid fossa should be treated as shoulder injuries, with treatment designed to retain shoulder motion. If the displacement is minimal, simple partial immobilization is all that is required. If there is marked displacement or comminution into the joint, traction is the treatment of choice.

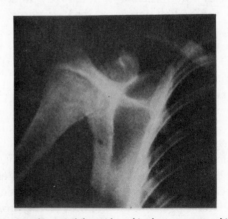

FIG. 2. This minibike rider, hit by an automobile, sustained multiple injuries including an undisplaced fracture of the scapula. Notice the pneumothorax present despite an inability to identify any rib fractures.

CLAVICLE. Fractures of the clavicle can almost always be treated by pulling the shoulders back and holding them in that position with a figure-of-eight bandage. With this bandage the axillae must be well padded to prevent compression injury of the brachial plexus and axillary artery. Open reduction should be avoided.

ACROMIOCLAVICULAR DISLOCATION. Acromioclavicular dislocation or shoulder separation is a common injury and is usually due to a fall on the shoulder. The extent of this injury may range from a slight subluxation, with only a tear of the acromioclavicular capsule, to a complete dislocation, with complete tearing of the coracoclavicular ligaments and stripping of the deltoid and trapezius muscles from the outer third of the clavicle. The outer third of the clavicle will be prominent on physical examination, and the patient will be tender directly over the acromioclavicular joint.

X-rays taken with the patient holding a heavy weight while his arms are hanging at his side will reveal any abnormal gap at the acromioclavicular joint. Treatment for this injury varies widely and may include only adhesive strapping or, for the most severe separations, surgical intervention with open reduction and repair of the coracoclavicular ligaments.

DISLOCATION OF THE SHOULDER. Dislocations of the shoulder usually result in displacement of the head of the humerus anterior to the shoulder joint. Dislocations in other directions may occur but are less common. The severity of the injury and the age of the patient often determine the degree of soft-tissue trauma. In general, more force is required to dislocate the shoulder in younger patients than in older people, and consequently they tend to have more tissue damage.

There are several methods of reduction. One of the simplest techniques involves having the patient lie prone on the table with the involved arm hanging straight down over the edge with a weight strapped

to the hand and wrist. The weight gradually tires and finally relaxes the muscles surrounding the neck of the humerus so that the head of the humerus can fall back into the joint. There are also several manipulative methods of reduction, but all must be used gently so that neurovascular damage or concomitant fracture does not occur during the reduction. At times, especially in older patients, a hairline fracture at the neck of the dislocated humerus may be overlooked on the initial x-rays but can be displaced at the time of reduction (Figs. 3, 4). Occasionally a concomitant displaced fracture of the greater tuberosity will reduce spontaneously at the time of reduction of the shoulder dislocation; however, if the greater tuberosity is still markedly displaced after closed manipulation, open surgical reduction of the greater tuberosity may be indicated.

Once the shoulder dislocation has been reduced, the patient's arm should be immobilized for four to six weeks; range-of-motion exercises should then be instituted. In older patients, these exercises should be started earlier to prevent development of a frozen shoulder. Recurrent dislocations of the shoulder usually occur in younger patients who have had severe injuries to the surrounding tissues. If the dislocations are frequent, surgical intervention should be done to tighten up the supporting ligaments and tissue.

Upper Extremity

FRACTURES OF THE PROXIMAL HUMERUS. Fractures of the proximal humerus, including the surgical neck, are common in older individuals. If the shaft is completely displaced from the head, manipulative reduction can usually bring it into an acceptable position which can be maintained in a hanging cast. In younger individuals with surgical-neck fractures with marked displacement that cannot be reduced by manipulation, either traction or open reduction may be utilized.

AXIOM

ULTIMATE FUNCTION OF A JOINT IS MUCH
MORE IMPORTANT THAN ANATOMIC REDUC-
TION OF THE FRACTURE FRAGMENTS.

If an older individual's upper arm is immobilized until the fractured humerus is healed, the shoulder will almost always become frozen. It is, therefore, wise to start these patients on pendulum exercises within two or three days after injury, even if a marked deformity results.[6,7]

FRACTURES OF THE HUMERAL SHAFT. Fractures of the humeral shaft can usually be treated by the hanging-arm-cast method. For this method to work, however, the patient should let the arm hang at all times; he should even sleep sitting in an upright position. Since the most common cause of

nonunion is distraction because the cast is too heavy, the fractures should be checked frequently with x-rays. If distraction does occur, the cast should be lightened; at times the cast may have to be completely removed and only a collar and cuff used. In all instances, exercises should be instituted within a few days to prevent a frozen shoulder.

SUPRACONDYLAR FRACTURES OF THE HUMERUS. The most serious complication with supracondylar fractures of the humerus is Volkmann's ischemic contracture resulting from compression or damage to the brachial artery. Severe swelling develops rapidly in this area, and the brachial artery is apt to be compressed if the elbow is flexed too much in an effort to provide an accurate reduction of the distal fragment. If there is any question about the circulation to the

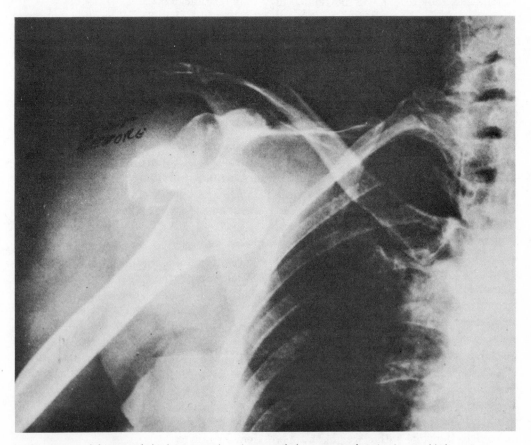

FIG. 3. Anterior dislocation of the humerus with a fracture of the greater tuberosity in an elderly patient.

forearm and hand, the arm should be taken out of flexion, placed in traction and closely observed. Skin color and temperature, pulses in the wrist, and blanching of the nailbeds all must be evaluated frequently. If circulatory embarrassment persists, arteriography should be undertaken immediately to determine the cause of the vascular obstruction. Appropriate measures, either surgical or nonsurgical, should then be taken to relieve the cause.[8]

In the adult, true supracondylar fractures are infrequent, and fractures of the distal humerus usually extend into the joint. If anatomic reduction cannot be obtained by manipulation or by traction, open reduction should be performed.[9]

DISLOCATION OF THE ELBOW. Dislocation of the elbow usually results in posterior displacement of the ulna. The coronoid process may be fractured or intact, depending upon the angle of the elbow at the time of dislocation. The dislocation should be reduced as soon as possible and immobilized at 90° of flexion with frequent careful checks on the circulation. Since a great amount of swelling usually occurs with this injury, vascular complications due to compression of the vessels, especially after the elbow has been reduced and immobilized, must be watched for closely.

FRACTURES OF THE RADIAL HEAD. If the fracture of the radial head involves one third or less of the articular surface and is nondisplaced, the fracture may be splinted for ten days and early motion instituted thereafter. If more than one third of the head is fractured or if the fracture is comminuted, early excision of the radial head should be performed.[10]

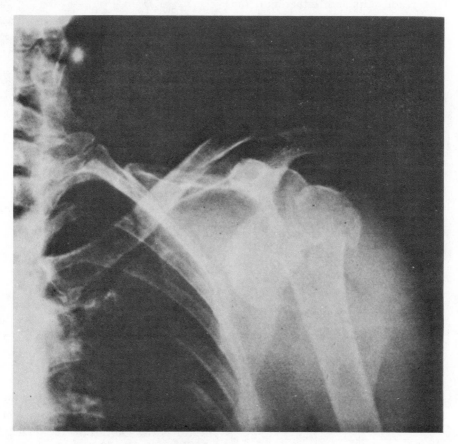

FIG. 4. After gentle traction, an unnoticed fracture of the humeral neck is displaced.

FRACTURES OF THE OLECRANON. If the fragment of fractured olecranon is large and can be reduced anatomically, it should be reduced and internally fixed. If the fragment is comminuted or cannot be reduced anatomically, the fragment should be excised and the triceps mechanism repaired and reattached.

FRACTURES OF THE FOREARM. In the adult, fractures of the forearm which are displaced usually require open reduction and internal fixation. If there is some contraindication to surgery, the fracture should be reduced by manipulation and casted in the neutral position, with no pronation or supination and with the elbow flexed to 90°.

Isolated fractures of the ulna are usually due to direct trauma and are frequently associated with dislocation of the radial head. The dislocation of the radial head is often not readily apparent; therefore the elbow should be closely inspected and x-rays obtained to rule out this injury. If

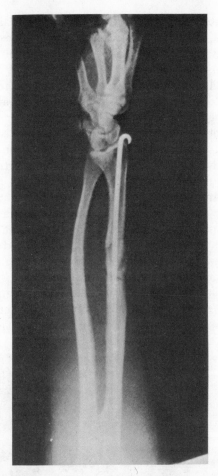

FIG. 6. Open reduction with medullary rod fixation maintains the interosseous space in this fracture.

there is marked displacement of the ulnar fragments, open reduction should be undertaken to maintain the interosseous space. Isolated displaced fractures of the radial shaft should also be treated with open reduction to maintain the interosseous space (Figs. 5, 6).[11]

FRACTURES OF THE WRIST. Fracture of the distal radius is probably the most common fracture seen and is usually due to a fall on the open hand. The deformity generally consists of shortening with dorsal displacement of the distal fragment. Reduction can usually be obtained under local anesthesia by traction and levering of the distal fragment over the shaft of the radius. The wrist and forearm should then be immobilized

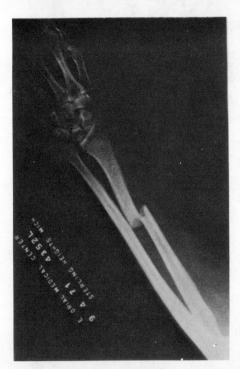

FIG. 5. A displaced fracture of the radius with the interosseous space compromised. If the fracture healed in this position it would limit pronation and supination.

in pronation, slight flexion and ulnar deviation. In elderly patients the distal fragment is often severely comminuted; with such injuries, treatment may include traction to maintain length or K-wire percutaneous fixation of the distal fragment to maintain reduction.[12]

Pelvis

As in any bony ring, fracture at one point in the pelvis is usually associated with a second fracture or dislocation elsewhere in the ring; unless the examination is careful, the other injury is often overlooked. Fractures of the pelvis in themselves are seldom of great consequence; they may, however, be associated with very severe concomitant visceral injuries.[13,14]

FRACTURES OF THE ILIAC CREST. A fracture of the iliac crest is usually due to a direct blow; however, unless the bone is markedly displaced by the force of the trauma, the fragments are usually held well in place by the numerous muscle attachments. The

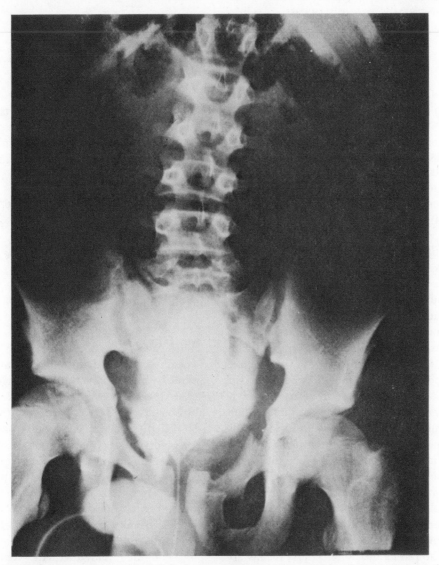

FIG. 7. This is a 14-year-old boy with multiple fractures of the pelvis. A cystogram demonstrates dye leaking out of the bladder. Multiple tears of the bladder were found at surgery.

main dangers in this type of fracture are associated intra-abdominal damage and local and retroperitoneal bleeding. Since a great amount of cancellous bone is present in this area, large quantities of blood can be lost from the raw bony surface. The hemorrhage may not be apparent, and patients have exsanguinated from what appear to be relatively simple fractures. The fracture itself can be treated by placing the patient at bed rest until he is comfortable. Ambulation with or without crutches is begun later as the pain disappears.

ISOLATED FRACTURES OF PUBIC OR ISCHIAL RAMI. Fractures of the pubic and ischial rami are quite common, and of themselves are usually little problem. If both rami on one side are fractured, the injury is usually caused by a direct blow from the side. Such trauma may drive the spikes of bone far enough inward to puncture the bladder, but after the force of the trauma is expended the fragments often spontaneously reduce, producing the appearance of a rather innocent-looking fracture (Fig. 7). All patients with pelvic fractures, especially if the pubic or ischial rami are involved, must have a rectal examination and a urinalysis looking for red cells. These patients should be put at bed rest until the acute pain subsides. Ambulation can then be begun without weight bearing on the involved side until fracture healing occurs.

DIASTASIS OF THE PUBIC SYMPHYSIS. This injury is usually due to severe trauma and is associated with either a rupture of the sacro-iliac ligaments or a posterior pelvic ring fracture. Tears of the urethra are apt to occur and should be looked for carefully with urinalysis and urethrograms.

Reduction can usually be obtained with the use of a pelvic sling, which will bring the two innominate bones together. If this method is not successful, skeletal traction on the lower extremities, with the extremities internally rotated, will usually accomplish the reduction. Where these means are unsuccessful, open reduction with fixation of the symphysis pubis may be required.

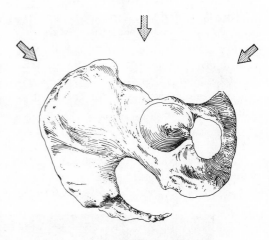

FIG. 8. In addition to the standard anterior posterior radiograph of the pelvis, two views at 45° will demonstrate the displacement of the pelvis.

UNSTABLE FRACTURES OF THE PELVIS. After severe direct force, double fractures of the pelvis may result in gross displacement of the fragments, including internal and external rotation (like the handle of a pail). Three radiologic views are required to determine the actual deformity (Fig. 8). These fractures can usually be reduced either by closed manipulation or by skeletal traction on the lower extremity, using whatever rotation is necessary to correct any bony deformity. Occasionally, open reduction with internal fixation is required.

Lower Extremity

FRACTURES OF THE HIP. Fractures of the proximal femur about the hip joint can be classified as cervical, intertrochanteric, or subtrochanteric. Cervical and intertrochanteric fractures most commonly occur in older individuals. Because of associated diseases and the problems of recumbency in older patients, specialized treatment is required. Initial treatment may consist of applying skin (Buck's) traction to the involved extremity to relieve pain. Special efforts are also made to encourage movement, coughing and adequate ventilation in these patients.[15]

Experience with 789 fractures about the

hip treated at Detroit General Hospital between 1962 and 1970 led to the policy of rapid surgical intervention to stabilize the fracture, followed by early mobilization. While prophylactic anticoagulation has been advocated in some centers, we have found that our mortality rate following meticulous wrapping of the lower extremities with Webril and Ace bandages was comparable with that obtained using anticoagulants. In addition, this meticulous wrapping has also reduced the incidence and severity of decubiti on the heels of these elderly patients.

Cervical or Neck Fractures. Fractures of the femoral neck in elderly individuals are often treated with removal of the femoral head and replacement with a prosthesis; this allows early movement of the patient and obviates problems related to aseptic necrosis of the femoral head. The recent literature, however, indicates that there is an increased morbidity with this type of treatment. Consequently in most patients we prefer to retain the femoral head and fix it internally with nails or multiple pins; the femoral-head prosthesis is used only in severely medically disabled individuals.[16,17]

Intertrochanteric Fractures. These fractures tend to occur in even older individuals, who are likely to have complications similar to or worse than those seen in patients with cervical fractures of the hip. They are treated with early internal fixation using a nail-and-plate combination.

Subtrochanteric Fractures. Subtrochanteric fractures are more common in younger individuals. The treatment of choice, however, is still early open reduction and internal fixation with a nail-and-plate combination.

DISLOCATION OF THE HIP. In traumatic dislocation of the hip, the femur is usually displaced posteriorly to the hip joint, causing the leg to be internally rotated and shortened. Associated fractures of the posterior aspect of the acetabulum are not uncommon. The sciatic nerve which runs just posterior to the hip joint may be damaged at the time of dislocation; when such nerve injuries occur, the peroneal portion is the most apt to suffer.

To ensure adequate relaxation of the involved muscles, reduction of a dislocated hip should usually be done under general anesthesia; simple direct traction with the thigh in 90° flexion will then generally be all that is required. If there is a fracture of the posterior aspect of the acetabulum, the stability of the hip joint should be determined before and after reduction. If the hip is unstable and the acetabular fragment is large, the fragment should be reduced and fixed surgically.

The incidence of aseptic necrosis of the femoral head after dislocation of the hip is rather high because the tearing of the capsular vessels and artery of the ligamentum teres removes much of its blood supply. Periodic x-ray examinations should, therefore, be done for at least a year after the injury to look for any increasing opacification of the femoral head.

FRACTURES OF THE SHAFT OF THE FEMUR. Fractures of the shaft of the femur are usually the result of tremendous violence and are generally associated with severe damage to adjacent muscles. Damage to nearby vessels is also not uncommon, and the status of the peripheral circulation must be evaluated very closely. If the femoral artery is damaged, the fracture should be reduced and fixed internally and the vessel repaired. If the fracture is not comminuted, open reduction and intramedullary fixation with a Schneider rod are usually performed. If the fracture is comminuted, the reduction and fixation are best accomplished with skeletal traction.[18]

PITFALL

IF THE KNEE LIGAMENTS IN PATIENTS WITH FEMORAL-SHAFT FRACTURES ARE NOT EVALUATED CLOSELY, ESPECIALLY AT THE TIME OF SURGERY, AND TREATED ACCORDINGLY, SERIOUS KNEE PROBLEMS MAY NOT BE APPRECIATED UNTIL THEY ARE VERY DIFFICULT TO TREAT.

A recent study at Detroit General Hospital emphasizes that patients who are hit by automobiles and who have sustained fractures of the femoral shaft often have concomitant injuries to the ligaments of the knees.[19] Although it is assumed that this injury to the knee occurs on the side of weight bearing at the time of automobile impact, the other knee is also often damaged (Fig. 9).

Unfortunately, examination of the knee is extremely difficult when the shaft of the femur is fractured, not only because of the instability of the distal femur but also because of the pain. Furthermore, discoloration and effusion at the knee are usually not evident until several days after injury. Consequently, the knee should always be checked for injury at the time of surgery after the intramedullary rod has been secured in the femoral shaft.

SUPRACONDYLAR FRACTURES OF THE FEMUR. Supracondylar fractures of the femur can be treated either by open reduction and internal fixation or by skeletal traction; however, if there is a T component to the fracture or if the fracture extends into the joint, open reduction is desirable so that anatomic restoration of the knee-joint surfaces can be obtained.

FRACTURES OF THE PATELLA. Fractures of the patella may be due either to direct trauma or to indirect violence from muscle pull. If the fracture is undisplaced, it can be adequately treated with a cylinder cast until healed; however, if the fracture is comminuted or if the fracture fragments are displaced, surgical intervention is required. If two large fracture fragments are present and can be anatomically reduced, the fracture can be handled with open reduction and a cylinder cast. If one of the fragments is small, it can be excised; if there are several fragments, we prefer to do a total patellectomy and repair the quadriceps mechanism.

FRACTURES OF THE TIBIAL PLATEAU. Fractures of the tibial plateau are usually associated with marked comminution of the fracture fragments and widening of the proximal tibia. Because this joint must bear weight, anatomic restoration of the joint surfaces is important and usually must be done surgically. The depressed fragments are elevated and held in place with a bone graft. If the fragments are displaced laterally or medially, they should be replaced in anatomic position and fixed with a Webb bolt.[20]

DISLOCATIONS OF THE KNEE. Dislocations of the knee are usually caused by severe trauma. The tibia is usually displaced anteriorly, tearing all of the ligaments about the knee and the posterior capsule. The popliteal vessels and nerves which are relatively confined in this area are also often damaged with this injury. Because of the

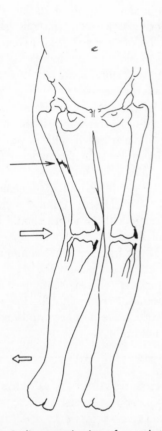

FIG. 9. A diagrammatic view of a pedestrian hit by an automobile and sustaining a fractured femur. The mechanism of the injury may also disrupt the medial collateral ligament of the same leg or a lateral collateral ligament of the opposite leg.

tremendous pressure that may be exerted by the displaced bone on vessels and nerves in this space, reduction should be accomplished as soon as possible. This is usually quite easily done under general anesthesia using traction on the leg with countertraction on the thigh. The neurovascular status should then be checked again after reduction and immobilization of the leg. If there is any question about the distal circulation, an arteriogram should be performed immediately, and surgical correction undertaken if any defect is noted. Popliteal-artery injury is extremely serious and is associated with a high incidence of distal gangrene (Chap. 26). If necessary, the ligaments may be surgically repaired a few days later, after the neurovascular status of the leg is assured.

ATHLETIC INJURIES OF THE KNEES. With the increasing popularity of football, injuries about the knee joint are being seen with increasing frequency. Depending upon the nature and severity of the trauma, the patient may exhibit a traumatic synovitis, a sprain, or a complete tear of the ligaments or menisci of the knee. If seen shortly after injury, an adequate examination of the knee can usually be performed. After a few hours, however, swelling, pain and muscle spasm make examination extremely difficult. The history is important in the evaluation of any acute or recurrent knee injury, and in many instances the diagnosis can be made on this basis alone. Examination is aided if the other knee is normal and can be used as a guide to the normal laxity of the ligaments and menisci. After the history and physical examination have been completed, AP and lateral x-rays should be taken. In many instances it is also useful to get tunnel, patellar, and oblique views of the knee.

Meniscal Injuries about the Knee. Meniscus injuries of the knee are usually due to rotational trauma and are apt to involve the medial meniscus. A history associated with a tear of the right medial meniscus might be as follows: The running football player's right foot touches the ground. At this time his cleats fix his tibia securely to the ground, and the knee is slightly flexed. If he tries to cut to the left, the femur rotates internally on the tibia and tends to force the medial meniscus toward the center of the joint. On extension of the knee, the meniscus may then be caught between the femur and tibia and torn longitudinally. If this longitudinal tear continues anteriorly, a classic bucket-handle tear occurs. Tears of the lateral meniscus tend to occur with vigorous external rotation of the femur on the tibia with the knee in partial flexion. If the history is taken carefully and the athlete's exact movements at the time of injury are known, the diagnosis can be made quite accurately, and physical examination may be only confirmatory.

To evaluate the medial meniscus specifically, the patient lies supine and the involved knee is fully flexed. The tibia is then externally rotated on the femur and the knee is slowly extended to 90° flexion. The flexion and external rotation tend to force the torn segment of meniscus into the joint. On extension of the knee a pop or click may be heard and the patient may also feel pain as the femur and tibia catch the torn fragment. To evaluate the lateral meniscus, the tibia is internally rotated while the knee is flexed and then extended. This test is diagnostic of meniscus injuries only between full flexion and 90° of flexion. Clicking with more extension is usually due to other causes (the patella going over the femoral condyles). At times the torn meniscus may be caught between the femur and tibia, thus preventing full extension. This must be differentiated from incomplete extension due to contraction of the hamstrings by the patient to protect his knee. There is usually also some effusion, and the knee is often tender on the side with the meniscal injury.

Treatment of a torn meniscus is surgical, with removal of the meniscus; a torn cartilage will not heal unless only the peripheral attachment is involved.

Injuries of the Collateral Ligaments. The medial collateral ligament tends to be torn by a valgus stress and the lateral collateral ligament by a varus stress. Since tremendous force is generally required to cause a complete rupture of the collateral ligaments, there is usually a great deal of swelling and ecchymosis about the knee after the injury; this makes examination extremely difficult. It may be helpful, under such circumstances, to inject 1% Xylocaine into the joint; at times it may even be necessary to put the patient to sleep to get an adequate examination.

The collateral ligaments are examined by stressing the knee medially and laterally; if a collateral ligament is torn, the

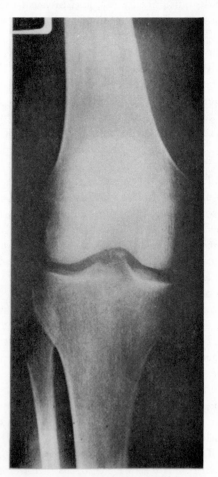

knee joint will open up like a book on the side of the injury. To examine the medial collateral ligament, one hand is placed on the lateral surface of the knee joint, the other hand grasps the lower leg and a valgus strain is placed on the knee. If the medial collateral ligament is completely torn, the knee will open up on the medial side and the defect can be palpated. The opposite maneuver is done to test the lateral collateral ligament. The knee should be slightly flexed when doing this, since with the knee fully extended the tibia rotates on the femur and is locked in place so that, even with complete tears, the knee joint may not open up. If the patient is large and it is difficult to handle the knee and palpate at the same time, x-rays may be taken while the stress is applied (Figs. 10, 11). Treatment for complete tears of the medial or lateral collateral ligament should consist of surgical repair and immobilization until the ligament has healed.

Cruciate Ligaments. Tears of the anterior and posterior cruciate ligaments usu-

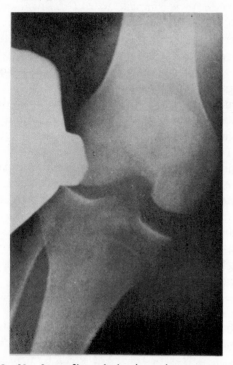

FIG. 10. This patient sustained a clipping injury to the knee while playing football. Routine anterior posterior radiograph reveals a fracture of the tibial spine.

FIG. 11. Stress films of the knee demonstrate complete tear of the medial collateral ligament.

ally occur in combination with collateral ligament injuries; however, tears of the anterior cruciate ligament may occasionally occur as isolated injuries of hyperextension. The anterior cruciate ligament runs from the lateral femoral condyle posteriorly to the anterior aspect of the tibial spines and prevents anterior displacement of the tibia on the femur. Consequently, to examine for the anterior cruciate ligament the knee is flexed, the foot is fixed and the tibia is then pulled forward on the femur. If the anterior cruciate ligament is torn, the tibia will displace farther anteriorly than the normal side. Conversely, the posterior cruciate ligament runs anteriorly from the medial femoral condyle to the posterior tibial spine and prevents posterior displacement of the tibia on the femur. To test for injury to this ligament, the knee and foot are positioned as described above and the tibia is pushed posterior on the femur. If the posterior cruciate ligament is torn, the tibia will displace posteriorly farther than in the opposite normal knee. Because these maneuvers are similar to opening and closing a drawer, they are referred to as the drawer test. Treatment for complete tears of the cruciate ligaments is usually surgical repair.

FRACTURES OF THE TIBIA AND THE FIBULA. Isolated fractures of the fibula, except at the ankle joint, are usually the result of direct trauma. The fracture itself is of little significance, and the only treatment necessary is symptomatic relief of the pain. The patient is often more comfortable with a compression dressing and crutches than with a cast. Since the peroneal nerve is commonly injured in fractures of the proximal fibula, the function of this nerve should be checked before and after any reduction or immobilization.

Isolated fractures of the tibial shaft may be due either to torsion or direct trauma. Displacement is usually minimal because of the splinting effect of the intact fibula. This fracture can thus usually be treated quite adequately in a long leg cast without manipulation or surgery.

Combined fractures of both the tibia and fibula are usually due to severe trauma and, because of the subcutaneous position of most of the tibia, these fractures are often open. As with all open fractures, thorough debridement and irrigation should be carried out as soon as possible. When the open wound is large or when there is excessive soft-tissue swelling, relaxing incisions may be necessary to close the primary wound. The neurovascular status of the lower extremity, as after all severe trauma, should be checked closely both before and after treatment.

If the fracture is treated with open reduction, it is extremely important to align the ankle and knee joints properly. If there is any residual angulation or malrotation, degenerative arthritic changes will develop in these joints in later years. The patient should be informed that these fractures often heal slowly, and that it may be six months to a year before union is complete.

INJURIES ABOUT THE ANKLE. Rotational and abduction or adduction injuries about the ankle are quite common. Depending on the severity of the injury and the strength of the ligaments and bone, the patient will suffer a strain, a sprain, or a fracture.

Lateral Collateral Ligament and Lateral Malleolus. The most common ankle injury seen after trauma is a tear of the anterior fibulotalar portion of the lateral collateral ligament. This injury can usually be adequately handled by a compression dressing and crutches. Increased force may cause a complete tear of the lateral collateral ligament, which can be demonstrated by stress films; these injuries should be immobilized in a short leg cast until the ligament has healed.

External rotation injuries about the ankle will, if severe enough, cause an oblique spiral fracture of the distal fibula. These fractures can almost always be treated adequately by closed reduction and a short leg cast.

Deltoid Ligament and Medial Malleolus. Abduction injuries of the ankle may cause a tear of the deltoid ligament or a fracture of the medial malleolus at or below the joint line. If the tear of the deltoid ligament is complete, some physicians feel that surgical repair should be undertaken; however, if the ankle mortice is undisturbed, others feel that the tear can be adequately treated by cast immobilization until the ligament is healed. If the medial malleolus fracture is undisplaced, it may be treated by immobilization until the fracture is healed; however, if it is displaced, open reduction and fixation with a screw should be performed.

Fracture Dislocation. Dislocation of the ankle may be due to abduction or to adduction injuries and may be associated with bimalleolar or trimalleolar fractures. Neurovascular complications are not uncommon with these injuries and there may also be great pressure exerted on the skin laterally or medially where the distal shaft presses against the skin.

PITFALL

IF REDUCTION OF SEVERE ANKLE DISLOCATIONS IS DELAYED UNTIL X-RAYS ARE OBTAINED, THE INCIDENCE AND SEVERITY OF SKIN NECROSIS AND NEUROVASCULAR COMPLICATIONS WILL BE INCREASED.

For medicolegal reasons, it is often felt that x-rays should be obtained before any form of treatment is directed to the injured extremity; however, if the foot is left dislocated for any period of time, the skin over the area where the pressure is occurring may slough. Consequently, the foot should be placed in as normal alignment as possible and splinted before the patient is sent to x-ray. These fractures are usually quite unstable and difficult to reduce and fix by closed techniques; however, once the medial malleolus has been reduced surgically and secured by internal fixation, the other fractures can usually be aligned quite easily. If the fracture of the posterior malleolus involves a third or more of the ar-

ticular surface of the distal tibia, open reduction with internal fixation of this fragment is also necessary.

Occasionally a diastasis of the ankle joint may occur as a result of tearing of the interosseous ligament and separation of the distal tibia and fibula. If an adequate closed reduction cannot be obtained, open reduction with screw fixation of the fibula to the tibia may be necessary. The screw, however, must be removed before ambulation is begun. It must be remembered that the articular surface of the talus is wider anteriorly than it is posteriorly; therefore, if the foot is not placed in a neutral position when the screw is secured, the ankle mortice will be narrowed.

FRACTURES IN CHILDREN

Remodeling and Growth

AXIOM

IN CHILDREN, ANGULATION AND OVERRIDING OF FRACTURE FRAGMENTS WILL OFTEN BE CORRECTED BY GROWTH, BUT ROTATION WILL NOT.

Healing of fractures in children, because of their growth and remodeling potential, is quite different from that in adults. The younger the child and the closer the fracture is to the growth center of the bone, the greater the degree of remodeling that will take place, and the greater the degree of deformity and angulation that can be accepted; this is especially true if the fracture angulation is in the plane of the joint. Overriding with bayonet apposition is also acceptable in a child; the shortening that occurs will usually correct itself because of overgrowth of the involved extremity. It must be remembered, however, that rotation is not affected by remodeling and must be corrected at the time of the reduction of the fracture.[21]

Injuries to Growth Centers

A fracture peculiar to children and occurring commonly in young adolescents is a fracture through the physis or growth center. Often a triangular fragment of metaphysis remains attached to the growth center and epiphysis and may be the only evidence of a fracture, especially if the fragments are not displaced. With this type of fracture, especially if it is due to crushing, the growth center may be damaged; early closure may take place, with later shortening of the extremity. An even greater problem may occur with partial damage to the growth center. Under these circumstances, one portion may close and the other continue to grow; angular deformities of the extremity result. Because of the problems associated with growth-center injuries, parents should always be warned that the involved extremity must be followed for at least several months after healing so that the status of the growth center can be evaluated properly.[22]

Pulled Elbow

"Pulled elbow" is an injury which usually occurs in children three to five years of age after a sudden pull or jerk on the arm. The child usually keeps the elbow flexed and pronated and the x-rays are completely normal. It was once felt that this injury was due to a subluxation of the radial head which occurred because in the child the radial head is smaller than the neck of the radius. The size of the radial head in the child, however, is comparable to that in the adult, and dislocation of the radial head does not appear to be the cause of this problem. This injury is now thought to be related either to a tear of the distal attachment of the annular ligament or to an internal derangement of the radial humeral joint, with a synovial fold pinched in the joint. Treatment is simply supination of the child's forearm while the elbow is flexed. A slight click is usually heard, and then the child can use the arm normally. If any pain persists, the child's arm may be placed in a sling for a few days.[23]

SPECIAL PROBLEMS RELATED TO ORTHOPEDIC TRAUMA

Fat Embolism

Fat embolism is a clinical syndrome consisting of depression of the central nervous system and respiratory difficulty associated with fractures or surgical procedures involving long bones. The symptoms classically begin approximately 24 to 48 hours after injury. The main clinical findings consist of fever, tachycardia, tachypnea, drowsiness and mental confusion, progressing to coma and respiratory failure. Petechiae may develop on the chest, in the axilla, and on the oral mucosa and the conjunctiva. These petechiae must be searched for frequently because they usually last for only a short period of time.

Several nonspecific laboratory abnormalities may occur. The hemoglobin level may fall, and free fat may be found in the urine or sputum in approximately 50% of cases. The serum lipase may become elevated, but usually not for several days. The chest x-ray may reveal diffuse fluffy infiltrates.

The pathogenesis of fat embolism is still controversial, but two theories of its etiology have been proposed. One theory suggests that intravasation of the fat into vascular channels occurs after trauma to a long bone; the other postulates that there is an alteration of the plasma colloidal dispersion of chylomicrons which may be brought about by a lipid-immobilizing hormone released from the pituitary.

Since most of the symptoms appear to be direct results of respiratory failure, ventilator assistance should be instituted immediately (Chap. 31). Additional treatment varies from one investigator to the next, and the literature contains many conflicting reports. Currently steroids appear to be advocated strongly. Some feel that heparin is valuable because it may facilitate the passage of chylomicrons into the tissues and because it activates lipoprotein lipase, which hydrolyzes unesterified fatty acids making them soluble. Low-molecular-weight dextran may help by reducing the intravascular aggregation of red blood cells, thereby increasing capillary flow and tissue perfusion. I.V. alcohol has also been tried, but without definite objective benefit.[24]

Volkmann's Ischemic Contracture

This clinical entity, consisting of severe contractures due to ischemic necrosis of muscle and later fibrosis, is treated by prevention. It is most commonly seen in children with trauma about the elbow joint, but it may also occur in the lower extremities after the use of improper skin traction or in any condition which may interfere with blood flow, especially to the anterior compartment of the lower leg.

Whenever there is increased pain after reduction and immobilization, an ischemic problem may have developed. Any vascular problem must be corrected immediately. Any immobilization and acute flexion should be relieved and the extremity placed in either skeletal or skin traction. If the circulation returns to normal after these maneuvers, traction may be continued or, after a few days when the swelling has subsided, closed reduction can again be attempted. If the signs of ischemia persist after these maneuvers, immediate surgical intervention should be undertaken. Arteriograms may be helpful before vascular surgery to pinpoint the exact cause of the circulatory problem.[25,26]

During surgery the fascial compartments are widely incised and the brachial artery is exposed. If an area of vascular narrowing is found, some authorities advocate immersion of the vessel in warm saline or procaine or the topical application of papaverine sulfate solution. Others favor stripping of the adventitia. If these measures fail or if a defect was demonstrated on the arteriogram, the involved segment should be excised and continuity reestablished with a graft or an end-to-end anastomosis. Once severe necrosis of the muscle bellies of the forearm or lower extremity has occurred, contractures are inevitable. Multiple recon-

structive procedures are then required, with poor results.

REFERENCES

1. Davis, G. L.: Management of open wounds of joints during the Vietnam war. A preliminary study. Clin. Orthop., 68:3, 1970.
2. Witschi, T. H., et al.: The treatment of open tibial shaft fractures from the Vietnam war. J. Trauma, 10:105, 1970.
3. Forsyth, F.: Extension injuries of the cervical spine. Instructional Course Lecture. J. Bone Joint Surg., A46:1792, 1964.
4. Holdsworth, F.: Fractures, dislocations and fracture-dislocations of the spine. J. Bone Joint Surg., A52:1534, 1970.
5. Smith, W., and Kaufer, H.: Patterns and mechanism of lumbar injuries associated with lap seat belts. J. Bone Joint Surg., A51:239, 1969.
6. Neer, C. S.: Displaced proximal humeral fractures (Part I). J. Bone Joint Surg., A52:1077, 1970.
7. Neer, C. S.: Displaced proximal humeral fractures (Part II). J. Bone Joint Surg., A52:1090, 1970.
8. Lipscomb, P. R., and Burleson, R. J.: Vascular and neural complications in supracondylar fractures of the humerus in children. J. Bone Joint Surg., A37:487, 1955.
9. Riseborough, E., and Radin, E.: Intracondylar T fractures of the humerus in the adult. J. Bone Joint Surg., A51:130, 1969.
10. Bakalim, G.: Fractures of radial head and their treatment. Acta Orthop. Scand., 41:320, 1970.
11. Sage, F. P.: *Fractures of the Shafts and Distal Ends of the Radius and Ulna.* AAOS Instructional Course Lectures, Vol. XX: 91. St. Louis, C. V. Mosby, 1971.
12. Scheck, M.: Long term followup of treatment of comminuted fractures of the distal end of the radius by transfixation with Kirschner wires and cast. J. Bone Joint Surg., A44:337, 1962.
13. Holm, C. L.: Treatment of pelvic fractures and dislocations. Clin. Orthop., 97:97, 1973.
14. Sullivan, L. R.: *Fractures of the Pelvis.* AAOS Instructional Course Lectures, Vol. XVIII:96. St. Louis, C. V. Mosby, 1961.
15. Friedenberg, Z. B., et al.: Fracture of the hip: A review of 200 consecutive fractures. J. Trauma, 10:51, 1970.
16. Metz, C. W., Jr., et al.: The displaced intracapsular fracture of the neck of the femur. Experience with the Deyerle method of fixation in sixty-three cases. J. Bone Joint Surg., A52:113, 1970.
17. Simon, W. H., et al.: Femoral neck fractures. A study of the adequacy of reduction. Clin. Orthop., 70:152, 1970.
18. Blichert-Toft, M., et al.: Treatment of fractures of the femoral shaft. Acta Orthop. Scand., 41:341, 1970.

19. Pedersen, H. E., and Serra, J. B.: Injury to the collateral ligaments of the knee associated with femoral shaft fractures. Clin. Orthop., 60:119, 1968.

20. Hohl, M., and Luck, V.: Fractures of the tibial condyle. J. Bone Joint Surg., A38:1001, 1956.

21. Godfrey, J.: Trauma in children. Instructional Course Lecture. J. Bone Joint Surg., A46:422, 1964.

22. Rogers, L. F.: The radiography of epiphyseal injuries. Radiology, 96:289, 1970.

23. Ryan, J. R.: The relationship of the radial head to radial neck diameters in fetuses and adults with reference to radial-head subluxation in children. J. Bone Joint Surg., A51:781, 1969.

24. Berk, J. P., and Collins, J. A.: *Theoretical and Clinical Aspects of Posttraumatic Fat Embolism Syndrome.* Instructional Course Lectures, Vol. XXII:38. St. Louis, C. V. Mosby, 1973.

25. McQuillan, W. M., and Nolan, B.: Ischemia complicating injury. J. Bone Joint Surg., B52:3, 1968.

26. Willhotte, D. R., et al.: Early recognition and treatment of impending Volkmann's ischemia in the lower extremity. Arch. Surg., 100:11, 1970.

Suggested Reading

1. Solheim, K., and Vaage, S.: Delayed union and nonunion of fractures: Clinical experience with the ASIF method. J. Trauma, 13:121, 1973.

2. Chan, D., et al.: Patterns of multiple fracture in accidental injury. J. Trauma, 13:1075, 1973.

3. Burri, C., et al.: Treatment of posttraumatic osteomyelitis with bone, soft tissue, and skin defects. J. Trauma, 13:799, 1973.

18   AMPUTATIONS FOLLOWING TRAUMA

J. R. KIRKPATRICK
R. F. WILSON

In patients below the age of 55 years, almost 50% of all amputations result directly from some type of trauma.[1] Even when the injury itself is relatively mild, complications related to an inadequate blood supply or infection may so compromise the viability or function of the extremity that a portion of the limb must be removed.

An amputation is seldom an emergency where there is doubt of its need. In general, one can be conservative in this regard. However, when it becomes apparent that removal of a portion of a limb may be necessary, the decision should be governed by a number of principles:

1. Do not amputate unless you are certain that an amputation is essential.
2. Conversely, do not persist in attempts to salvage a limb if the effort would endanger the patient's life or overall welfare.
3. Amputate as little tissue as possible initially; the first procedure need not be definitive.
4. Consider the patient's physical condition and his potential ability to utilize a prosthesis.
5. Keep in mind the stump that will allow the patient to use the optimal prosthesis.
6. Rehabilitation, both mental and physical, begins at the time of amputation.
7. Do not close amputation wounds if infection is present or likely to occur.

AXIOM

FOR BEST RESULTS, AN AMPUTATION SHOULD BE CONSIDERED AS PART OF A TOTAL REHABILITATION PROGRAM.

All too often, physicians have considered an amputation as a last resort and an acknowledgment of failure. Moreover, the surgeon will often perform the amputation without considering future goals of rehabilitation and without a clear understanding of the type of prosthesis which will provide optimal function. The surgeon's responsibility to the patient does not end with the amputation; rather, he must be prepared to restore the patient to maximal function using appropriate prosthetic devices. It is in this regard that the help of an experienced prosthetist is invaluable. Many amputations that were poorly tolerated in the past can now be managed with excellent prostheses that can restore much of that limb's previous function.

INDICATIONS FOR AMPUTATION

The main indications for amputation include (1) loss of tissue viability and (2) loss of function. Unfortunately, the status of the viability and function of an injured extremity is not alway clear, especially in the early post-traumatic period.

AXIOM

LOSS OF SKIN, MUSCLE, OR BONE ALONE IS VIRTUALLY NEVER AN INDICATION FOR EARLY AMPUTATION.

In attempting to establish objective criteria for defining nonviability and nonfunction, every extremity can be thought of as possessing five basic components or structures: skin, muscle, bone, nerve, and blood vessels. Obviously, if all five components are lost or destroyed, the amputation has already occurred or is unavoidable. On the other hand, if all five structures are viable and functioning, there is no need for amputation, unless complications develop later. Unfortunately, it can be extremely difficult to assess accurately the status of each of these components immediately after injury, and many days of treatment and observation may be needed before a proper decision can be made.

SKIN. Loss of skin alone is almost never an indication for amputation. Even an extremity with a total degloving loss of skin, such as that caused by a washer or wringer, can, with proper treatment, regain good function and viability.

MUSCLE. Amputation rarely results from excessive loss of muscle alone and this type of injury seldom occurs without loss of other vital structures. However, it is important in the early assessment to determine the viability of the traumatized muscle so that an adequate debridement can be performed. Unfortunately, the classic indications of muscle viability—irritability, bleeding, and color change—are not always reliable. A better approach is daily debridement, excising only the tissue which is obviously dead.

BONE. Bone loss alone is almost never an indication for early amputation. In most instances, the main determinants of amputation are the associated vascular and neurologic injuries. In injuries associated with severe tissue loss, such as those caused by close-range shotgun blasts and high-velocity missiles, stabilization of the bone, by appropriate means, is essential to the success of any vascular or neurologic repairs.

VASCULAR STRUCTURES. Prior to World War II, injuries to the main arteries of an extremity were the prime indications for early amputation. Injured major vessels such as the popliteal, common femoral, or axillary arteries were usually ligated to prevent continuing hemorrhage; this resulted in a high incidence of gangrene and amputation. Today, every effort should be made to repair all injured large arteries as soon as possible, particularly if they are the major supply to the extremity. Even though the lumen may ultimately thrombose, injured large veins should be repaired because even a slightly impaired venous drainage during the initial postoperative period may jeopardize a limb which has a marginal blood supply.

NERVE INJURY

AXIOM

IF NERVE FUNCTION TO AN EXTREMITY IS LOST, THAT LIMB IS USELESS.

Restoration of nerve function is usually the primary limiting factor in reimplantation or reconstruction of a severely injured extremity. Since the first successful reimplantation of an extremity 20 years ago, it has become increasingly apparent that the final result is measured by the degree of nerve regeneration.

As a general rule, when four of the five main components or structures of a limb are severely injured, but the nerve injury is minimal, every effort should be made to reconstruct and salvage the extremity. If the nerve injury is so severe that it is unlikely that the extremity will have any function, the most prudent course to follow, particularly in a young individual, is immediate amputation and early fitting with a prosthesis. This not only decreases hospital time but markedly reduces the likelihood of proximal contractures or muscle atrophy which can defeat or greatly retard the rehabilitation of the patient.

Late Amputations

Most frequently, if the viability of an extremity deteriorates after initial therapy, it does so as a result of infection, vascular occlusion, or severe edema. However, even if the extremity is viable, late amputation is also indicated where the muscle or nerve loss is so extensive that the extremity is nonfunctional.

PITFALL

IF A SURGEON ATTEMPTS TO RECONSTRUCT A SEVERELY INJURED LIMB THAT WILL PROBABLY HAVE NO FUNCTION, HE MAY PLACE THE PATIENT'S LIFE AND THE FUNCTION OF THE REMAINDER OF THE EXTREMITY IN UNNECESSARY JEOPARDY.

Before he embarks upon a prolonged series of complicated procedures, he should consider the patient's loss of time from work, the pain and inconvenience, and the probability of eventual failure with resultant amputation. He must also consider whether his attempts at reconstruction may compromise some future level of amputation.

AXIOM

IN HIS ZEAL TO PRESERVE A PORTION OF A LIMB, THE SURGEON MUST NOT JEOPARDIZE THE MORE PROXIMAL SEGMENTS BY UNWISE PERSISTENCE.

It would be deplorable if attempts at reconstruction converted a below-knee or below-elbow amputation to one at a higher level. This is an especially serious consideration because of the great importance that the knee and elbow have in the eventual function and usefulness of the extremity.

The surgeon must also consider whether the rehabilitation is apt to be complicated by deterioration of the patient's general health during the long hospitalization and numerous surgical procedures that may be required to salvage the extremity. To put all these considerations in their proper context, it is imperative that the responsible surgeon also understand the great strides that have been made in the rehabilitation of patients with early amputations.

TYPES OF AMPUTATIONS

Two major types of amputations are performed: open and closed. Both are usually performed with proximal tourniquet control, except in the presence of arteriosclerotic vascular disease when the tourniquet may damage or occlude the major vessels.

Open or Guillotine Amputations

Open amputations are interim lifesaving procedures in which no attempt is made to close or approximate any of the tissues. A guillotine amputation is an open amputation through a circular incision in which all the tissues (skin, muscle, and bone) are cut straight across. The muscle is cut at the level of the retracted skin and the bone is cut at the level of the retracted muscle. These are usually performed when spreading infection or wet gangrene is established. This amputation provides maximal exposure and open drainage of the tissues. Postoperatively, skin traction can be applied through a stockinette glued to the skin. Since a circular scar eventually develops and adheres to the bone with inadequate soft-tissue cover, the amputation must be revised before a prosthesis can be applied.

Closed or Flap Amputation

When no infection is present, primary closure of the amputation site may be performed. The incision is made to produce two flaps of skin, attempting, except with above-knee amputation, to keep the scar from the end of the stump. The flap with the tougher skin and better blood supply is fashioned to be longer. The muscle is cut at the level of the retracted skin and the bone at the level of the retracted muscle. The arteries and veins are ligated separately to prevent A-V fistula formation. The nerves are divided under traction so that they cannot adhere to the scar and produce stump pain. The deep fascia is sutured to allow proper muscle attachment to the bone and to prevent muscle ends from adhering to the skin. Some surgeons will insert drains or Hemovacs in the corners of the wound and remove them in 48 to 72 hours, while others will use no drains at all.

Postoperative Care

If drains are used, the dressings may have to be changed every two to three days to be kept dry; if drains are not used, the dressings need to be changed only every four to six days. The outer elastic dressings are adjusted as often as needed to maintain uniform pressure on the stump. The stump usually heals slowly, and the skin sutures should be left in place for at least two weeks. Since there is a tendency to flexion contractures, splints may be applied over the dressings.

Exercises to strengthen and prevent contracture of the muscles of the extremity should be begun early—even before the extremity has healed completely. Care must be taken, however, not to traumatize the end of the stump.

SPECIFIC AMPUTATIONS

Lower-extremity Amputations

Although 80% of all civilian amputations involve the lower extremity, the number of upper- and lower-extremity amputations resulting from trauma is almost equal.[2] Of 172 lower-extremity amputations performed at the University of Washington between May 1964 and September 1968, only 34 resulted directly from trauma or post-traumatic complications. In contrast to the other 138 patients, these 34 were almost invariably less than 50 years of age and they were able to attain their preamputation level of activity in a much higher percentage of cases[2] (Table 1).

The main factors in rehabilitation of the patient with a lower-extremity amputation include: (1) preservation of the knee, (2) preservation of maximum length of bone, (3) salvage of an end-weight-bearing stump, and (4) reliance, if possible, on full-thickness covering of the stump.

TABLE 1. PATIENTS WITH BELOW-KNEE AMPUTATIONS
May 1964 through September 1968

Distribution of Cases by Age and Etiology
N = 172

Age group in years	Vascular with diabetes	Vascular without diabetes	Infection	Tumor	Trauma and post-trauma complications	Congenital	TOTAL
1–12	0	0	0	0	3	4	7
13–24	0	1	1	0	8	1	11
25–50	4	9	15	0	19	0	47
51–75	38	30	17	1	4	0	90
76–100	8	8	1	0	0	0	17
TOTAL	50	48	34	1	34	5	172

From Ernest M. Burgess, M.D. Prepared by Prosthetic and Orthotic Studies, New York University Post-Graduate Medical School, for the Subcommittee on Child Prosthetics Problems of the Committee on Prosthetics Research and Development, under a special grant from the Children's Bureau, Department of Health, Education, and Welfare.

PITFALL

Every effort should be made to salvage a functional knee or elbow and no reconstructive procedures should interfere with or compromise the viability or function of these two structures.

DIGITAL AMPUTATION. For severe combined bony and soft-tissue injuries to the middle three digits of the foot, early amputation is the preferred method of management. Attempts should be made, however, to salvage the little toe and the great toe whenever possible, because they are extremely important in "push off" during the stance phase of gait. No prosthetics are required for the amputation of a digit and no real disability results unless the great toe is lost. In this event, rehabilitation will usually require a padded toe within the shoe and a steel shank to help the patient during push off.

TRANSMETATARSAL AMPUTATIONS. Transmetatarsal amputations are particularly suitable in lawn-mower or power-mower injuries where the toes are either traumatically amputated or severely lacerated. Other situations where transmetatarsal amputations may be required are crush injuries such as those which may occur when an automobile either falls or rolls over the distal portion of the foot.

This is a very useful amputation site. Little power or balance is lost in walking or standing and there is little or no limp. It is the highest level of amputation at which no special prosthesis is required; however, for this stump to have good long-term function, it is preferable to conserve maximum skin length posteriorly and create an anterior suture line at the time of amputation. Following healing, the patient usually does well with a padded shoe with a steel shank.

TARSAL-METATARSAL DISARTICULATION (Chopart's amputation). Following trauma, the prime indication to perform a Chopart type of amputation is failure of a transmetatarsal amputation. Here, as with a transmetatarsal amputation, great care should be taken to preserve maximum skin and soft tissue to pad the stump.

This particular amputation has the advantages of preserving not only equal length of the extremities but also an end-weight-bearing stump in which an immediate postoperative prosthesis can be utilized. It has been condemned for many years because of the poor prostheses that were available and because the imbalance in the remaining muscles tends to produce an equinovarus deformity of the foot. In recent years, the prosthetists have made this level of amputation more functional. Attempts to correct the equinovarus deformity by arthrodesis of the ankle joint have not been very successful; the balance of the foot is lost and there is no active push-off phase during walking.

SYME'S AMPUTATION (Fig. 1). This is the highest level of amputation in which equality of lower-extremity length can be maintained and should be used whenever the amputation is to be carried through the ankle joint. To be successful, the amputation should provide a heel flap free from infection and scarring and possessing adequate sensation and circulation. Proper centering and stability of the heel flap over the distal tibia are also crucial to the successful function of the amputation. In addition, the malleoli should not be trimmed except to eliminate the rough and sharp edges of the distal tibia and fibula.

Previously, this procedure was not utilized extensively in this country; however, the stability of the present postoperative prosthesis is much improved over that of those utilized in the past and it is being advocated with increasing frequency. It is

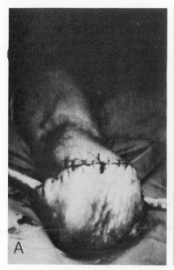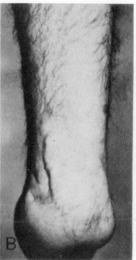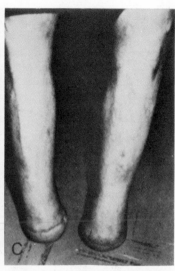

FIG. 1. *A:* Completed Syme's amputation. *B:* Patient demonstrates the appearance of a well-healed amputation site. *C:* Bilateral Syme's amputation: Note the equality of length and weight-bearing properties of this amputation. (Courtesy of Ernest M. Burgess, M.D., Robert L. Romano, M.D., and Joseph H. Zettle, C.P.)

now possible to get a tailored Syme's or Chopart's socket that has total contact and provides good functional support.

The two most attractive features of this level of amputation are the retention of extremity length and the maintenance of an end-weight-bearing stump. Retention of length is especially helpful in the elderly patient who is spared the difficulties of applying a prosthesis prior to ambulation. Maintenance of end weight bearing is an important aid in balance.

During the swing and stance phases of walking, the lower extremity rotates internally and externally on its long axis, causing the stump to tend to rotate inside the prosthesis. If the prosthesis does not fit properly, the friction and irritation can cause pain and breakdown of the stump.

BELOW-KNEE AMPUTATION (Fig. 2). When an amputation must be performed above the ankle, the site of election should provide a stump five to seven inches long below the knee joint. Longer stumps are difficult to fit to a prosthesis and are apt to have circulatory problems. If the knee is preserved even in "doubtful" cases, approximately 80 to 85% of trauma patients can be success-

fully managed with a below-knee amputation. The single overriding reason for taking this position is that, despite marked improvements in above-knee prosthetic devices, it is virtually impossible for an A-K amputee to achieve 100% rehabilitation unless he is a young, healthy individual who utilizes a hydraulic knee. With a below-knee amputation, it is possible for many rehabilitated persons to achieve an almost totally normal life style which can include cycling, running, and climbing of steps. Any amputation level above this carries a high likelihood of limitation of motor function.

Surgical Technique. The goals of this technique include: (1) creation of a long posterior flap, because this contains the major portion of the blood supply to the calf, (2) provision for some degree of myodesis or myoplasty (i.e. complete covering of bone with muscle), and (3) early ambulation, whenever possible. Postoperatively, there should be immediate application of a rigid dressing. If for some reason a rigid dressing is not used, fluffs and Telfa are applied to the anterior suture line and a stump sock is pulled over the dressings

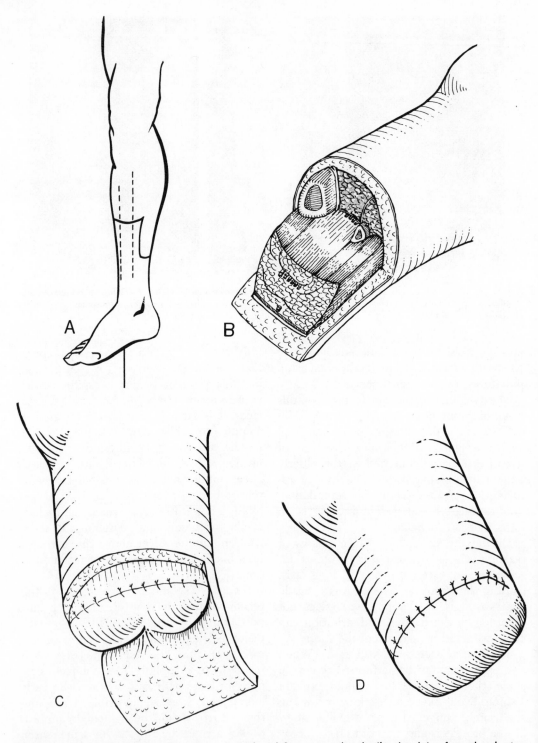

FIG. 2. *A:* Schematic drawing of skin incision. *B:* Myofascial flap contoured and tailored to bring forward and suture anteriorly. *C:* Myoplasty completed and ready for skin closure. *D:* Final closure, lateral view. (From Burgess, Ernest M., Romano, Robert L., and Zettle, Joseph H.: *Management of Lower-extremity Amputations.* Seattle, Prosthetics Research Study, 1969.)

up to the level of the groin, where it is held in place by nonallergic tape.

Postoperative Care and Prosthetic Fitting. Complete wound healing of a lower-extremity amputation has often been felt to be a prerequisite to the fitting of a prosthetic device. For many years now, however, the early application of a temporary prosthesis has been used in patients with questionable stump healing.

PITFALL

IF APPLICATION OF A RIGID DRESSING AND IMMEDIATE FITTING OF A PROSTHESIS ARE UNDERTAKEN WITHOUT AN EXPERIENCED THERAPIST AND PROSTHETIST AS PART OF THE TEAM, BREAKDOWN OF THE STUMP AND FAILURE OF HEALING ARE APT TO RESULT

Irrespective of the immediate method of management of the stump, at approximately six weeks to three months following amputation, if all goes well, the patient will be ready for a prosthesis. The preferred prosthesis for the B-K amputee is the PTB model, which incorporates the concept of a horizontal loading of force through the patellar tendon. This prosthesis contains a total contact socket as opposed to the pre-1950 version which has a so-called plug-fit type of socket. The suspension for the patellar tendon-weight-bearing (PTB) prosthesis can include a variety of supportive mechanisms ranging from a thigh corset (not recommended in the young healthy person) to the more elaborate supracondylar-suprapatellar wedge that is becoming increasingly popular. Frequently, however, a simple suspension cuff is quite satisfactory. The foot utilized should almost always be of the SACH (solid ankle, cushioned heel) variety. This type of foot is basic for all types of prosthetic devices currently in use and has supplanted the single axis foot because of ease of construction, durability, and simplicity of design.

It should be stressed that, in the motivated B-K amputee with a properly fitted prosthesis, physical therapy can restore close to 100% of his preoperative exercise tolerance. Anything less than this represents a compromise with the ideal.

THROUGH-KNEE AMPUTATIONS. Through-knee amputations are rarely used in the trauma patient unless there is a traumatic avulsion directly through the knee joint. This amputation is distinctly unpopular in this country because the added length of femur makes construction of a knee assembly difficult; moreover, the prostheses that are available are not as functional as those used for above-knee amputees. It does, however, have the advantages of a longer lever that is controlled by undamaged muscles and an end-bearing stump.

ABOVE-KNEE AMPUTATION. Since most trauma patients have good arterial inflow, above-knee amputation should be reserved for those patients who clearly demonstrate one of the following criteria: (1) traumatic amputations above the level of the knee, (2) frank gangrene extending above the knee, and (3) documented nonambulation prior to injury.

The surgical technique for the above-knee amputation is available in many other standard textbooks; however, it should be emphasized that (1) in contradistinction to the below-knee amputation, the position of the suture line is not of major concern and the classic "fish-mouth" incision is quite suitable, (2) the femur should be amputated at least two to three inches higher than the skin closure, preferably just above the condyle flare, and (3) the utilization of an immediate rigid dressing and prosthesis is generally not indicated.

HIP DISARTICULATIONS. Hip disarticulation is rarely required in the trauma patient except with severe avulsions in pedestrian accidents or when a patient develops a severe synergistic type of infection or gas gangrene.

Upper-extremity Amputations

Because of the frequency with which the upper extremity is exposed to trauma in factory workers and farmers, injuries have been the main cause of upper-extremity amputation. Amputations because of vascular disease, congenital anomalies, and tumors are much less frequent.

DIGITAL AND HAND AMPUTATIONS

AXIOM

NEVER SACRIFICE VIABLE TISSUE IN THE HAND UNTIL THE FINAL DECISION HAS BEEN MADE AS TO THE DEGREE OF FUNCTIONAL RESTORATION THAT IS POSSIBLE.

Early amputation in the upper extremity is almost never indicated unless it involves the distal tip of a phalanx. Preservation of the hand is of paramount concern. With severe hand injuries, one should attempt to: (1) preserve the thumb at all costs, since it is virtually impossible adequately to restore function to the hand without retention of thumb-finger opposition, (2) preserve at least two other digits, and (3) accept a nonfunctioning digit which later may be made functional by using a tendon transfer. If it is possible to salvage a thumb and two digits, the individual can regain almost total functional capacity of his hand, including writing, lifting, turning, and playing sports. With the thumb and only one digit, this is much more difficult and many of these activities are not possible.

Even though a small amount of length may be lost, any excision through the base of the nail to revise the amputation site should include all the matrix to prevent the later growth of a painful nail. If the amputation is through a joint space, the distal cartilage should be removed so that the skin over the stump will be less mobile. It is also often wise to trim the condyles of the phalanx to narrow the tip of the stump to a more functional shape. Tendons should never be sutured over the end of a stump, since this limits the motion of the adjoining fingers. The stump must be covered with nonsensitive durable skin; thus, if the

pulp of the fingertip is still present, it should be covered with a split-thickness skin graft. If the pulp is damaged or absent, however, a pedicle graft is preferred. If the middle and ring fingers are amputated, an attempt should be made to preserve the base of their proximal phalanges. The metacarpal heads of these two digits maintain the transverse arch of the hand and ensure a broad grasping surface for the palm. Removal of one metacarpal head results in a decrease in work area of approximately 25% with a corresponding reduction in both leverage and appearance.

The index and little fingers are vital, and even a markedly shortened fifth digit will be of considerable value to a worker using hand tools. Removal of the entire little finger decreases stabilization of the hand, places a strain on the middle digits, and causes the balancing effect of a broad palm to be lost. If the little finger absolutely cannot be salvaged, the head of the fifth metacarpal should be removed so that the fourth digit then can become the terminal digit. The hypothenar muscle mass can be brought over the obliquely transected head of the fifth metacarpal to act as padding.

The index finger is the key digit in pinching and picking movements; therefore, if the normal ratio between the length of the thumb and the length of the index finger is not maintained, loss of these motions occurs. Loss of the index finger past the distal interphalangeal joint makes these two motions exceedingly difficult and loss past the middle interphalangeal joint makes them impossible. In most cases, a very short index finger stump is more of a handicap than an aid.

WRIST DISARTICULATION. Although amputation through the carpal bones is occasionally possible, it is seldom practical; disarticulation at the radiocarpal joint is much more practical. This site was avoided in the past because of difficulty with poor wound healing and difficulty with fitting a prosthesis. Because of newer prostheses, if the stump can be covered with good palmar skin, it has many advantages—including preservation of full pronation and supination and maintenance of a strong forearm lever.

FOREARM AMPUTATIONS. If a wrist disarticulation cannot be done, the level of choice is the junction of the middle and lower thirds of the forearm. These amputations are similar in some respects to the below-knee amputations previously discussed. If the "hinged mechanism" (elbow) is retained, the functional capabilities are good; however, since weight bearing is not required, the surgeon may concentrate on preservation of function. To obtain good function, maximum length is required. Since the newer prostheses rely on local functional muscles to perform pronation and supination, retention of maximum length is important to maintaining good function. As a result of improvements which allow the prosthesis to slide over the widened end of the stump, carpal disarticulation, which was once considered a poor amputation, is now acceptable.

KUKENBERG AMPUTATION. This is historically an interesting and unique type of forearm amputation in which a cleft is created between the radial and ulnar portion of the forearm, and the two sides of the stump work together in an up-and-down pincer movement rather than by rotation. This type of procedure can be performed only if six to eight inches of radius and ulna are available below the elbow. Skin with good tactile sensation should be placed over the two contact surfaces. The radial cleft is covered completely with normal skin while the ulnar portion is covered with split-thickness skin or a pedicle graft. The resultant stump is not cosmetic; however, many patients are pleased because sensation and strength are both retained. Furthermore, it is possible to fit a standard prosthesis over this type of amputation. Double amputees benefit from this amputation since emphasis can be placed on retaining strength in the major (dominant)

extremity. Occasionally, it is also indicated in a single amputation when the dominant extremity is removed and the individual must do heavy labor.

ABOVE-ELBOW AMPUTATIONS. The standard amputation at this level should retain 50 to 90% of the total length of the humerus, and is very similar in technique to an above-knee amputation; the prime concern is to obtain healing and to preserve shoulder function. A well-padded stump is recommended, and the suture line may lie at any point on the stump that is convenient.

When a patient has an above-elbow amputation, he is faced with a much more difficult program of rehabilitation since none of the mechanical elbows currently available provides normal function. The usual prosthesis has a total contact socket with a cross-chest suspension system. The standard elbow joint allows motion from 5 to 135° of flexion and has multiple locking positions within this range. The locking device is controlled through a suspension system which allows positioning of the elbow at the desired amount of flexion. The cable system of the prosthesis can then transfer power directly to the terminal device (a hook or a hand) which is connected to a forearm shell by means of a mechanical wrist joint. The mechanical wrist joint is usually an oval or round friction device which allows for prepositioning in either pronation or supination. Other available wrist joints include the flexion and quick-change wrist units, both of which are more complicated than the simple friction wrist joint.

The terminal device for an above-elbow prosthesis is usually a split hook, made of steel or aluminum. All are voluntary opening devices in that the power is transmitted to the hook which works against a series of rubber bands. The grasping power of the hook is related to the elasticity of the restraining rubber bands. Thus, it is possible to predetermine the amount of rebound built into the prosthesis and to change it as the patient desires. This type of terminal device is the most popular and functional and is especially appreciated by patients who must do manual labor.

The artificial hands currently available are cosmetically more pleasing than a hook, but functionally are very poor. They are usually suitable only for patients who do work requiring minimal strength or grasping power. A force of 15 to 25 pounds is required to open the fingers, but, because of the complicated gears required to operate the fingers, the actual force transmitted from the fingers to an object is considerably less.

THE IMMEDIATE POSTSURGICAL PROSTHESIS

The concept of fitting a patient with a prosthesis immediately after surgery and initiating ambulation the day of surgery originated with Berlemont in the late 1950s.[3] His procedure was then modified by Wise,[4] Burgess[5] and others and is currently being utilized in various centers throughout the United States. About 1,500 of these procedures have been performed in this country with a success rate of about 90%.

For practical purposes, the term "immediate postsurgical prosthesis fitting" has become almost synonymous with below-knee amputations for several reasons: (1) below-knee amputations are the most common type of amputations in which this technique is used, (2) the rigid dressing is the easiest to apply at this level, and (3) early ambulation is best achieved in the below-knee amputee. To make the system work properly, it is necessary to develop a protocol which begins with a thorough preoperative evaluation and continues through definitive limb fitting. It should also be em-

phasized that this technique is seldom applicable to the initial or emergency amputation after trauma; it is strictly an elective procedure to be used during the definitive or final amputation.

The surgical portion of the procedure can be divided into three steps: (1) amputation, (2) application of a rigid dressing, and (3) the addition of a walking pylon to the dressing. The principles involved in the amputation itself have already been discussed.

The Rigid Dressing

It is important to recognize that the application of a rigid dressing to any amputation site has distinct advantages regardless of whether or not early ambulation is achieved. This dressing acts as a plaster prosthetic socket which, if properly applied, provides fixation for the stump and permits controlled pressure which in turn reduces postamputation edema. Shaping or maturation of the stump begins immediately when the rigid dressing is applied. With proper pressure to the end of the stump and good local tissue immobilization, the amputee also enjoys greater freedom of movement and comfort.

Some surgeons feel that the most important accomplishment of the rigid dressing has been to redefine criteria for choosing the level of amputation. Traditionally, the level of lower-extremity amputation was dictated by the status of the circulation and pulses and an estimate as to where optimal healing might occur. However, with the advent of the rigid dressing and its greater applicability in below-knee amputees, attention was directed toward preserving the knee whenever possible. The increased success with B-K amputations should probably not be attributed to the rigid dressing alone; it seems more likely that the importance of the collateral circulation around the knee was not fully recognized. Many authors in the past were unaware that a below-knee amputation could be supported on collaterals alone without any direct popliteal artery blood flow.

The technique for applying the rigid dressing is not complicated. Following amputation, a Telfa dressing is applied over the suture line and several fluffs of lamb's wool are placed over the end of the stump. A tightly contoured elastic stump sock is then applied from stump to groin. This is held in place by an assistant who applies upward traction on the stump sock at all times. Soft felt pads are pasted to the stump sock with surgical glue to protect the patella and tibial and fibular flares. Elastic plaster is then applied to the stump with maximum pressure over the distal end of the stump and decreasing pressure toward the groin until a molded semirigid cast is in place. The cast is molded above the knee to prevent instability during ambulation. With the knee kept in 15° flexion, a conventional plaster cast is applied to support the rigid inner dressing. A suspension strap is molded into the outer layer of plaster, and the rigid dressing is kept in place by an outer elastic belt worn around the waist.

If early ambulation is desired, a standard prosthetic four-way socket attachment plate is applied to the surface of the stump and held in place with several additional layers of plaster. The early-ambulation pylon and foot are then attached to the socket plate and adjusted to the length of the opposite extremity.

Postoperatively, the patient is monitored on a daily basis for fever, excessive pain, or odor from the dressing. If any of these problems occurs, the cast is removed and the stump is inspected. If the postoperative course is uneventful, cast changes are programmed according to the subsequent shrinkage of the tissue in the stump. Some patients require a second rigid dressing at ten days, while others with minimal tissue shrinkage can go up to three weeks without a dressing change. The skin sutures are removed at the time of the second dressing. At three weeks the patient is converted to a temporary prosthesis, and at six weeks to three months he is fitted to a permanent prosthesis.

Early Ambulation

This is the most controversial part of the program; many centers have modified their approach and are becoming more conservative. At New York University,[6] for example, the surgeons permit no weight bearing at all for the first four to five days and full weight bearing on the stump is not allowed until at least three weeks. Our own preference is to allow ambulation according to each patient's motivation and ability.

PITFALL

IF THE PATIENT DOES NOT LEARN CRUTCH WALKING AND FOUR-POINT BALANCE PREOPERATIVELY, HE IS UNSUITABLE FOR EARLY AMBULATION.

All patients selected for early ambulation are sent to physical therapy for five to seven days prior to surgery to learn crutch walking and four-point balance, which are essential to early ambulation. An interested physical therapist is an absolute necessity in this portion of the program. The application of a weighted stocking to the leg to be amputated also helps the patient to adjust to the extra weight that he will encounter with rigid dressing and attached prothesis.

Highly motivated patients can begin crutch walking the night of surgery. By the first or second postoperative day, all patients are encouraged to begin crutch walking, applying up to 25 pounds of weight bearing on the amputated side. By the fifth day they are walking between parallel bars. Progress from this point is individualized; however, several of our patients have left the hospital at ten days walking on their protheses without crutches.

REIMPLANTATION OF SEVERED LIMBS

The conditions permitting reimplantation of extremities are rare and few individuals or teams are likely to develop an extensive experience. It is imperative, therefore, that a detailed systematic approach to the patient and his severed limb be understood.

AXIOM

CONSIDER REIMPLANTATION WHENEVER THE UPPER EXTREMITY IS COMPLETELY AMPUTATED BY TRAUMA.

The usual treatment when the distal portion of an extremity has been completely amputated is closure of the proximal stump and rehabilitation with a prosthesis. No prosthesis, however, can completely replace the functions of an intact limb, especially sensation; accordingly, there has been interest in the reimplantation of severed limbs under certain selected circumstances.

Since the first successful human limb reimplantation in 1962 by Malt and Mc-Kahnn,[7] several well-documented series have been published. However, since the postoperative care and rehabilitation of these patients are often prolonged and complicated and since the eventual function is often poor, it is now clear that this procedure should be attempted only under the most ideal conditions. The results with lower-extremity implantations have been poor; thus, reimplantation of legs or feet should not be attempted. Although all patients with upper-extremity amputations might be considered candidates for functional reimplantation, few actually meet the required criteria. The patient should have no serious preexisting disease or other significant injuries and the trauma to the severed extremity should be a clean laceration with minimal additional tissue damage. He should also be young, preferably less than 40 years, and highly motivated. Some surgeons have suggested that the patient should be evaluated by a psychiatrist preoperatively.

Preparation of the Patient and Severed Limbs

For optimal results reimplantation should be performed by a two-team approach,

with one team responsible for the patient and the other responsible for the severed extremity. The teams should include at least a vascular surgeon, a neurosurgeon, and an orthopedic surgeon. It is extremely important to keep the ischemia time of the severed limb to an absolute minimum, and certainly the implantation should be completed within six to twelve hours of the injury.

The patient must be treated rapidly and aggressively so that he can be brought into optimum preoperative condition manifested by stable vital signs and good urine output. Hemorrhage from the stump should be controlled with broad even compression, such as that provided by a blood pressure cuff. If the severed extremity was not brought in with the patient, the ambulance team should be sent back for it immediately. The amputated limb should be cleansed, and the vessels infused with cold heparinized saline as soon as possible.

PITFALL

IF ONE CONCENTRATES ON REIMPLANTING THE SEVERED LIMB AND FORGETS THE PATIENT, ONE MAY LOSE BOTH THE PATIENT AND THE LIMB.

In the midst of the preparation of the limb for reimplantation, one must not forget about the patient. Malt has noted that at least one patient has lost his life after a successful reimplantation because of an unrecognized rupture of an abdominal organ.

After the initial resuscitation, the patient is moved to the operating room where the wound is irrigated and meticulously debrided. Malt has pointed out that the debrided tissue from the limb and stump should be sent for cultures and sensitivity studies. The structures to be anastomosed are identified at this time and may be tagged with sutures.

The team responsible for the severed limb should cleanse and debride it carefully in the operating room and aspirate the major arteries and veins. Following this they should irrigate the limb through the main artery or arteries with cold heparinized saline, lactated Ringer's or Rheomacrodex. The veins are gently milked during the irrigation to remove as much blood and clot as possible. The last portion of the irrigating fluid should contain antibiotics, e.g. 2,000,000 units of penicillin per liter.

Technique of Reanastomosis

The actual procedure of anastomosis is carried out in the following steps:

The bone is approximated and stabilized, preferably with internal fixation. Although there is some objection to an intramedullary nail because it may interfere with endosteal blood supply, application of plates and screws causes much more soft-tissue dissection. Wires or pins that protrude through the skin should be avoided because of the danger of infection.

The main veins are anastomosed, and then the main arteries. In many respects establishment of an adequate venous return is more important than the arterial inflow. To be absolutely certain that clots are removed from the distal vessels, it may be wise to pass Fogarty catheters after complete irrigation. If there is any question about the patency of the distal vessels after the anastomoses are performed, an intraoperative arteriogram should be performed.

Primary repair of the main nerve trunks is performed whenever possible. A magnifying lens or a dissecting microscope may help obtain a more meticulous anastomosis. If the amputation has been associated with muscle damage, as with blunt trauma, delayed nerve repair is preferable.

Muscles and tendons are repaired to the extent possible. By the time bone fixation and vascular and nerve anastomoses have been completed, any residual devitalized tissue will usually be readily apparent. The goals of the muscle repair are to provide adequate coverage for all anastomotic sites and to rejoin maximal areas of well-vascularized tissue for optimal capillary and lymphatic regeneration.

The skin is sutured wherever possible without tension; partial-thickness skin grafts may be applied to any remaining open areas. The tissues in the severed portion of the limb will almost always swell significantly, increasing the tendency to ischemia at the wound edges if the sutures are too tight.

A fasciotomy of the forearm should be performed at the end of the procedure in virtually all patients. If the fascial compartments are intact, the severe muscle swelling which almost always occurs can cause pressure necrosis of the muscle and occlusion of the major vessels.

Postoperative Care

Low-molecular-weight dextran in doses of 500 ml every 12 hours by slow I.V. infusion postoperatively may help maintain perfusion of the limb. The severed limb should be elevated for at least six days to help reduce edema. No constrictive or compressive dressings should be applied. Inhalation of high concentrations of oxygen may help to provide oxygen to the hypoxic tissues if the extremity is cyanotic.

If there is any question about the arterial circulation to the reattached limb, arteriography should be performed. Fluid must be administered to maintain a normal blood pressure and normal or high cardiac output to keep blood flow to the limb at a maximum. Overloading with crystalloids, however, may increase swelling. Urinary output must be kept above 50 ml per hour to ensure adequate handling of any myoglobin that may be washed out of the severed limb into the patient. Massive parenteral antibiotics should be used; a combination of penicillin, Staphcillin, and gentamicin might be appropriate.

If signs of gross nonviability develop, the limb must be amputated immediately. Although one may be reluctant to sacrifice a reimplanted limb after many hours of operative attempts to save it, the patient's life cannot be jeopardized.

Rehabilitation

PITFALL

IF EFFORTS AT REHABILITATION ARE INTER-MITTENT OR SHORT-LIVED, THE REPLANTED LIMB WILL PROBABLY BE FUNCTIONLESS.

Even if the limb survives, its eventual usefulness will depend primarily on the rehabilitative phase of treatment, which is extremely time consuming and may go on for many years. It should include maintenance of the limb in a position of function, protection of the limb from trauma, special attention to joint function and galvanic stimulation of the denervated muscle.

REFERENCES

1. Mital, M. A., and Pierce, D. S.: *Amputees and Their Prostheses.* Boston, Little, Brown, and Co., 1971.
2. Burgess, E. M., Romano, R. L., and Zettle, J.: *Management of Lower Extremity Amputations.* Prosthetic Research Study. Superintendent of Documents, Washington, 1971.
3. Berlemont, M.: Notre experience de l'appaorellage precoce des amputes des membres influeas aex etroblessements helio-marins de bluk. Ann. Med. Physep. 4:4, 1961.

4. Weis, M.: Myoplasty—immediate fitting—ambulation. Session of World Commission on Rehabilitation, Weisbaden, 1966.
5. Burgess, E. M., and Romano, R. L.: The management of lower extremity amputees using immediate post-surgical prostheses. Clin. Orthop., 57:137, 1968.
6. New York University Manual on Prosthetics and Orthoptics. New York, 1971.
7. Malt, R. A., and McKhann, C. F.: Replantation of severed limbs. JAMA, 189:716, 1964.

Suggested Reading

1. Boyes, J. H.: *Bunnell's Surgery of the Hand,* 5th ed. Philadelphia, J. B. Lippincott, 1970.
2. Burgess, E. M.: *The Management of Lower Extremity Amputations.* Prosthetic Research Study. Superintendent of Documents, Washington, 1971.
3. Mital, M. A., and Pierce, D. S.: *Amputees and Their Prostheses.* Boston, Little, Brown and Co., 1971.
4. Utterback, T. D., and Rohren, D. W.: Knee disarticulation as an amputation level. J. Trauma, 13:116, 1973.
5. McNamara, J. J., et al.: Vascular injury in Vietnam combat casualties: Results of treatment at the 24th evacuation hospital 1 July 1967 to 12 August 1969. Ann. Surg., 178:143, 1973.
6. Silverstein, M. J., and Kadish, L.: A study of amputations of the lower extremity. Surg. Gynec. Obstet., 137:579, 1973.
7. Warren, R., et al.: The Boston interhospital amputation study. Experience with a community service in immediate postoperative amputation prosthetic fitting. Arch. Surg. 107: 861, 1973.

19 INJURIES TO THE NECK

Injuries to the neck may be caused by penetrating or blunt trauma. Because these two types of injuries are so different in their presentation and management, penetrating injuries to the neck and blunt trauma to the larynx will be discussed separately.

Section 1

PENETRATING WOUNDS OF THE NECK

S. SANKARAN
C. E. LUCAS
A. W. WEAVER
S. FROMM

AXIOM

ALL PENETRATING NECK WOUNDS MAY BE DANGEROUS.

Since the neck is so compact and contains such a great number of large vessels and other vital structures, it is imperative that every penetrating neck wound be considered as a potential life-threatening injury, even if there is no immediate evidence of severe hemorrhage or respiratory embarrassment. Until World War II penetrating wounds of the neck were rarely seen in civilian medical practice except in large metropolitan hospitals. With the rapid increase in our population densities and the use of handguns, the incidence of these injuries has risen sharply.

EMERGENCY ROOM MANAGEMENT

Ventilation

Any patient with a penetrating wound of the neck must be quickly evaluated for the adequacy of his airway and control of internal or external bleeding. If the airway is compromised in any way, it must be reestablished immediately. Endotracheal intubation is generally far superior to an emergency tracheostomy. Following intubation, gentle tracheal aspiration and irrigation with small amounts of saline will aid in clearing blood or other material from the tracheobronchial tree.

If the patient has a wound of the pharynx or mouth with excessive bleeding which is obscuring the endoscopist's view of the larynx, it is usually safer to perform an immediate coniotomy (cricothyroidotomy), or tracheostomy. Coniotomy is used only rarely in most emergency departments, but may be lifesaving in selected cases. Whenever an airway must be established rapidly and an endotracheal tube cannot be readily inserted, coniotomy should be considered as it can be performed safely and speedily. The most superficial portion of the airway in the neck is just above the cricoid cartilage. An anterior transverse incision in this area, through the cricothyroid membrane, is relatively safe as the vocal cords are above the incision and the posterior portion of the cricoid cartilage protects the esophagus (Fig. 1). An endotracheal or tracheostomy tube is then passed down into the trachea through the coniotomy incision. This procedure can be especially useful for establishing an airway in someone choking on a bolus of food. It must be stressed that a coniotomy should be used only as a temporary measure. A standard tracheostomy should be performed as soon as the patient's condition has been stabilized.

Blood Volume Replacement

Necessary fluid and blood replacement is given through large venous catheters.

PITFALL

IF VEINS OF THE UPPER EXTREMITY ARE USED TO TREAT HYPOTENSION FROM A WOUND OF THE THORACIC INLET, THE FLUIDS MAY EXTRAVASATE INTO THE MEDIASTINUM.

In those patients in whom injury to the innominate or subclavian vein is suspected, leg veins should be used for fluid administration. The rate and volume of fluid and blood given will be determined by the patient's clinical condition, vital signs, CVP and his response to treatment.

Examination of the Wound

As soon as the adequacy of the airway has been established and large I.V. lines

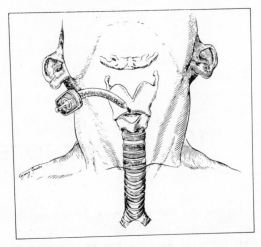

FIG. 1. An airway can be quickly established below the vocal cords through a transverse incision in the cricothyroid membrane (coniotomy).

inserted, the patient's wound is carefully examined for the presence of internal or external bleeding, hematoma formation, and subcutaneous emphysema. The probable direction of the missile tract or lacerating injury should also be noted; attempts to blindly probe the wound beyond the depth of the platysma muscle should be discouraged. It is much better to follow these tracts by enlarging and examining the wound under direct vision using local anesthesia.

PITFALL

PROBING NECK WOUNDS UNDER UNFAVORABLE CONDITIONS MAY PRECIPITATE EXSANGUINATING HEMORRHAGE FROM PREVIOUSLY SEALED VASCULAR INJURIES.

Damage to the brachial plexus or spinal cord, although a frequent cause of severe morbidity or mortality, is often overlooked during the initial examination. It must be emphasized repeatedly that the entire patient must be examined thoroughly to avoid overlooking any extracervical injuries. When absent motor and sensory functions in the upper and lower extremities are first noted in the postoperative period, it may be difficult to rule out intraoperative injury.

Intrathoracic injuries accompany neck wounds so frequently that this association must always be suspected. Under such circumstances a lethal pneumothorax or hemothorax may develop unrecognized while efforts are being concentrated on achieving hemostasis in the neck. In a few instances the thoracic injury has been missed because it was on the opposite side of the neck wound.

Control of Bleeding

External bleeding from small penetrating wounds can usually be controlled by direct pressure applied over a sterile dressing. The veins and arteries in long superficial lacerations can be ligated safely and adequately in the emergency room. However, bleeding from deeper vessels should be controlled by direct digital pressure. These vessels should not be clamped except under the unusual circumstance when digital pressure cannot effectively control bleeding.

PITFALL

IF BLEEDING VESSELS ARE CLAMPED DEEP IN THE NECK, THE CAROTID ARTERY MAY BE IRREVOCABLY DAMAGED AND PERMANENT BRAIN DAMAGE MAY ENSUE.

If a clamp must be applied because massive bleeding cannot be controlled in any other way, a vascular clamp should be used so that there is minimal damage to the vessel.

X-rays

Following emergency examination and resuscitative measures, the situation should be reviewed. Occasionally the patient's condition is such that urgent surgical exploration must supersede additional diagnostic efforts. Eighteen (8%) of 211 patients with penetrating neck injuries seen at Detroit General Hospital had to be rushed to the operating room before x-rays could be obtained because of severe persistent shock.

ROUTINE NECK AND CHEST FILMS. Routine diagnostic studies should include AP and lateral radiographs of the neck and chest. Retropharyngeal air or anterior displacement of the air-filled pharynx or trachea on the lateral film can be a particularly important finding and often indicates pharyngeal or esophageal injury. Interstitial emphysema or air in the fascial planes of the neck, however, is frequently misleading because air can also enter the neck along the tract of the injury (Table 1).

In 5 of 14 patients with interstitial emphysema in our recent study, no injuries to any major structures were found. On the other hand, many of the 43 patients with injuries to the pharynx, larynx, trachea or esophagus showed no air in the soft tissues.

GASTROGRAFIN SWALLOW. Contrast studies with Gastrografin should be performed if there is any suspicion of pharyngeal or esophageal injury; careful fluoroscopy dur-

---

TABLE 1.   SUBCUTANEOUS AND INTERSTITIAL EMPHYSEMA AND STRUCTURES INJURED

Subcutaneous & interstitial emphysema	Structures injured					
	None	Pleura	Pharynx	Esophagus	Trachea	Larynx
Present (14 patients)	5	3	3	2	2	1
Absent (43 patients)		12	8	10	10	6

Number of patients

ing this procedure may be required to locate the exact site of perforation.

PITFALL

IF A NORMAL GASTROGRAFIN STUDY IS RELIED ON TO RULE OUT INJURY TO THE PHARYNX OR ESOPHAGUS, IMPORTANT INJURIES TO THESE ORGANS WILL OFTEN BE OVERLOOKED.

False-negative results with this technique are so frequent that no assurances can be drawn from a negative Gastrografin swallow.

ANGIOGRAPHY. If there is a possibility of injury to the internal carotid artery, vertebral artery, or internal jugular vein near their cranial foramina, it is wise to obtain angiography to determine if a combined surgical-neurosurgical procedure may be required. Aortography may be employed where injury to structures at the root of the neck is suspected and the condition of the patient is stable enough to allow for this procedure.

Endoscopy

If the patient's condition is stable and the location and direction of the wound or the x-ray findings make one suspect an injury to the larynx, pharynx, trachea or esophagus, preoperative endoscopy is indicated. Obviously any impairment of the airway or voice is also an indication for direct or indirect laryngoscopy. In some instances, blood in the esophagus on esophagoscopy may be the only indication of an esophageal injury, especially if the perforation is below the thoracic inlet.

SURGICAL MANAGEMENT

Traditionally the management of penetrating injuries of the neck has been largely influenced by military surgeons who for centuries had treated most of these wounds nonsurgically, except for control of hemorrhage. As early as the Civil War, however, surgical exploration of neck wounds with accurate hemostasis, debridement and

drainage began to become the accepted practice.[1] Tracheostomy also gained increasing recognition as a lifesaving procedure for wounds of the larynx and upper trachea. Nevertheless, disagreement still exists among surgeons as to whether immediate exploration of all wounds of the neck that penetrate the platysma is indeed essential.[2-5]

Although it has been our stated policy that all wounds that penetrate the platysma should be explored, of 221 patients with such injuries seen from 1964-68, 43 were not explored because the surgeon felt the wound was directed posteriorly away from the major vessels, larynx, pharynx, trachea and esophagus. Of these 43 patients, two died from spinal cord injuries, which would not have benefited from surgery. Three other patients did, however, require subsequent surgical treatment, including incision and drainage of a neck abscess, repair of a pseudoaneurysm of the carotid artery and closure of an arteriovenous fistula. In 84 patients in whom no significant injury was found, there was little morbidity and no mortality. It is felt, however, that the improved hemostasis and debridement of damaged muscle following exploration in these cases probably resulted in better wound healing. Most of these patients were discharged from the hospital within 72 hours and showed no complications on follow-up examinations.

AXIOM

ALL WOUNDS IN THE ANTERIOR TRIANGLE OF THE NECK MUST BE EXPLORED.

The carotid arteries, internal jugular veins, larynx, trachea and esophagus are situated in the anterior triangle and center of the neck and are particularly susceptible to damage by any wound in this area. Injuries to these structures, moreover, are frequently found in patients with deceptively unimpressive skin wounds. Wounds in this area should always be explored as it is not possible to predict with accuracy the precise path taken by a knife or missile. Posterior wounds, on the other hand, may be observed with less danger. The surgeon who chooses to "observe" his patient must do so with the recognition of the hazards involved. The risk of missing a major injury is great, whereas there should be essentially no mortality and little morbidity from a negative exploration of the neck by competent surgeons in a well-equipped hospital.

PITFALL

IF THE NEED FOR SURGICAL EXPLORATION IS OBVIOUS, ELABORATE DIAGNOSTIC STUDIES MAY ONLY DELAY THE OPERATION AND INCREASE THE CHANCES OF SEVERE REBLEEDING.

Exploration of the neck, if indicated, should be performed as soon as possible and certainly within six hours from time of injury. In practice, however, there is not infrequently a time lag of many hours between the time of injury and the admission of the patient to the hospital. In addition, many of these patients are deeply intoxicated, making the risks of aspiration and intolerance to anesthesia significant. In these circumstances, close observation of the clinically stable patient with no evidence of vascular injury is often the desirable approach. If the patient has shown no deterioration after 24 hours, he will need operation only if a subsequent arteriovenous fistula develops. Where any doubt as to the integrity of the cervical vessels exists, arteriography may be helpful. If it is apparent that surgical exploration will be required regardless of what diagnostic studies may reveal, the diagnostic studies should usually not be performed.

Anesthesia

The surgeon should always be with the patient during induction and should be poised to provide hemostasis or perform a coniotomy or tracheostomy. Surgical explor-

ation is best performed under general endotracheal anesthesia with the head of the table slightly elevated. Intubation in conscious patients is generally discouraged because it may be extremely difficult, and any associated straining may reactivate bleeding which had previously been controlled. For the same reason it may be unwise to attempt to pass a nasogastric tube prior to the anesthetic.

There are some differing opinions about the value of elevation of the head during operation. We feel that slight elevation helps reduce blood loss from the neck wound. Others feel that this is unnecessary and may increase the chances of air embolism.

PITFALL

HIGH ELEVATION OF THE HEAD IN A HYPOVOLEMIC PATIENT WITH INJURED NECK VEINS INCREASES THE RISK OF AIR EMBOLISM.

While positive-pressure anesthesia will help prevent air embolism, it may also increase the chances of producing or increasing a pneumothorax if the lung has been punctured. The chest should, therefore, be examined carefully prior to and after induction. A pneumothorax may sometimes develop very gradually and this possibility should be considered strongly if the patient unexpectedly becomes hypotensive or develops increased resistance to ventilation.

Incisions

Proximal and distal control of the injured vessels is the keystone of the immediate surgical management of hemorrhage. The thoracic inlet provides potential difficulty because its anatomic relationships sometimes preclude easy access to the injured vessel. Valuable predictors of the probable need for intrathoracic exposure of the vessels include unequal radial pulses, a widened mediastinum, hemopneumothorax, and certain angiographic abnormalities. In most instances, the neck can be adequately explored through a standard incision along the anterior border of the sternocleidomastoid muscle. This approach provides excellent exposure to the major structures in the neck and can be easily extended transversely above the sternal notch (Fig. 2) or extended downward to join a midline sternal-splitting incision (Fig. 3). The operating surgeon should not hesitate to alter or extend his incision as necessary.

Low transcervical wounds and injury at the thoracic inlet can be particularly troublesome. Proximal control through the thorax is often essential to control exsanguinating hemorrhage from major vascular injury in this region. For most major vessels in the upper chest and thoracic inlet, a median sternotomy is the preferable surgical approach. If troublesome hemorrhage is encountered low in the neck, the bleeding should be controlled with direct digital compression while the sternum is split from below upward. This will provide ample exposure for proximal control of most major vessels in the area. Injury to the left subclavian artery near its take-off from the aorta is best approached through a high left lateral thoracotomy incision (Fig. 4). However, since the source of bleeding fol-

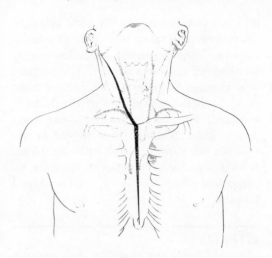

FIG. 3. The anterior sternocleidomastoid incision can easily be extended downward to join a sternal-splitting incision if the injury involves vessels in the upper anterior thorax.

lowing a gunshot wound of the neck is usually not apparent initially, this area can often be approached by extending the sternal-splitting incision along the left fourth intercostal space (Fig. 5).

Specific Injuries

VASCULAR. *Veins.* Major veins are the vessels most apt to be injured by penetrating neck wounds (Table 2). Ligation is the procedure of choice for injuries of the

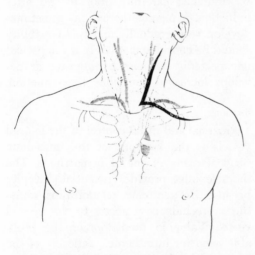

FIG. 2. The anterior sternocleidomastoid incision which provides excellent exposure to most structures in the anterior or lateral neck can be easily extended transversely above and across the clavicle to expose the distal portions of the subclavian vessels.

TABLE 2. ANATOMIC DISTRIBUTION OF INJURIES IN PENETRATING NECK WOUNDS

Vascular	68
Arteries ....(22)	
Veins ....(46)	
Neurological	24
Spinal cord .....(10)	
Peripheral	
nerve ....(14)	
Vertebrae	16
Pleura	15
Esophagus	12
Trachea	12
Pharynx	11
Larynx	7
Thyroid gland	7
Thoracic duct	2

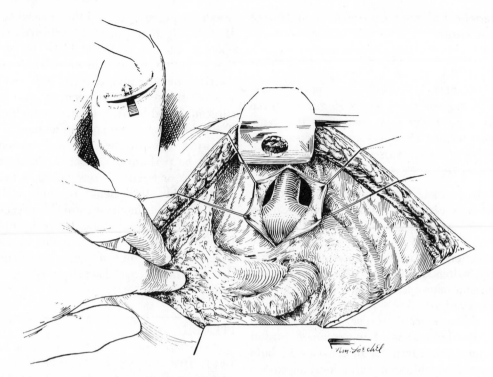

FIG. 4. If the injury involves the proximal portion of the left subclavian artery or the adjacent distal arch or descending portion of the thoracic aorta, a left lateral thoracotomy usually provides optimal exposure.

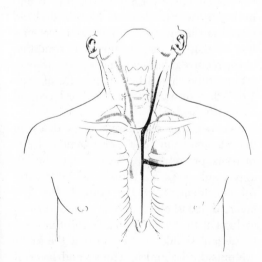

FIG. 5. If an injury to the proximal left subclavian artery or upper descending thoracic aorta is found after a sternal-splitting incision has been performed, that area may be exposed by extending the incision laterally along the fourth intercostal space.

smaller veins and for severe through-and-through perforations of the large veins. Simple lacerations of the internal jugular and subclavian veins, however, should be repaired. All venous holes should be covered as soon as they are exposed and then ligated or closed rapidly to reduce the chances of air embolism.

Arteries. The management of arterial injuries varies with the vessel involved. Arteries other than the common carotid, internal carotid, or subclavian arteries should be ligated. The vertebral artery when injured in its more inaccessible segments may be best occluded by the use of a silver clip. The use of internal shunts during surgical repair of the common or internal carotid arterial injuries remains controversial. They are often recommended but are usually unnecessary. In general, where collateral circulation is inadequate, the time lapse from injury to operation will have determined whether irreparable brain damage will ensue.

PITFALL

IF THERE IS A NEUROLOGIC DEFICIT, RES-TORATION OF BLOOD FLOW TO THE INVOLVED AREA OF BRAIN MAY COMPOUND THE CERE-BRAL INJURY BY INCREASING THE DISRUPTION OF THE INFARCTED TISSUE.

If a patient develops a neurologic defect from a cerebral infarct following carotid artery injury, repair of the vessel and restoration of blood flow will not improve function but may cause hemorrhage into the softened infarcted tissue. Under such circumstances it is preferable to ligate the involved vessel.

If the injury or surgery is in the region of the bifurcation of the common carotid artery, the adventitia of the carotid bulb should be infiltrated with a local anesthetic to prevent hypotension caused by reflexes originating in the pressor receptors in the carotid sinus. Atropine may also help to counteract hypotension from such vagal-mediated reflexes.

Once the carotid artery is exposed, the damaged area must be quickly repaired. If direct repair of the internal carotid will significantly reduce its lumen, a venous patch-graft should be used. If the internal carotid artery is severely damaged, the external carotid artery may be separated from its distal branches and anastomosed to the distal internal carotid artery. Injuries at the base of the skull present a special problem. If the patient is not bleeding excessively, an arteriogram should be performed. If the artery is found to be damaged, it should be repaired, ligated, or plugged. If the artery is not involved, the fascia and skin are sutured and pressure is maintained over the area.

In the patient who is bleeding excessively, immediate surgery is mandatory. Unfortunately, direct repair of the vessel in this area is rarely possible and ligation is usually required to control the hemorrhage. If distal ligation cannot be effected, the opening into the skull should be plugged tightly with wax, muscle or other sterile material and the area covered with tissue which is sutured over the opening. A neurosurgeon should be ready to do a craniotomy if the bleeding continues intracranially.

LARYNX AND TRACHEA. A tracheostomy should be performed as soon as injury to the larynx or trachea is recognized. Whenever possible, this should be done while ventilation is maintained through an endotracheal or coniotomy tube. However, time should not be wasted in attempting to pass an endotracheal tube if there is evidence that the trachea may have been disrupted by the injury.

PITFALL

PERSISTENT EFFORTS TO VENTILATE A PA-TIENT THROUGH AN ENDOTRACHEAL TUBE WHICH SEEMS TO BE PARTIALLY OBSTRUCTED MAY FORCE AIR INTO THE TISSUES OF THE NECK OR MEDASTINUM RATHER THAN INTO THE LUNGS.

With an airway established, the wound in the larynx or trachea can be debrided and closed in the operating room, with close attention paid to the location and condition of the recurrent laryngeal nerve. The tracheostomy tube should be retained for at least 5 to 7 days or until the tracheal or laryngeal wound is healed.

PHARYNX AND ESOPHAGUS. Any delay in debridement and repair of wounds of the pharynx or esophagus will almost invariably result in fistula formation. After careful debridement of the wound, the first layer of absorbable sutures should turn in at least 2 to 3 mm of viable full-thickness tissue and should be tied so that the knots are outside the lumen. The second layer of nonabsorbable sutures just reinforces the first layer. Soft rubber drains should then be left near, but not on, the site of repair to prevent accumulation of secretions and later abscess formation if there is any leak from the site of repair.

If a pharyngeal or esophageal injury is suspected but cannot be found at the time of surgery, the anesthetist can force air into the mouth with a tube or mask while the wound is filled with saline. Bubbles escaping from the wound can then readily disclose the exact site of injury.

NEUROLOGIC INJURIES

PITFALL

FAILURE TO DO A COMPLETE NEUROLOGIC EXAMINATION PRIOR TO EXPLORATION OF A PENETRATING NECK WOUND CAN EASILY LEAD TO MISSING IMPORTANT NERVE DAMAGE WHICH MIGHT LATER BE CONSIDERED TO BE OF IATROGENIC ORIGIN.

Brachial Plexus. It is extremely important to perform a complete neurologic examination as soon as possible after admission. This examination should systematically include the brachial plexus, phrenic nerves and cranial nerves. Damage to the cranial nerves in the neck is often overlooked unless gagging (IX), vocal cord function (X), shoulder shrugging (XI), and tongue motion (XII) are checked specifically. The sensory and motor function of the hand is especially important and each of the three main nerves (ulnar, median, and radial) must be checked separately. Although thorough exploration of all structures that could have been damaged is always indicated, those roots, trunks, branches, or cords which appear to have impaired function are inspected with extra care. In some instances contusion or pressure from a hematoma may temporarily impair function of a nerve, and conservative management, therefore, is warranted unless there is an obvious laceration.

Spinal Cord. Spinal cord injury is a frequent cause of death in patients with penetrating wounds of the neck (Table 3). Since

TABLE 3.   CAUSES OF DEATH (221 PATIENTS TREATED)

Spinal cord injury	5
Vascular injury	5
Cerebral infarct (3)	
Hemorrhage (2)	
Esophageal injury	2
Undetermined	1
Total	13 (6%)

many of these patients arrive with severe shock and are often poorly responsive, it may be difficult to perform a complete and accurate neurologic examination. In some instances the neurologic lesion may only be suspected from x-ray evidence of damage to the cervical vertebrae or a foreign body within or adjacent to the spinal cord.

The care of patients with neurologic injury is discussed in Chapter 14. Most of the patients with high spinal cord injuries die of respiratory failure. Consequently, as soon as such a lesion is recognized, a tracheostomy should be performed and the patient given ventilatory assistance.

Injuries to the thyroid gland itself are seldom a major problem; they are, however, often associated with injuries to the trachea or larynx. In controlling the bleeding from the thyroid gland with suture ligatures, one should be careful not to damage the recurrent laryngeal nerves which are closely associated with the branches of the inferior thyroid artery and the posterior surface of the thyroid gland.

THORACIC DUCT. In all instances of injury near the junction of the subclavian and internal jugular veins, any injuries of the thoracic duct or other major lymphatics should be identified and carefully ligated. Fistulae from such lymphatic wounds can be troublesome; however, most of these leaks eventually close spontaneously.

Wound Closure

Shotgun wounds with large areas of missing skin and muscle can be extremely difficult to treat. After careful debridement has been performed and complete hemostasis obtained, the main vessels and nerves are covered with muscle or fascia. Forty-eight hours later the dressing is changed in the operating room and, with adequate quantities of blood available for transfusions, further debridement is performed as needed. The wound is then covered with a dry dressing consisting of an inner layer of fine mesh gauze which is covered by multiple fluff dressings. If large vessels are exposed, porcine skin heterografts are applied and changed daily. Debridement, if necessary, and dressing changes are then performed daily until the wound is clean. Split-thickness skin grafts are then applied when the wound surface is healed. The patient is sent home. A knowledge of the skin flaps utilized to cover large defects in cancer surgery can be extremely valuable for later reconstruction of the neck. Some of the more useful flaps include laterally based deltopectoral flaps, flaps from the nape of the neck, and medially based chest flaps.

REFERENCES

1. Fogelman, M. J., and Stewart, R. D.: Penetrating wounds of the neck. Amer. J. Surg., 91:581, 1956.
2. Jones, R. F., et al.: Penetrating wounds of the neck; an analysis of 274 cases. J. Trauma, 7:228, 1967.
3. Shirkey, A. L., et al.: Surgical management of penetrating wounds of the neck. Arch. Surg., 86:955, 1963.
4. Stein, A., and Seaward, P. D.: Penetrating wounds of the neck. J. Trauma, 7:238, 1967.
5. Stone, H. H., and Callahan, G. S.: Soft tissue injuries of the neck. Surg. Gynec. Obstet., 117:745, 1963.

Suggested Reading

1. Boruchow, I. B., and Teachey, W.: Control of severe hemorrhage from stab wound of the neck: A case report. J. Trauma, 12:174, 1972.
2. Knightly, J. J., et al.: Management of penetrating wounds of the neck. Amer. J. Surg., 126:575, 1973.
3. Williams, J. W., and Sherman, R. T.: Penetrating wounds of the neck: Surgical management. J. Trauma, 13:435, 1973.

Section 2

TRAUMA TO THE LARYNX

J. McKENNA
H. J. JACOB

AXIOM

DELAY IN DIAGNOSIS OF LARYNGEAL INJURIES IS DANGEROUS.

Early diagnosis and treatment of any laryngeal injury are essential, regardless how minor the trauma or symptoms. The initial examining physician has a great responsibility in this regard. It is his high index of suspicion that is most apt to lead to early diagnosis and prompt treatment of this often overlooked injury. Too often it is not until the signs and symptoms of laryngeal fibrosis and stenosis set in that attention is directed to the injured larynx. Treatment begun at this late date will give results markedly inferior to those obtained following early treatment.

DIAGNOSIS

AXIOM

SEVERE LARYNGEAL INJURY MAY BE ASSOCI-
ATED WITH MINIMAL INITIAL SYMPTOMS.

The presenting signs and symptoms of laryngeal injury may be extremely deceptive and often correlate poorly with the severity of the damage. In some instances laryngeal edema gradually obstructing the airway may not become evident for up to 48 hours. It can, therefore, be extremely difficult to make an early diagnosis unless the examining physician has a high index of suspicion.

The most obvious evidence of laryngeal trauma is airway obstruction. The resulting signs and symptoms may range from minimal dyspnea to severe respiratory embarrassment requiring an immediate tracheostomy. Frequently, hematoma and swelling about the neck serve to direct attention to the possibility of a laryngeal injury; however, even when the larynx is severely fractured, with marked displacement of all laryngeal structures, there may be only minimal external evidence of injury. Patients with separation and malfunction of the vocal cords may show only minimal hoarseness, which may remain stable or progress rapidly to acute aphonia. Thus, the quality of the voice is not necessarily a good indication of the severity of the underlying laryngeal damage.

If an emergency tracheostomy is performed on a severely injured patient soon after his arrival in the emergency department, many of the signs and symptoms of laryngeal injury may be missed. When the physician suspects laryngeal damage, he should, if possible, perform a full laryngeal examination before the tracheostomy. If this is not done, subcutaneous emphysema may mistakenly be attributed to the tracheostomy rather than to the underlying laryngeal or tracheal damage. Later, when

attempting to decannulate the patient, destructive scarring of the larynx may make phonation and ventilation difficult or impossible.

AXIOM

IF THERE IS ANY DIFFICULTY WEANING A PA-
TIENT FROM HIS TRACHEOTOMY, A SEARCH
SHOULD BE MADE FOR UNDERLYING LARYNGEAL
DAMAGE.

Examination of the neck externally may reveal subcutaneous emphysema (often beginning in the anterior infrathyroid region of the neck), palpable laryngeal fractures, or loss of the normal external architecture of the larynx. The thyroid notch and prominence which are usually readily felt and identified in the male may not be palpable. In the female this area of the thyroid cartilage may be difficult to evaluate because the angle of the thyroid prominence is more obtuse. The loss of the cricoid prominence is a significant finding in either sex.

Special Studies

If there is any suspicion of injury to the larynx, it should be examined thoroughly by indirect mirror laryngoscopy, soft-tissue x-rays, and, if indicated, laryngograms and direct laryngoscopy.

INDIRECT MIRROR LARYNGOSCOPY. Specific features that should be looked for include: hemorrhage or hematoma formation, false passages, the position of the arytenoids, the size and shape of the laryngeal and tracheal lumen, and any exposed cartilage. Hematomas are most apt to involve the false cords, true cords, and aryepiglottic folds. False passages in short-necked individuals are more apt to be infraglottic, whereas long-necked patients tend to have supraglottic injuries. Ogura reports that he has never seen a supraglottic injury in a short-necked individual.[1] If the arytenoids are dislocated by blunt trauma, these are usually displaced posteriorly and superiorly.

When the larynx is disrupted, the lumen will usually seem to end abruptly. Exposed cartilage within the lumen is prima facie evidence of laryngeal fracture.

AXIOM

LARYNGEAL TRAUMA CAN CAUSE BILATERAL VOCAL CORD PARALYSIS WITHOUT OBVIOUS AN- ATOMIC EVIDENCE OF EXTERNAL OR INTERNAL DAMAGE.

The mobility of the vocal cords should be noted carefully whenever the larynx is examined. Bilateral cord paresis suggests a thyrocricoid disarticulation with either entrapment or avulsion of the recurrent laryngeal nerves. Unilateral cord paralysis often indicates a cricoid-arytenoid joint dislocation. If there is any abnormality of vocal cord function, the arytenoids and their location should be assessed carefully. If the arytenoids are not fractured and are in their normal position, the prognosis is excellent; over 95% of these patients will have spontaneous return of normal cord mobility.

SOFT-TISSUE X-RAYS. Soft-tissue x-rays of the neck and chest should be obtained on all patients with suspected laryngeal trauma. The laryngotracheal shadow should be evaluated along its entire length for any evidence of disruption. Interstitial emphysema along the fascial planes of the neck or mediastinum following blunt trauma is virtually diagnostic of a tear in the pharyngeal or laryngotracheal mucosa. In addition, these x-rays may reveal a fracture of either the thyroid, cricoid or hyoid cartilages, especially if these structures are calcified.

LARYNGOGRAMS. The use of laryngograms to diagnose laryngeal trauma has been controversial. Some feel that the extravasation of dye into the perilaryngeal tissues increases the possibility of infection and delayed wound healing. As Ogura has noted, however, extravasation of dye is an indication for immediate exploration of the neck and larynx. In his series of over 20 cases, there has been no evidence of increased infection or delayed healing following laryngograms.

DIRECT LARYNGOSCOPY AND BRONCHOSCOPY

PITFALL

IF DIRECT LARYNGOSCOPY IS PERFORMED ON A PATIENT WITH LARYNGEAL TRAUMA, IT MAY DISLOCATE FRACTURE FRAGMENTS OR CAUSE DAMAGE THAT MAY REQUIRE IMMEDIATE COR- RECTION.

These direct diagnostic techniques are indicated whenever a fracture of the larynx is suspected but not proven or ruled out by the above workup. The use of direct laryngoscopy and bronchoscopy, however, should be reserved for those physicians who are completely familiar with the techniques to be used and the injuries that may be encountered. The examiner should also be fully capable of proceeding with the immediate surgical reconstruction of the larynx.

Whenever possible, the laryngoscopy should be performed within three to four hours of the initial injury. If the patient's condition does not allow immediate examination, however, a waiting period of three to four days is advised to allow some of the edema and hematoma to subside.

At the time of direct laryngoscopy, the cervical esophagus, hypopharynx and endolarynx should be completely evaluated. The obvious presence of exposed cartilage, false passages, or other disruption of the normal endolaryngeal architecture demands open reduction and correction of the abnormality. The mobility of the cords can also be tested by having the anesthetist lighten the patient to the point of having the patient cough.

PITFALL

IF DIRECT LARYNGOSCOPY IS NOT PER-
FORMED WITHIN 12 TO 24 HOURS OF INJURY,
THE NORMAL LANDMARKS MAY BE OBSCURED
BY LARYNGEAL EDEMA AND HEMATOMAS
WHICH MAY BE GREATLY AGGRAVATED BY THE
PROCEDURE.

ETIOLOGY

Trauma to the larynx may be caused by
blunt external forces or internal manipulation at the time of endoscopy, tracheal intubation, or tracheostomy.

External Trauma

Today, with the increased use of seat
belts, external laryngeal trauma is more frequent. In a high-speed collision with sudden deceleration, the seat belt firmly an-
chors the passenger's pelvis to the back of
the seat while the upper body is propelled
forward with the neck in hyperextension
(Fig. 6). Upon impact with the dashboard,
the larynx is compressed against the cervical spine. In addition to the large hematomas and laryngeal fractures which may
occur with this trauma, the larynx may
tear away from the upper trachea as it is
displaced upward. Where shoulder straps
are worn they may constitute a hazard if

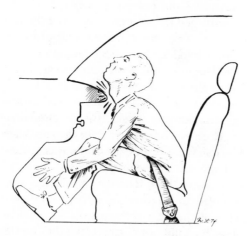

FIG. 6. In high-speed automobile collisions, the patient's hyperextended neck may strike the dashboard
with great force, causing severe laryngeal damage.

the patient slips under them, allowing the
straps to act as a direct shearing force on
the neck.

Internal Trauma

ENDOTRACHEAL INTUBATION. *During Insertion*

PITFALL

IF AN ENDOTRACHEAL TUBE IS TOO LARGE
OR IS INSERTED ROUGHLY, IT CAN CAUSE SEVERE
DAMAGE TO THE LARYNX OR TRACHEA.

A wide variety of laryngeal and tracheal
injuries may occur at the time of intubation. A tube which is too large may
damage the anterior commissure with subsequent anterior web formation. Where a
tube is manipulated excessively, the vocal
cords may become torn or ulcerated with
subsequent scar or nodule formation. If the
tube is inserted or pushed too vigorously,
it can cause arytenoid dislocation and post-
cricoid ulceration and scarring. Because of
the resultant scar and laryngeal web and
stricture formation, the patient may then
develop aphonia and progressive respiratory embarrassment.

Prolonged Intubation

AXIOM

ALTHOUGH ENDOTRACHEAL TUBES MAY BE
LIFESAVING, THEIR PROLONGED USE MAY DAM-
AGE THE LARYNX AND TRACHEA, ESPECIALLY
IF A HIGH-PRESSURE BALLOON CUFF IS USED.

Even if the initial intubation is completely atraumatic, prolonged endotracheal
intubation can cause severe mucosal and
cartilaginous changes with eventual stricture formation in the larynx and trachea.
This is especially apt to occur in the trachea
if the tube incorporates a high-pressure
balloon cuff which is inflated completely to

seal the airway for more effective ventilation with a respirator. We recommend strongly that the new tubes, with "soft," very compliant balloon cuffs which automatically avoid excessive pressure, be used. They cause much less damage to the trachea, especially if they are not completely inflated and a small amount of air is allowed to escape during expiration.

In his classic study, Bryce showed that mucosal changes may develop in the trachea within three hours after insertion of an endotracheal tube.[2] With more prolonged intubation, the superficial ulcerations extend into the underlying cartilage producing a perichondritis and subsequent chondromalacia. After removal of the endotracheal tube, the fibrosis and scar formation can cause progressive narrowing of the trachea with eventual stricture formation. Consequently it has been the policy of many physicians to avoid the use of endotracheal tubes for more than 48 to 72 hours. If more prolonged airway support is needed, a tracheotomy is performed.

Because their larynx and trachea are so much narrower than those of adults, children are much more prone to develop airway damage from endotracheal intubation. Foreign bodies are also a significant cause of laryngeal damage in the younger age groups.[3] In children over the age of 12 years, the incidence of external trauma to the larynx, usually from automobile accidents, baseball bats, and bicycle injuries, approaches that of the adult age group.

TRACHEOTOMY. The performance of a tracheotomy over an endotracheal tube makes the procedure much easier and safer, especially when there is established respiratory distress. Cardiac arrest all too often occurs while a tracheotomy is being performed on a struggling dyspneic patient. Under these conditions, the surgical procedure may be extremely difficult and prolonged; hemorrhage may be increased due to raised venous pressure and the patient is likely to become progressively hypoxic

and hyperactive. It is only rarely that a tracheotomy should have to be performed rapidly as an emergency; the prior insertion of an endotracheal tube through the nose, mouth, or cricothyroid membrane (coniotomy) usually allows adequate ventilation during the operation and often helps to define the tracheal anatomy, especially in children.

PITFALL

IF A TRACHEOTOMY IS NOT PERFORMED AS IF IT WERE A DELICATE, POTENTIALLY DANGEROUS MAJOR OPERATION, SEVERE AND OCCASIONALLY LETHAL COMPLICATIONS MAY BE CAUSED.

A tracheotomy, although often lifesaving, is not a simple harmless procedure. If done poorly, it may itself cause death or severe respiratory problems. Some of the more frequent immediate complications of tracheotomy include hemorrhage, pneumothorax, and inadequate ventilation during the procedure. Careful attention to hemostasis, restriction of the dissection to the immediate area of the second, third, and fourth rings of the trachea in the midline, and insertion of an endotracheal tube prior to the tracheotomy all help to reduce the incidence and severity of the complications.

Prolonged use of a tracheotomy tube produces many of the same tracheal problems as prolonged endotracheal intubation. The most frequent site of stricture formation in the trachea is the tracheotomy stoma itself. The next most frequent site is the middle of the trachea where the inflated cuff can cause pressure necrosis of the cartilages. The combined incidence of stenosis at these two sites in patients requiring ventilator support for more than two weeks has been reported to be as high as 20%.[4] The strictures at the tracheotomy stoma are generally triangular and can often be treated adequately by dilations or various plastic surgical procedures. Strictures at the cuff site, however, are often circumferential, respond poorly to dilations and frequently require segmental resection of the stricture and reanastomosis of the uninvolved trachea.

TYPES OF LARYNGEAL INJURIES

Vertical Midline Thyroid Fracture (Fig. 7)

This injury, generally due to a direct frontal blow to the larynx, is the most common laryngeal fracture, occurring in 81% of patients explored for laryngeal trauma in Middleton's series.[5] In about 50% of these patients, the epiglottis was displaced posteriorly with herniation of the periepiglottic contents into the larynx. In about 25% the cords were separated. It is significant that the mucosal tears were recognized in only about half these patients at the initial examination.

Avulsion of the Larynx from the Trachea (Fig. 8)

Avulsion of the larynx from the trachea occurred in 18% of patients explored for laryngeal trauma.[5] This injury occurs when the force of impact is directed in a posterior-superior direction. Since the airway is apt to be rapidly obstructed by this injury,

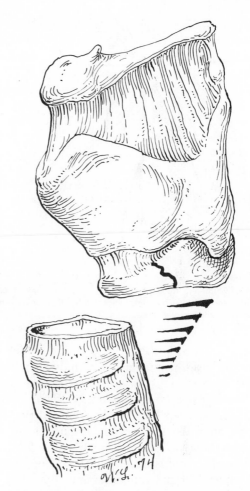

FIG. 8. The larynx may be avulsed from the trachea just below the cricoid cartilage by severe trauma to the lower neck, particularly if the force of impact is direct posteriorly and superiorly. In this instance, the cricoid cartilage is also fractured.

an immediate tracheostomy or coniotomy may be required.

Because of the position of the recurrent laryngeal nerves where these enter the larynx close to the cricothyroid articulation posteriorly, bilateral vocal cord paralysis may occur with the initial trauma or in the course of surgical attempts to deal with the injury.

Lateral Thyroid Ala Fracture (Fig. 9)

This fracture results from lateral forces against the thyroid cartilage and generally causes arytenoid dislocation with displace-

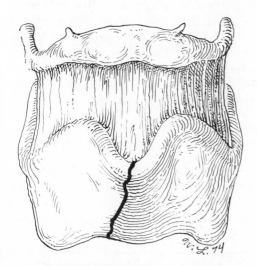

FIG. 7. A direct frontal blow to the larynx may cause a vertical midline fracture of the thyroid cartilage. This is the most frequent laryngeal fracture.

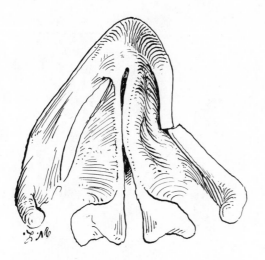 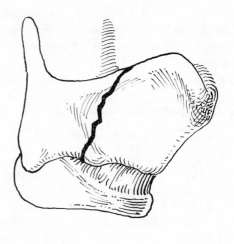

FIG. 9. Severe trauma to the side of the neck may result in fracture of the lateral thyroid ala. Occasionally these fragments will snap back into place, leaving little or no external evidence of the severe internal damage that may have occurred concurrently.

ment of the ipsilateral vocal cord which can be readily appreciated on indirect mirror laryngoscopy. On occasion, because of the resilience of the thyroid cartilage, the fragments snap back to their normal position after the force of the trauma is expended without any evident fracture; however, the vocal cord itself may still be dislocated. Without mirror examination, this injury might never be appreciated.

Soft-tissue Injuries

Hemorrhagic infiltration or hematoma of either the aryepiglottic folds, false cords or true cords may occur with or without associated fractures. The hallmarks of this injury are pain and tenderness in the area of the larynx and some airway obstruction; there is usually no hemoptysis or crepitation over the laryngeal cartilages, and vocal cord mobility seems to be normal in the absence of fracture or dislocation of the cartilage.

TREATMENT

Hematomas

In general, regardless of the type of laryngeal injury, the patient should be placed on steroids and penicillin or a broad-spectrum antibiotic. The dose of steroids should be the equivalent of 200 mg of hydrocortisone daily for an average adult male, with appropriate reduction in dosage for small children. In cases of pure hematoma with no fracture, humidification, steroids, and antibiotics are usually the only treatment needed. Good return of the laryngeal function in virtually all cases can be anticipated. If open reduction is needed to correct laryngeal abnormalities, a tracheotomy should be left in place postoperatively for at least three weeks and the antibiotics and steroids continued until the tracheotomy tube is removed.

Laryngeal Fractures

PITFALL

IF LARYNGEAL INJURIES ARE NOT CORRECTED WITHIN 7 TO 10 DAYS, THE RESULTANT SCARRING MAY MAKE CORRECTION EXTREMELY DIFFICULT AND RETURN OF FUNCTION INCOMPLETE.

Early diagnosis and treatment of laryngeal fractures can prevent most of the potential crippling sequelae and will usually provide a satisfactory voice, patent airway, and good protection of the lower respiratory system. Exploration and reduction of laryngeal fractures, however, should be undertaken only by those who are thoroughly familiar with the anatomy, physiology, and operative techniques required. In the recently fractured larynx the landmarks may be so distorted that even in the hands of the experienced laryngeal surgeon using the binocular microscope it may be difficult to identify definite residual normal laryngeal structures.

INDICATIONS FOR OPERATION. The main indications for immediate exploration and surgical correction of the traumatized larynx include:

1. exposed cartilage
2. false passages
3. obvious palpable fracture
4. loss of architectural landmarks
5. displacement of the arytenoid
6. posterior displacement of the epiglottis
7. presence of cervical or mediastinal emphysema.

SPECIFIC INJURIES. *Thyroid Cartilage Fractures.* Number 32 stainless-steel sutures are used to reapproximate large fragments into their normal position. If comminution of the fracture is present, an endolaryngeal stent is recommended for a period of approximately four to six weeks.

Arytenoid Dislocation. Unilateral arytenoid dislocation is treated by replacement of the arytenoid onto the cricoid articulation and stabilization with stainless-steel sutures or an endolaryngeal stent. However, if the arytenoid cartilage is badly dislocated with concomitant thyroid cartilage fracture, Ogura recommends a vertical hemilaryngectomy.[1] Using this technique, he reports satisfactory voice and lower airway protection in 48 of 150 patients with this injury.

Laryngotracheal Separation. In most instances of laryngotracheal separation, the cricoid cartilage must be resected and the trachea must be anastomosed directly to the thyroid cartilage. The disparity in size

of the trachea and thyroid cartilage, however, makes this a particularly delicate procedure. This is also a potentially hazardous operation because it may cause recurrent laryngeal nerve injury with vocal cord paralysis. If this does occur, a simultaneous unilateral or bilateral arytenoidectomy may be necessary. In the event that the cricoid cartilage can be spared, it is recommended that a T-tube stent or an endolaryngeal stent be left in place for approximately six weeks to prevent stenosis at the anastomotic site.

Epiglottic Displacement. If the epiglottis is displaced posteriorly, the base of the epiglottis may be amputated and sutured anteriorly to the remnant of the thyroid cartilage. In more severe epiglottic injuries with associated thyroid cartilage fractures, Ogura has found that a supraglottic laryngectomy often results in good return of voice and protective function of the larynx.[1]

Tracheal Fractures. The tracheal fracture site should generally be removed and an end-to-end primary anastomosis performed. The mucosa is sutured with absorbable material with the knots left extraluminally. This layer of sutures is usually sufficient to allow adequate healing, but stainless-steel retention sutures above and below the anastomosis may help by relieving tension on the suture line. All denuded areas of trachea must be covered either by means of mucosal flaps or split-thickness skin grafts. The use of split-thickness skin grafts, however, necessitates the use of a splint to prevent subsequent stenosis from scar formation. The neck is then sutured in flexion by means of a heavy silk stitch from the sternum to the chin.

Treatment in the Pediatric Age Group

PITFALL

IF RECONSTRUCTION OF LARYNGEAL INJURIES IN CHILDREN IS DELAYED, THE RESULTANT EXCESSIVE SCARRING MAY PREVENT NORMAL GROWTH OF THE LARYNX.

If it is impossible to perform an immediate repair in a child, it is Hollinger's recommendation that the stenotic areas be treated by dilatation and conservative treatment. Definitive repair should then be delayed until the conclusion of puberty, thus giving the larynx an opportunity to achieve maximal adult growth and maturity. Beyond puberty the treatment is the same as for adults.

CONCLUSION

Trauma to the larynx is becoming an increasingly frequent problem. It demands a high index of suspicion on the part of the examining physician so that prompt and proper treatment may be instituted to prevent the crippling sequelae of laryngeal and tracheal stenosis. Immediate open reduction of these fractures usually results in adequate laryngeal function with satisfactory voice and airway protection.

REFERENCES

1. Ogura, J. H., and Biller, H. F.: Reconstruction of the larynx following blunt trauma. Ann. Otol., 80:492, 1971.
2. Bryce, D. P.: The surgical management of laryngotracheal injury. J. Laryng., 85:547, 1972.
3. Hollinger, P. H., and Schield, J. A.: Pharyngeal, laryngeal, and tracheal injuries in the pediatric age group. Ann. Otol., 81:538, 1972.
4. Pearson, F. G., and Andrews, M. J.: Detection and management of tracheal stenosis following cuffed tube tracheostomy. Ann. Thorac. Surg., 12:359, 1971.
5. Middleton, P.: Traumatic laryngeal stenosis. Ann. Otol., 75:139, 1966.

Suggested Reading

1. Fitz-Hugh, G. S., Wallenborn, W. M., and McGovern, F.: Injuries of the larynx and cervical trauma. Ann. Otol., 71:419, 1962.
2. Pennington, C. L., Jr.: Glottic and supraglottic laryngeal injuries and stenosis from external trauma. Laryngoscope, 74:317, 1964.
3. Ogura, J. H., and Powers, W. E.: Functional restitution of traumatic stenosis of the larynx and pharynx. Laryngoscope, 74:1081, 1964.
4. Montgomery, W. W.: Surgical management of supraglottic and subglottic stenosis. Ann. Otol., 76:786, 1967.
5. Shumrick, D. A.: Trauma of the larynx. Arch. Otol., 86:691, 1967.
6. Miller, L. H.: Laryngo-tracheal trauma in combat casualties. Ann. Otol., 79:1088, 1970.
7. Harris, H. H., and Tobin, H. A.: Acute injuries of the larynx and trachea in 49 patients. Laryngoscope, 80:1376, 1970.
8. Polayes, I. M., and Kirchner, J. A.: Septal reconstruction of the human larynx. Trans. Amer. Acad. Ophthal. Otolaryng., 75:56, 1971.
9. Olson, N. R., and Miles, W. K.: Treatment of acute blocked laryngeal injuries. Ann. Otol., 80:704, 1971.
10. Pennington, C. L., Jr.: External trauma of the larynx and trachea. Immediate treatment and management. Ann. Otol., 81:546, 1972.

20 THORACIC INJURIES

R. F. WILSON
Z. STEIGER
D. HIRSCH
N. THOMS
A. ARBULU

Chest trauma is increasing as a cause of death in our society and accounts directly for over 25% of the 50,000 to 60,000 fatalities that result annually from automobile accidents.[1] Not only is the number of thoracic injuries increasing, but also the severity; more rapid transportation by better-trained ambulance personnel brings to the emergency room many critically injured patients who previously would have died before arriving at the hospital.

If treatment under such circumstances is to be successful, it must be applied vigorously and accurately according to procedures which have been formulated and practiced prior to their actual need. Important tools to have at hand in the emergency room for the management of these patients include laryngoscopes, endotracheal tubes, respirators, chest tubes and thoracentesis sets.

PITFALL

FAILURE TO OBTAIN A CHEST X-RAY SOON AFTER ADMISSION AND AGAIN WITHIN 4 TO 8 HOURS MAY RESULT IN SIGNIFICANT INTRATHORACIC INJURIES BEING OVERLOOKED.

The presence of a chest injury is often readily apparent from the history and physical examination; however, accurate assessment of the damage, especially to the intrathoracic organs, often requires serial chest x-rays (Fig. 1).

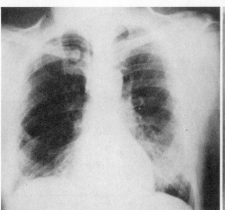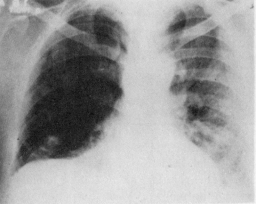

FIG. 1. Initial PA chest radiograph of a patient stabbed in the right anterior chest is shown on the left. Film taken four hours later shows a 20% pneumothorax.

SYMPTOMS

The most frequent symptoms of chest trauma are pain and shortness of breath. The pain is usually well localized to the involved area of the chest wall, but not infrequently it is referred to the abdomen, neck, shoulder, or arms. Dyspnea and tachypnea are important symptoms of lung and chest-wall damage but are often non-specific and may be caused by anxiety or pain from superficial and relatively mild injuries.

PHYSICAL EXAMINATION

PITFALL

EXCESSIVE RELIANCE ON CHEST X-RAYS MAY LEAD TO DIAGNOSTIC ERRORS.

Unfortunately, many physicians when confronted with a patient with chest trauma spend relatively little time on the physical examination. After a brief auscultation of the anterior chest, they may send the patient directly to the x-ray department. A thorough physical examination, however, can be performed rapidly and may provide valuable information to help confirm or rule out any equivocal findings on the x-rays.

Inspection

CHEST WALL

PITFALL

WITHOUT CAREFUL INSPECTION OF THE CHEST WALL, CONTUSIONS, FLAIL CHEST, INTRATHORACIC BLEEDING, AND OPEN OR "SUCKING" CHEST WOUNDS MAY BE OVERLOOKED.

In some patients a contusion may be the only external evidence of severe thoracic trauma. The paradoxical motion of a flail chest may be minimal when the patient is first seen, especially if it involves the lateral or posterior thorax. Although external bleeding is easily recognized, it may be difficult to determine if the source is intrathoracic or from the chest wall itself. Most chest wounds that communicate with the pleural cavity are readily apparent because of the noise made as the air passes through the tissue in the chest wall; some of these wounds, however, are open only intermittently and may be discovered only in retrospect.

NECK. Distended neck veins, especially when the patient is sitting upright, may indicate the presence of severe pericardial tamponade or congestive heart failure. If the face and neck are cyanotic and swollen, severe damage to the superior mediastinum with occlusion or compression of the superior vena cava should be suspected. Severe subcutaneous emphysema from a torn bronchus or laceration of the lung may cause much swelling of the neck and face, quickly obliterating landmarks and, in some instances, shutting the eyelids.

ABDOMEN. A scaphoid abdomen, particularly in infants, may indicate a diaphragmatic injury with herniation of abdominal contents into the chest. Excessive abdominal movement with respiration, especially in males, may indicate chest-wall damage that might not otherwise be apparent.

Palpation

Palpation should begin with determining if the trachea is in its normal position, which is in the midline or slightly to the right. Palpation of the chest wall may reveal areas of localized tenderness or crepitation from fractured ribs or subcutaneous emphysema.

PITFALL

A FRACTURED STERNUM CAN BE EASILY MISSED UNLESS THE STERNUM IS PALPATED CAREFULLY OR SPECIAL X-RAY VIEWS ARE OBTAINED.

Motion of a portion of the sternum or severe localized tenderness may be the only objective evidence of a fractured sternum. When a patient is coughing or straining, the physician can sometimes palpate abnormal motion of an unstable portion of the chest wall better than he can see it.

Percussion

Percussion of the chest wall is of great help in differentiating between hemothorax and pneumothorax. Dullness to percussion over one side of the chest following trauma may be the first and only evidence that a hemothorax is present; hyperresonance, on the other hand, may indicate the presence of a pneumothorax. If the pericardial cavity is greatly distended by an effusion or tamponade, the area of cardiac dullness may extend far beyond the midclavicular line on the left or the sternal border on the right. This sign is especially helpful if the point of maximal impulse is located more than an inch inside the left border of cardiac dullness.

Auscultation

Whenever possible, the chest should be auscultated systematically and thoroughly, anteriorly, laterally, and posteriorly at both the bases and apices. If the breath sounds are equal bilaterally, the upper airway, trachea, and major bronchi are probably intact. Decreased breath sounds on one side usually indicate the presence of hemothorax or pneumothorax, but occasionally may also occur with a foreign body or ruptured bronchus. The presence of bowel sounds high in the chest may be the first indication of a diaphragmatic injury.

TREATMENT

Most patients with chest injuries can be treated nonoperatively or at most by insertion of a chest tube connected to water-seal drainage, with or without suction. An emergency thoracotomy is occasionally needed, however, for release of cardiac tamponade, control of severe continuing bleeding or a massive air leak, or repair of the diaphragm or esophagus.

Acute Emergencies

The problems most apt to be rapidly fatal following chest trauma are: (1) inadequate ventilation, (2) massive bleeding, (3) cardiac tamponade, (4) rupture of the thoracic aorta.

INADEQUATE VENTILATION. Rapidly lethal ventilatory problems following chest trauma may be caused by: airway obstruction, open chest wounds, tension or severe pneumothorax, severe flail chest, or diaphragmatic injury or herniation.

Airway Obstruction. If the patient is making an effort to breathe, but there is little or no movement of air, an airway obstruction can be assumed to be present. The mouth and oropharynx must be rapidly cleared of any blood, dentures, or vomitus, using a finger and a large suction catheter. If the tongue tends to fall back and occlude the pharynx because of mandibular injury or severe intoxication, the chin should be pulled forward until an oral airway can be inserted. If the patient is still not breathing properly, a face mask and Ambu-bag should be used for ventilation until an endotracheal tube can be inserted or a coniotomy or tracheostomy performed. One must then listen carefully to both sides of the chest anteriorly, laterally and posteriorly to be sure that both lungs are being ventilated adequately.

Open ("Sucking") Chest Wounds. Small open chest wounds can act as one-way valves, allowing air to enter the pleural cavity during inspiration but preventing its exit during expiration. Thus, a progressively larger pneumothorax may develop with each breath, not only reducing the tidal volume and vital capacity but also interfering with venous return to the heart. Larger openings in the chest wall further reduce the effective tidal volume by allowing air to move in and out through the opening rather than the tracheobronchial tree. If the chest wall opening is larger than the trachea, effective ventilation of the lungs may cease.

Open or sucking wounds of the chest should be covered immediately by a sterile air-tight dressing such as Vaseline gauze. Since a pneumothorax almost invariably accompanies these wounds, a chest tube should also be inserted and connected to a water-seal and controlled (10 to 30 cm H_2O) suction or a Heimlich valve. If these are not available, a simple one-way valve may be constructed from a finger cot or the finger of a rubber glove by securing the open end to the end of the chest tube and incising it distally. Air is prevented from entering the chest during inspiration because the sides of the glove finger or finger cot collapse together as soon as the pleural cavity develops any negative pressure.

Pneumothorax. Collections of air or blood within the pleural cavity reduce vital capacity and raise intrathoracic pressure, thereby reducing the ventilation of the lung and venous return to the heart. During inspiration, the negative intrathoracic pressure increases the tendency for air or blood to leak into the pleural cavity through any

wound in the lung or chest wall; if there is any obstruction to the airway, or if the patient has obstructive lung disease, additional air may be forced into the pleural cavity during expiration, causing a tension pneumothorax (Fig. 2).

PITFALL

CARDIAC ARREST MAY OCCUR SUDDENLY AND RAPIDLY IF THERE IS ANY DELAY IN RELIEVING A SUSPECTED TENSION PNEUMOTHORAX IN A HYPOTENSIVE PATIENT. X-RAYS ARE NOT NEEDED BEFORE TREATMENT UNDER SUCH CIRCUMSTANCES.

If a tension pneumothorax is suspected because the patient is in severe respiratory distress and has decreased breath sounds and hyperresonance on one side of the chest, insertion of a large needle into the involved side can quickly confirm the diagnosis and offer some temporary relief until a chest tube can be inserted. Under such circumstances the delay involved in obtain-

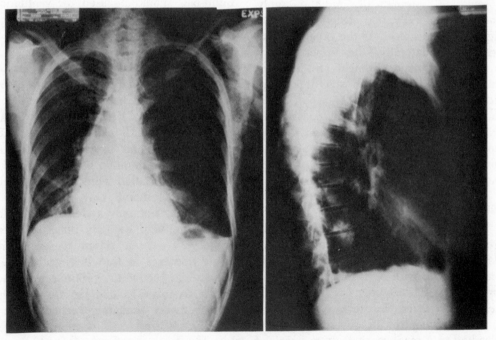

FIG. 2. PA and lateral chest radiographs show a tension pneumothorax with a small hemothorax indicated by the air-fluid level. Tension is recognized by a shift of the mediastinum away from the side of the pneumothorax.

ing a chest x-ray before treatment may be fatal. The catheter or chest tube is usually connected initially to simple water-seal drainage; if the air leak is large, 10 to 20 cm H_2O suction is added to the water seal. A high-flow system such as that provided by Emerson chest-suction machines generally works well for this purpose.

Although a small pneumothorax which is unchanged on two chest x-rays taken 4 to 6 hours apart in an otherwise healthy individual can usually be treated by observation alone, chest tubes or small catheters should probably be inserted as a precautionary measure; large 15- or 18-gauge intravenous catheters are easy to insert and when attached to a water seal or to suction can often remove the air very effectively.

PITFALL

INSERTING A CHEST TUBE WHILE THE PATIENT IS LYING FLAT INCREASES THE CHANCES OF INJURY TO THE DIAPHRAGM.

If at all possible, chest tubes should be inserted only while the patient is sitting upright. When the patient is lying down, the diaphragm may rise as high as the second or third intercostal space. At Detroit General Hospital, most chest tubes for relieving a hemothorax are inserted in the fifth intercostal space in the midaxillary line. If only a pneumothorax is present, the chest tube or I.V. catheter may alternatively be inserted in the second or third intercostal space in the midclavicular line.

The skin incision for the chest tube should be at least an inch below the interspace through which the tube will be placed; this oblique tunnel through the chest wall usually closes promptly, thereby reducing the chances of an air leak along the tube tract after the tube is removed. Once the tube has been inserted, the physician should ascertain that it is functioning properly and then secure it in position with heavy sutures and tape. The intrathoracic position of the chest tube and the amount of air or fluid remaining in the pleural cav-

ity should then be checked with an upright chest x-ray as soon as possible. While the patient is en route to the x-ray department the chest tube should *not* be clamped, because a continuing air leak can collapse the lung or cause a tension pneumothorax; however, when the tube is unclamped, the water-seal bottle should be kept 1 to 2 feet lower than the patient's chest.

Serial chest x-rays and careful recording of the amount of blood loss and the size of the air leak are important guides to the functioning of the chest tubes. If a chest tube becomes blocked and a significant pneumothorax or hemothorax is still present on the x-ray, the tube should be replaced; this can often be done very easily through the same hole that the previous chest tube occupied.

PITFALL

IF AN AIR LEAK AND PNEUMOTHORAX SPACE ARE ALLOWED TO PERSIST TOGETHER, THE PATIENT IS APT TO DEVELOP AN EMPYEMA OR BRONCHOPLEURAL FISTULA.

In general, patients can tolerate a small or moderate-sized pneumothorax space without complications as long as there is no continuing air leak. Likewise, an air leak will usually stop if the lung can be completely expanded. However, if a combination of pneumothorax space and continued air leak is not corrected within 24 to 48 hours, the incidence of empyema and bronchopleural fistula is greatly increased.

The most frequent reasons that a pneumothorax cannot be rapidly and completely evacuated are (1) improper position of the tubes, (2) an inadequate number of tubes, (3) an inadequate amount of suction, and (4) retained bronchial secretions. An air leak and pneumothorax space which persist in spite of several well-placed chest tubes attached to 20 to 30 cm H_2O suction are generally due to occlusion of bronchi with secretions, a large tear of the lung parenchyma or a leak from one of the larger bronchi. Under such circumstances, an emergency bronchoscopy should be performed to clear the bronchi and to identify any damage to the tracheobronchial tree, with particular attention directed to the origins of the main stem bronchi. In some instances, bronchograms may be needed to identify the site of the air leak. If a tear of a larger bronchus or the trachea is found, early repair is the treatment of choice. Conservative management of such injuries is seldom successful; furthermore, a delay of 48 to 72 hours or longer is associated with a greatly increased risk of infection, bronchial stenosis or breakdown of any repair.

After repairing the trachea or a major bronchus, it is important to prevent any accumulation of secretions distal to the suture line. Nasotracheal suctioning or bronchoscopy, preferably with a flexible fiberoptic bronchoscope, should be judiciously performed when necessary, taking care not to traumatize the anastomosis.

Flail Chest. If two or more adjacent ribs have segmental fractures (fractures at two or more sites on the same rib), the involved portion of chest wall may be so unstable that it will move paradoxically or opposite to the rest of the chest wall while the patient is breathing (Fig. 3). Thus, during inspiration the unstable or "flailing" segment will move inward while the rest of the chest wall is expanding; the opposite occurs during expiration. The flail chest may be especially severe if it is associated with a transverse fracture of the sternum. In general, because there is much less muscular support over the anterior and lateral chest, segmental fractures in these areas tend to cause a much more severe flail than similar injuries posteriorly. In addition, the posterior chest is supported by the bed or stretcher when the patient is lying on his back.

Pendeluft, a ventilatory phenomenon referring to movement of air from the lung on the side with the flail to the lung on the uninjured side during inspiration and vice versa during expiration, is not likely to be a problem unless there is partial obstruction of the upper airway (Fig. 4).

Immediately after the injury, while the lung compliance is still relatively normal, the pressure differential between the atmospheric and intrathoracic pressures may be so small that there is little or no apparent flail. Later, as lung compliance falls, more

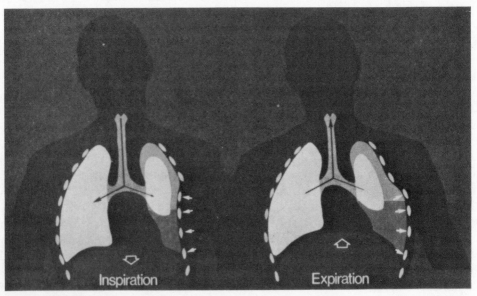

FIG. 3. The paradoxical notion of the left anterolateral chest in a patient with "flail chest" is shown. The area that flails moves paradoxically inward during inspiration and outward on expiration.

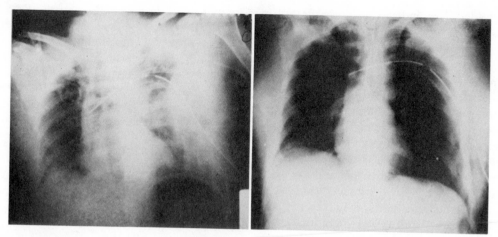

FIG. 4. "Pendeluft" is suggested by a PA radiograph of a patient with a large left anterolateral flail and an obstructed upper airway. The radiograph on the left shows that the left-sided flail falls inward as the air flows from the left lung into the right lung which has an intact hemithorax. The radiograph on the right shows that removing the airway obstruction decreased the left sides retraction and elevated "Pendeluft" (right). The gastric dilatation seen on the first radiograph has been relieved by a nasogastric tube.

pressure is needed to inflate the lungs. The differential between the intrathoracic and atmospheric pressures may then become large enough to overcome the resistance of the muscles attached to the fractured ribs, thereby allowing the involved chest wall to move paradoxically. Increasing bronchial secretions, by partially occluding the bronchi, will also increase the effort needed to ventilate. In addition, because of the decreased efficiency of ventilation and the increasing muscle effort, the patient may quickly become fatigued, beginning a vicious cycle of decreasing ventilation and increasing fatigue and oxygen needs.

A severe flail chest can be most quickly managed initially by applying a sandbag or pressure over the unstable portion of the chest wall. Although this reduces the vital capacity, it increases the efficiency of ventilation and the effective tidal volume.

PITFALL

IF A PATIENT WITH MULTIPLE INJURIES WHICH INCLUDE A FLAIL CHEST IS NOT GIVEN VENTILATORY ASSISTANCE WITH A RESPIRATOR SOON AFTER ADMISSION, HE IS APT TO DIE OF RESPIRATORY FAILURE.

In general, a patient with a flail chest should be given ventilatory assistance immediately if three or more of the following conditions or problems are present: shock, three or more associated injuries, severe head injury, previous pulmonary disease, fracture of eight or more ribs, or age greater than 65 years.[2] Such patients require assisted ventilation for at least 7 and usually 10 to 14 days before they can be weaned from the respirator. If respiratory failure is allowed to develop, treatment is extremely difficult; it is far easier to prevent respiratory failure with early ventilator assistance than it is to correct it later.

There appears to be a good correlation between physiologic shunting in the lungs, alveolar-arterial oxygen differences (A-aDO$_2$) on room air and early or impending respiratory insufficiency.[3] Where the need for respirator assistance is not clear, it is important to study the patient's blood gases at least every 12 to 24 hours. If the physiologic shunting in the lung exceeds 40% or is above 30% and rising, the patient should be put on a respirator. An A-aDO$_2$ on room air which is greater than 55 mm Hg or is above 45 mm Hg and rising should also be considered an indication for respirator assistance.

Diaphragmatic Damage. Since 60 to 80% of normal ventilation may depend upon proper function of the diaphragm, damage to this structure can cause serious respiratory problems. In addition, if the injury occurs on the left side away from the protection of the liver, the abdominal contents may herniate into the chest, compressing the lungs and mediastinum and reducing the vital capacity and venous return to the heart. If the opening is small, the negative intrathoracic pressure may gradually pull the intra-abdominal contents into the chest

through the diaphragmatic defect over a period of several weeks, months or years. In some respects, a diaphragmatic hernia is like a time bomb; even after having been stable for several years, it can suddenly enlarge, causing respiratory failure, shock due to an impaired venous return or strangulation of the herniated bowel.[4]

PITFALL

IF A DIAPHRAGMATIC INJURY IS NOT SUSPECTED AND LOOKED FOR IN ALL PATIENTS WITH CHEST TRAUMA, THE DIAGNOSIS WILL PROBABLY BE MISSED.

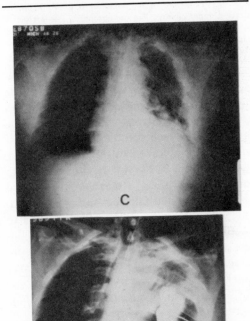

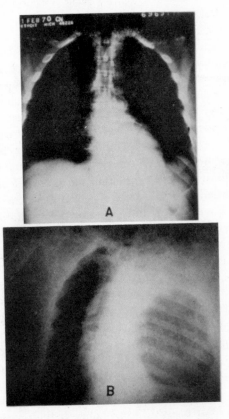

FIG. 5. A, B: A 56-year-old man, involved in a car accident, hit the steering wheel with his chest, and sustained a dislocated right hip. The initial x-ray of the chest (A), although not ideal because it was overpenetrated, was considered normal. The chest x-ray taken, unfortunately, with the patient in the supine position (B), was thought to show a tension hemopneumothorax on the left. C, D: A chest tube was inserted (C). The patient was somewhat relieved but gastric content came out of the tube. A Gastrografin injection through a Levin tube confirmed the diagnosis of a herniated stomach into the chest (D). The hernia was immediately repaired through a left thoracotomy. A tear in the tendinous portion of the diaphragm was found. The patient had an uneventful recovery.

The diagnosis of diaphragmatic injury is seldom made when the patient is first seen. The initial chest x-rays are generally non-specific (Fig. 5); however, this problem should be suspected if any abnormal shadows are noted in the left lower lung field, if the left diaphragmatic outline is unclear, or if the mediastinum is pushed to the right. Insertion of a nasogastric tube may confirm the diagnosis; if the end of the tube passes from the abdomen up into the left chest, it is apparent that the stomach has herniated through the diaphragm. Upper and lower gastrointestinal x-rays can also provide a definitive diagnosis by demonstrating loops of bowel within the chest.

Diaphragmatic injuries or herniations should be repaired as soon as the patient's condition allows. Many surgeons prefer to use the abdominal approach to the diaphragm, especially if there is a suspicion of concomitant intra-abdominal injury. If it is difficult to pull the bowel back from a chronic hernia into the peritoneal cavity, it may be helpful to slip a small catheter alongside the bowel into the hernia sac, thus allowing air to enter the sac and prevent the development of negative pressure as the bowel is reduced.

MASSIVE BLEEDING. *External Bleeding.* Bleeding from the chest wall may be quite heavy, especially if the wound transects several of the larger muscles. These external bleeding sites are usually easily controlled by direct pressure, direct clamping or suture ligatures.

PITFALL

IF IT IS ASSUMED THAT BLEEDING FROM THE CHEST WOUND IN A HYPOTENSIVE PATIENT IS SUPERFICIAL IN ORIGIN, THE DIAGNOSIS AND TREATMENT OF SEVERE INTRATHORACIC BLEEDING MAY BE DELAYED.

The physician should always suspect that bleeding from the chest may be intrathoracic in origin, especially if the blood wells or pulsates out with each breath or heart beat. Under these circumstances, pressure must be applied directly over the wound and the patient brought immediately to the operating room. Although preventing the escape of blood from the chest may cause a hemothorax or pericardial tamponade to increase, these problems are generally less serious than the hypovolemia that may rapidly develop if the bleeding continues unhindered.

Internal Bleeding. A hemothorax should be suspected following trauma if the breath sounds are reduced and the chest is dull to percussion on the involved side. Confirmation of the diagnosis and a more accurate estimation of the size of the hemothorax, however, depend upon x-ray examination. Fluid collections greater than 200 to 300 ml can usually be seen on good upright x-rays of the chest (Fig. 6). Occasionally, however, a large quantity of blood collecting between the lung and diaphragm may not be appreciated on a routine upright chest x-ray; the only abnormality noted under such circumstances may appear to be an elevation of the diaphragm. An x-ray taken with the patient in the decubitus position, however, may show a large quantity of fluid layering out against the dependent lateral chest wall.

PITFALL

REPEATED ATTEMPTS TO COMPLETELY ASPIRATE A SMALL HEMOTHORAX WITH A NEEDLE AND SYRINGE MAY CAUSE A PNEUMOTHORAX OR EMPYEMA.

A small hemothorax which is not increasing on serial x-rays does not have to be removed, but it should be carefully observed. In general, we have avoided needle aspiration of the smaller fluid collections and have relied primarily on chest tubes if drainage seemed indicated. On several occasions, repeated needle aspiration has resulted in a pneumothorax or infected hemothorax.

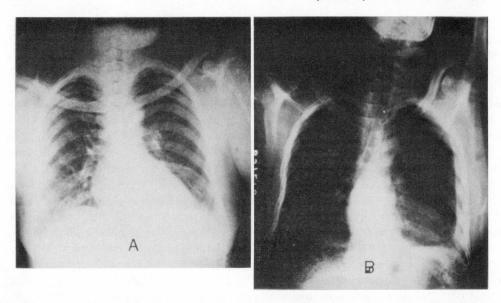

FIG. 6. The initial chest radiographs (A) of a patient who was stabbed in the left chest were considered normal even though the left diaphragm was slightly higher than normal and there was minimal blunting of the left costo-phrenic angle. The left lateral decubitus, however, confirms the presence of a significant hemothorax.

The ideal chest tubes for draining a hemothorax are 28 or 32 French rubber or Argyle plastic catheters. If the hemothorax persists and there is minimal chest-tube drainage, the chest tube is probably occluded or was inserted in the wrong position. Under these circumstances, the tube should be replaced or additional tubes should be inserted. If there is still minimal drainage, the hemothorax is probably partially clotted or loculated. If decubitus films of the chest show any fluid shift, some of the blood is unclotted and may be partially removed by a careful thoracentesis. This should not, however, be continued after more than two or three unsuccessful attempts.

If the hemothorax involves most of one pleural cavity and cannot be removed with chest-tube drainage, it may be wise to perform an early thoracotomy to remove the clots and control the bleeding site(s). A thoracotomy is also indicated if the hemothorax appears to be infected. In general, however, a stable hemothorax will gradually disappear spontaneously in 4 to 6 weeks.

Continued severe bleeding following a penetrating chest wound or rib fracture is generally due to damage to a systemic vessel, usually an intercostal artery. Bleeding into the pleural cavity from the lung parenchyma is generally limited by the lower intravascular pressure in the pulmonary circuit, the large concentrations of thromboplastin in the lungs and the tamponading effect of the hemothorax; however, in some patients, bleeding from the lung may be severe and extremely difficult to control. If the patient is hypotensive and rapid infusion of 2 to 3 liters of fluid and blood does not restore the blood pressure to normal, lacerations of larger arteries such as the internal mammary or branches of the aortic arch should be suspected. Under such circumstances, the patient should have an immediate thoracotomy to control the bleeding.

Occasionally, blood will drain out of the chest tube so rapidly that the patient appears to be exsanguinating. If the patient's respirations and vital signs improve while blood is being removed, the suction and drainage should be continued. However, if the patient's condition deteriorates, the patient may be bleeding from a large vessel which was temporarily tamponaded by the hemothorax. Under these circumstances, the chest tube should be clamped and the patient taken directly to surgery.

It should be stressed that most patients with intrathoracic bleeding can be treated quite adequately by administration of intravenous fluids and evacuation of the hemothorax with a chest tube; it is infrequent that a thoracotomy is required except for massive continuing hemorrhage. If the patient's vital signs are unstable, if the drainage of blood from the chest exceeds 200 ml per hour for 4 hours or longer, or if the hemothorax is increasing rapidly, a thoracotomy is generally indicated. Bleeding less than 200 ml per hour will usually subside spontaneously.

Ligation or repair of the injured vessels is the usual treatment for massive bleeding from any site; however, if a torn major pulmonary vessel cannot be repaired, the involved lobe or lobes should generally be removed. In a rare patient in extremely poor condition, ligation alone may have to be resorted to, especially if extensive pleural adhesions are present. Large bleeding lacerations of the lung parenchyma away from the hilum can sometimes be extremely difficult to manage. Where feasible, it is preferable to directly ligate or suture the larger bleeding points and bronchioles; however, in most instances, deep through-and-through sutures incorporating 1 to 2 cm of parenchyma on both sides of the laceration are needed to control the hemorrhage and air leaks. Unfortunately, large intrapulmonary hematomas may occasionally develop deep to such sutures. These hematomas usually resolve spontaneously, but occasionally they become infected and form lung abscesses. Bleeding and air leaks from superficial lung lacerations can usually be controlled quite readily with a continuous parenchymal suture.

In patients with penetrating chest wounds, use of high ventilatory pressures to inflate the lungs may force air from an injured bronchus into an open pulmonary vein, producing a systemic air embolus. This is probably more apt to occur if a large or tension pneumothorax is also present. Such a bronchovenous fistula may account for some of the severe arrhythmias and sudden deaths that occur soon after induction of a general anesthetic or use of a volume respirator in patients with severe penetrating chest wounds.

Later, when the patient is recovering, chest tubes can generally be removed 48 hours after the air leak stops and the drainage of fluid or blood from the chest falls to less than 100 ml per day. In most patients, any residual hemothorax will gradually disappear during the next few weeks. If after 4 to 6 weeks x-ray still shows a hemothorax involving more than half of one hemithorax, a thoracotomy should be performed to evacuate the hemothorax and decorticate the lung. During the decortication, great care must be taken to avoid causing any air leaks and to be certain that the lung can expand completely, especially on its basal surface. Occasionally, a relatively small hemothorax may trap a large portion of the lower lung, causing a persistent significant atelectasis. Where this is suspected, a bronchogram should be performed; if crowding of bronchi indicating a significant atelectasis is found, a decortication should be performed.

CARDIAC TAMPONADE. The rapid accumulation of blood or fluid in the pericardial cavity raises the filling pressure of the heart and may greatly reduce venous return and cardiac output. Any stab wound of the chest or upper abdomen between the mid-clavicular line on the right and the anterior axillary line on the left should be considered as a stab wound of the heart until proven otherwise. If there is any evidence of shock, tamponade, or severe hemothorax following such a wound, the patient should be brought immediately to the operating room. Management of cardiac injuries and tamponade is discussed in Chapter 21.

RUPTURE OF THE THORACIC AORTA. Approximately 80 to 90% of the patients with traumatic rupture of the thoracic aorta die within a few minutes of injury. Of the 10 to 20% who reach a hospital alive, approximately 30% die in six hours and 49% in 24 hours.[5] Unfortunately, although early diagnosis and repair are often successful, the diagnosis is usually not made until autopsy.

Diagnosis. Diagnosis of traumatic rupture of the thoracic aorta depends upon a high index of suspicion. Although great force is usually needed to tear the aorta, about a third of these patients have little or no external evidence of chest trauma. Furthermore, most of them have multiple severe extrathoracic injuries which tend to distract the physician. Consequently, if this problem is to be diagnosed early, it must be suspected in all patients who have had severe chest trauma or have been in automobile accidents at speeds exceeding 45 miles per hour.

Findings which suggest the diagnosis of traumatic rupture of the aorta include: (1) a systolic murmur over the precordium or on the back, medial to the left scapula, (2) hoarseness because of pressure of the hematoma on the left recurrent laryngeal nerve, (3) hypertension in the upper extremities, or (4) hypotension or weak pulses in the lower extremities. In the rare instances in which the injury involves the ascending aorta, the resulting aneurysm or hematoma may produce a clinical picture of superior vena caval obstruction.

Although the circumstances of the accident and the physical findings are occa-

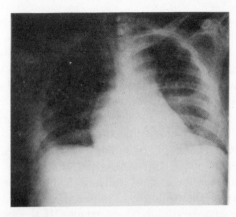

FIG. 7. This 23-year-old male was a passenger in a severe two-car auto collision. On chest x-ray the superior mediastinum was widened, particularly near the aortic knob, and there is a slight haziness over the left chest suggesting mild contusion of the lung in that area. The heart may appear widened because the x-ray was taken in an anterior-posterior direction, or because of myocardial contusion.

sionally helpful, the diagnosis is usually made or suspected from findings on the routine chest x-ray. Since over 90% of these injuries involve the aorta near the attachment of the ligamentum arteriosum, the characteristic x-ray finding is widening of the superior mediastinum adjacent to the aortic knob (Fig. 7). Occasionally, downward displacement of the left main stem bronchus will also be noted. A left hemothorax is present in many of these patients and helps to draw attention to this area. Unfortunately, the mediastinal widening may not be apparent on the chest x-rays of some patients for several hours or days.[6] Consequently, serial chest x-rays should be taken in any patient with severe chest trauma at 4- to 8-hour intervals during the first day and then daily for at least the next three days.

Once the diagnosis is suspected because of physical findings or the chest x-ray, the physician is forced to provide rapid answers to a series of crucial questions. Should the patient have an aortogram? What is the quickest way to obtain a reliable aortogram? Is the patient's condition such that he can tolerate the delay inherent in an aortogram? Can the patient tolerate a thoracotomy at this time? Is there an advantage to waiting until his condition improves? How long can one safely wait? Will cardiopulmonary bypass be needed? How rapidly can it be set up?

Aortography. In general whenever the diagnosis of rupture of the thoracic aorta is suspected, aortography should be performed, using either a percutaneous right axillary or retrograde femoral arterial approach (Fig. 8). If it is difficult to obtain arterial aortograms, intravenous or forward aortograms using two large catheters in the superior vena cava can sometimes provide good visualization of the thoracic aorta and may be safer to perform.

PITFALL

FAILURE TO OBTAIN AN AORTOGRAM WHEN THERE IS SUPERIOR MEDIASTINAL WIDENING FOLLOWING BLUNT CHEST TRAUMA MAY RESULT IN AN INACCURATE DIAGNOSIS AND AN UNNECESSARY THORACOTOMY.

There is some question as to whether aortography should be performed on all patients with suspected aortic injury, especially if the patient is in shock or has a rapidly expanding mediastinal hematoma. Under these circumstances, the delay of surgery by the aortography may be lethal. Other concerns have been the possibility that the catheter used or the pressure of the injection of the contrast material might tear the remaining adventitia at the site of aortic injury; however, no catheter trauma to the damaged area has been reported, and the pressure of the injection is dissipated rapidly. Furthermore, we have had several instances in which mediastinal widening was not associated with aortic injury and a thoracotomy in these critically injured patients might have been lethal.[6] As a consequence, unless the hematoma is expanding rapidly or the patient remains hypotensive in spite of liberal fluid and blood replacement, we insist on an aortogram to provide a precise diagnosis.

Treatment. EXPECTANT. The main fac-

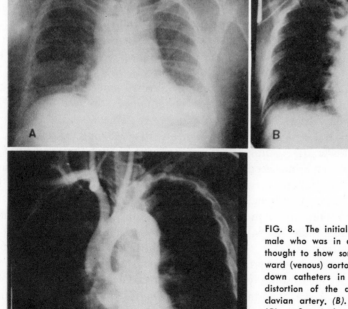

FIG. 8. The initial chest x-ray (A) on a 38-year-old male who was in a severe automobile accident was thought to show some mediastinal widening. The forward (venous) aortogram through bilateral venous cutdown catheters in the arms showed widening and distortion of the aorta just distal to the left subclavian artery. (B). A retrograde femoral aortogram (C) confirmed the presence of a ruptured thoracic aorta which was corrected surgically.

tors affecting the chances of successful management of a rupture of the thoracic aorta are the number and severity of the associated injuries. The judgment as to whether to attempt immediate repair of the thoracic aorta in the poor-risk patient with multiple injuries is difficult and must be individualized. A period of careful preoperative preparation may greatly reduce the risk of surgery; in addition, the longer the injury has been present the less likely it is to rupture suddenly. Keeping this in mind, it may be preferable, in very poor-risk patients with multiple severe injuries, to observe them carefully, in or adjacent to the operating room, until the risk of surgery is reasonable.

SURGERY WITHOUT CARDIOPULMONARY BYPASS. On occasion a patient will require surgery immediately before cardiopulmonary bypass can be set up, because of a rapidly expanding hematoma or evidence of continuing blood loss into the left chest. Under such circumstances, intravenous Arfonad is infused into the upper portion of the body while the aorta is clamped. The surgery, however, must be rapid and precise because clamping of the descending aorta for more than 20 minutes without perfusion of the distal aorta invites serious risk of spinal-cord and abdominal visceral damage.

Another alternative is to bypass the area of the aortic injury with special tubing or a graft. The proximal end of the tubing can be inserted in the ascending aorta or the aortic arch, and the distal end can be inserted in the middle or lower descending thoracic aorta. If special heparin-coated polyvinyl tubing is used, the patient does not have to be exposed to the additional risks of systemic heparinization; this consideration is especially important in patients with severe head injuries.

SURGERY WITH CARDIOPULMONARY BYPASS. Cardiopulmonary bypass is not absolutely essential for repair of the thoracic aorta distal to the arch, but it does allow increased time for a meticulous unhurried re-

pair and does reduce the risk of ischemic damage to the spinal cord and abdominal viscera. If the patient's condition is stable, transfer to a hospital where cardiopulmonary bypass is available appears to be wise.

Traumatic Aneurysms. Traumatic aneurysms of the thoracic aorta which are first noticed several weeks or months after the initial trauma are usually stable. However, even if they remain unchanged for several years, they always retain the potential for suddenly increasing in size and rupturing fatally.

Once the diagnosis is confirmed by aortography, the aneurysm should be excised and the normal ends of aorta anastomosed with a graft under left-atrial-femoral or femoral-artery femoral-vein cardiopulmonary bypass.

Less Urgent Problems

Some of the more frequent but less urgent problems following chest trauma include: (1) soft-tissue injuries, (2) subcutaneous emphysema, (3) fractured ribs, (4) pulmonary contusion and hematomas, (5) esophageal injury, and (6) thoracic-duct injury.

SOFT-TISSUE INJURIES OF THE CHEST WALL. Probing of penetrating chest wounds is seldom done, but if done carefully may occasionally provide useful information on their depth and direction. If the wound can be thoroughly cleaned and complete hemostasis can be obtained, the wound may be closed in layers; otherwise the skin and subcutaneous tissue should be left open.

Injuries caused by high-powered rifles or shotguns at close range may destroy such large quantities of tissue that it may be extremely difficult to close and stabilize the chest wall. All such open "sucking" chest wounds must be immediately covered or closed. In many patients, ventilatory support through an endotracheal tube may also be required. Chest tubes must also be inserted to control the air leak that may continue for several days.

Some large chest-wall defects are extremely difficult to manage. Because of the anticipated problems with closure, the surgeon is often too conservative in his initial debridement, thereby greatly increasing the risk of infection and breakdown at the suture lines. With some of the larger defects, it may be necessary to rotate muscle flaps into the wound. If the muscle flap which is developed for closing the defect is too large or narrow, the edges may become ischemic with similar results. These muscle flaps heal better and are less apt to flail if properly supported either by Marlex mesh or a latticework of pericostal nonabsorbable sutures. Even if there is little or no flail, it is wise to support the patient's ventilation with a respirator for 10 to 14 days or longer. Although any prosthetic material used in these wounds can become infected, it will usually continue to provide some support until the chest and abdominal wall are healed. In some instances, the infection can be handled by local drainage and irrigation with antibiotic solutions without removing the prosthetic material.

SUBCUTANEOUS EMPHYSEMA. Severe progressive subcutaneous emphysema develops when air from an injured lung or one of the major bronchi gains access to the chest wall through an opening in the parietal pleura. The air may also reach the chest wall by dissecting along the pulmonary vessels or bronchi back into the hilum and mediastinum and then into the extrapleural spaces. During inflation with a respirator or positive expiration, air continues to be forced between the layers of the chest wall, especially between the subcutaneous tissue and the muscles. Occasionally the swelling from the subcutaneous emphysema can reach massive proportions, extending up to the eyelids, which may be swollen shut, and down to the scrotum, which may become several times normal size. Although the patient's appearance may seem very serious, and he may have moderate to severe discomfort, the subcutaneous emphysema itself does not cause any significant ventilatory or hemodynamic problem un-

less there is an associated pneumothorax. Even if a pneumothorax is not apparent on x-ray, a chest tube should be inserted on the injured side because of the problems of accurately evaluating the chest under these circumstances. However, a major bronchial injury must be suspected in all patients with severe or rapidly expanding subcutaneous emphysema; bronchoscopy and bronchography under such circumstances are usually diagnostic. If a tear in a major bronchus is identified, it should be repaired surgically as soon as possible.

Once the initiating cause is controlled, the swelling usually disappears gradually over a period of several days. If there is any respiratory difficulty, a tracheostomy serves to maintain adequate ventilation and also allows a route for the air to escape from the subcutaneous tissue. It would appear wise, nevertheless, to give antibiotics to these patients.

FRACTURED RIBS. Fractured ribs, even if they do not damage the underlying lung tissue or cause a hemopneumothorax, can greatly interfere with ventilation because of the pain produced by motion of the fracture fragments. The adjacent muscles, in an effort to splint that portion of the chest wall, may develop severe spasm which causes additional pain. If the patient cannot ventilate properly because of the chest pain, atelectasis will often develop and progress to severe pneumonitis.

Strapping the chest with adhesive tape may be effective in young athletic individuals, but in less vigorous patients may significantly reduce ventilation to the underlying lung. If some sort of external support is indicated, rib belts are much more pleasant to use; they do not blister the skin, and the patient can adjust them as needed. Mild to moderate chest-wall pain is best treated by 0.5 to 1.0 grains of codeine every 3 to 4 hours; this will relieve the pain but will usually not interfere with the patient's ventilation or ability to cough. More severe pain from multiple rib fractures is best controlled with intercostal nerve blocks, injecting 1 to 2 ml of 0.5 to 1.0% Xylocaine with epinephrine around the intercostal nerves at the lower borders of the involved ribs in the midscapular line. In many instances, to achieve adequate relief of pain, the intercostal block must include two intercostal nerves above and two below the injured ribs. This will usually produce dramatic relief from pain for several hours. Since it is easy to puncture the lung accidentally while performing an intercostal block, it is wise to obtain a chest x-ray after the procedure to be sure the patient has not developed pneumothorax.

PITFALL

HYPOTENSION FOLLOWING BLUNT CHEST TRAUMA IS FREQUENTLY DUE TO INTRA-ABDOMINAL BLEEDING.

If the patient with fractured ribs following blunt trauma becomes hypotensive and does not have a large hemothorax or pneumothorax, it should be strongly suspected that he has intra-abdominal bleeding.[7] In general, it is wise to admit any patient with two or more fractured ribs to the hospital for at least 24 to 48 hours, especially if the ninth, tenth, or eleventh ribs are involved. This will usually provide ample time to observe the patient for additional injuries that might not be apparent initially; it also allows the physician more time to determine what measures must be taken to provide adequate ventilation and pain relief for the patient.

PULMONARY CONTUSION AND HEMATOMAS. Blunt or penetrating trauma to the lung characteristically causes an accumulation of blood and edema fluid in the involved interstitial tissue, alveoli, and small bronchi. The reduced vital capacity and pulmonary compliance, together with increased secretions from the injured lung, tend to cause an increasing atelectasis. This combination of atelectasis, disrupted tissue and extravasated blood and plasma provides an ideal site for severe pneumonitis and eventual abscess formation.

Treatment includes maintenance of ventilation to all parts of the lung and prophylactic antibiotics. If the patient becomes septic and an abscess develops, resection of the involved tissue may be indicated, especially if it responds poorly to intensive antibiotic therapy and repeated bronchoscopy.

Recently, questions have been raised as to the preferred initial management of large pulmonary hematomas following gunshot wounds of the chest. If there is no reason to perform a thoracotomy, these should be treated conservatively; however, if a thoracotomy is required for some other reason, some members of our staff now feel that, because of the high incidence of severe persistent infection in these hematomas, the involved lobe should be resected. Further evaluation of this approach is required.

ESOPHAGEAL INJURY. If esophageal injury is suspected, an esophagogram with a water-soluble radiopaque material (Gastrografin) or barium should be performed. Unless the fluoroscopy is done very carefully, however, the exact site of perforation may be missed. The esophagogram is performed before esophagoscopy to warn the endoscopist of any unusual injury, constriction, or anomaly that may be present.

PITFALL

DELAY IN CLOSURE OR DRAINAGE OF ESOPHAGEAL INJURIES RESULTS IN A HIGH MORBIDITY AND MORTALITY; HENCE, EARLY DIAGNOSIS AND TREATMENT ARE VITAL.

Ideally, esophageal perforations should be repaired primarily within 6 to 12 hours of injury; however, the ability to do this is dependent on early diagnosis. If treatment is delayed beyond 24 hours, a primary closure is not advisable because the local edema, tissue necrosis and infection make secure suturing and primary healing unlikely. In the distal esophagus, a Thal gastric fundic patch may help protect the anastomosis.[8] Whether or not a repair is attempted, drainage of the stomach, preferably with a gastrostomy tube, and the adjacent mediastinum is extremely important and may be necessary for several weeks or longer. Massive antibiotics should be given in all cases.

The esophagus can also be injured by foreign bodies which perforate the wall at the time of swallowing or which may, if left in situ, cause deep ulcerations with later perforation. Impacted meat can be removed endoscopically, or it can, occasionally, be dissolved with papain or similar enzymes.

THORACIC-DUCT INJURY. Although the thoracic duct is seldom damaged by the initial trauma itself, there is a significant risk of injury by the surgeon if he is forced to perform extensive dissection in the posterior mediastinum. If the leakage from the injured thoracic duct is watery, it is not likely to be recognized at the time of injury. Many of these injuries are diagnosed later when the patient develops a chylothorax.

Many thoracic-duct injuries will close spontaneously, but, if the leak is large and persistent, surgery may be required. Unfortunately, it is usually extremely difficult to identify the torn ends at the time of surgery. Occasionally, however, lymphangiograms preoperatively may help to locate the site of the injury. At surgery, the duct injury can occasionally be visualized after running normal saline solution subcutaneously into both thighs. After a few minutes, a trickle of fluid may be seen at the site of the injured duct. Injection of dyes usually discolors the operative area very quickly and makes it difficult to identify the duct.

General Measures

Some of the general measures and drugs which are important in the management of thoracic injuries include: 1) tracheobronchial toilet, (2) oxygen, (3) bronchodilators, (4) inhalation therapy, (5) ventilators, (6) fluid therapy, (7) digitalis, (8) diuretics, (9) nasogastric suction, (10) antibiotics, and (11) steroids.

TRACHEOBRONCHIAL TOILET. The early establishment of an airway in the patient with chest trauma is only the initial skirmish in a long-drawn-out battle to keep the tracheobronchial tree open and clear. The patient can help himself immensely in this regard if he is able and willing to breathe deeply and to cough. However, if the patient cannot adequately handle his secretions, the judicious use of nasotracheal catheter suctioning and bronchoscopy, especially with the new flexible fiberoptic models, is indicated (Chap. 31).

OXYGEN. Because the function of the lungs is impaired by most types of trauma and the oxygen requirements are increased, it is important to supply enough oxygen to keep the arterial Po_2 above 60 mm Hg and preferably at 80 to 100 mm Hg. If at all possible, however, the inhaled oxygen concentration should be kept below 40%; use of higher concentrations for more than 48 to 72 hours may cause additional damage to the lungs.

BRONCHODILATORS. Bronchodilators are used if there is any evidence of bronchospasm. Aminophylline and isoproterenol are the most frequent choices (Chap. 31).

INHALATION THERAPY. After the patient's initial respiratory problems have been corrected, he can be assisted in his efforts to ventilate deeply, cough and bring up secretions by judicious inhalation therapy, using intermittent positive pressure breathing (IPPB) and nebulizers. The IPPB can help the patient cough and propel various drugs into the tracheobronchial tree to produce bronchodilation or liquefy thick secretions. Nebulizers that provide droplets of water less than 5 microns in diameter can moisten the tracheobronchial tree down to the level of the respiratory bronchioles (Chap. 31).

VENTILATOR ASSISTANCE

PITFALL

ANY DELAY IN PROVIDING ADEQUATE VENTILATORY SUPPORT GREATLY INCREASES THE RISK OF IRREVERSIBLE RESPIRATORY FAILURE.

If there is any question about the adequacy of the patient's ventilation after the airway has been opened and the pleural cavities have been emptied of any collections of air or blood, an endotracheal or tracheostomy tube should be inserted and the patient placed on a ventilator. The tidal volume should generally be maintained at 10 to 15 ml/kg and enough oxygen should be given to maintain a Po_2 of 80 to 100 mm Hg (Chap. 31).

FLUID THERAPY

PITFALL

EXCESSIVE ADMINISTRATION OF CRYSTALLOIDS GREATLY INCREASES THE RISK OF RESPIRATORY FAILURE.

While excessive administration of crystalloids may produce pulmonary edema in any patient, those with pulmonary contusions are at special risk. Even minimal overloading with crystalloids can increase pulmonary capillary congestion, interstitial edema, and intra-alveolar fluid. During the initial resuscitation, the CVP response should be checked frequently and the lungs auscultated at the bases for any evidence of fluid overload. At least a fourth of all the fluids given to the patient should be either blood or colloidal solutions, such as albumin or plasma. While many physicians are content to keep the hemoglobin above 10.0 gm/100 ml, we believe that there is an advantage in keeping the hemoglobin at 12.5 to 14.0 gm/100 ml and the serum albumin above 2.5 gm/100 ml.

DIGITALIS. Digitalis preparations are used if there is any evidence of congestive heart failure, if the CVP seems inappropriately high, if rales develop bilaterally, or if the patient maintains a tachycardia above 130/min. Many elderly patients with arrhythmias, except atrioventricular block, bradycardia, or premature ventricular contractions, can benefit from digitalis (Chap. 32).

DIURETICS. If the patient appears to be developing respiratory failure and oliguria simultaneously, the judicious use of fluids and diuretics is extremely important. Whereas fluid restriction may be important in the treatment of pulmonary congestion and respiratory failure, it can also cause oliguria and renal failure in critically injured patients. On the other hand, increased use of fluids, especially crystalloids, may improve the urine output, but will also tend to increase pulmonary congestion. However, use of small amounts of diuretics, to maintain a urine output greater than 50 ml per hour in spite of mild fluid restriction, may help solve this problem (Chap. 30).

MEMBRANE OXYGENATORS. Persistent hypoxia (Po_2 less than 40 to 50 mm Hg) in spite of maximal ventilatory support, aggressive dehydration, and 100% oxygen may be an indication for partial extracorporeal venoarterial bypass using a membrane oxygenator. The membrane oxygenator may not only increase the arterial oxygen content but may also improve the patient's lungs by reducing the pulmonary artery flow and congestion.[9]

NASOGASTRIC SUCTION

PITFALL

FAILURE TO EMPTY THE STOMACH WITH A TUBE SOON AFTER CHEST TRAUMA GREATLY INCREASES THE RISK OF ASPIRATION AND SEVERE ILEUS.

A large number of patients with chest trauma will vomit and aspirate gastric contents or will develop ileus later because of associated abdominal injuries or as a nonspecific response to severe trauma. Not infrequently, aerophagia due to dyspnea and nervousness further increases the gastrointestinal distension.

Early emptying of the stomach with a nasogastric tube reduces the chances of aspiration and also decreases the tendency for the stomach and intestine to distend and press upward against the diaphragm. Once severe ileus has developed, it can seriously interfere with ventilation and is extremely difficult to correct (Chap. 33).

ANTIBIOTICS. When the thoracic injury warrants a chest tube or thoracotomy, the patient should be given antibiotics. If a prosthetic graft is inserted at the time of surgery, the consequences of an infection are especially grave. When used, prophylactic antibiotics should be given preoperatively, intraoperatively and for at least 2 to 3 days postoperatively.

STEROIDS. Steroids should be considered if the patient has aspirated gastric contents or has inhaled smoke in a confined space for more than a few minutes. In both these conditions the findings on chest x-ray and physical examination may be minimal for 12 to 36 hours. Once the severe inflammatory reaction develops in the bronchi and alveoli, however, a picture of patchy pneumonitis may develop, followed by a severe confluent pneumonia. If a steroid such as hydrocortisone is begun early, in doses of 200 to 300 mg daily (or an equivalent amount of Solu-Medrol or Decadron), the pulmonary changes usually tend to be less severe. If the steroids are started after the pulmonary changes are apparent, they are less effective.

If severe progressive respiratory failure develops in spite of vigorous ventilatory assistance and dehydration of the patient, massive steroids in doses equivalent to 150 mg hydrocortisone per kg body weight should be given intravenously every 4, 6, 8 or 12 hours, depending on the patient's response (Chap. 31).

SUMMARY

Diagnosis of most intrathoracic injuries depends upon a high index of suspicion and serial chest x-rays. Most patients with chest trauma can be treated conservatively by maintaining adequate ventilation and by judicious use of chest tubes to remove any air or blood that may have accumulated in the pleural cavity. Adequate ventilation can usually be maintained by relieving pain and keeping the airway clean through frequent coughing by the patient, nasotracheal suction, or bronchoscopy. If there is any indication that a respirator will be needed, either because of the clinical situation or the patient's blood gases, it should be used early.

Emergency thoracotomy is rarely needed for the management of chest trauma. When it is required for certain specific problems such as cardiac penetration, severe continuing intrathoracic bleeding, rupture of the thoracic aorta, or injury to a major bronchus, the esophagus or diaphragm, the surgery must be performed promptly and expeditiously.

REFERENCES

1. Blair, E., et al.: Major blunt chest trauma. In Current Problems in Surgery (Rewich, M. M., Ed.). Chicago, Year Book Medical Publishers, 1969.
2. Sankaran, S., and Wilson, R. F.: Factors affecting prognosis in patients with flail chest. J. Thorac. Cardiov. Surg., 60:402, 1970.
3. Wilson, R. F., et al.: Physiologic shunting in the lung in critically ill or injured patients. J. Surg. Res., 12:571, 1970.
4. Fromm, S. H., and Lucas, C. E.: An unusual complication of chronic diaphragmatic hernia in an adult patient. J. Thorac. Cardiov. Surg., 61:654, 1971.
5. Parmley, L. F., et al.: Nonpenetrating traumatic injury of the aorta. Circulation, 17:1086, 1958.
6. Wilson, R. F., et al.: Acute mediastinal widening following blunt chest trauma. Arch. Surg., 104:551, 1972.
7. Bassett, J. S., et al.: Blunt injuries to the chest. J. Trauma, 8:418, 1968.
8. Wilson, R. F., et al.: Spontaneous perforation of the esophagus. Ann. Thorac. Surg., 12:291, 1971.
9. Lefrak, E. A., et al.: Current status of prolonged extracorporeal membrane oxygenation for acute respiratory failure. Chest, 63:773, 1973.

Suggested Reading

1. Carrasquilla, C., et al.: Management of massive thoraco-abdominal wall defect from close-range shotgun blast. J. Trauma, 11:715, 1971.
2. Olson, R. O., and Johnson, J. T.: Diagnosis and management of intrathoracic tracheal rupture. J. Trauma, 11:789, 1971.

3. Nahum, A. M., et al.: The biomechanical basis for chest impact protection: I. Force-deflection characteristics of the thorax. J. Trauma, 11:874, 1971.

4. Erickson, D. R., et al.: Relationship of arterial blood gases and pulmonary radiographs to the degree of pulmonary damage in experimental pulmonary contusion. J. Trauma, 11:689, 1971.

5. Nahum, A. M., et al.: The biomechanical basis of chest impact protection II. Effects of cardiovascular pressurization. J. Trauma, 13:443, 1973.

6. Relihan, M., and Litwin, M. S.: Morbidity and mortality associated with flail chest injury: a review of 85 cases. J. Trauma, 13:663, 1973.

7. Mulder, D. S., et al.: Posttraumatic thoracic outlet syndrome. J. Trauma, 13:946, 1973.

8. Wise, L., et al.: Traumatic injuries to the diaphragm. J. Trauma, 13:946, 1973.

9. Katz, S., et al.: Traumatic transection associated with retrograde dissection and rupture of the aorta. Recognition and management. Ann. Thorac. Surg., 17:273, 1974.

10. Neugebauer, M. K., et al.: Traumatic rupture of the trachea and right main stem bronchus. J. Trauma, 14: 265, 1974.

11. Fischer, R. P., et al.: Pulmonary resections for severe pulmonary contusions secondary to high-velocity missile wounds. J. Trauma, 14:293, 1974.

12. Urschel, H., Jr., and Razzuk, M. A.: Management of acute traumatic injuries of the tracheal broncheal tree. Surg. Gynec. Obstet., 136:113, 1973.

21 CARDIAC INJURIES

R. F. WILSON
Z. STEIGER
N. THOMS
A. ARBULU

The incidence of penetrating injuries to the heart, especially those due to gunshot wounds, has been steadily rising in our cities.[1] A similar or even greater rise in the incidence of blunt cardiac injuries can also be expected because of the speed and number of automobiles on our highways. Since the presentation and treatment of these two types of cardiac trauma are very different, they will be discussed separately.

Section 1

PENETRATING WOUNDS OF THE HEART

It has been estimated that only about 50% of patients with stab wounds of the heart and 10 to 15% of those with gunshot wounds of the heart reach the hospital alive.[2]

PITFALL

ANY DELAY IN TREATING A PENETRATING CARDIAC WOUND MAY BE FATAL.

In few other injuries is the outcome of the patient so directly dependent on the speed and accuracy of diagnosis and treatment. The margin of safety may be so small that even a slight delay in definitive therapy may be fatal. It is essential, therefore, that

TABLE 1. THE MOST FREQUENT ERRORS MADE IN THE TREATMENT OF PATIENTS WITH PENETRATING CARDIAC INJURIES

1. Not suspecting the diagnosis in a patient with a penetrating chest wound.
2. Delay in opening the chest in the emergency room if the patient has a cardiac arrest.
3. Failure to attempt pericardiocentesis if the patient is deteriorating.
4. Failure to infuse adequate quantities of fluid if the patient is severely hypotensive.
5. Delay in getting the patient to the operating room.
6. Stopping for a chest x-ray when the patient is hypotensive or unstable.
7. Elaborate prepping and positioning of the patient prior to opening the chest.

the emergency physician have a clear understanding of both the potential pitfalls and essential actions in the treatment of these wounds (Table 1).

DIAGNOSIS

Any penetrating injury of the chest, especially if it is between the midclavicular line on the right and the anterior axillary line on the left, should be considered as involving the heart until proven otherwise. In general patients will exhibit the clinical picture of either tamponade or severe blood loss. At surgery approximately a third will have tamponade without bleeding from the cardiac wound, a third will have tamponade and bleeding, and a third will have bleeding without tamponade.[4]

Tamponade

In 1935, Beck[3] described the clinical triad of hypotension, distended neck veins, and decreased or muffled heart sounds which is apt to be associated with a sudden accumulation of blood or fluid in the pericardial cavity.

PITFALL

BLIND INSISTENCE THAT THE COMPLETE BECK'S TRIAD OR DISTENDED NECK VEINS BE PRESENT BEFORE MAKING A DIAGNOSIS OF PERICARDIAL TAMPONADE MAY RESULT IN DANGEROUS DELAYS IN PERICARDIOCENTESIS AND CARDIORRHAPHY.

Although the signs in Beck's triad may be of great help in making the diagnosis of acute cardiac tamponade, they are not as reliable as might be expected. On examining our own records on 200 patients with penetrating wounds of the heart seen between 1949 and 1965, we found that of 63 patients with tamponade who had complete descriptions of the neck veins or venous pressure, blood pressure, and heart tones, the complete Beck triad was present in only 26 (41%) and no clinical evidence of tamponade was present in three (5%)[4] (Table 2).

HYPOTENSION. Hypotension was present in the great majority of patients with penetrating cardiac wounds and was an important indication for early thoracotomy; however, it was of no value in differentiating between tamponade and continued hemorrhage.

CENTRAL VENOUS PRESSURE. While classically the central venous pressure (CVP) should be elevated in the presence of tamponade, it may be low or within normal limits if there has been concomitant severe blood loss. Under such circumstances, the CVP may not rise until the hypovolemia is at least partially corrected. On the other hand, the CVP is occasionally elevated when there is no tamponade or cardiac wound, possibly because of straining by the patient at the time of the examination.

DECREASED HEART SOUNDS. While the pa-

TABLE 2.   BECK'S TRIAD IN 91 PATIENTS WITH PENETRATING CARDIAC INJURIES[4]

Clinical sign	Incidence in patients with			
	Tamponade and no bleeding	Tamponade and bleeding	Bleeding without tamponade	Total
Elevated venous pressure	21/31 = 68%	24/32 = 75%	15/28 = 54%	60/91 = 66%
Hypotension	27/31 = 87%	27/32 = 84%	27/28 = 96%	81/91 = 89%
Abnormal heart sounds	17/31 = 55%	18/32 = 56%	18/28 = 64%	53/91 = 58%
Complete Beck's triad	14/31 = 45%	12/32 = 38%	13/28 = 46%	39/91 = 43%
Partial Beck's triad	15/31 = 48%	19/32 = 59%	14/28 = 50%	48/91 = 55%
None of Beck's triad	2/31 = 7%	1/32 = 3%	1/28 = 4%	4/91 = 4%

tient should be routinely examined for heart size and the loudness and characteristics of the heart sounds, these signs correlate poorly with the surgical findings. In many instances, patients with normal heart size and tones had severe tamponade whereas others noted to have enlarged quiet hearts had no tamponade. It was also found that the examining physicians not infrequently disagreed with each other on the description of the physical findings.

X-RAYS

The urgency of the need for x-ray examination of the chest must be individualized. If the diagnosis is clinically obvious and the patient's condition is critical, films are not needed. Less than 200 ml of blood in the pericardial cavity can cause tamponade, but it often takes much more blood to make the heart shadow appear enlarged on x-ray. Thus, it is not surprising that the cardiac shadow appeared normal in over half of the patients with tamponade.[4]

Hemorrhage

The patients with hemorrhage and little or no tamponade rarely reach the hospital alive. Cardiac tamponade, in the presence of an open cardiac wound, may be lifesaving by reducing the amount and rate of bleeding, even though this is achieved at the cost of a reduced cardiac output. Although the signs of severe blood loss from the heart are similar to those seen with other exsanguinating injuries, these are often modified by any tamponade that may be present.

MANAGEMENT

Initial Management

Immediately upon the arrival of a patient with a penetrating wound of the heart, a standard rapid aggressive outline of management should be followed (Table 3).

TABLE 3. OUTLINE OF INITIAL MANAGEMENT OF PATIENTS WITH PENETRATING CARDIAC WOUNDS

1. Insert *endotracheal tube* and use Ambu-bag or *respirator* if necessary to maintain adequate ventilation.
2. Start 2 to 3 large *I.V. catheters* (including CVP).
3. Draw blood for *CBC* and *type and cross-match*.
4. Infuse 2 to 3 liters of 5% *G/RL* rapidly.
5. Insert *nasogastric tube* and *Foley catheter*.
6. Perform *pericardiocentesis* if deterioration or persistent hypotension.
7. Move rapidly to the *operating room*. This may be done by way of the x-ray department only if the patient is stable.

VENTILATION If there is any question about the adequacy of ventilation, the mouth and pharynx are cleared of any secretions or foreign bodies. If the ventilation is still inadequate, an endotracheal tube is inserted and ventilatory assistance is given with an Ambu-bag or respirator.

VOLUME REPLACEMENT. Two or three large (14- to 16-gauge) intravenous catheters are inserted percutaneously or by cutdown into the veins of the upper extremity or the subclavian veins. One of these catheters is advanced into the superior vena cava to monitor the central venous pressure. Blood samples are obtained for complete blood count and a type and cross-match for at least four units of blood. Five percent dextrose in lactated Ringer's solution is infused rapidly, followed by group O negative or preferably type-specific blood, depending upon the urgency of the situation and the response of the CVP and blood pressure.

PITFALL

IF FLUIDS AND BLOOD ARE WITHHELD FROM A HYPOTENSIVE PATIENT BECAUSE HIS NECK VEINS ARE DISTENDED, THE CARDIAC OUTPUT MAY FALL TO LETHAL LEVELS.

NASOGASTRIC TUBE AND FOLEY CATHETER. A nasogastric tube and a Foley catheter are inserted to decompress the stomach and to monitor urine output. Many patients have full stomachs and tend to vomit, especially later during the induction of anesthesia. Constant monitoring of the urine output is a valuable guide to the overall adequacy of tissue perfusion.

PERICARDIOCENTESIS. If there is any evidence of tamponade or if the patient's condition is deteriorating in spite of rapid volume replacement, a pericardiocentesis should be performed immediately. Removal of 5 to 10 cc of nonclotting blood is virtually diagnostic of a hemopericardium; it may also, by increasing the stroke volume an equivalent amount, improve cardiac output and blood pressure dramatically, seemingly greatly out of proportion to the small amount of blood removed. It must be remembered, however, that a negative tap does not rule out the presence of a cardiac tamponade. Many technical problems, including the presence of clots in the pericardium, may interfere with a successful tap.

AXIOM

A PHYSICIAN EQUIPPED TO PERFORM IMMEDIATE PERICARDIOCENTESIS MUST ACCOMPANY THE PATIENT WITH A SUSPECTED PENETRATING CARDIAC WOUND AT ALL TIMES UNTIL THE INJURY IS REPAIRED.

Even if the patient's condition appears to be well stabilized, a physician with a long 18-gauge needle and 20-cc syringe (preferably Luer-Lok) must accompany the patient to the x-ray department or to the operating room. Such a patient can deteri-

orate suddenly, and, unless a pericardiocentesis is performed immediately when this occurs, he is likely to have a cardiac arrest. Not infrequently this problem develops while the patient is en route to the x-ray department or the operating room when minimal personnel and equipment are immediately available. Repeated aspirations of the pericardial cavity may provide time until the tamponade can be released under direct vision in the operating room; however, pericardiocentesis should never delay the operation.

DRUGS. Drugs are of very limited value in the initial management of a patient with a penetrating wound of the heart. A patient with persisting hypotension in spite of adequate pericardiocentesis and volume replacement may benefit from the administration of sodium bicarbonate to combat severe acidosis. Isoproterenol improves the contractions of a slow weakly beating heart, and digoxin or Cedilanid can be valuable if there is evidence of heart failure. If the patient has had massive transfusions, 10% calcium chloride (2.5 ml for each unit of blood) may also improve myocardial contractions. It must be emphasized, however, that attempts to improve the patient's condition with drugs should not delay surgery. Complete release of the tamponade and direct cardiorrhaphy will correct the cardiovascular problems much more rapidly and completely than any combination of drugs.

MOVEMENT TO THE OPERATING ROOM WITH OR WITHOUT X-RAYS. As soon as adequate ventilation is provided and the intravenous catheters, nasogastric tube, and Foley catheter are in place, the patient is moved to the operating room. If his condition is stable, chest x-rays are rapidly obtained on the way to the operating room; if not, the x-rays are dispensed with because delay under these circumstances may be fatal.

OPEN CARDIAC MASSAGE. If a cardiac arrest occurs in a patient with a penetrating chest wound while he is in the emergency room, an endotracheal tube is rapidly inserted and open cardiac massage is begun (Chap.

11). If the patient responds to resuscitation, he is moved to the surgical suite for completion of the operation.

PITFALL

CLOSED CARDIAC MASSAGE IN THE PATIENT WITH A PENETRATING CHEST INJURY IS USUALLY FUTILE AND CAN CAUSE DANGEROUS DELAYS.

The results of closed cardiac massage in patients who have had a cardiac arrest following a penetrating wound of the chest are generally poor. In these circumstances, external massage usually only increases the tamponade or bleeding and may be completely ineffective if the patient is severely hypovolemic or the pericardium is open. Open cardiac massage allows the surgeon to directly evaluate cardiac filling and contractions and to control active bleeding sites. In addition he can compress or clamp the descending thoracic aorta to improve coronary and cerebral blood flow.

Definitive Treatment

Until 1896, the only surgical treatment available for penetrating wounds of the heart was pericardiocentesis or phlebotomy. In that year Rehn successfully relieved the tamponade and sutured the myocardial laceration of a patient who had been stabbed with a table knife on the previous day.[5]

For the next 30 to 40 years, cardiorrhaphy was felt by many surgeons to be the preferred method for managing such wounds. In 1930, however, Blalock and Ravitch[6] reported their success with pericardiocentesis alone. Since then, the definitive management of penetrating cardiac wounds has been controversial.[4,7,8] In our own hands, early cardiorrhaphy has been the treatment of choice for over 20 years and has resulted in survival rates of 83% for 179 patients with stab wounds[4] and 74% for 27 patients with gunshot wounds of the heart.[1] This experience concurs with the present majority

view and suggests that virtually all penetrating injuries of the heart, especially large stab or gunshot wounds, should be treated by immediate thoracotomy and cardiorrhaphy.[10–12]

PERICARDIOCENTESIS. *Indications.* Some authors consider pericardiocentesis to be

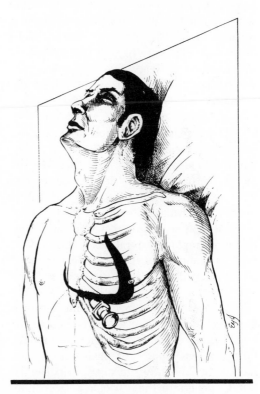

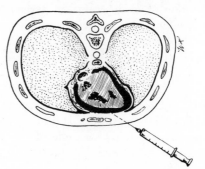

FIG. 1. The technique for precordial pericardiocentesis is shown. The 3-inch 18-gauge needle is angled 45° medially from a point 1 inch lateral to the left sternal border, carefully aspirating every 1 or 2 mm until the pericardium is entered. Any blood aspirated should be saved and observed for clotting. If the blood clots, the blood was probably aspirated from the heart rather than the pericardial cavity.

the preferred definitive method of management for most penetrating wounds of the
heart, especially small stab wounds, resorting to a thoracotomy only if the patient
does not improve after the pericardial tap
or if he deteriorates later in spite of repeated taps. The patients most likely to
respond to pericardiocentesis are those
with minimal or no hypotension and small
wounds such as those caused by ice picks
or very narrow knife blades. Unfortunately,
a few of our patients who responded very
well to pericardiocentesis initially later de-
teriorated suddenly and almost died.

Techniques. PRECORDIAL APPROACH (Fig.
1). The precordial approach to pericardiocentesis is made through the fifth intercostal space about one inch outside the
lateral sternal border. With the tip angled
45° medially, a long (3-inch) 18-gauge
needle is advanced carefully through the
chest wall, 1 to 2 mm at a time, with frequent attempts at aspiration. If this is done
with a continuous EKG or cardioscope
monitoring, PVCs, S-T changes, or a different rhythm may be noticed when the
needle contacts the myocardium. Record-
ings from a precordial lead attached to the
needle may show abrupt changes in the
QRS complex when the epicardium is contacted. Occasionally the needle tip can be
felt to penetrate the parietal pericardium.

Aspiration of blood from the pericardial
cavity is seldom marked by the same steady
flow which occurs if blood is being aspirated directly from the atrium or ventricle.
Any blood that is obtained should be set
aside and observed for clotting. Blood in
the pericardial cavity will also often have
a low hematocrit because it is diluted with
some pericardial fluid and some of the red
cells become incorporated in the clots that
are present.

One disadvantage of the precordial approach is the ease with which the anterior
descending coronary artery can be damaged. Although this complication is rather
infrequent, it can have serious consequences.

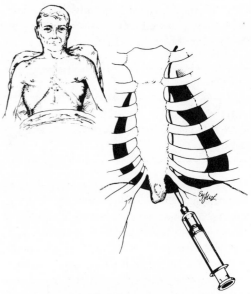

FIG. 2. The paraxiphoid approach to pericardiocentesis
can be performed rapidly by experienced physicians and
is generally safer than the precordial approach.

PARAXIPHOID APPROACH (Fig. 2). The
paraxiphoid approach is made to the left
of the xiphoid process, advancing the needle
with its point directed posteriorly, laterally,
and cephalically. For best results the patient should be in a semisitting position so
that the blood will be apt to pool on the
diaphragmatic surface of the pericardium;
if the patient is lying flat, the blood will
tend to accumulate posteriorly and may be
missed. The same general precautions
should be followed as mentioned in the
precordial approach.

SUBXIPHOID APPROACH (Fig. 3). Recently
we have used a direct surgical subxiphoid
approach to the pericardium on several
occasions to establish the presence of hemopericardium under local anesthesia.[9] The
xiphoid process is resected through a vertical or left subcostal incision. The pericardium which then comes into view is opened
between clamps or sutures. If blood is present, we proceed with a left anterior thoracotomy. If no hemopericardium is found,
the wound is closed. This procedure seems
to be safe, fast and foolproof in the relatively stable patient.

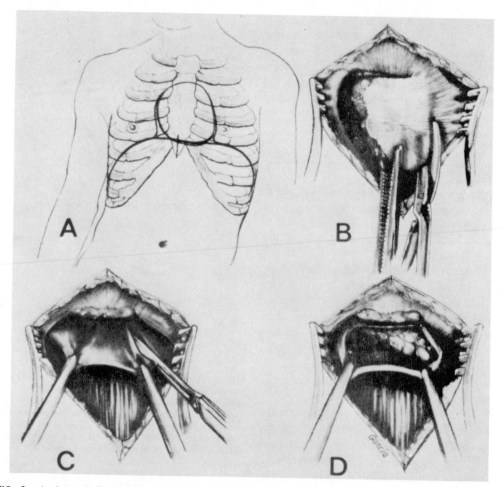

FIG. 3. A: Anatomic location of the incision. B: Excision of xiphoid process. C: Incised pericardium. D: Pericardial window. (From Fontenelle, L. J., et al.[6])

INTRA-ABDOMINAL APPROACH (Fig. 4). Not infrequently a patient with an upper abdominal wound or multiple injuries involving the chest and abdomen will have a heart wound which is not suspected clinically. This is most apt to occur if the wounds are more than an inch or two from the precordium, if examination of the heart is normal, and if the central venous pressure is low.

If sudden unexplained deterioration of the patient occurs while the abdomen is being explored, the surgeon should immediately extend the incision to the xiphoid and open the pericardium from below. In a thin patient, the diaphragmatic pericar-

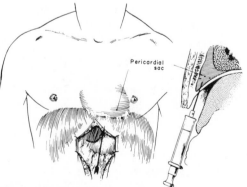

FIG. 4. The intra-abdominal or transdiaphragmatic approach to the pericardial sac is shown. The central diaphragm anterior to the left lobe of the liver may be punctured with our 18-gauge needle prior to making an incision directly into the pericardial cavity through the diaphragm.

dium can be grasped directly with an Allis clamp and incised; in more obese patients, the xiphoid may have to be quickly excised and the anterior portion of the pericardium incised. Depending upon what is found, the surgeon may or may not need to make a second incision in the chest.

CARDIORRAPHY

PITFALL

ELABORATE ANESTHETIC PREPARATIONS IN THE PATIENT WITH SEVERE TAMPONADE OR BLEEDING ONLY DELAY NEEDED SURGERY.

Most patients with penetrating cardiac wounds are severely hypotensive and generally little or no anesthesia is required during the early stages of the operation. The main requirement initially is enough paralysis or sedation to insert an endotracheal tube so that adequate ventilation with high concentrations of oxygen can be maintained during the operation.

We favor a left anterolateral thoracotomy through the fourth intercostal space for most cardiac wounds (Fig. 5). This incision provides rapid access to the heart and can be enlarged either to the right by dividing the sternum transversely or to the left by extending the incision to the left posteriorly in the intercostal space. Wounds of the right side of the heart can be approached from either side; although it is easier to repair right-sided injuries through the right chest, cardiac massage is performed more rapidly from the left. The midline sternal-splitting incision provides the best overall exposure of the heart, but because it requires much more time than the other incisions, its use is seldom warranted under emergency conditions.

The pericardium is opened parallel to and 2 to 3 cm anterior to the phrenic nerve. Bleeding from the cardiac wound is controlled with the tip of one finger while a 2-0 or larger nonabsorbable suture is passed under the finger through the muscle on

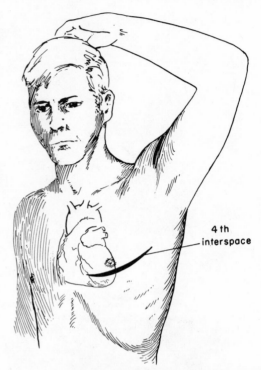

FIG. 5. A fourth intercostal space anterolateral thoracotomy incision provides excellent exposure to the left ventricle for repair of cardiac wounds and for cardiac massage. This incision may be carried across the sternum if needed to expose the right side of the heart. The arm should be secured over the head for this incision so that the incision can be extended laterally into the axilla if needed.

either side of the injury and then back again as a horizontal mattress suture (Fig. 6). If the myocardium is friable or is torn by the initial sutures, pledgets of Teflon felt or a similar material should be incorporated with the suture on both sides of the wound so that the suture pulls against the pledgets instead of the myocardium as it is tied.

PITFALL

FAILURE TO SUTURE A CARDIAC WOUND WHICH IS NOT BLEEDING MAY ALLOW THE WOUND TO BLEED LATER WHEN THE BLOOD PRESSURE RISES OR THE PATIENT AWAKENS FROM THE ANESTHETIC AND BEGINS TO COUGH OR STRAIN.

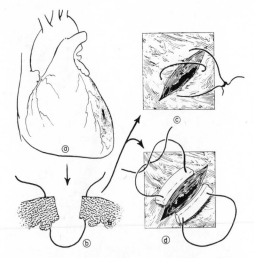

FIG. 6. A stab wound of the left ventricle (a) is shown (b) repaired by the standard simple interrupted suture and (c) figure-of-eight suture. The insert (d) illustrates our preferred technique for repair of large cardiac wounds. The pledgets on the horizontal mattress suture greatly reduce the risk of the sutures pulling out off the myocardium as they are tied down.

Certain cardiac wounds may be extremely difficult to repair because of their location and the severity of the bleeding. Injuries near the junction of the inferior vena cava and right atrium, for example, bleed profusely and are easily enlarged by any sutures which are poorly placed or are tied under tension. In addition, the coronary sinus can be easily closed or narrowed if the sutures are placed too deeply. Under such circumstances, a very useful technique for controlling the bleeding is to pass a Foley catheter through the cardiac wound and, after inflating the balloon, pull it gently up against the wound edges so that the opening is sealed (Fig. 7). A purse-string suture can then be placed around the wound, being careful not to perforate the balloon. This method produces minimal distortion of the heart and allows suture of the cardiac wound in a dry operating field.[13]

After the tamponade has been relieved and any obvious penetration repaired, the surgeon should look carefully for a posterior or lateral exit wound, especially if the injury has been caused by a bullet. If the bullet is lodged deeply in the myocardium, it is probably best to leave it in place until its exact position can be evaluated later by further x-rays and cardiac catheterization. Superficial bullets can usually be removed safely at the initial operation, especially if a cardiac surgeon and cardiopulmonary bypass team are readily available should complications develop.

CARDIOPULMONARY BYPASS. Because of the urgency with which surgery must be performed, most penetrating wounds of the heart will be treated by noncardiac surgeons. For the most part these injuries are easily managed if an orderly outline of management is followed. There are, however, some special circumstances in which the services of a trained cardiac surgeon and cardiopulmonary bypass team are required. These situations should be recognized as soon as possible by the initial attending surgeon. In most instances, bleeding can be controlled and cardiac activity maintained until proper help and equipment can be obtained.

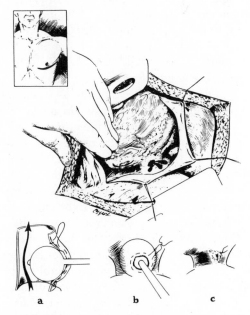

FIG. 7. The drawings show the balloon catheter technique for the repair of a "difficult-to-reach" major vessel or cardiac injury.

PITFALL

IF A LACERATION OF A MAJOR CORONARY
ARTERY, ESPECIALLY ON THE LEFT, IS NOT RE-
PAIRED OR BYPASSED, THE PATIENT MAY DE-
VELOP SERIOUS ARRHYTHMIAS OR PUMP FAIL-
URE AS A RESULT OF MYOCARDIAL INFARCTION.

Coronary Artery Lacerations. The mortality rate following coronary artery lacerations is high both immediately and in the
postoperative period.[14] Damage to larger
coronary arteries, especially the left main
coronary or proximal anterior descending
coronary artery, is particularly lethal. Such
injuries should be treated by direct arterial-
repair saphenous vein patch or a saphenous
vein graft between the aorta and the distal
portion of the injured coronary, preferably
under cardiopulmonary bypass.[15] Although
these operations can often be performed
without special equipment, cardiopulmonary bypass and anoxic cardiac arrest
greatly increases the speed and accuracy
of the repair and may be essential to maintain adequate systemic perfusion if the
myocardial ischemia causes persistent arrhythmias or pump failure. A femorocoro-
nary shunt may be improvised in order to
perfuse the distal portion of the injured
coronary artery while the aortocoronary
bypass is being performed[16] (Fig. 8).

Septal Defects. Occasionally a penetrating or blunt injury will result in an interventricular or, rarely, an interatrial septal
defect or aorto-right ventricular fistula. The
murmur of the interventricular defect is a
characteristic holosystolic murmur which
sounds close to the ear and radiates from
the precordium toward the right chest. If
the septal defect is confirmed on cardiac
catheterization, it should be closed under
cardiopulmonary bypass 4 to 6 months later
unless the development of intractable cardiac failure makes earlier repair mandatory.

Injuries to the Conducting System. Severe
blunt damage or direct penetrating injury
to the heart may result in partial or complete atrioventricular block in the conduct-

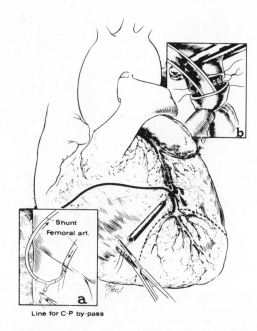

Line for C-P by-pass

FIG. 8. The diagrams show two methods of repairing a
lacerated coronary artery while perfusing the distal coronary artery: by direct repair when the artery is large
enough or saphenous aortocoronary bypass when the
artery is too small for direct end-to-end repair. In both
techniques the femoral arterial cannulation provides distal
coronary artery perfusion while the coronary artery is
repaired.

ing system. Complete A-V dissociation or
RBBB with left anterior hemiblock should
be treated by insertion of a permanent
demand pacemaker as soon as possible.

Postoperative Management

Intravenous antibiotics to cover gram-
positive and gram-negative organisms are
usually administered intra-operatively and
are generally continued for at least 3 to
5 days postoperatively. Although a number
of patients have had their thoracotomies
begun in the emergency room with minimal
sterile precautions, wound infections are
extremely rare.

Postoperatively these patients are handled much as those following any elective
cardiac procedure. The endotracheal tube,
nasogastric tube, and Foley catheter can
usually be removed on the day following
surgery. Coughing is encouraged and naso-

tracheal suction and flexible bronchoscopy are used as needed to remove excessive bronchial secretions. Ambulation is usually begun cautiously by the third or fourth day with a gradual increase in activity thereafter.

Recurrent pericardial effusion has been reported in up to 22% of patients with penetrating cardiac injury.[17] This phenomenon has been compared to the postpericardiotomy syndrome following elective surgery on the heart. The pain from these effusions can usually be managed symptomatically with salicylates. If cardiac tamponade develops, pericardicentesis or a pericardial window may be required.

Section 2

BLUNT INJURIES TO THE HEART

Blunt injuries to the heart may consist of myocardial rupture, myocardial contusion, pericardial effusions or hemorrhage, and septal or valvular disruptions. Virtually all patients with rupture of the myocardium die before they can be brought to a hospital, and septal and valvular disruptions are rare.[2] Significant pericardial effusions or hemorrhage following blunt trauma are uncommon, seldom require drainage, and are usually associated with myocardial contusion.

ETIOLOGY

In our experience motor vehicle accidents are by far the most common cause of blunt trauma to the heart. The physical forces that can cause nonpenetrating injury to the heart have been classified by Parmley and Mattingly[2] into six mechanisms which may act separately or in combination: (1) unidirectional force against the chest, (2) bidirectional or compressive force against the chest, (3) increases in intravascular pressure due to compression of the abdomen and lower extremities, (4) decelerative forces, (5) blast forces and (6) concussive forces.

DIAGNOSIS

PITFALL

IF A MYOCARDIAL CONTUSION IS NOT SUSPECTED, THE DIAGNOSIS WILL USUALLY BE OVERLOOKED.

Myocardial contusion should be suspected after any severe blunt injury to the anterior chest, especially when associated with steering-wheel trauma in high-speed automobile accidents. Unfortunately, however, this diagnosis is often missed because the associated musculoskeletal, craniocerebral, and abdominal injuries tend to dominate the clinical picture (Table 4).

TABLE 4. THE MOST FREQUENT ERRORS MADE IN THE TREATMENT OF PATIENTS WITH NONPENERATING CARDIAC INJURIES

1. Not suspecting the diagnosis in patients with blunt chest trauma.
2. Not obtaining an EKG and enzyme studies soon after admission.
3. Not admitting a patient with suspected cardiac injury even if the initial EKG is normal.
4. Failure to observe the patient's vital signs and cardiac rhythm closely.
5. Failure to obtain serial EKGs and enzyme levels.

Although the circumstances of the trauma and the presence of chest pain should alert the clinician to the possible diagnosis of myocardial contusion, this problem is seldom suspected except by EKG. Even the EKG, however, may be misleading because it can be "normal" for the first 6 to 36 hours and, when nonspecific S-T segment changes do develop, they may be attributed to changes in cardiac position, hypoxia, or hypotension. In addition, these EKG changes are often interpreted quite differently by various cardiologists depending on the past history of the patient and the evolution of the S-T segment changes.

PITFALL

IF SERIAL ELECTROCARDIOGRAMS ARE NOT OBTAINED ON A PATIENT WITH SUSPECTED MYOCARDIAL CONTUSION, THE SERIOUSNESS AND EXTENT OF THE INJURY MAY NOT BE SUSPECTED.

Persistent S-T abnormalities or changes similar to those produced by myocardial infarction are usually considered to be evidence of extensive myocardial contusions. Enlargement of the cardiac shadow on x-ray due to ventricular dilatation or accumulation of pericardial fluid or blood may also suggest the diagnosis.

Elevations of various enzymes, especially creatinephosphokinase (CPK) and serum glutamic oxaloacetic transaminase (SGOT), may also be helpful, but such changes can also be caused by injury to skeletal muscle and liver. If a new or unusual murmur is heard, or if cardiac failure develops, a complete heart catheterization should be performed to accurately identify the anatomic abnormality.

TREATMENT

The patient with suspected myocardial contusion should be treated similarly to the patient with an acute myocardial infarction. Careful monitoring for the development of any arrhythmias is important during the first 24 to 48 hours. If arrhythmias develop, they should be treated with the appropriate drugs and endocardial pacing as needed. If the EKG changes are mild and transient, the patient's activity may be increased rapidly. If pericardial effusion develops, pericardicentesis or a pericardial window may be required to treat any signs or symptoms of tamponade.

The valve most likely to be damaged by blunt chest injury is the mitral valve. If the patient goes into progressive severe heart failure in spite of good medical management, the valve should either be repaired or replaced under cardiopulmonary bypass. Tricuspid and pulmonic valvular insufficiency is usually well tolerated unless the patient has moderate to severe pulmonary hypertension or a diseased left side of the heart.[18]

PROGNOSIS

The prognosis for most patients with myocardial contusion or pericardial effusion is excellent; most deaths in patients with these injuries are caused by associated noncardiac damage.

REFERENCES

1. Carrasquilla, C., et al.: Gunshot wounds of the heart. Ann. Thorac. Surg., 13:208, 1972.
2. Parmley, L. F., and Mattingly, T. W.: Traumatic heart disease. Less common diseases of the heart. In: *The Heart, Arteries and Veins* (Hurst, J. W., and Logue, R. B., Eds.). New York, McGraw-Hill Book Company, 1966.
3. Beck, C. S.: Two compression cardiac syndromes. JAMA, 104:714, 1935.
4. Wilson, R. F., and Bassett, J. S.: Penetrating wounds of the pericardium or its contents. JAMA, 195:513, 1966.
5. Rehn, L.: Ueber Penetriren der Herzwunden und Herznaht. Arch. Klin. Chir., 55:315, 1897.
6. Blalock, A., and Ravitch, M. M.: A consideration of the nonoperative treatment of cardiac tamponade resulting from wounds of heart. In: *Current Surgical Management* (Mulholland, J. H., Ellison, E. H., and Friesen, S. R., Eds.). Philadelphia, W. B. Saunders, 1957.
7. Bahnson, H. T., and Spence, F. C.: Pericardial aspiration in treatment of acute cardiac tamponade from penetrating wounds of heart. In: *Current Surgical Management* (Mulholland, J. H., Ellison, E. H., and Friesen, S. R., Eds.). Philadelphia, W. B. Saunders, 1957.

8. Boyd, T. F., and Strieder, J. W.: Immediate surgery for traumatic heart disease. J. Thorac. Cardiov. Surg., 50:305, 1969.

9. Fontenelle, L. J., et al.: Subxiphoid pericardial window. J. Thorac. Cardiov. Surg., 62:95, 1971.

10. Beall, A. C., et al.: Penetrating wounds of the heart: Changing patterns of surgical management. J. Trauma, 12:468, 1972.

11. Sugg, W. L., et al.: Penetrating wounds of the heart: an analysis of 459 cases. J. Thorac. Cardiov. Surg., 56:531, 1968.

12. Borja, A. R., Lansing, A. M., and Ramsdell, H. I.: Immediate operative treatment for stab wounds of the heart. J. Thorac. Cardiov. Surg., 95:662, 1970.

13. Arbulu, A., and Thoms, N.: Control of bleeding from a gunshot wound of the inferior vena cava at its junction with the right atrium by means of a Foley catheter. J. Thorac. Cardiov. Surg., 63:427, 1972.

14. Rea, W. J., et al.: Coronary artery lacerations. Ann. Thorac. Surg., 7:518, 1973.

15. Tector, A. J., et al.: Coronary artery wounds treated with saphenous vein bypass grafts. JAMA, 225:282, 1973.

16. Arbulu, A., and Wheeler, R.: Direct aorto-left coronary vein graft anastomoses without cardiopulmonary bypass. Chest, 58:292, 1970.

17. Tabatznik, B., and Isaacs, J. P.: Postpericardiotomy syndrome following traumatic hemopericardium. Amer. J. Cardiol., 7:83, 1961.

18. Arbulu, A., et al.: Total tricuspid valvulectomy without replacement in the treatment of pseudomonas endocarditis. Surg. Forum, 22:593, 1971.

Suggested Reading

1. O'Sullivan, M. J., Jr., et al.: Rupture of the right atrium due to blunt trauma. J. Trauma, 12:208, 1972.

2. Beckman, D. L., and Friedman, B. A.: Mechanics of cardiothoracic injury in primates. J. Trauma, 12:620, 1972.

3. Selmonosky, C. A., and Ellison, R. G.: Traumatic incompetence: Case report. J. Trauma, 12:632, 1972.

4. Shoemaker, W. C., et al.: Hemodynamic monitoring for physiologic evaluation, diagnosis, and therapy of acute hemopericardial tamponade from penetrating wounds. J. Trauma, 13:36, 1973.

5. Bartlett, H., et al.: Bullet embolism to the heart. J. Trauma, 13:476, 1973.

6. Payne, D. D., et al.: Surgical treatment of traumatic rupture of the normal aortic valve. Ann. Thorac. Surg., 17:223, 1974.

7. Trinkle, J. K., et al.: Management of the wounded heart. Ann. Thorac. Surg., 17:230, 1974.

22 GENERAL CONSIDERATIONS IN ABDOMINAL TRAUMA

A. J. WALT
R. F. WILSON

About 20 to 30% of patients with intra-abdominal trauma who die subsequent to reaching a hospital do so because of delayed, inadequate or inappropriate treatment; the incidence of avoidable morbidity is probably even higher. Physicians in emergency departments are required to be much more sophisticated in their approach to abdominal trauma now than in the past. On the one hand, more decisive diagnosis without undue reliance on radiologic and laboratory data is expected for those who require urgent surgery; on the other hand, a conservative approach to surgery in selected cases is increasingly advocated as a means of reducing a morbidity rate of about 30% and a mortality of up to 6.3% in those patients who undergo negative laparotomy. Nance et al., following a policy of selective observation of 393 stab wounds, reduced the percentage of patients subjected to exploration from 95% to 45% with clear improvement in overall results.[1] A similar policy has been strongly advanced for gunshot wounds, with no complications occurring in 52 patients observed but not operated upon.[1] A clear understanding of the potential clinical spectrum of abdominal injuries is therefore essential.[2,3]

PITFALL

IF IT IS FELT THAT INTRAPERITONEAL PENETRATION IS ALWAYS ASSOCIATED WITH VISCERAL DAMAGE, A SUBSTANTIAL NUMBER OF UNNECESSARY AND POTENTIALLY HARMFUL LAPAROTOMIES WILL BE PERFORMED.

The physician faced with a patient who has suffered abdominal trauma must ask certain critical questions: (1) Are any organs injured? (2) If so, is surgery required? (3) If surgery is required, what is the optimal time for operation? (4) Is there extra-abdominal injury which takes priority?

The causes of intra-abdominal injury may vary considerably not only in different parts of the country but also in different hospitals in a single metropolitan community. This factor, together with the variations in time which may elapse between injury and initial treatment, makes comparison of results between specific institutions and between rural and urban regions difficult and often unrealistic. However, the fundamental principles of treatment are universal, and form the basis for this chapter.

DIAGNOSIS

Early diagnosis of intra-abdominal injuries may severely tax the clinical acumen of the most experienced physician. The multiplicity of organs within the peritoneal cavity and the varied symptoms which may arise from injuries to these structures provide numerous potential pitfalls. Severity of impact or size of missile often fail to reflect the degree or extent of internal damage. Blunt trauma is particularly deceptive as the clinical manifestations of the injury may be delayed for hours, days or, rarely, weeks, even though the internal visceral damage is serious and sometimes lethal. Much depends on the position of the patient, the tension of the abdominal wall and the degree of energy applied at the moment of impact. Paradoxically, some patients with serious abdominal trauma from high-speed automobile accidents may have virtually no abnormal physical findings initially, only to deteriorate rapidly in subsequent hours. Conversely, some patients develop extensive guarding and rebound tenderness after ostensibly minimal trauma.

AXIOM

IT IS ESSENTIAL TO VIEW THE PATIENT WITH ABDOMINAL INJURY AS A WHOLE AND NOT TO BE DISTRACTED FROM RECOGNIZING CONCOMITANT EXTRA-ABDOMINAL LESIONS.

Severe blunt trauma to the abdomen is often associated with extra-abdominal damage. About 75% of patients with nonpenetrating intra-abdominal visceral damage have concomitant injuries of the head, chest or extremities which not only alter prognosis but also profoundly affect the timing of any projected operation. Injury to a single intra-abdominal organ is unlikely to be fatal, but the mortality rate rises sharply with the number of associated injuries.

Not infrequently, extra-abdominal inju-ries may cause severe hypovolemia or inadequate ventilation from a tension pneumothorax or airway obstruction—manifestations which have very high priority in treatment and usually take temporary precedence over abdominal injury. Unfortunately, in some patients the need for rapid transfusion and immediate laparotomy for massive intra-abdominal hemorrhage may allow little or no time for an optimal clinical examination or routine roentgenograms.

History

A careful history, when available, is important for providing valuable clues not only to the diagnosis of the patient's injury but also to any underlying medical problems, and should be accurately recorded both for medical and for medicolegal reasons. Changes in symptoms with time or with posture may be diagnostically significant and should be sought by direct questioning. For example, while pain which develops over the shoulder may be due to injury of that area, it may also be referred to this region from a diaphragm irritated by blood or bile.

Unfortunately, the history is often unobtainable, incomplete, inaccurate or misleading. The patient may be under the influence of alcohol or drugs, or may have injuries to the head, neck or chest which prevent adequate communication. Severe emotional stress may profoundly influence the interpretation of the event by the patient and bystanders. Occasionally, the history may be deliberately falsified because of anticipated legal action by police or by projected plans for the claiming of future compensation. Whenever possible, however, inquiries should be made and recorded about: (1) the details of the accident, (2) the time of onset, location, severity, and any changes in symptoms, (3) past and current disease and medications, (4) drug allergies, (5) bleeding tendencies, and (6) previous operations.

Physical Examination

AXIOM

CAREFUL REPEATED EXAMINATION OF THE
PATIENT IS THE KEYSTONE TO THE EARLY
ACCURATE DIAGNOSIS OF INTRA-ABDOMINAL
INJURIES.

In most cases of abdominal trauma, the
physical examination is the most informative portion of the diagnostic evaluation
and should be as complete as time and the
condition of the patient permit. A systematic approach is highly desirable, leaving
the obviously injured areas until last. The
more frequently and carefully these examinations are performed in cases of doubt,
the earlier and more accurately the diagnosis can be made and treatment instituted.

AXIOM

NARCOTICS SHOULD NOT BE GIVEN DURING
THE PERIOD OF OBSERVATION, AS THE EFFECTS
MAY COMPLETELY OBSCURE THE CLINICAL
PICTURE.

Even with similar visceral injuries, striking variations in the signs and symptoms
may exist in different patients. Hematoma
or rupture of the rectus abdominis muscle,
fractures of the ribs or pelvis, extreme
obesity and an altered sensorium due to
head injury, alcohol, or drugs may make
physical examination difficult to interpret
and even grossly deceptive at times.

AXIOM

ALL PATIENTS HAVE A BACK AS WELL AS
A FRONT.

The initial examination of a patient with
suspected abdominal trauma is no time for
excessive social niceties. The patient should
be stripped completely. In patients with
penetrating injuries, one must look carefully for entrance and exit wounds, es-

pecially in skin creases around the buttocks or perineum. The internal damage
does not necessarily reflect the extent of
the external wounds, which may be only
small punctures but nevertheless lethal.
Patients with blunt trauma from automobile accidents must be carefully examined
for tire marks, abrasions, bruises or disruption of abdominal muscles resulting
from seat belts.

Occasionally, dissection of blood into the
abdominal wall from retroperitoneal tissues may cause ecchymosis or purplish discoloration of the umbilicus (Cullen's sign)
or flanks (Grey-Turner sign). Such discoloration, however, usually requires at
least several hours to develop.

Increasing abdominal distension can also
be a valuable sign of intra-abdominal damage. If reliance is placed on subjective
evaluation, increasing distension, when
gradual, may not be appreciated until it
is well established. Consequently, measurement of the abdominal girth at the umbilical level should be made soon after the
patient's admission to provide a baseline
from which subsequent significant changes
can be determined early and objectively.

PALPATION. Palpation of the abdomen
should be done gently and with the patient as relaxed as possible. The extent and
severity of any guarding or tenderness, the
location of any referred or rebound tenderness, and the presence of any masses or
subcutaneous emphysema are specifically
recorded.

Abdominal rigidity and tenderness are
important signs of peritoneal irritation by
blood or intestinal contents but may also
be caused by fractured lower ribs or contusions. While rigidity is a variable sign
and sometimes difficult to assess, it is always a dangerous sign to ignore. In cases
of doubt, infiltration of local anesthetic
below or at the site of broken ribs may
relieve the pain of associated rib fractures
but will not abolish abdominal guarding or
rigidity which is due to concomitant intra-
abdominal injury. Further, it may also be

difficult to differentiate pain caused by severe contusion of the abdominal wall from the pain of intra-abdominal visceral injury. In contrast to the patient whose main injury is in the abdominal wall, the patient with visceral damage will tend to have less pain on palpation when his head is raised. Where doubt exists, however, it must be assumed that the guarding or rigidity is caused by intra-abdominal intraperitoneal injury.

An abdominal mass following blunt trauma is an uncommon but extremely important finding. Such masses generally represent hematomas of the liver, spleen, mesentery or omentum. A fixed mass or fixed area of dullness (Ballance's sign) in the left upper quadrant is generally due to a subcapsular or extracapsular hematoma of the spleen and may develop only over many days. Dependence on physical examination is less absolute today than formerly, with the acceptance of emergency paracentesis and with the availability of angiography and other radiographic techniques.

Subcutaneous emphysema is an uncommon finding after abdominal trauma, but is always highly significant. Crepitation in the abdominal wall is most likely to result from intrathoracic injury with downward dissection of air, but may also result from injury of the retroperitoneal duodenum or the distal colon or rectum.

A rectal examination should be an integral part of the general examination and is essential if it is even remotely possible that damage may have occurred in the region of the pelvis or perineum. In women, a vaginal and bimanual examination should be added. In a few patients the most suggestive indication of peritoneal irritation may be tenderness high anteriorly in the rectum. Occasionally, gross blood in the rectum is the only early evidence of rectal damage from a penetrating wound or pelvic fracture.

AUSCULTATION. The presence of bowel sounds is a reassuring indicator of peristalsis but is by no means totally reliable in determining whether or not visceral injury has occurred. Active bowel sounds can be heard in the presence of intraperitoneal bleeding or rupture of hollow abdominal viscera in about 30% of patients who have such lesions. Conversely, about 30% of patients who have no bowel sounds preoperatively are subsequently shown to have no visceral damage. While the presence or absence of bowel sounds may be deceptive, these should nevertheless be sought carefully as they serve as a clinical guide.

Although only rarely present, a bruit, often heard better over the back than over the anterior abdomen, may be a valuable sign of an intra-abdominal arterial injury such as a false aneurysm or arteriovenous fistula.

INITIAL CARE

Maintenance of Respiratory and Cardiovascular Function

As with all injuries, the most important initial consideration is maintenance of adequate respiratory and cardiovascular function (Chap. 7). Depending upon the extent of the injury and potential blood loss, two or more large-gauge intravenous catheters should be inserted, with one of the catheters in the superior vena cava for CVP monitoring. Leg veins should be avoided because the inferior vena cava may have been damaged by the abdominal trauma. Blood is drawn for type- and cross-matching, hematocrit and hemoglobin measurements and any other tests suggested by the location or extent of the injury or the patient's other medical problems. Fluids are administered to maintain adequate tissue perfusion and vital signs. The failure of 2000 to 3000 ml of rapidly administered fluid such as Ringer's lactate to restore adequate blood pressure and tissue perfusion strongly suggests that the patient is bleeding massively and may require urgent surgical exploration.

12

Monitoring of vital signs in patients who have multiple injuries in addition to the abdominal trauma is especially important. If enough fluid and blood to replace losses from fractures or lacerations have been administered, further deterioration, often gradual, of the vital signs may be the only clue to continued intra-abdominal bleeding. The margin between the blood volume deficit that can cause hypotension and that which can be lethal may be as little as 1000 to 1500 ml. Consequently, the monitoring of the patient must be done frequently and carefully. This is especially essential in elderly patients who have a reduced margin of reserve and are prone to myocardial infarction due to reduced coronary perfusion.

Nasogastric Tube

PITFALL

FAILURE TO INSERT A NASOGASTRIC TUBE IN ANY PATIENT WHO HAS AN INJURY WHICH MAY CAUSE VOMITING OR A SEVERE ILEUS MAY RESULT IN SUBSEQUENT ASPIRATION AND A HIGH MORTALITY.

Early insertion of a nasogastric tube is particularly important where there is a possibility of intra-abdominal visceral damage or when the patient may have eaten or drunk recently. While the nasogastric tube is of value in diagnosing an injury to the stomach when bright-red blood is found, its role in decompressing the gastrointestinal tract and preventing aspiration of gastric contents is far more important. Aspiration of gastric contents occurs more frequently than is usually recognized. The pulmonary damage following aspiration occurs so quickly that even immediate bronchoscopy and lavage may be of relatively little benefit except for the removal of large solid particles of food. In many instances, aspiration is not suspected until a diffuse bilateral pneumonic process is noted on the chest roentgenograms 48 to 72 hours later. The mortality rate of aspiration is very high, and has been estimated at 70%.[4]

Nasogastric tubes are also invaluable in the removal of excessive air from the stomach. Injured patients tend to swallow air, especially if they are extremely anxious or have any respiratory distress. The patient resuscitated with a face mask may have a great amount of air forced into the stomach. The resulting distension of the stomach not only increases the chances of vomiting and aspiration but also raises the diaphragm, increasing the resistance to ventilation. Air which has entered the small bowel is much more difficult to remove and hinders exploration and subsequent closure of the abdomen. In addition, distended bowel interferes with the return of peristalsis in the postoperative period.

Foley Catheter

Urinalysis should be performed on all patients with suspected abdominal or pelvic damage as a guide both to possible injury of the urinary tract and to the detection of diabetes or concomitant renal parenchymal disease. A spontaneously voided specimen is preferable, as the trauma of insertion of a catheter may in itself cause spurious hematuria. If injury of the urinary tract is suspected, an intravenus pyelogram or cystogram, or both, should be performed as soon as possible. This may be achieved by the addition of 150 ml of Renografin-60 to the balanced salt solution being administered intravenously, resulting in a drip infusion.

The Foley catheter is also valuable as a means of monitoring the urinary output closely, especially where there is evidence of shock or severe hemorrhage. A sustained urinary output of 50 ml or more per hour in a patient who is not receiving a diuretic is sound evidence of satisfactory tissue perfusion in most cases.

Laboratory Studies

The number and type of laboratory studies requested will depend upon the type of surgery contemplated and the urgency of the operation.

COMPLETE BLOOD COUNT. The hemoglobin and hematocrit levels present initially do not usually reflect the amount of recent hemorrhage that has occurred and tend to be deceptively high. Several hours are often required for the customary hemodilution to be accurately reflected in the hematocrit. Nevertheless, these values can serve as a baseline and are important if a general anesthetic is necessary. In general, a hemoglobin level of less than 10.0 gm/100 ml may not provide adequate oxygen transport during anesthesia, especially if the patient is elderly or has a relatively low cardiac output. Trauma usually causes some leukocytosis but injury to the spleen should be suspected in the well-hydrated patient in whom the leukocyte and platelet counts rise rapidly to about 20,000/cu mm and 600,000/cu mm respectively.

SERUM AMYLASE. Serum amylase levels must be interpreted with caution following abdominal trauma. A rising level of serum amylase and subsequent high persistent hyperamylasemia is suggestive but not pathognomonic of pancreatic injury. In a series of 179 patients with blunt abdominal trauma, only 20% had hyperamylasemia and suprisingly few (only 3 of the 36 patients with hyperamylasemia) had pancreatic injuries proven at operation.[5] Equally important, it was reconfirmed that some patients with pancreatic injury may have no rise in serum amylase. Consequently, a raised serum amylase must be placed in proper perspective following abdominal trauma, with the recognition that many patients with hyperamylasemia do not have pancreatic injuries and may in fact have no demonstrable visceral damage. Presumably, in this latter group, spasm of the sphincter of Oddi occurs, especially when certain narcotic drugs such as morphine have been given.

X-rays

When the condition of the patient permits, important information may be derived from radiologic examinations, particularly in patients with gunshot wounds and multiple injuries. In patients with abdominal trauma, flat and upright films of the abdomen and an upright film of the chest are desirable; not infrequently, however, upright films may be precluded by the poor clinical condition of the patient and, in such circumstances, a lateral decubitus film of the abdomen may be substituted. In the presence of severe hemorrhage and shock, it is necessary to exercise judgment in the use of x-rays. Volume replacement and laparotomy obviously have priority when the patient fails to respond to intravenous infusions.

PITFALL

THE DELAY AND EXTRA MOVEMENT OCCASIONED BY AN INSISTENCE ON "ROUTINE" RADIOLOGIC EXAMINATIONS MAY BE DANGEROUS AND EVEN ON OCCASION FATAL.

X-RAYS OF THE CHEST. X-rays of the chest should always be obtained where the patient's condition permits in order to identify any associated intrathoracic disease or injury. In addition to the usual careful examination of the lung parenchyma and pleural cavities, it is important in trauma that the area of the diaphragm be examined very carefully to rule out the possibility of a diaphragmatic rupture. Even minimal abnormalities, especially in the dyspneic patient, may provide the significant clue. Very occasionally, passage of the stomach or the intestines into the left chest may be clearly evident with the patient supine but difficult to determine with the patient upright if the organs have passed back into the abdominal cavity.

X-RAYS OF THE ABDOMEN. Flat films of the abdomen are of most help in locating or discovering radiopaque foreign bodies such as bullets, separation of loops of intestine by fluid, and loss of the psoas muscle outlines, and should be taken in two planes whenever possible. The entrance and exit wounds of any penetration should be covered with radiopaque markers so that the trajectory of the missile or weapon can be determined. A general haziness or ground-glass appearance of the abdomen on x-ray may be caused by the accumulation of fluid or blood in the peritoneal space; however, this generally requires a considerable quantity of fluid and is a late sign of intra-peritoneal hemorrhage. Fractures of lower ribs, spine or pelvis should direct attention to injuries likely to be associated with adjacent organs such as the liver, spleen, small intestine or bladder. Changes in the outline or position of the liver, spleen, kidneys, gastric air bubble and intestine should be noted.

Undue reliance upon upright and lateral decubitus films of the abdomen to demonstrate free air is unwarranted. The most reliable results are obtained when the patient is able to remain upright or on his side for at least ten minutes prior to the radiologic examination to allow air to accumulate under the diaphragm or along the flank. Absence of free air does not, however, rule out intraperitoneal rupture of a hollow viscus, especially of the more distal small bowel.

INTRAVENOUS PYELOGRAPHY. An I.V.P. should be obtained if there is any possibility of renal injury as suggested by the location or severity of the trauma or the presence of hematuria (Chap. 24).

ABDOMINAL ANGIOGRAPHY. Freeark[6] and others[7] have used abdominal angiography as a major diagnostic tool to evaluate abdominal injuries. Angiography has its greatest value in poor-risk patients in whom there is some question about the need for abdominal exploration and in patients suspected of having intravisceral hematomas.

Using the retrograde femoral Seldinger technique, selective arterial studies give maximal information. Where experienced angiographers are not readily available, however, a central aortic flush of about 50 ml of appropriate contrast material (such as Hypaque-M 75 or Renografin-76) at approximately 20 ml/sec may give valuable information. In patients with marked atherosclerosis or in whom pelvic or femoral fractures make access to the femoral arteries difficult, the transbrachial route may be used.

Abdominal Paracentesis

In the 1950s, the technique of four-quadrant needle aspiration of the abdomen was introduced as a diagnostic tool in cases of suspected intra-abdominal hemorrhage. The recovery of nonclotting blood, bile, intestinal fluid or fluid with a high amylase content is highly suggestive of intra-abdominal bleeding or organ damage. This approach was used in comatose patients and in those with multiple severe injuries for whom an unnecessary laparotomy might tip the scales against survival. Unfortunately, false-negative results are so common with simple needle aspiration that a negative tap has no diagnostic significance. As an improvement on this technique, tube paracentesis (without lavage) using a polyethylene catheter through a #15 short-bevel needle has been advocated and a false-negative result of only 1% is claimed.[8]

AXIOM

ALTHOUGH A POSITIVE ABDOMINAL TAP IS OF GREAT DIAGNOSTIC VALUE, A NEGATIVE TAP MUST NEVER BE REGARDED AS DEFINITIVE.

Peritoneal Lavage

In a search for a more accurate diagnostic test of intraperitoneal bleeding following trauma, the concept and technique of peritoneal lavage were popularized in 1965.[9] This procedure has virtually superseded the four-quadrant tap and is most useful in comatose or semicomatose patients with multiple injuries when it may be difficult or impossible to determine whether hypotension is caused by intraperitoneal bleeding or by some other injury.

To perform a peritoneal lavage, a peritoneal dialysis catheter is inserted via a small subumbilical incision after the bladder has been emptied. If no blood, bile, or intestinal fluid can be aspirated through the catheter, the abdominal cavity is irrigated with 500 to 1000 ml of saline through the catheter and, if feasible, the patient is moved from side to side to be sure that the saline reaches all parts of the abdominal cavity. The fluid is then allowed to drain out by gravity.

Some controversy exists about the amount of blood that must be present to constitute a positive test. One criterion has been the ability to read newsprint through a test tube containing the fluid.[10] Others feel that the presence of 100,000 RBC/ml is sufficient to make laparotomy mandatory. Using these criteria, 95% accuracy has been achieved. Since false-negative results occur in about 5% of cases, laparotomy should not be delayed if the patient's clinical state suggests the possible presence of an intra-abdominal lesion.

Stabograms

As long as it was accepted practice to perform a laparotomy for all wounds which penetrated into the peritoneal cavity, even in the absence of clinical evidence of visceral damage, the determination of the depth of any penetrating injury was extremely important. To facilitate this determination and thereby avoid unnecessary laparotomy, Cornell et al. developed the technique of introducing 60 to 80 ml radiopaque contrast material into a Foley catheter sutured tightly into the anesthetized wound.[11] Anterior, posterior and lateral roentgenograms were taken to reveal whether or not the peritoneal cavity contained the contrast material. This technique has been generally abandoned because of an unacceptable number of false-negative results. We prefer to explore these apparently superficial wounds digitally under local anesthesia, even if enlargement of the wound is necessary to provide adequate visualization of the depths. Alternatively, close clinical observation may be sufficient.

Radioisotope Scanning

Scanning is a relatively simple noninvasive technique for outlining certain intra-abdominal organs, especially the liver and spleen.[12] However, whether due to necrosis or subcapsular hematoma, defects of the liver or spleen must be at least 2 cm in diameter to be visualized. More frequent use of this technique will undoubtedly reveal a number of clinically occult lesions in the solid organs following trauma. This information automatically poses fresh problems, especially in dealing with hepatic injuries where it is known that substantial defects may return to normal without operation.

INDICATIONS FOR LAPAROTOMY (Table 1)

Significant intra-abdominal bleeding and visceral damage are the main indications

TABLE 1. INDICATIONS FOR EXPLORATORY LAPAROTOMY FOR ABDOMINAL TRAUMA

Any gunshot wound which, because of its entrance wound, exit wound, or location on x-ray, might have entered the peritoneal cavity.

Penetration of the peritoneum as demonstrated by direct vision or radiographic studies.

Evidence of severe or continuing blood loss which cannot be readily explained by other injuries.

Increasing or severe abdominal tenderness or rigidity.

Deterioration of the patient's general condition and evidence of peritonitis.

Free air demonstrated within the peritoneal cavity or along retroperitoneal tissue planes by x-ray.

Abdominal paracentesis or irrigation revealing blood, bile, air, or intestinal fluid.

An enlarging intra-abdominal or pelvic mass, especially in the absence of pelvic or vertebral fractures.

for laparotomy following trauma. Intra-abdominal bleeding should be strongly suspected when persistent or recurrent hypotension occurs despite ostensibly adequate replacement of blood and fluid. The presence of intra-abdominal bleeding may be confirmed by the demonstration of blood on abdominal paracentesis or peritoneal irrigation or by delineation of damage to the liver, spleen or major vessels on arteriography or scintiscanning.

A progressive fall in the hemoglobin level and hematocrit in the absence of hypotension may also serve as a warning signal of continuing bleeding but 24 to 48 hours are often required for this hemodilution to be apparent. Significant intra-abdominal visceral damage in the absence of hypotension is suspected or diagnosed primarily on the basis of increasing abdominal pain, tenderness, rigidity or evidence of free air. Great potential variation in the development of these signs and symptoms must always be anticipated.

An increasingly conservative approach to penetrating wounds of the abdomen has become apparent in recent years. In addition to the various techniques which aim to provide definitive criteria for operation, physicians must ultimately rely heavily on their clinical judgment and their ability to observe changing clinical signs once the patient is under careful observation in the hospital. Even the presence of protruding omentum is no longer regarded by some as an absolute indication for laparotomy, provided the patient is clinically stable. In selected cases, good results have been claimed for amputation of the protruding omentum with return of the proximal portion to the abdomen.[13]

EXPLORATORY LAPAROTOMY

Preoperative Preparation

Once the decision to perform an exploratory laparotomy has been made, surgery should not be unduly delayed. However, concomitant medical problems such as electrolyte imbalance, acidosis, or diabetes should be corrected prior to surgery wherever feasible. On the other hand, excessive delay tends to cause deterioration of the clinical situation and increases the operative risk.

Although patients obviously respond better to anesthesia and surgery if adequate replacement of the blood volume can be accomplished preoperatively, excessive delay through attempts to restore the blood volume while severe hemorrhage continues may be disastrous. In these circumstances, the infusion of blood and fluid is closely monitored as anesthesia is induced. The surgeon is well advised to stand by the operating table during this critical period. Most general anesthetics cause vasodilatation and an increase in vascular capacitance. Consequently, additional replacement of volume may be required during and just after induction if the chance of further hypotension is to be reduced.

Fractures should be splinted, casted or otherwise immobilized so that the patient may be transported safely to the operating room. Although an endotracheal tube can usually provide an adequate airway, it may be necessary occasionally to perform a tracheostomy preoperatively to assure adequate ventilation in patients with severe associated maxillofacial injuries.

Antibiotics should be started intravenously or intramuscularly preoperatively if there is a suggestion of intra-abdominal contamination so that adequate blood levels may be achieved during operation when hypotension and further disruption of protective mechanisms against the invasion of bacteria may be present[14,15] (Chap. 29). Various antibiotic combinations are available, with some of the current favorites including ampicillin, methicillin, cephalosporins or gentamicin if renal function is adequate. When significant peritoneal contamination from injury to the colon or distal small bowel is present, clindamycin may be added to help control or prevent infection by anaerobic organisms, notably the Bacteroides (Chap. 29).

Anesthesia

The initiation of general anesthesia is potentially an extremely dangerous phase for the patient and the team should be prepared to deal with aspiration, sudden hypotension or cardiac arrhythmias during this time. Since electrocautery may be necessary to obtain hemostasis rapidly, the anesthetist should give preference to the use of a nonexplosive anesthetic. In patients who are in shock, minimal anesthesia may be supplemented by muscle relaxants. In some instances, it may be advantageous to begin the procedure under local anesthesia. This is especially true in poor-risk patients with whom there is doubt as to whether or not a wound has penetrated the peritoneal cavity.

Incisions

Stabs in the flanks or lateral abdomen can often be approached satisfactorily through a transverse or oblique incision in the area of injury. In general, however, a midline incision is preferred because it is relatively bloodless, can be performed rapidly, and allows good exposure to virtually all parts of the abdomen. For gunshot wounds, the midline incision is most desirable because the bullet may ricochet unpredictably and cause widely separated injuries. Occasionally the incision may have to be extended into the left or right side of the chest to obtain adequate exposure to structures immediately under the diaphragm or to concomitant thoracic injuries. More recently, in severe hepatic trauma involving the hepatic veins, extension of the midline incision proximally, splitting the distal end of the sternum, has become popular as a quicker and more effective approach to control of the hepatic veins and supradiaphragmatic inferior vena cava.

Where the patient has a distended abdomen and is in profound shock in spite of rapid infusion of large quantities of fluid and blood, the incision into the abdominal cavity is not uncommonly followed by cardiac arrest within a minute or two. Release of an abdominal tamponade in the severely hypovolemic patient can result in sudden reduction in the venous return to the heart as the previously compressed intra-abdominal veins are permitted to distend. In addition, release of the tamponade may be followed by torrential intra-abdominal bleeding which may not be easy to control immediately. In such seriously injured patients, placement of an adequate number of intravenous cannulas, ready availability of sufficient blood and fluid, and suitable vascular instruments, including an aortic compressor, at the operating table must be assured preoperatively. Furthermore, consideration must be given to the possible desirability of obtaining control of the thoracic aorta through a left thoracotomy before the abdominal incision is made. Once the peritoneal cavity has been opened, blood is rapidly evacuated with large sponges or suction so that the bleeding sites can be quickly controlled. If the source of massive hemorrhage cannot be controlled rapidly, the aorta should be compressed manually at the esophageal hiatus with a large sponge or compressor until more proximal control can be obtained and the sites of bleeding identified.

Technique of Exploration

Once the significant bleeding has been controlled, an orderly exploration of the abdomen should be performed. It is usually advisable to repeat this exploration at the conclusion of the operation as a double check to ensure that no area of injury has been overlooked.

PITFALL

IF AN ODD NUMBER OF HOLES IN THE INTESTINE ARE ATTRIBUTED TO A TANGENTIAL INJURY, A SMALL WOUND ON THE MESENTERIC ASPECT MAY BE EASILY OVERLOOKED.

The bowel must be inspected systematically and meticulously; if a penetrating injury is present, one must demonstrate an even number of holes or prove that the injury to the small intestine is tangential. This concept is extremely important as a small perforation in the mesentery of the small intestine might otherwise be overlooked, resulting in subsequent leakage and peritonitis. Once an intestinal injury is recognized, it should be closed temporarily by a nontraumatic clamp while the initial inspection of the abdomen is completed. Failure to do this often results in the continuing escape of intestinal content and avoidable widespread peritoneal contamination. If there is any suspicion of injury in the lesser sac, this area should be examined by making an opening in the gastrocolic omentum. The transverse colon, posterior wall of the stomach and pancreatic region can then be thoroughly inspected.

Single holes in blood vessels must also be viewed with much skepticism. Where the second hole is not observed, subsequent hemorrhage, false aneurysm or arteriovenous fistula may be anticipated. If only one hole can be found in a vessel, a distal search must be made to ensure that the missile has not migrated down the involved vessel, occluding it or a branch peripherally. It is also important to exclude the possibility of an arteriovenous fistula through an opening into an adjacent vessel which is not immediately apparent.

Whenever a hematoma surrounds the aorta and inferior vena cava, this area should be carefully opened after the blood volume is restored and proximal and distal control of the vessels is obtained.

Peritoneal Irrigation

With the intra-abdominal portion of the operation concluded, some surgeons lavage the peritoneum with large quantities of saline to reduce the bacterial load. The addition of antibiotics is often recommended but their usefulness remains to be proven. Furthermore, neomycin or other aminoglycosides in the irrigating solutions may result in respiratory depression in some patients, and the hazards attendant on their use in this manner often outweigh any potential value.

Drains

The indications, numbers, and types of drains used for any particular intra-abdominal injury vary greatly from surgeon to surgeon. As drains may serve as conduits for infection into the peritoneal cavities, produce erosion of vessels and adjacent organs on occasion and provide egress of blood, pus or other material from a limited area only, the placement should have a specific objective. The principal justifications for the use of drains include pancreatic and extensive hepatic injury and the presence of a grossly contaminated peritoneal cavity. Drains should be soft, accurately placed, intermittently moved, carefully dressed and brought through stab wounds of adequate size in the abdominal wall. Drains should not be used routinely and should not be left in situ once they cease to function.

Closure

The method of closure of the abdomen is also a matter of personal preference. Special precautions, however, are taken in patients with extensive trauma in whom it is anticipated that peritonitis, ileus or respiratory failure may develop. Many surgeons prefer to close the linea alba with a single layer of interrupted figure-of-eight or near-far, far-near #28 wire because such a closure is stronger and less likely to become infected. Unfortunately the use of wire tends to be associated with a high incidence of injury to the surgeon's gloves and hands, increasing the risk of wound infection to the patient and hepatitis to the surgeon. Consequently, most surgeons continue to use nonabsorbable sutures. Large full-thickness retention sutures tied over dental rolls or rubber tubing may add considerable strength to the closure. Where there has been gross contamination of the peritoneal cavity and subcutaneous tissue, as with massive colonic wounds, the skin should not be closed primarily.

SUMMARY (Table 2)

Although increasingly sophisticated techniques are available for the diagnosis of abdominal injuries, decisions for surgery are largely dependent on careful continuous clinical observation and should be individualized. Care must be taken not to limit attention to the abdominal problems, with resultant inadequate appreciation of serious extra-abdominal lesions. A systematic approach to preoperative diagnosis and preparation, intraoperative inspection and repair, and postoperative care and observation for complications is essential for optimal results.

TABLE 2. TEN FREQUENT ERRORS IN THE MANAGEMENT OF ABDOMINAL TRAUMA

1. Failure to observe clinical progress carefully, with consequent failure to recognize the need for emergency surgery at an early stage.
2. Performance of a laparotomy on all patients with penetrating abdominal wounds with little attention to or regardless of the signs, symptoms, or duration of the injury.
3. Concentration on an abdominal injury to the extent that serious or life-threatening extra-abdominal injuries are overlooked.
4. Insistence on "routine" preoperative radiologic studies in the rapidly deteriorating patient.
5. Failure to appreciate the high incidence of aspiration after abdominal trauma and to adequately guard against it.
6. Delayed and incorrect use of antibiotics.
7. Unsystematic examination of the abdomen during laparotomy, thereby increasing the likelihood of missing lesions.
8. Early discontinuation of nasogastric suction in patients recovering from severe abdominal trauma.
9. Insistence on performing a one-stage operation, including skin closure, where a staged procedure would be safer.
10. Inappropriate use of intraperitoneal drains.

REFERENCES

1. Nance, F. C., et al.: Surgical judgement in the management of penetrating wounds of the abdomen: Experience with 212 patients. Ann. Surg., 179:639, 1974.
2. Freeark, R. J.: Penetrating wounds of the abdomen. New Eng. J. Med., 291:185, 1974.
3. Jordan, G. L., and Beall, A. C.: *Diagnosis and Management of Abdominal Trauma, Current Problems in Surgery.* Chicago, Year Book Medical Publishers, 1971.
4. Cameron, J. L.: Aspiration pneumonia: A clinical and experimental review. J. Surg. Res., 7:44, 1967.
5. Olsen, W. R.: The serum amylase in blunt abdominal trauma. J. Trauma, 13:200, 1973.
6. Freeark, R. J.: Role of angiography in the management of multiple injuries. Surg. Gynec. Obstet., 128:761, 1969.
7. Lim, R. C., et al.: Angiography in patients with blunt trauma to the chest and abdomen. Surg. Clin. N. Amer., 52:551, 1972.
8. Montegut, F. J.: Tube pancreatitis without lavage. J. Trauma, 13:142, 1973.
9. Root, H. D., et al.: Diagnostic peritoneal lavage. Surgery, 57:633, 1968.
10. Olsen, W. R., and Hildreth, D. H.: Abdominal paracentesis and peritoneal lavage in blunt abdominal trauma. J. Trauma, 11:824, 1971.
11. Cornell, W. P., et al.: A new nonoperative technique for the diagnosis of penetrating injuries to the abdomen. J. Trauma, 7:307, 1967.
12. Little, J. M., et al.: Radioisotope scanning of liver and spleen in upper abdominal trauma. Surg. Gynec. Obstet., 125:725, 1967.
13. Stein, A., and Lisoos, I.: Selective management of penetrating wounds of the abdomen. J. Trauma, 8:1014, 1968.
14. Fullen, W. D., et al.: Prophylactic antibiotics in penetrating wounds of the abdomen. J. Trauma, 12:287, 1972.
15. Thadepalli, H., et al.: Abdominal trauma, anaerobes and antibiotics. Surg. Gynec. Obstet., 137:271, 1973.

23 SPECIFIC ABDOMINAL INJURIES

A. J. WALT
R. F. WILSON

Whereas the previous chapter was designed to provide an overall approach to the diagnosis and management of abdominal trauma, this section deals with specific abdominal injuries. Since there is an extensive literature available to the interested reader, the main objective here is to draw attention to the more common pitfalls and problems of management rather than to provide a detailed clinical picture of each individual injury.

The relative incidence of organs injured in abdominal trauma varies in different series. In a state-wide study of major abdominal trauma in Connecticut in 1971, 67% of the cases were due to blunt injury, 17% to knife wounds, 14% to gunshots and the remainder to other penetrating trauma.[1] Since blunt trauma is caused mainly by automobiles, tractors, snowmobiles and athletic injuries, it is relatively more common in suburban and rural areas. In contrast, in most urban centers penetrating wounds predominate.

In a consecutive group of 307 patients with blunt abdominal trauma treated at Detroit General Hospital, splenic injury was present in 30%, hepatic injury in 19%, and pancreatic injury in 9%.[2] The small intestine, liver and colon are the organs most frequently injured by penetrating wounds, as reflected in the overall experience of the Ben Taub Hospital where these were involved in 38%, 33%, and 32% of patients respectively.[3]

Certain distinctive constellations of injuries should also be kept in mind because they occur frequently together, especially in blunt trauma. Falls from heights may rupture the pelvis and bladder in addition to fracturing the os calcis and lumbar spine; seat-belt injuries are often associated with damaged lumbar pedicles and tears of the distal ileum or sigmoid; steering-wheel injuries not infrequently damage the liver and spleen in addition to the right lung and ribs.

PITFALL

IF INDIVIDUAL INJURIES ARE VIEWED IN ISO-LATION RATHER THAN AS PARTS OF A PAT-TERN, CERTAIN LESIONS MAY NOT BE APPRE-CIATED UNTIL THEY ARE DIFFICULT TO COR-RECT.

ABDOMINAL WALL

Blunt Injury

Many of the symptoms and signs seen with injury to intra-abdominal organs (nausea, vomiting, tenderness, guarding and rigidity) may also be produced by hematoma of the abdominal wall. The hematoma usually results from hemorrhage into the rectus muscle caused by rupture of the muscle with or without tears of the epigastric vessels. The clinical picture may be difficult to differentiate from intraperitoneal injury. Diagnosis may be aided by the demonstration of a mass which is palpable when the patient sits up tensing his rectus muscle and which cannot be moved from side to side. If an intraperitoneal injury cannot be excluded or if the hematoma is very large and painful, exploration of the abdominal wall and evacuation of the hematoma are indicated. Disruptions of muscle, which are increasingly encountered among wearers of seat belts, should be repaired and the area drained for a day or two if any potential dead space is present or if continued oozing occurs.

Penetrating Injuries

Penetrating injuries of the abdominal wall which are superficial to the peritoneum are usually easy to treat. After thorough debridement and cleansing under local anesthesia, these may be sutured or left open and drained, depending upon the size, nature and duration of the wound.

Less attention has been paid to the large defects of the abdominal wall, such as those which occur with shotgun blasts at close range. These destructive injuries are increasingly met with in civilian life and present some unique problems. In some patients the abdominal wall defect may be so large as to preclude closure with the patient's own tissues. As a further complication, underlying organs, particularly the colon, are so severely damaged that sepsis is almost inevitable. These wounds must be thoroughly debrided after any intraperitoneal injuries have been treated. Many strategies have been advocated where flaps of various size are rotated into the defect; however, many flaps become necrotic because of sepsis or an inadequate blood supply.

The simplest, but not necessarily the most efficient, technique for closing such wounds is the suturing of omentum to the edges of the defect which is then covered with Vaseline gauze and a firm dressing of Owen's cloth or similar material. After a healthy base of granulation tissue forms on the omentum, split-thickness skin grafts can be applied. The ultimate objective is skin closure, which may be speeded by the use of pigskin as a biologic dressing which is changed every 24 to 48 hours. Used in this manner, pigskin may be very helpful in establishing granulations which will accept skin grafts more rapidly. Recently, Silastic sheets have been sewn to the edges of the defect at the time of the initial debridement, with good success. Other surgeons, seeking definitive repair of the defect, have preferred the immediate use of Marlex mesh with coverage provided by a full-thickness skin flap or, where this is not possible, by split-skin grafts. Local antibiotics such as kanamycin or bacitracin may be helpful in reducing the surface bacterial load. Whatever temporary technique is employed, thorough debridement of the area and reduction of sepsis are essential prerequisites.

SPLEEN

The spleen is the intra-abdominal organ most frequently injured by blunt trauma. If damage is confined to the spleen, the mortality rate is only about 1 to 2%.[4] When the spleen is injured with other organs, the mortality rate rises to about 10%. Most splenic injuries are due to automobile accidents but splenic tears or ruptures may also occur during athletic activities, fights and bicycle accidents when trauma is slight or unnoticed. Relatively minor tears of the friable vascular parenchyma can cause severe bleeding.

It has been estimated that 10 to 20% of blunt splenic injuries are followed by delayed rupture.[5] About 75% of these occur during the first two weeks after injury, but some occur only after many months. The hemorrhage may be sudden and sufficiently severe to produce hypovolemic shock rapidly, or it may increase slowly over a period of a few days. Some patients will develop delayed rupture of the spleen following minimal and unappreciated trauma often sustained while drunk. The possibility of delayed rupture must always be explained to the patient and his family before he is discharged from the hospital. In addition, a note of this warning and the instructions given should be made in the chart.

Signs and Symptoms

The signs and symptoms of a torn spleen are principally due to peritoneal irritation and blood loss and reflect the severity and rapidity of hemorrhage, the presence of other injuries and the time between injury and examination. The usual symptoms caused by a ruptured spleen include pain, tenderness, guarding, nausea and vomiting, with about 75% of the patients developing some hypotension. Pain referred to the tip of the left shoulder (Kehr's sign) occurs in about 20% of patients. Rebound tenderness in the upper abdomen is often greater and sometimes more significant than direct tenderness, but pain due to associated fractured ribs may cause clinical confusion. Rarely, when a large extra- or subcapsular splenic hematoma is present, a tender mass can be palpated below the left costal margin or an area of fixed dullness on the left

(Ballance's sign) and shifting dullness on the right may be percussed.

AXIOM

ANY PATIENT—EVEN WITHOUT SYMPTOMS— WHO HAS BEEN IN A SEVERE ACCIDENT OR HAS HAD SIGNIFICANT TRAUMA TO THE ABDOMEN SHOULD BE OBSERVED FOR AT LEAST 6 TO 12 HOURS, WITH FREQUENT AND CAREFUL EXAMINATION OF THE ABDOMEN.

During a period of 6 to 12 hours of observation, most patients in whom the spleen has ruptured will have developed one or more of the clinical symptoms outlined above.

Laboratory Studies

The white blood cell count usually rises rapidly after splenic injury and a leukocytosis of 12,000 to 30,000/cu mm may be present. The hemoglobin level may not fall significantly for 6 to 12 hours even with a fairly substantial blood loss. Occasionally, the platelet count will rise abruptly and associated injury to the pancreas may cause a raised serum amylase.

X-ray Studies

About 40% of patients with ruptured spleens have fractures of the lower left ribs, especially the 9th, 10th or 11th. Other suggestive radiologic findings include an enlarged splenic shadow, distortion of the gastric bubble, loss of definition of the normal outline of the left kidney, the left psoas muscle or the properitoneal fat, and the presence of a left pleural effusion. One or more of these findings are present in about 50% of patients.

Abdominal Angiography

Levi[6] and others have advocated the use of abdominal angiography as a major diagnostic tool in the evaluation of abdominal injuries. Angiography has its greatest value in poor-risk patients in whom the need for abdominal exploration is not clear and for whom an unnecessary laparotomy may constitute an unwarranted risk to life; it seldom must be performed during the phase of acute bleeding, however. In the nonacute phase, angiography by delineating distortions of the splenic vessels has been shown to reflect the type and degree of splenic damage, with few if any false-negative results; occasional false-positives may occur but are rare. Angiography may also be decisive in revealing occult injuries of the liver and kidneys.

Scintiscanning

In patients suspected of having a subcapsular or intraparenchymal hematoma, scintiscanning may be an invaluable technique for the visualization of subcapsular hematomas or filling defects greater than 2 cm, particularly the latter. Identification of minor splenic lesions in the asymptomatic patient poses serious decisions for the surgeon, as it is now well recognized that many minor splenic injuries heal spontaneously. Where small occult lesions are demonstrated, watchful waiting may be a reasonable clinical approach.

Splenectomy

Where reasonable suspicion of splenic rupture exists, exploratory laparotomy should be performed as expeditiously as possible and the spleen removed if it is damaged. The mortality for early splenectomy when the spleen alone is injured is about 1%, but rises above 10% in patients with a delayed rupture. Splenectomy per se is not an indication for drainage. This should be reserved for patients in whom there is continued oozing, associated pancreatic damage or contamination from intestinal wounds.

Complications after splenectomy are not uncommon. Of these, a left subphrenic abscess is the most frequently encountered. Postoperatively, pancreatitis may occur but is usually mild and subsides spontaneously. The dangers of thrombocytosis have probably been overemphasized, but temporary anticoagulation therapy with heparin should be considered if the platelet count rises above 1,000,000/cu mm. Splenic vein thrombosis with extension into the portal vein, causing portal hypertension, is rare.

Splenosis results from the implantation and growth of pieces of disrupted splenic tissue upon various peritoneal surfaces and organs. Although splenosis is usually harmless, intestinal obstruction may occur if implants on adjacent loops of bowel become adherent.

LIVER

In spite of the protection provided by the lower ribs, the size, weight, consistency, location and mobile ligamentous attachments of the liver make this organ particularly susceptible to injury of all types. In a series of 891 patients with liver injuries treated at Detroit General Hospital between 1961 and 1971, the mortality rates of patients with stab wounds was 2.4%, with gunshot wounds, 16.7%, and with blunt injuries, 29.7%.

The outcome of these injuries is related to the nature of the wounding agent, the age and general health of the patient, the delay before treatment is instituted, the degree of shock, and the number and extent of associated injuries. Stab wounds are seldom lethal unless a major vessel is injured concomitantly or the patient has cirrhosis which prevents normal hemostasis. Furthermore, most stab wounds have ceased bleeding by the time they are explored. In contrast, gunshot wounds and blunt injuries have a potentially wide spectrum of complex intrahepatic and extrahepatic damage which can usually be correlated with the type of missile and the speed of impact. The final lesion may range from a neat track with little adjacent ischemic tissue, necessitating little if any debridement, to severe shattering of an entire lobe or more.

In blunt trauma, the pattern of injury may reflect the type of force applied. In falls from heights, a large pulpified segment of liver with an intact Glisson's capsule may be present. With direct blows, a subcapsular hematoma of variable size may occur and enlarge with time. In crush injuries, a lobe—usually the right—is deeply fissured and may be the site of multiple fractures, especially in the posterior superior subdiaphragmatic area. More than 90% of blunt hepatic injuries are accompanied by damage to other intra-abdominal organs, most notably the spleen, kidney and intestine. With penetrating injuries, while any organ may be involved, the diaphragm is injured in more than 50% of patients and pulmonary complications may be anticipated.

The clinical picture may be deceptive, especially in the first few hours after injury. In patients suspected of having possible hepatic injury, the primary objectives are (1) diagnosis, (2) operation, (3) prevention or management of complications.

Diagnosis and Clinical Picture

The diagnosis of hepatic injury after penetrating trauma is made by study of the entrance and exit wounds and the clinical picture, remembering that the dome of the liver extends to the fourth right intercostal space and that the left lobe may extend well to the left of the midline. It should also be noted that missiles may describe a bizarre course, especially when they have ricocheted off bony structures. In blunt trauma, the presence of fractured ribs or abrasions over the chest or abdomen must always alert the physician to the possibility of associated hepatic injury.

When first admitted to the emergency department, patients with liver injuries subsequently proven to be serious will not necessarily be in any unusual distress and may have very few symptoms. There may be little or no hypotension, tachycardia or abdominal distension. Tenderness may be minimal. Over the ensuing hours, however, deterioration may develop gradually or may occur very suddenly as a contained hematoma leaks or ruptures. Rarely, the overt

signs of intra-abdominal hemorrhage and acute pain may appear only after two or three days and, unless a history of injury is elicited, may result in erroneous diagnoses such as ruptured ectopic pregnancy, strangulated intestinal obstruction or acute pancreatitis. A careful history, watchful clinical monitoring and abdominal lavage will usually point to the diagnosis and the need for operation. Angiographic or isotopic scanning studies are of value in the infrequently encountered patient with blunt trauma, hepatomegaly, upper abdominal discomfort and grossly deranged biochemical studies who is nevertheless in a stable clinical condition. Angiography is invaluable where hemobilia or other injury to the hepatic portal vessels is suspected.

Operation

PREOPERATIVE PREPARATION. Laparotomy is essential for hepatic injuries except where delay beyond about 12 to 18 hours has occurred for whatever reason and yet the patient is virtually asymptomatic. Appropriate preparation for operation may determine whether the patient ultimately lives or dies. Certain specific if not unique preoperative features in dealing with hepatic injury are (1) the use of multiple cannulas inserted into the arm veins in the case of sudden torrential hemorrhage, (2) avoidance of leg veins as the inferior vena cava may have been injured, (3) restoration of blood volume and urinary output whenever possible, and (4) assurance that all instruments needed to achieve hemostasis are available. These include instruments to perform sternotomy, thoracotomy, and vena caval or aortic occlusion where necessary.

Special attention is paid to the patient with an abdomen distended by blood who remains hypotensive despite vigorous efforts to restore blood volume. Loss of the tamponading effect of the intact abdominal wall leads to catastrophic bleeding, hypotension and, not infrequently, sudden cardiac arrest when the peritoneum is opened.

In these circumstances, preliminary precautions to provide immediate aortic occlusion through the chest or abdomen must be made and an adequate supply of blood ensured. It has increasingly been the practice on our emergency surgical services to perform a left thoracotomy and supradiaphragmatic aortic occlusion before opening the abdomen to reduce the chances of a sudden cardiovascular collapse and to produce relative hemostasis and a clear field while the pattern of injury is being assessed during the critical initial minutes.

AXIOM

IN BLUNT INJURIES ASSOCIATED WITH FRACTURED RIBS AND IN PENETRATING WOUNDS WHERE THE MISSILE HAS ENTERED THE THORACIC CAVITY, SERIOUS CONSIDERATION SHOULD BE GIVEN TO THE INSERTION OF A CHEST TUBE BEFORE ANESTHESIA IS INDUCED, WHETHER OR NOT A PNEUMOTHORAX IS RADIOLOGICALLY VISIBLE.

When "prophylactic chest tubes" are not inserted in patients with possible penetrating lung damage, the chances of an unrecognized tension pneumothorax developing, particularly during surgery, are substantial.

SURGICAL PROCEDURE. In serious cases, a long midline incision is made to gain rapid access and wide exposure.

Control of Bleeding. Of the deaths following hepatic injury, 75% are due to hemorrhage and a substantial number are due to failure to obtain adequate early control. Direct or manual pressure on a sponge over the injured area is usually effective in producing hemostasis, at least as long as the compression is continued. The blood in the peritoneal cavity is then evacuated and the area of injury inspected. While the hepatic lesion is being tamponaded, associated injuries (splenic laceration, perforated intestine) can be given attention.

If direct pressure fails to control the bleeding, the portal triad is occluded digitally or by a vascular clamp. If this is ef-fective, the bleeding point in the liver can often be identified and transfixed selectively. Where this maneuver fails, consideration must be given to the possibility that the liver may have an abnormal arterial supply. This occurs in about 10 to 20% of patients and usually arises from the superior mesenteric artery or the left gastric artery. More dangerous and more common possibilities to be considered, however, are lacerations of hepatic veins or the retrohepatic inferior vena cava.

Adequate exposure for control of bleeding liver wounds is vital. When the bleeding is arterial, the appropriate hepatic artery may be occluded, temporarily at first or permanently if necessary. Where bleeding originates from the posterior-superior surface of the liver or the hepatic vein-vena caval complex, extension of the incision may be essential. Until recently, the midline incision was usually extended into the right side of the chest; today splitting of the lower half of the sternum is favored as quicker, easier and more efficient in providing direct access to the intrapericardial inferior vena cava and to the hepatic veins.[7] Injuries of these veins are associated with an extremely high mortality rate, but successful salvage of a few patients with such injuries has been effected by the introduction of a temporary intracaval shunt through the right atrium or through the subdiaphragmatic vena cava.[8]

Whenever the bleeding is so excessive that the site of hemorrhage cannot be identified, temporary occlusion of the abdominal or thoracic aorta may be invaluable. When this is necessary, the period of occlusion should be carefully noted. Precautions must be taken to ameliorate potential ill effects on renal function by intermittently releasing the aortic clamp at 15-min intervals while fluids and diuretics are provided in amounts aimed at producing a urinary output of approximately 50 ml/hr.

About 85% of penetrating hepatic injuries are easily managed. Most stab wounds and many low-caliber shotgun wounds have ceased bleeding by the time the laparotomy is performed. Those still bleeding need careful hemostasis by undersewing of the individual bleeding points with or without local debridement, depending on the wounding agent and the degree of parenchymal damage. In some circumstances, approximation of the damaged liver margins by widely placed catgut sutures on liver needles, rather than ligation of individual vessels in the depths of the laceration, may be selected as the more practical method of hemostasis. If this is done, care should be taken not to tie these sutures too tightly. The use of Oxycel pledgets as baffles on the surface may reduce the tendency for the liver sutures to pull through the liver tissue.

AXIOM

SPECIAL ATTENTION MUST BE GIVEN TO ENSURE THAT BLEEDING IS NOT CONTINUING IN THE DEPTHS OF LIVER WOUNDS THAT ARE BEING CLOSED, AS THIS MAY RESULT IN THE FORMATION OF LARGE INTRAHEPATIC HEMATOMAS, SUBSEQUENTLY LEADING TO DELAYED HEMORRHAGE, ABSCESSES OR HEMOBILIA.

Through-and-through bullet wounds are thoroughly drained by the careful positioning of Penrose drains with or without sump tubes near the entrance and exit wounds. If they are not bleeding, these tracts are not disturbed unless they are near the surface where they can be opened to form a trough and then adequately debrided under direct vision. Some surgeons favor the placement of a catheter attached to low suction into the track but this would seem to be unnecessary and potentially harmful.

Debridement. All identifiable ischemic liver tissue is removed as it is a potential source of subsequent sepsis. It is possible to remove hundreds of grams of liver tissue in piecemeal fashion and to produce effective hemostasis subsequently by carefully undersewing the parenchymal vessels and bile radicles. In rare cases, the liver injury consists of a large intrahepatic hematoma with a variable amount of pulpified parenchymal tissue, and resection may be inadvisable where the patient is very ill with multiple injuries or impossible when the lesion involves both lobes. In these circumstances, an effective compromise may be achieved by the insertion into the softened area of a large catheter which is led out of the abdomen through a separate stab wound and attached to gentle suction. The intrahepatic necrotic tissue may gradually drain through the catheter and the intrahepatic defect will hopefully close spontaneously in a few weeks. Formal emergency lobectomy carries a mortality of 30 to 80% in most hands and should not be embarked upon except by experienced teams and with well-defined indications.

Hepatic Artery Ligation

AXIOM

HEPATIC ARTERY LIGATION SHOULD BE CONSIDERED IF BLEEDING FROM A DEEP HEPATIC WOUND CANNOT BE CONTROLLED BY DIRECT SUTURE.

A substitute for lobectomy in severe hepatic bleeding may be found in ligation of the hepatic artery. This technique warrants special attention as a maneuver which at minimal cost is often dramatically effective in achieving hemostasis in large wounds. Mays[10] has advocated this as a safe procedure which, contrary to previous surgical dogma, produces only temporary hepatic dysfunction and is compensated for by development of collateral vessels to the deprived hepatic segment within about 10 hours. Ideally, the right or left hepatic artery should be ligated but, where necessary, the common hepatic artery may be ligated with relative impunity. Our own experience and that of others confirms the efficacy of hepatic artery ligation in selected cases. Subsequent hyperbilirubinemia and enzymatic derangement are generally only moderate and transient, seldom lasting for more than a week. In conjunction with hepatic artery ligation, however, strenuous efforts must be made to maintain normal blood pressure, adequate portal oxygenation and reduced intestinal metabolic activity in the postoperative period. Success is best achieved by fresh blood transfusions, the maintenance of blood volume, adequate ventilation through an endotracheal tube or tracheostomy if necessary, normothermia, antibiotics, and continuous gastric aspiration. Madding[11] has advocated the use of 2 mg of glucagon I.V. as a bolus followed by 2 mg/hr as a method of increasing the splanchnic blood flow during the first critical 72 hours.

Packing. For physicians with relatively little experience who are forced to operate on patients with hepatic injury as grave emergencies and in whom the methods described fail to produce complete hemostasis, the insertion of a large-gauze pack prior to transferring the patient to an appropriate center may be lifesaving. Although properly discouraged because of the poor results obtained with this technique during World War II, such packs are much more likely to be effective under conditions of civilian life. The pack should be carefully removed in 4 to 6 days with all preparations made for further exploration to achieve hemostasis if necessary. By this time, however, the patient should be in a stable condition and attended by an experienced team.

AXIOM

PACKING OF LARGE MASSIVELY BLEEDING LIVER WOUNDS BY THE SURGEON WITHOUT EXPERIENCE IN LIVER RESECTIONS MAY BE LESS DANGEROUS THAN A DESPERATE ATTEMPT AT FORMAL HEPATIC LOBECTOMY.

Drainage. Most surgeons feel that all liver wounds should have some type of external drainage. Whenever hepatic tissue is injured and requires debridement,

suture repair or resection, the possibility of subsequent necrosis of liver tissue and consequent sepsis and fever is to be anticipated. It is, therefore, of vital importance that adequate drainage be provided; in the more severe injuries, removal of the twelfth rib may be necessary to achieve this.

External Biliary Drainage. Over the past decade there has been controversy about the need for routine drainage of the biliary tract following moderate to severe liver injuries. In a prospective randomized study of 189 patients with hepatic trauma, Lucas et al. demonstrated that the presence of a T tube in the common bile duct was associated with a significant increase in morbidity and no decrease in mortality.[12] In the light of these and other reports, there appears to be no indication for routine T-tube drainage except in the presence of damage to the extrahepatic biliary apparatus.

Complications

Complications are frequent in patients with severe liver injury. In many cases the clinical picture may be difficult to decipher initially. For example, transient fever due presumably to necrosis of small amounts of liver tissue frequently occurs during the first week or two and transient jaundice is not uncommon. Hemorrhage from acute erosive gastritis, persistent ileus and wound problems often occur among the more specific complications, of which the following warrant special mention.

SUBPHRENIC AND SUBHEPATIC ABSCESSES

AXIOM

SEPSIS FOLLOWING LIVER TRAUMA IS DUE TO A SUBPHRENIC ABSCESS UNTIL PROVEN OTHERWISE.

Subphrenic and subhepatic abscesses are common following major liver trauma. Such collections, particularly in the subhepatic areas, are difficult to diagnose but should be suspected whenever sepsis develops following liver trauma. Pus or infected hematomas immediately beneath the diaphragm may interfere with movement of the diaphragm and may be associated with atelectasis and collections of pleural fluid. Liver scans, arteriograms, and sonograms may help to confirm the diagnosis of subphrenic or subhepatic collections. Efficient drainage is vital and care must be taken to ensure that the stab wound through which the drains emerge is of adequate size. If the abscess is posterior on the right, drainage is usually best done through the bed of the twelfth rib. Anterior collections and collections on the left are more conveniently approached through an anterior incision, with the position of the drains depending on the location of the abscess.

AXIOM

THE ADMINISTRATION OF ANTIBIOTICS DOES NOT SUBSTITUTE FOR ADEQUATE SURGICAL DRAINAGE.

VENTILATORY INSUFFICIENCY. Liver injuries are often accompanied by pulmonary parenchymal damage, fractured ribs, diaphragmatic injury, postoperative ileus, massive transfusions, associated fractures with some degree of fat embolism and infection. The net result is clearly reflected in the increased physiologic shunting and inadequate ventilatory exchange which characterize these patients. Failure to retain the endotracheal tube and to assist ventilation during the first 48 to 72 hours after a serious hepatic injury or, in selected cases, to perform a tracheostomy results in an increased morbidity and an occasional avoidable mortality.

PITFALL

PREMATURE EXTUBATION AND FAILURE TO PROVIDE VENTILATORY SUPPORT INVITE SEVERE PULMONARY COMPLICATIONS FOLLOWING HEPATIC INJURY.

HEMOBILIA. Hemobilia is not a common complication—only 0.3% in the Wayne State University series—but it may result in preventable mortality. Classically, this entity is characterized by the development of jaundice, discomfort in the upper abdomen and melena with or without hematemesis. About 75% of patients with this complication have their first episode of bleeding more than two weeks after injury and consequently may well be at home when this occurs. The hemorrhage is seldom catastrophic initially and will consist of small quantities of blood intermittently. In some cases these episodes may extend over many weeks and may incorrectly be attributed to a peptic ulcer. As any bleeding may suddenly develop into an exsanguinating hemorrhage, early diagnosis and prompt surgical intervention are essential.

While hemobilia is self-evident where a T tube is in place, the rarity of this complication does not justify the use of prolonged common duct drainage for the purpose of early diagnosis. The diagnosis of hemobilia should be entertained in any patient who develops unexplained anemia, hematemesis or melena and has had a hepatic injury within the past year. If there is active bleeding, a hepatic arteriogram is usually diagnostic; in the nonbleeding patient, the liver scan may be highly suggestive.

When hemobilia is established as the cause of bleeding, surgical treatment consists, where possible, of the unroofing of the intrahepatic cavity, ligation of the bleeding artery and appropriate drainage. In many cases, ligation of the hepatic artery branch outside the liver should be added or may suffice in itself. Occasionally, hepatic lobectomy may be unavoidable, but there appears to be no justification for this approach as the routine procedure.

CLOTTING DEFECTS. Most clotting defects after hepatic trauma are related to platelet deficiencies caused by multiple transfusions of banked blood which contains few, if any, functional platelets. Following destruction or surgical removal of liver tissue, falls in the levels of prothrombin, Factor V, Factor VIII and fibrinogen often occur but seldom to a degree responsible for excessive bleeding. Nevertheless, the freshest blood possible and fresh frozen plasma are most desirable in treating massive injury.

LIVER FAILURE. Hepatic regeneration is possible if only 20% of normal liver tissue remains following elective resection. In trauma, with its prelude of associated injuries, shock, multiple transfusions and gross bacterial contamination, the results of large resections are far less satisfactory. The most strenuous efforts must be directed toward the maintenance of hepatic perfusion, perihepatic drainage, control of sepsis, intestinal rest, and the provision of albumin and 200 gm or more of glucose daily to afford maximal protection against hepatic failure.

EXTRAHEPATIC BILIARY TRACT

Free bile anywhere in the abdomen suggests injury to the liver, extrahepatic biliary tract, or duodenum and demands thorough exploration of all these structures. Where there is associated hemorrhage from the portal vein or hepatic artery, the bleeding points can usually be controlled by direct digital compression until a rubber-shod or soft clamp can be applied to the structures proximal to the site of injury. If avoidable, hepatic blood flow should not be occluded for more than 15 minutes in these patients, who are often hypovolemic and hypotensive.

Failure to identify injuries to the extrahepatic biliary tract or adjacent structures may be lethal. Acute complications include hemorrhage and bile peritonitis. More chronic problems include jaundice, ascites, acholic stools, hepatic failure and general deterioration. Bile staining without an obvious source after thorough exploration makes an intraoperative cholangiogram mandatory.

Gallbladder and Cystic Duct

Injuries to the gallbladder or cystic duct are usually treated by cholecystectomy. In poor-risk patients, or when other injuries suggest some advantage to biliary tract drainage, a cholecystostomy might be considered as an alternative.

AXIOM

NO STRUCTURE IN THE PORTAL TRIAD SHOULD BE LIGATED UNTIL ITS ANATOMY HAS BEEN CLARIFIED.

Common Bile Duct

Isolated injuries of the common bile duct are rare and occur almost exclusively as a result of blunt trauma. The usual site of disruption is at the junction of its mobile and fixed segments just above the pancreas. Transection may be complete or partial.

The clinical picture reflects the severity of any associated injuries. When these injuries are extensive, attention may be drawn from the biliary tree and biliary leakage may be recognized only postoperatively when the patient develops a bile peritonitis. When the common bile duct alone is injured, the mild initial symptomatology may be deceptive in that the extravasating bile may be small in volume and rapidly diluted, temporarily loculated, or predominately confined to the retroperitoneal tissues. Consequently, rebound tenderness, pain, fever, and jaundice may develop only after a few days. Very rarely, when damage to the duct is primarily ischemic, gradual stenosis may occur and produce the signs of biliary obstruction many months after the injury.

At operation, the site of injury can be established by intraoperative cholangiography or by the injection of saline or diluted methylene blue. Most cases of disruption after blunt trauma do not lend themselves to primary repair and are best treated by a Roux-en-Y choledochojejunostomy. In the unusual circumstance where a localized segment of the wall has been injured by perforating trauma, limited resection with repair over a T tube inserted above or below the anastomosis may be feasible. It is essential to avoid excessive tension, as this interferes with healing and may lead to later stenosis.

Hepatic Ducts

Injuries to the right or left hepatic ducts are even rarer than those of the common bile duct following trauma and cause more difficult problems by virtue of the small size of the ductal structures. In desperate circumstances, the severed duct may be drained externally or ligated with the knowledge that the possibility of subsequent hepatic sepsis is substantial. Where possible, however, repair is carried out over a small ureteral catheter which may be left as a stent for many months. Occasionally, a Roux-en-Y hepaticojejunostomy may be required.

Hepatic Artery and Portal Vein

If a hepatic artery is injured in such a manner that repair is feasible, it should be done. Alternatively, ligation may be performed (see *Liver Injuries*). Injury to the portal vein may be hidden in a retroperitoneal hematoma, and massive hemorrhage may occur only when the tamponade is released. Where possible, direct repair should be performed. Where this is not possible, a portacaval or mesocaval shunt may be unavoidable but the chances of operative success in these circumstances are minimal. Moreover, patients with normal livers may have severe problems of "meat intoxication" following a portacaval shunt.

DUODENOPANCREATIC INJURIES

Injuries of the duodenum and pancreas should be considered both singly and in combination as the damage to one may profoundly influence both the clinical picture and the management of the other.

Blunt Duodenal Injury

The mortality rate from blunt duodenal injury has fallen from about 90% in 1910 to approximately 15% today, but this figure may be reduced still further if diagnosis and treatment are approached systematically. Unfortunately, the 25% of patients who have isolated blunt duodenal injuries often present relatively mild or vague symptoms. Duodenal injury itself seldom results in death if recognized and appropriately treated within 24 hours. When patients are neglected beyond that time, the mortality rate rises precipitously.[14] Complications in patients who reach the hospital alive are most often from associated injuries, especially to the pancreas.

CLINICAL PICTURE. The history is important in that most of the blunt injuries to the duodenum are due to automobile accidents or direct blows to the upper abdomen. Most of the victims have been driving automobiles and have been struck in the right upper quadrant of the abdomen by the steering wheel. Apparently minor blows may cause serious injury to the duodenum. Unlike patients who suffer blunt trauma to the liver, relatively few with isolated duodenal injuries have associated chest or pulmonary damage.

Initially, the patient may not experience any pain, especially if he is intoxicated. With time, pain develops in the right upper quadrant and nausea, vomiting and fever follow. With further neglect, an ileus may develop and signs of frank peritonitis or septicemia may appear.

ANATOMY OF THE INJURY. Duodenal injuries are most common in the second part of duodenum but about 25% are found in fourth part, close to the ligament of Treitz. Consequently, this latter area must always be carefully inspected by incising the peritoneum and working gently under the lower border of the pancreas. Unless this is done, a tear may be easily missed in this area. The size of any associated hematoma does not necessarily reflect the severity of the injury. Most duodenal lacerations are transverse in direction. The majority involve less than 50% of the diameter, but many are greater than this. The mucosa tends to pout widely and, consequently, special care should be taken in repairing the rent. Occasionally, associated injuries, particularly to the liver, pancreas, inferior vena cava, right kidney and mesenteric vessels, may dominate the picture. In penetrating injuries, no organ in the peritoneal cavity is immune from injury. Therefore, a laparotomy must always be extremely thorough.

Unfortunately, about half the patients with duodenal injuries have associated pancreatic damage of varying degree, ranging from severe contusion to laceration or rupture. Very occasionally the pancreas may be intact but separated in part from the medial border of the duodenum, causing concern about the status of the common bile and pancreatic ducts. Associated pancreatic injuries raise the mortality rate of duodenal injuries from about 5% to 40%.

INVESTIGATION

PITFALL

IF AN INTENT SEARCH FOR RETROPERITONEAL AIR IS NOT MADE ON PLAIN X-RAYS OF THE ABDOMEN, THE DIAGNOSIS OF TRAUMATIC RUPTURE OF THE DUODENUM WILL GENERALLY BE GREATLY DELAYED AND THE MORTALITY RATE WILL BE EXTREMELY HIGH.

The diagnosis of an isolated rupture of the duodenum is often very difficult. X-rays of the abdomen may provide the only early clue by demonstrating retroperitoneal air along the right psoas muscle, duodenum or kidney, or obliteration of the right psoas shadow. Retroperitoneal air can be easily missed unless a careful search is made for a series of tiny bubbles in those areas and to the right of the transverse processes of T-12 and L-1. Even in retrospect, however, the plain films are not helpful in about half the cases. Where uncertainty still exists, administration of a water-soluble radiopaque material through the nasogastric tube, which is then clamped, may demonstrate the duodenal leak. Because the ultimate prognosis is largely dependent on the time

lag between injury and surgical correction, this technique should be used without hesitation.

AXIOM

SERUM AMYLASE LEVELS CAN BE EXTREMELY DECEPTIVE IN PATIENTS WITH ABDOMINAL TRAUMA.

Serum amylase levels may be elevated in patients without pancreatic injury and may be normal in others with severe pancreatic damage. In fact, the highest levels of serum amylase have been found in patients with rupture of the duodenum with leakage of duodenal content into the peritoneal cavity. In patients with continuing abdominal pain, paracentesis with careful examination of the returning fluid for bile or blood may be of great value. A disappointing number of negative results, however, have been obtained in patients subsequently shown to have lesions requiring urgent surgery. This is most apt to occur in patients in whom the duodenal tear and leakage are confined to the retroperitoneal space. Arteriography has been recommended as a further method of investigation. Where there is sufficient suspicion to arouse conjecture, a laparotomy rather than further radiologic studies is called for in most cases.

OPERATION

PITFALL

IF RETROPERITONEAL HEMATOMAS OVERLYING THE DUODENUM ARE NOT OPENED SO THAT THE BOWEL CAN BE EXAMINED CAREFULLY, SERIOUS TEARS MAY BE COMPLETELY MISSED.

At operation, retroperitoneal tears of the duodenum are recognized by the associated retroperitoneal hematoma which may also contain obvious air, bile, chyme or pancreatic juice. Consequently, all hematomas in this area must be opened and the structures carefully inspected. Isolated duodenal injuries, which make up less than half the cases, seldom present serious problems if they are diagnosed and repaired in less than 24 hours. A two-layer suture closure of the laceration with nonabsorbable sutures and good drainage of the area will usually be adequate. In the delayed or more complex cases, a tube inserted into the duodenal loop to decompress the damaged bowel may be added, but this is seldom necessary.

Duodenal fistulae frequently occur as a sequel to a delayed repair of a recognized lesion or failure to diagnose the injury at the initial operation. This complication is obvious if drains are still in situ. When no drain is present, the signs and symptoms, such as pain which may be referred to the back, fever and other signs of sepsis with some degree of ileus, are relatively nonspecific. These side fistulae rarely close spontaneously. The general approach to this serious complication, which carries a mortality rate of about 50%, includes restoration of blood volume, administration of antibiotics, intravenous hyperalimentation and subsequent operative repair of the lesion. Approaches which have been advocated for treating traumatic duodenal fistulae include the use of direct suture (which is usually not feasible), an onlay graft of jejunum, an exclusion procedure, or pancreaticoduodenectomy (Whipple procedure). The most effective and safest operative approach is usually jejunoduodenostomy using a Roux-en-Y loop sutured directly over the fistula.

Combined Pancreatic and Duodenal Injuries

In combined duodenopancreatic injuries, three degrees requiring increasingly extensive procedures may be recognized.

1. Duodenal laceration with mild pancreatic contusion is treated by local repair of the duodenum, with or without reinforcement by an onlay graft of jejunum, gastrostomy and duodenal decompression, thorough drainage of the area and delayed or secondary closure of the abdominal wound.

2. Where the damage to the duodenum is extensive but amenable to local repair and the pancreas is damaged but not completely smashed, a more extensive operation must be considered. The basic aim in these circumstances is to put the injured bowel at physiologic rest. The technical features of the operation may be summarized as follows;
   a. The injured duodenum is converted to a controlled end-fistula by creation of a tube duodenostomy rather than placing the patient at risk from the development of a large side fistula.
   b. A gastrojejunostomy is constructed to bypass the duodenal repair and to decrease pancreatic stimulation.
   c. The distal stomach is removed to reduce gastric acid.
   d. A vagotomy is added to reinforce the acid reduction and to decrease the chances of a stomal ulcer developing.
   e. Bile is diverted from the duodenum by a T tube placed in the common bile duct.
   f. Extensive drainage of all areas is ensured.

3. Where a large segment of duodenal wall is destroyed and local repair is not possible or where the head of the pancreas is so grossly disrupted or pulpified that any procedure short of resection would predictably fail, there is no alternative to pancreaticoduodenectomy. Many of these patients are young and healthy immediately prior to operation and a number of survivors have been reported.[15] Pancreaticoduodenectomy for trauma should not be confused with the same operation performed in the debilitated individual suffering from malignancy. While controversy exists as to whether the remaining pancreas should be resected or implanted into the jejunum, with or without duct ligation, we have preferred simple implantation.

Intramural Hematomas of the Duodenum

Intramural hematomas of the duodenum are being recognized with increasing frequency and merit special consideration. These lesions may occur at any age but are more common in children. In adults, many of the patients are alcoholics and fail to give a clear history of trauma. The full symptom complex frequently takes time to unfold and nausea and vomiting may appear only after a few days. Nevertheless, there is almost invariably progressive discomfort in the right upper quadrant from the start, ranging from a dull ache to severe pain. A palpable mass is seldom present but local guarding is frequently observed. Depending on the site and extent of the hematoma, the vomitus may or may not be blood stained but, since most cases occur in the distal portion of the duodenum or in the upper region of the jejunum, bile is frequently seen. The diagnosis, once entertained, is easily confirmed following the oral administration of water-soluble radiopaque materials. These reveal the lumen to be partially and eccentrically obstructed with a characteristic "coiled-spring" appearance. In a few patients, obstruction may be complete but this rapidly regresses. Where doubt exists, peritoneal lavage may help to exclude the possibility of other intraperitoneal injuries.

As most of these hematomas resolve spontaneously within 5 to 14 days, a nonsurgical approach, using nasogastric suction and intravenous fluid replacement, should be tried. Even with retroperitoneal perforation excluded by clinical and radiologic observations, close supervision is essential as delayed perforation may occur within the first week, presumably through a partially ischemic area of the duodenal wall. In the few cases in which surgical treatment is deemed to be necessary, a thorough laparotomy with delineation of the extent of the hematoma and meticulous confirmation that there is no concomitant duodenal laceration is essential. Treatment may then consist of transverse incision of the serosa and muscularis of the duodenum, as nearly complete evacuation of the hematoma as is possible, closure of the incision in two layers of interrupted silk, and thorough drainage of the paraduodenal area. In some cases there may be understandable but probably not well-founded concern about the viability of the bruised bowel. Where this occurs a loop of jejunum can be sewn to the surrounding uninjured duodenal wall as an onlay graft to provide added insurance. The addition of a gastrojejunostomy—which in turn demands a vagotomy—is very rarely justifiable.

Pancreatic Injuries

ETIOLOGY AND ANATOMIC LESIONS. The incidence of pancreatic trauma is increasing and comprehensive reports are available.[16,17] About two thirds of the injuries are caused by penetrating lesions and about one third by blunt trauma. The spectrum of the injury is wide and the pancreas may be contused, lacerated, fractured, or totally disrupted. The damage may be minor, as in many stab wounds, or massive as with gunshot wounds. Blunt trauma may cause contusions and hematomas only but may also produce severe shattering from direct compression of the pancreas between the striking force and the retroperitoneal tissues. Fractures usually occur at the junction of the body and head of the pancreas where the pancreas overlies the vertebral column.

Isolated injuries of the pancreas are uncommon.[18] In blunt trauma, certain unique patterns of associated visceral damage are well recognized[19] and must be looked for, as such injuries, initially occult, may ultimately cause severe morbidity or death. Where the right upper quadrant is the epicenter of the blow, the organs situated in the area of the pancreatic head are pushed upward into the chest or downward into the lower abdomen. As the liver is displaced upward and the duodenum and pancreas downward, the gastroduodenal artery and common bile duct may tear at their relatively fixed connection to the pancreas. These tears may be complete, in which case severe symptoms develop immediately, or incomplete, in which a slowly evolving and often confusing clinical picture is produced. In these circumstances, the liver is apt to tear along its suspensory ligaments while the downward movement of the transverse colon may cause disruption of the mesentery and its vessels.

PITFALL

IF A LACERATION OF THE MAIN PANCRE-
ATIC DUCT IS NOT RECOGNIZED AND TREATED
PROPERLY, A LARGE CHRONIC FISTULA OR
PSEUDOCYST WILL ALMOST INVARIABLY DE-
VELOP.

In all pancreatic injuries, the integrity of
the pancreatic ducts is extremely important
but may be very difficult to assess in the
presence of a large overlying hematoma.
While immediate pancreatography through
a duodenotomy or through the transected
tail has been advocated,[20] this is difficult
to accomplish in emergency circumstances
and will frequently increase the risk to the
severely injured patient. Adequate drainage of the area is a much safer approach,
accepting the chance of a subsequent controlled pancreatic fistula or pseudocyst. The
former will usually close spontaneously
within three to six weeks; the latter can be
safely dealt with later. In either event, direct visualization of the ductal pattern can
be obtained in the convalescent patient by
means of sinograms or peroral endoscopic
pancreatography.

The mortality rate for pancreatic injury
varies with the causative lesion. Stab
wounds carry a mortality rate of less than
10%, whereas gunshot wounds have a mortality rate of about 25% and shotgun
wounds have a mortality rate in excess of
60% because of the more extensive damage
to both the pancreas and adjacent structures. Isolated blunt injury of the pancreas
is seldom lethal, but when combined with
injury to associated organs has a mortality
rate of approximately 50%. Injury to the
pancreatic head is more lethal than injury
to the body and tail, as these latter are far
more easily managed.

DIAGNOSIS. Pancreatic trauma must be
suspected in any patient who has suffered
middle or upper abdominal blunt or penetrating injury. An elevated serum amylase
in the order of 500 to 600 Somogyi units is
highly suggestive where the patient has not

received narcotics or does not have perforated bowel. In an appreciable number
of cases, however, the amylase is normal
or only transiently elevated in the first 24
hours. In such circumstances, some help
may be obtained by the measurement of
urinary amylase or by measurement of the
amylase in fluid obtained by abdominal
paracentesis. Prolonged elevation of the
serum amylase suggests the development
of a pseudocyst. Hyperamylasemia alone in
association with abdominal trauma does not
constitute an indication per se for abdominal exploration.

AXIOM

HYPERAMYLASEMIA IN AND OF ITSELF IS
NOT AN INDICATION FOR LAPAROTOMY WHEN
THE CLINICAL SIGNS OF PANCREATIC OR IN-
TESTINAL INJURY ARE NOT PRESENT.

PATHOPHYSIOLOGY. The high mortality
rates associated with trauma to the pancreas reflect the fact that this organ is extremely vascular, contains a vital duct
which is susceptible to trauma and is closely
surrounded by a large number of organs
and large vessels. In addition, significant
concomitant damage to the duodenum,
spleen, kidneys and liver and overlying intestine is frequently encountered. Damage
to the pancreatic duct results in extravasation of pancreatic enzymes into the parenchyma of the pancreas and surrounding
tissues. These enzymes when activated may
cause severe local digestion, inflammation
and necrosis of tissue with a large loss of
fluid and blood into the area. The resultant
hypovolemia may in itself be extensive
enough to cause shock; however, the vasoactive substances (e.g. bradykinin) which
are released can produce a severe vasodilatation which may account for a large
portion of the severe systemic hemodynamic changes.

Long-term severe complications can be
caused by the continued loss of the exocrine pancreatic secretions through pan-

creatic fistulae or by the development of a pancreatic pseudocyst. The main cause of death, however, is postoperative hemorrhage or infection, which may occur locally or in the subphrenic areas. Knowledge of the pathophysiology should influence decisively the type of surgical treatment adopted.

TREATMENT. Thorough hemostasis in the pancreatic area and efficient drainage are the two most important principles of treatment. Bleeding from simple stab wounds of the pancreas can usually be managed easily by suture ligation and external drainage. Adequate drainage of all pancreatic injuries cannot be overstressed. Penrose drains with or without sump tubes may be used but, where the latter are employed, great care should be taken to place these accurately so that they do not press or lie against adjacent bowel or vessels.

PITFALL

IF A RIGID SUMP TUBE IS ALLOWED TO LIE AGAINST BOWEL OR LARGE VESSELS, IT MAY ERODE INTO THESE STRUCTURES.

Drains are left in situ as long as drainage continues but for not less than a week. Most fistulae, if well drained, will close spontaneously within a few weeks unless they involve the major pancreatic duct.

At surgery it is sometimes very difficult to determine the extent and severity of the pancreatic injury, as the area in question may be covered by a large hematoma. This hematoma should always be opened and the area gently explored. Where a laceration of the pancreatic parenchyma has occurred, it is not necessary to insist on obtaining a cosmetic approximation of the tissue and capsule of the pancreas. Meticulous hemostasis is the primary aim following cautious debridement of any tissue which is obviously nonviable. Lacerated pancreatic tissue should be suture-ligated using nonabsorbable suture, and thorough hemostasis should be obtained. An attempt

is made by gentle dissection to delineate the area of the main pancreatic duct, but care should be taken to avoid occlusion of the duct by a suture because the presence of hematoma and contusion may make the anatomy of the area obscure. Careful judgment must be exercised as extensive exploration in the face of an obscuring retroperitoneal hematoma is difficult, sometimes hazardous, and often nonproductive. If only the small pancreatic ducts are disrupted, leakage of pancreatic juice will almost always cease spontaneously. When larger ducts are damaged, a continuing fistula may form; however, this can generally be satisfactorily and safely managed by current methods of support.

Postoperatively, essential therapy includes fluid and electrolyte replacement, intestinal rest, and, in selected cases, intravenous hyperalimentation to provide nutrition and to reduce the quantity of pancreatic secretions. Some have advocated the administration of atropine but this is probably of little benefit.

In those patients in whom the pancreas is found to be transected—and this usually occurs over the spinal column—the definitive treatment is distal pancreatectomy. Attempts to achieve direct end-to-end approximation of the duct and repair of the pancreatic parenchyma or to anastomose a Roux-en-Y loop of intestine to the two transected surfaces of the pancreas prolong the operation and are unnecessary and hazardous. Loss of up to 80% of the pancreas does not result in significant subsequent exocrine deficiency.

Decisions on the management of severe trauma to the head of the pancreas are much more difficult to make with confidence. In most cases, meticulous external drainage of the area produces the best results. The pancreas tends to heal slowly but steadily, and persistent or recurrent subsequent pancreatitis is very uncommon. On the whole, there has been an excessive fear about the morbidity associated with pancreatic fistulae following trauma, leading to ill-fated attempts to perform definitive procedures in the severely ill patient. Most fistulae, even when originating from the main duct, will heal over a period of two or three months. Where a fistula does not heal, subsequent elective operation with placement of a Roux-en-Y loop of jejunum over the point in the pancreas from which the fistula originates is much easier and safer in the patient who is metabolically and hemodynamically stable.

A number of successful cases of primary pancreaticoduodenectomy have been described. The indications are difficult to define but would include: (1) gross shattering of the head of the pancreas, as is occasionally encountered with shotgun injuries and very severe blunt trauma, (2) combined damage to the head of the pancreas and the duodenum, in which the vascular supply to one or the other organ has been completely disrupted or where continuity of a large section of the duodenal wall has been destroyed, and (3) damage to the retropancreatic portal vein. Surprisingly, pancreaticoduodenectomy in some cases of trauma may be easy, in that the hematoma has clearly defined the tissue planes for dissection.

COMPLICATIONS. Some of the more important complications of pancreatic damage include fistulae, pseudocysts, abscesses, and delayed hemorrhage. Occasionally a pseudocyst will rupture, causing pancreatic ascites. If much of the pancreas is destroyed, malabsorption may be caused by reduced pancreatic exocrine secretion and diabetes mellitus may rarely result because of a severe reduction in the number of functioning islets of Langerhans. The fistulae and pseudocysts can often be treated without surgery; however, large persisting pseudocysts should be treated with internal drainage where possible.

STOMACH

Although the stomach is frequently injured by penetrating wounds of the upper abdomen and lower chest, it is seldom torn as a result of blunt trauma. If vomitus or gastric aspirate is bloody, an injury to the stomach should be suspected. However, it is not uncommon to find small amounts of blood in the gastric aspirate even though laparotomy reveals no grossly apparent lesion. If there is any reason to suspect a gastric injury, the gastrocolic omentum must be widely opened at surgery so that the entire posterior surface of the stomach may be completely inspected. If there is any blood in the gastrohepatic ligament, the lesser curvature of the stomach must be examined particularly closely.

Wounds of the stomach generally heal very well and seldom leak, unless there is a distal obstruction or a severe infection develops in the area. If prolonged gastric decompression seems necessary and there is a strong likelihood that the patient will develop respiratory complications, a gastrostomy should be considered. If there has been any spillage of gastric or other intestinal contents into the peritoneal cavity, this should be completely removed and the soiled portions of the abdomen completely irrigated. Special attention should be given to cleansing and irrigating the subphrenic and subhepatic spaces and the pelvis.

SMALL BOWEL INJURIES

Etiology

Injuries of the small intestine following blunt trauma often occur at the junction of a mobile and a fixed segment of bowel. The fixity may be due to normal peritoneal attachments or adhesions from previous surgery or inflammation. Sudden deceleration which causes the mobile portion of bowel to move away from its point of fixation causes the tear. These injuries are frequently encountered near the ligament of Treitz and the ileocecal junction. Rarely, adhesions will involve a portion of the bowel in such a manner that during sudden compression of the abdomen a closed-loop phenomenon is created with a resultant blowout of the area. Occasionally, direct trauma from a blow or a seat belt[21] may be responsible for the damage which occurs at the point of impact.

Diagnosis

Most patients with perforated small intestine will exhibit some degree of abdominal rigidity. Where operation is delayed beyond 12 hours, the prognosis deteriorates steeply. Lacerations of the lower small bowel may be particularly deceptive, however, as surrounding loops may wall off the damaged area quickly and efficiently. In such cases, the patient may appear relatively well for many days apart from localized tenderness and a later mild ileus. Free air may never be visible radiographically and bowel sounds may persist. Such patients may eat and have bowel movements for a week or more before fever and other signs of intraperitoneal sepsis appear. In doubtful cases, paracentesis may be helpful by revealing the presence of blood, bile, intestinal contents, vegetable matter or organisms on gram smear. Occasionally, damage may occur to the mesentery without involving the bowel. Minor tears are of little significance, but large hematomas may ultimately compress the adjacent mesenteric vessels and cause intestinal ischemia with later perforation.

During any laparotomy for possible intra-abdominal injuries, the entire small bowel should be meticulously examined. Each hole, as it is encountered, should be clamped or partially sutured so as to prevent further leak and contamination of the peritoneal cavity during the remainder of the exploration. The wounds of entrance and exit on the abdominal wall cannot be used to predict the likely site of a small bowel injury because of the mobility of the small intestine and the variability of the patient's position at the time of injury.

PITFALL

IF THE MESENTERIC BORDER OF THE BOWEL IS NOT EXAMINED CLOSELY IN PATIENTS WITH PENETRATING ABDOMINAL WOUNDS, PARTICULARLY IF AN ODD NUMBER OF PERFORATIONS IS FOUND, UNOBTRUSIVE BUT POTENTIALLY LETHAL HOLES IN THIS AREA MAY BE OVERLOOKED.

Treatment

Lacerations of the small bowel are sutured in two layers after removal of any tissue which is even questionably nonviable. Care is taken to avoid excessive narrowing of the bowel by the repair. Where damage to the bowel wall is extensive, where multiple holes are situated fairly close to one another or where there is a large associated mesenteric hematoma, resection of the involved bowel rather than repair of the individual holes is preferred. Removal of the extensively damaged intestine is generally faster and safer, provided a sufficient length of viable bowel remains to permit adequate absorption of food later.

COLON, RECTUM AND ANUS

Etiology

About 90% of wounds of the colon and rectum are due to gunshots or stabs. Another 5% result from iatrogenic perforations following sigmoidoscopy, colonoscopy, biopsies, fulgurations or barium enemas, or accidental impalement or rupture by a jet of compressed air or a foreign body. Automobile seat belts, falls from heights and direct blows account for the 5% attributable to blunt injury. While the initial clinical picture may vary widely with the different etiologic factors, certain basic principles of management are broadly applicable.

The mortality rate in most large series is about 12 to 18%. Of cases treated at Detroit General Hospital over the past decade, 15.5% died, mostly from hemorrhage or sepsis and rarely from the colonic injury itself. This group had an average of two associated visceral injuries per patient; those who died on the operating table required about 13 units of blood each. The mortality rate among stab wounds was 2.2%, in contrast to 12.2% for gunshot wounds and 50% in shotgun injuries. Colonic wounds are seldom isolated and the ultimate mortality usually reflects the number and variety of extracolonic injuries. Whereas fewer than half of the stab wounds had damage to viscera other than colon, 80% of gunshots and 100% of shotgun wounds did.

Diagnosis

PITFALL

FAILURE TO CLOSELY EXAMINE THE ANAL AND GLUTEAL AREAS MAY RESULT IN OVERLOOKING IMPORTANT PENETRATING INJURIES.

With penetrating wounds near the pelvis, the anal and gluteal regions should always be carefully inspected in a good light, as small wounds may be hidden. These wounds may be associated with critical internal injuries. A rectal examination is essential and the color of the stool should be noted. Where blood is seen in the stool, proctoscopy and, where feasible, sigmoidoscopy should follow. Plain x-rays of the abdomen, with entrance and exit wounds marked, may be helpful in demonstrating the track of the missile, the presence of free air or associated fractures.

PITFALL

UNLESS ALL BULLETS ARE ACCOUNTED FOR, SERIOUS INJURIES MAY BE MISSED.

If no exit wound is visible, special attention must be given to the x-rays of the chest and limbs, as missiles sometimes pursue very unpredictable courses.

In view of the proximity and importance of the sacral plexus, a neurologic examination, including the state of the anal sphincter, should be recorded in case paralysis is present or occurs later. Skin abrasions or tears of the rectus muscle which may be attributable to injury by a seat belt should

be noted, especially as these lesions may have a prolonged and sometimes deceptive clinical unfolding.

Management

Whenever colonic or rectal injury is suspected, intravenous antibiotics effective against colonic bacteria should be started immediately. Penicillin and gentamicin and, in cases of unquestioned fecal spillage, clindamycin are the most effective combinations. If exploration subsequently proves to be negative, antibiotics are stopped. Despite some theoretical objections, administration of antibiotics for a short time has not been shown to be harmful to the patient.

If they have not been neglected to the point where peritonitis has resulted, most stab wounds are easily repaired by a one- or two-layered closure and local drainage. While sepsis sometimes occurs, death is unusual except where there is associated major injury to adjacent structures.

Gunshot wounds present the main challenge to judgment in civilian injuries. The central objective is to reduce the period of hospitalization without jeopardizing the safety of the patient. With the recognition that extrapolation to civilian conditions of military experience where high-velocity missiles dominate is not valid, an increased flexibility of management has been increasingly accepted.[22]

Decisions need to be tempered by the degree and duration of shock, the extent of peritoneal contamination, the character of any severe concomitant injuries and the age of the patient if over 50. All these factors adversely affect both prognosis and the healing of intraperitoneal anastomoses and thus encourage conservatism.

Where these factors do not pertain, small wounds of the bowel wall caused by low-velocity bullets may be trimmed, the adequacy of the blood supply confirmed, and a primary repair performed without a defunctioning colostomy. On the other hand, in the patient severely injured by a gunshot wound, the simplest, quickest and safest procedure is the time-honored exteriorization of the lesions where feasible, or resection, wide local drainage and the establishment of a proximal colostomy and distal mucous fistula.

In extensive damage to the right side of the colon, right hemicolectomy with primary anastomosis is usually easy to accomplish and ordinarily carries a low morbidity rate. It is vital, however, to avoid pursuing this approach at all costs in the determination to avoid ileostomy. Patients who have been in deep shock requiring massive transfusions, who have serious intra-abdominal injuries associated with gross contamination, or who have suffered severe residual retroperitoneal muscle damage are best served by removal of the injured area of colon, wide drainage of the retroperitoneal region, and the establishment of an ileostomy and colonic mucous fistula. With the patient fully resuscitated, free of sepsis and in a favorable metabolic state, definitive reestablishment of intestinal continuity can be safely performed in 2 to 12 weeks, depending on the patient's progress.

AXIOM

BLIND INSISTENCE ON PRIMARY ANASTOMOSIS OF THE COLON IN THE PRESENCE OF SHOCK INVITES DISASTER.

Although primary anastomosis is significantly more hazardous on the left side of the colon than on the right, a more aggressive approach to primary resection and anastomosis in this region has become evident in elective surgery in recent years. Transposing this concept to the field of emergency surgery, some surgeons, disappointed by the 20 to 30% morbidity and even occasional mortality of a defunctioning colostomy, are cautiously performing primary closures of highly selected gunshot wounds of the left colon.

Other surgeons, seeking to steer a middle course, have tried to avoid the morbidity and further surgery of a proximal colostomy by repairing the damaged bowel and exteriorizing the anastomosis.[23] This anastomosis can then be observed on the abdominal wall and, if healing is satisfactory, returned to the peritoneal cavity about the tenth postoperative day. When successful, this approach obviates the need for subsequent closure of the colostomy initially established to protect the intraperitoneal suture line. If the technique of extraperitonealization of the anastomosis is attempted, it is important that an adequate passage through the abdominal wall (about 8 cm) is established so that there is no kinking of the exteriorized sector with consequent iatrogenic obstruction of the already unavoidably edematous segment. Using this technique, Okies et al.[24] have avoided formal colostomy in 49% of a group of 37 patients. In contrast, Schrock et al.[25] reported a success rate of only 21%. In a prospective randomized study which included 29 cases in which the repaired colon was exteriorized for 10 days prior to return to the peritoneal cavity, Kirkpatrick[23] successfully avoided colostomy in 55% of these cases but surprisingly found that hospitalization was not significantly reduced, largely because of the delay in healing of associated injuries.

PITFALL

ATTEMPTS TO ACHIEVE PRIMARY REPAIR OF INJURIES TO THE RETROPERITONEAL RECTUM WITHOUT ADEQUATE DEFUNCTIONING OF THE PROXIMAL COLON AND DRAINAGE OF THE SURROUNDING AREA ARE HAZARDOUS AND ALMOST INVARIABLY UNSUCCESSFUL.

Special precautions are necessary in dealing with injuries of the extraperitoneal rectum.[26] Not infrequently the extent of the damage is virtually impossible to assess adequately at the initial operation, and in many cases the situation is further complicated by vesical or sacral injuries. Attempts to achieve initial definitive repair are hazardous and lead to high morbidity. While any easily accessible lacerations of the rectum should be repaired, the best results are obtained by (1) a proximal diverting sigmoid colostomy, (2) thorough cleansing of the bowel between the colostomy and the anus by saline irrigations at the time of operation to reduce the bacterial load and to obviate subsequent leakage of stool into the damaged extraperitoneal planes, (3) thorough debridement of the pelvic tissues, (4) extensive drainage of the extraperitoneal area with drains emerging through an adequate precoccygeal incision, (5) administration of systemic antibiotics, most often penicillin, gentamicin and clindamycin, (6) instillation of antibiotics such as neomycin or kanamycin into the defunctioned bowel, and (7) general supportive measures.

Whenever there has been gross contamination of the peritoneal cavity by intestinal content, the abdomen should be thoroughly washed with saline at the end of the operation and then widely drained.

PITFALL

IN PATIENTS WHO HAVE HAD IRRIGATION OF THE ABDOMINAL CAVITY WITH ANTIBIOTICS, ADEQUATE VENTILATION OVER SEVERAL HOURS MUST BE DOCUMENTED BEFORE REMOVAL OF THE ENDOTRACHEAL TUBE.

The insertion of irrigating catheters for the purpose of instilling antibiotics such as kanamycin or cephalosporin remains controversial. Neomycin and kanamycin should not be used until the effects of the muscle relaxants have been completely eliminated if the risk of prolonged respiratory paralysis is to be avoided with certainty. The subcutaneous tissues are best left open initially and closed by secondary suture after approximately 5 days in order to reduce the frequency of wound sepsis.

Rectal impalement by a wide variety of objects, such as pickets, broomsticks or hydraulic jacks, has been described. The wound may extend into any abdominal organ and even into the chest. The principles of treatment are the same as for all penetrating injuries with the additional caveat that the object of the impalement be left in situ and removed only at operation under direct vision with the abdomen open. This facilitates the identification of the injured organs, reduces fecal spillage and assists immediate control of hemorrhage which may otherwise be catastrophic on withdrawal of the responsible foreign body.

Perforation associated with barium enemas is far more serious as the mixture of barium and feces is a potentially virulent mixture causing severe infection. Most of these lesions are due to carelessness with the large balloon or enema tip and may take the form of extensive lacerations, often extraperitoneal. It is highly questionable whether a barium enema performed gently can be held responsible for the perforation of a diverticulum, as sometimes claimed. Immediate operation is always desirable.

Similar but more extensive lesions may result from the passage of a jet of compressed air up the anal canal. This injury usually follows a prank when the nozzle is held a few inches from the victim's buttocks and the pressure suddenly turned on. It has been estimated that about 4 lb/sq in of pressure is needed to rupture the bowel; compressed air jets may generate up to 125 lb/sq in. The laceration of the bowel usually occurs in the rectosigmoid area and may extend for 10 cm or more. Early operative treatment is essential.

SIGMOIDOSCOPY AND COLONOSCOPY PERFORATIONS. The incidence of perforation during the passage of these instruments or following biopsy with or without fulguration is not fully reflected in the literature. In many cases, the patient immediately experiences acute abdominal or shoulder tip pain, accentuated when air is insufflated. In others, discomfort and subsequent peritonitis may not develop for a number of hours. Free air in the peritoneal cavity on plain radiographs of the abdomen or direct visualization of the rent are pathognomonic.

In the past, mortality rates of as high as 50% were described following this complication. The outcome is largely related to the time which is permitted to elapse between the injury and formal operation. Where this is less than 6 hours, there should be virtually no deaths as the bowel is generally clean due to preparation preliminary to the endoscopy.

BLUNT TRAUMA. Blunt trauma to the colon poses special problems as its effects are very rarely recognized in the early stages. Isolated colonic injury occurs in only about 10% of these cases and concomitant head, chest or extremity injuries usually dominate the clinical picture. Twenty-two of our thirty-five patients were involved in automobile accidents either as pedestrians or passengers, while the remainder suffered falls or direct assaults. The responsible mechanism is most often a shearing injury or increased intraluminal bursting tension, but in a few cases seems to be a direct crush, especially when the patient is wearing a seat belt. Seat-belt injuries are being increasingly encountered, especially when the seat belt is incorrectly worn so that it is placed above the iliac crest or is so loose that the victim slides downward and forward at the time of impact. In addition to the colonic injury (usually sigmoid), the abdominal wall, the ileum, the mesenteries and the lumbar vertebrae may be damaged.

Symptoms and signs of serious intra-abdominal injury may be delayed for up to a week as the ischemic bowel becomes more necrotic before finally perforating into the free peritoneal cavity or, more rarely, into the retroperitoneal tissues with formation of a colocutaneous fistula. The severity of the blow is not necessarily reflected in the degree of intestinal damage and the ultimate colonic injury is greatly influenced by the degree of tension of the abdominal muscles at the moment of impact. Occasionally, the muscles may suffer a linear rupture along the line of the blow.

Intramural hematomas of the colon probably occur more often than has been recognized. Most of these will regress spontaneously but, in a few cases, sudden rupture with intraperitoneal hemorrhage or chronic inflammatory changes leading to later colonic stenosis may occur.

An uncommon form of crush injury may occur in pedestrians run over by a vehicle when the intra-abdominal pressure is raised and then suddenly released, resulting in rupture of the pelvic diaphragm. The anorectal apparatus may be left intact but torn from the levator ani sling. Blast injuries from below have been reported to produce similar lesions in some patients. This complex injury is recognized by the retraction proximally above the levators of the anal canal and the rectum or by the gross eccentric displacement of the anus in the perineum. The patient will often be in shock and may have associated genitourinary injuries. Such a patient requires early operation with debridement and drainage of the perineum, repair of the bowel where a laceration has occurred, anchoring of the anal canal, both to the levators and to the perineal skin, and, finally, the establishment of a proximal colostomy in most cases.

ABDOMINAL AORTA AND INFERIOR VENA CAVA

About 80% of patients with wounds of the abdominal aorta and the inferior vena cava (I.V.C.) or their major branches die before they reach the hospital. The survivors can be saved only by the most vigorous resuscitation and immediate surgery. All these patients are in shock and most have associated injuries. The fact that they are still living is usually attributable to substantial tamponade by the intact abdominal wall or surrounding structures such as the crura of the diaphragm or periaortic nerve plexuses and connective tissue. Only about 20 survivors with aortic injury have been reported in the literature[27] but it is safe to assume that many more have not been reported. If certain principles were routinely followed, the salvage rate would increase.

Resuscitation of patients with these vascular injuries requires the immediate administration of type-specific blood until cross-matched blood is available. This is best done in the operating room so that laparotomy can be performed without delay, should the patient deteriorate further or suffer cardiac arrest. The availability of an autotransfuser may be invaluable. Arteriographic or other radiologic evaluation is seldom feasible under these circumstances.

A prerequisite to success is a previously planned systematic approach to the problem. Identification, control and repair of any major vascular lesion should be approached as methodically as possible. When the abdomen is grossly distended with blood preoperatively and the patient fails to respond to the administration of large amounts of blood and fluid, left thoracotomy through the fifth intercostal space as a preliminary measure to obtain control of the thoracic aorta just above the diaphragm may be lifesaving. This maneuver improves cerebral and coronary perfusion, reduces intra-abdominal hemorrhage and, if performed low on the descending thoracic aorta, greatly reduces the danger of spinal-cord ischemia and subsequent paralysis.

The track of the missile may give a clue as to whether the aorta or I.V.C. has been injured. In the presence of an arteriovenous communication, a pathognomonic bruit may be heard preoperatively or felt at laparotomy. Proper control of such vascular injuries generally requires wide exposure, usually through a midline incision from xiphoid to pubis. With the higher caval injuries the duodenum and colon must be reflected to the left and with the more proximal injuries the spleen, pancreas, colon and perhaps the kidney must be reflected to the right. Bleeding is temporarily controlled by digital compression or sponge sticks, appropriate vascular clamps, or a special aortic compressor inserted through the lesser sac. The blind or agitated use of vascular clamps may produce additional damage, especially to the very fragile retroperitoneal veins. An alternative method advocated for rare occasions involves the insertion of an occluding balloon catheter transfemorally.

As soon as temporary control of the bleeding sites has been obtained, further surgical manipulation is discontinued until the intravascular volume has been restored. The occluding clamp is advanced as close to the injured segment as possible, with special attention being paid to the maintenance of a urinary output of at least 50 to 100 ml/hr by the administration of blood and fluids and mannitol and/or furosemide as needed.

Small defects in the aorta may be repaired by simple suture. Larger defects may require the insertion of a prosthetic graft, and successful results have been obtained with grafts, even in the presence of spillage from associated intestinal injuries, if local and systemic antibiotics are administered. In these circumstances, it may be of value to soak the graft in 1% neomycin prior to its insertion.

About 50% of patients with inferior vena caval injuries die. These injuries can be conveniently divided into those above and below the renal veins. Infrarenal lesions are obviously more accessible and control of the segment of involved vein and adjacent lumbar tributaries is best obtained manually or by pressure with sponge sticks. On occasion, the insertion of a Foley catheter using the inflated balloon for local tamponade may be a reasonable temporizing measure. Where possible, the tear is sutured. Tears of the posterior wall of the I.V.C. may be repaired by working through an incision in the anterior wall when it may be hazardous to rotate the vessel in the attempt to obtain exposure.

Most pericaval hematomas should be opened once adequate control and exposure have been obtained. In many cases, however, ligation of the I.V.C. may be the quickest and safest approach. In addition, ligation tends to reduce the risk of subsequent pulmonary embolism. When possible, the ligation should be placed just distal to a major tributary to avoid proximal venous stagnation. Swelling of the legs may occur in the postoperative period under these circumstances but long-term disability is uncommon where venous collaterals are intact and the veins in the legs are patent.

The suprarenal I.V.C. injury presents some of the most difficult problems in abdominal trauma, both because of its inaccessible position and because the liver is often injured concomitantly. It is probable that this segment of the vein is injured more often than is appreciated but that the tamponading effect on this low-pressure system by the liver anteriorly, the abdominal wall posteriorly, and the diaphragm above contains the hematoma until spontaneous healing occurs.

AXIOM

RETROPERITONEAL HEMATOMAS IN THE AREA OF THE SUPRARENAL I.V.C. ARE OFTEN BEST LEFT UNDISTURBED.

If it is necessary to open such a hematoma because of an associated duodenal, biliary, or hepatic injury, an orderly approach must be adopted. To gain exposure to the lesion, a relatively dry field is essential. This is best obtained by ensuring control of the intra-abdominal I.V.C. The abdominal incision may be extended proximally with splitting of the sternum. Um-

bilical tapes may then be placed around the intrapericardial portion of the I.V.C. with a tube in the I.V.C. as a temporary conduit for the return of venous blood to the heart. Details of the available surgical techniques have been well described.[8]

RETROPERITONEAL HEMATOMAS

Etiology and Incidence

Most retroperitoneal hematomas develop from tears of fragile small or medium-sized veins in the retroperitoneal space. Such injuries are common with both blunt and penetrating trauma. Not infrequently, there appears to be little or no relationship between the size of the hematoma and the severity of the trauma. In patients who have a laparotomy for blunt trauma, a retroperitoneal hematoma without associated injuries is found in only about 10%. In the others, the most frequent visceral injuries are those involving the kidney or pancreas. Fractures of the pelvis or lumbar spine make up most of the other associated injuries.

Diagnosis

The clinical picture is often extremely deceptive. The patient may have relatively few signs or symptoms on admission, but several hours later he may develop a progressive abdominal distension and ileus, with or without tenderness or rigidity, particularly if spinal fractures are present. Although visceral perforation is unlikely, peritoneal lavage may reveal blood, leading to laparotomy. At operation, there is sometimes no evidence of visceral injury, but a large bulging hematoma with leakage of blood through the posterior peritoneum is identified as the source of the bleeding. Conversely, hypovolemic shock may develop due to the loss of two, three or more liters of blood into the retroperitoneal space.

Treatment

In attempting to decide whether or not a laparotomy is indicated, a number of investigations may be helpful. These include serum amylase determinations, plain x-rays of the abdomen, and intravenous pyelogram. In some cases, arteriography, either pre- or intraoperatively, may be invaluable for delineating the site of a significant vascular injury, permitting accurate early control of the damaged vessel and subsequent repair if feasible. Alternatively, in the presence of a large expanding hematoma associated with a pelvic fracture, definitive occlusion of the vessel has been obtained by injection of autogenous clot or muscle through the angiographic catheter.[28] On a few occasions, control of the bleeding vessel has been obtained by using an occluding balloon catheter. Where these techniques are unavailable or are unsuccessful, attempts to control serious continuing pelvic bleeding may be made by ligation of the internal iliac arteries bilaterally. There is, however, no guarantee that this will succeed. In case of failure, there is no alternative to the insertion of tightly packed rolls of gauze as a temporizing measure. The pack is left in situ for 2 to 3 days before being slowly and gently removed, with all arrangements made for operative intervention if the bleeding recurs.

Absolute indications for the exploration of a retroperitoneal hematoma include: (1) visible enlargement or pulsation, (2) suspicion that a ruptured viscus, such as the duodenum, retroperitoneal colon or pancreas, lies within or behind the hematoma, (3) suspected perforation of a large vessel, such as the aorta, renal artery, or infrarenal vena cava, and (4) evidence of significant damage to the kidney, ureter or bladder.

AXIOM

NONEXPANDING RETROPERITONEAL HEMATOMAS IN THE PELVIS AND BEHIND THE RIGHT LOBE OF THE LIVER ARE GENERALLY BEST LEFT UNDISTURBED.

While some surgeons advocate the opening and evacuation of retroperitoneal he-

matomas routinely once the patient's condition is stable and adequate exposure has been obtained, there is little evidence to support such a diagnostic approach. Furthermore, two circumstances exist in which such an approach might be catastrophic. The more common dilemma is presented by the large hematoma associated with severe pelvic fractures. Opening of such pelvic hematomas may be followed by catastrophic hemorrhage which may be almost impossible to control except with a large pack. Caution and watchful waiting are preferable in most of these cases, as the contained hematoma will usually tamponade the vessel responsible for the bleeding. Laceration of the major iliac arteries or veins is seldom the cause of the bleeding in these patients, but angiographic studies are mandatory if such vascular injuries are suspected. Identification of the precise area of damage is invaluable to the surgeon forced to operate on such injuries.

The second type of retroperitoneal hematoma posing special difficulties is that which occurs high in the right upper quadrant of the abdomen behind the liver. Bleeding into this area is generally from small retrohepatic tributaries of the inferior vena cava which are extremely difficult to control. In some instances, when such a hematoma is opened, thoracotomy and temporary catheterization of the inferior vena cava through the right atrium may be required to control the bleeding. Where the hematoma and the patient are both stable and there are no associated organ injuries, conservatism is the preferred approach.

SUMMARY

The morbidity and mortality following injury to abdominal organs are largely determined by the number and severity of the associated injuries. The preoperative preparation and diagnostic workup should be as thorough as the situation allows, but cannot always be exhaustive. Hypotension and peritoneal contamination must be

TABLE 1. TEN FREQUENT ERRORS IN THE MANAGEMENT OF SPECIFIC ABDOMINAL INJURIES

1. Failure to consider the possibility of delayed splenic rupture in patients who have recently sustained blunt abdominal trauma.
2. Failure to protect against the development of a tension pneumothorax during anesthesia in patients with penetrating upper abdominal or lower chest wounds or with fractured ribs.
3. Attempts to control bleeding in the depths of a liver wound by the use of tightly tied sutures in the superficial liver substance which hides the bleeding rather than controls it.
4. Attempts by inexperienced surgeons to perform an emergency hepatic lobectomy in critically injured unstable patients when lesser measures may suffice.
5. Failure to examine plain x-ray films of the abdomen for retroperitoneal air in patients with blunt trauma and possible rupture of the duodenum.
6. Failure to open retroperitoneal hematomas over the pancreas and duodenum to rule out lacerations of the underlying viscera.
7. Failure to provide efficient safe and continuing abdominal drainage, often because of too tight an exit wound for the drain, or carelessly placed drains.
8. Failure to search adequately for perforations along the mesenteric border of the intestine following penetrating injuries, particularly if any odd number of holes is found.
9. Failure to examine the gluteal area and other skin creases closely for penetrating injuries, particularly following gunshot wounds of the lower abdomen.
10. Failure to exercise restraint in performing primary colonic anastomosis in the face of shock and sepsis.

kept to a minimum. The surgical management of each injured organ should be adjusted according to the patient's condition, remembering that in many instances definitive repair or anastomosis is best left for a later time when the patient is more stable hemodynamically and metabolically. Wide drainage is essential in any area of continued oozing, or where intestinal leakage or contamination has occurred. Table 1 summarizes some important major pitfalls encountered in our experience.

REFERENCES

1. Strauch, G. O.: State wide survey of trauma in Connecticut. Major abdominal trauma in 1971. Amer. J. Surg., 125:413, 1973.
2. Walt, A. J., and Grifka, T.: Blunt abdominal trauma: A review of 301 cases. In: *Impact Injury and Crash Protection* (Gurdjian, E. S., Lange, W. A., Patrick, W. M., and Thomas, L. M., Eds.). Springfield, Charles C Thomas, 1970.
3. Jordan, G. L., and Beale, A. C.: Diagnosis and management of abdominal trauma. Curr. Probl. Surg., 1:62, 1971.
4. Shires, G. T., et al.: Morbidity, mortality and injuries to the spleen. J. Trauma, 14:773, 1974.
5. Ayala, L. A., et al.: Occult rupture of the spleen. Ann. Surg., 179:472, 1974.
6. Levi, R. C., et al.: Angiography in patients with blunt trauma to the chest and abdomen. Surg. Clin. N. Amer., 52:551, 1972.
7. Miller, D. R.: Median sternectomy extension of abdominal incision for hepatic lobectomy. Ann. Surg., 175:193, 1972.
8. Bricker, D. L., et al.: Surgical management of injuries to the vena cava: changing patterns of injury and newer techniques of repair. J. Trauma, 11:725, 1971.
9. Walt, A. J.: Hepatic trauma. In: *A Forum on The Surgery of the Liver* (Smith, R., Ed.). In press.
10. Mays, E. T., and Wheeler, C. S.: Hepatic artery ligation. New Eng. J. Med., 290:993, 1974.
11. Madding, G. F., and Kennedy, P. A.: Hepatic artery ligation. Surg. Clin. N. Amer., 52:719, 1972.
12. Lucas, C. E., and Walt, A. J.: Analysis of randomized biliary drainage for liver trauma in 189 patients. J. Trauma, 12:925, 1972.
13. Fish, J. C., and Nippert, R. H.: Traumatic hemobilia: the dilemma of delay. J. Trauma, 9:546, 1969.
14. Lucas, C. E., and Ledgerwood, A.: Factors influencing outcome after blunt duodenal injuries. J. Trauma, in press.
15. Nance, F. C., and DeLoach, D. H.: Pancreatico-duodenotomy following abdominal trauma. J. Trauma, 11:577, 1971.
16. Northrop, W. F., III, and Simmons, R. L.: Pancreatic trauma: a review. Surgery, 71:27, 1972.
17. Steele, M., et al.: Pancreatic injuries, methods of management. Arch. Surg., 106:544, 1973.
18. Wilson, R. F., et al.: Pancreatic trauma. J. Trauma, 7:643, 1967.
19. Thal, A. P., and Wilson, R. F.: A pattern of severe blunt trauma to the pancreas. Surg. Gynec. Obstet., 119:773, 1964.

20. Bach, R. D., and Frey, C. F.: Diagnosis and treatment of pancreatic trauma. Amer. J. Surg., 121:20, 1971.

21. Ritchie, W. P., et al.: Combined visceral and vertebral injuries from lap type seat belts. Surg. Gynec. Obstet., 131:431, 1970.

22. Garfinkle, S. E., et al.: Civilian colon injuries. Arch. Surg., 109:402, 1974.

23. Kirkpatrick, J. R., et al.: Management of a high-risk intestinal anastomosis. Amer. J. Surg., 125:312, 1973.

24. Okies, J. E., et al.: Exteriorized primary repair of colon injuries. Amer. J. Surg., 124:807, 1972.

25. Schrock, T. R., and Christensen, N.: Management of perforating injuries of the colon. Surg. Gynec. Obstet., 135:65, 1972.

26. Wanebo, H. J., et al.: Rectal injuries. J. Trauma, 9:712, 1969.

27. Yeo, M. T., et al.: Penetrating injuries of the abdominal aorta. Arch. Surg., 108:839, 1974.

28. Ring, E. J., et al.: Angiography in pelvic trauma. Surg. Gynec. Obstet., 139:375, 1974.

24   TRAUMA TO THE URINARY TRACT

R. F. WILSON
J. M. PIERCE, JR.

The urinary tract may be damaged by a wide variety of blunt or penetrating traumas to the chest, abdomen or pelvis. In recent years, there has been a marked increase in the number of these injuries caused by gunshot wounds. The male genitalia are also subject to damage, usually from penetrating injuries such as knife or gunshot wounds but occasionally also from belt-driven machinery.

Ideally, every busy emergency room should have a trained urologist, who is readily available, to handle these problems. However, any physician who sees acutely injured patients should be able to make a reasonably accurate diagnosis and begin therapy if his approach to the problem is orderly and systematic. Although damage to the urinary tract per se is rarely fatal, it is often associated with other serious injuries and may contribute significantly to increased morbidity and mortality. Trauma is no respecter of organ systems or medical specialties. Multiple anatomic structures are often involved, and the physician managing trauma cannot allow himself to become so involved with one area that he fails to recognize what may be more serious associated injuries elsewhere.

PITFALL

IF THE PHYSICIAN CONCENTRATES HIS AT-TENTION ON POSSIBLE GENITOURINARY DAMAGE, OTHER UNTREATED INJURIES MAY CAUSE A SUDDEN DETERIORATION IN THE PATIENT'S CONDITION.

INJURIES TO THE KIDNEY

Diagnosis

HISTORY. The keystone to the diagnosis of renal injuries is a high index of suspicion based on the type and location of the trauma. Persistent, severe flank or upper abdominal pain following abdominal, pelvic or lower thoracic trauma should make the physician particularly suspicious of a genitourinary injury, especially of the bladder and kidney, and indicates a need for radiologic examination of the complete urinary tract.

PHYSICAL EXAMINATION. After the patient is completely examined and while careful monitoring of vital signs is continued, a more specific search can be made for possible renal injury. Flank or upper abdominal tenderness is a frequent finding after renal injury, and in some patients a flank mass may be palpable. An expanding mass may indicate that the renal injury is severe and has caused extravasation of blood or urine into the perirenal tissue and perhaps through Gerota's fascial capsule.

PITFALL

IF THE PHYSICIAN FAILS TO AUSCULTATE
OVER THE LOWER BACK FOLLOWING SEVERE
BLUNT TRAUMA, HE MAY MISS RENAL VASCU-
LAR INJURIES THAT MIGHT NOT OTHERWISE
BE APPARENT.

Occasionally a bruit heard in the posterior midline near the first and second lumbar vertebrae may be the only indication
of damage to the renal vessels. In penetrating injuries in the upper abdomen or flank,
a bruit may suggest an acute arteriovenous
fistula involving the renal artery and vein
or the renal artery and vena cava.

LABORATORY STUDIES. *Urinalysis.* If the
patient can void, a urinalysis should be obtained and, ideally, examined by the physician. The presence of microscopic or gross
hematuria in such a specimen is strongly
suggestive of a urinary tract injury.

PITFALL

INSERTION OF A FOLEY CATHETER BEFORE
OBTAINING A URINE SPECIMEN GREATLY RE-
DUCES THE VALUE OF THE URINALYSIS.

Since the insertion of a urethral catheter
can itself cause hematuria, the urine to be
examined should, whenever possible, be
collected without catheterization. Unfortunately, seriously injured patients often
cannot urinate within the first 15 to 30 minutes and a Foley catheter must be inserted
so that the urine output may be monitored
properly. In the menstruating female a
catheterized specimen may be more accurate, especially when it is important to ascertain the presence or absence of hematuria. If only a few red cells are present in
a catheterized specimen, clinical judgment
must be exercised as to whether further investigation is necessary. In cases of doubt,
it is probably safer to obtain the appropriate studies.

Although hematuria strongly suggests the
presence of a urologic injury and is an indication for complete urologic examination,
the absence of hematuria is of less diagnos-

tic value. Approximately 5 to 10% of patients with proven renal injuries have no
hematuria at the time of the initial examination. The urinalysis is most likely to be
normal in the face of severe renal injury if
the vascular pedicle has been transected.
The observation of hematuria may also be
prevented if the ureter is occluded by a
large expanding hematoma from a ruptured
kidney or other retroperitoneal damage.

BUN and Creatinine. A rising blood urea
nitrogen (BUN) or serum creatinine may
indicate impaired renal function following
trauma. These changes, however, are not
usually apparent for at least 24 to 48 hours.
The BUN, moreover, may rise without renal
disease or damage. Blood in the intestinal
tract, for example, may increase the BUN up
to 50 mg/100 ml, even in patients with normal renal function. Furthermore, the blood
urea nitrogen may vary, in a given laboratory, from 7 to 21 mg/100 ml, which is actually a threefold variation. The serum creatinine varies far less; it is less influenced by
exogenous creatinine in the diet, and it is
affected very little by blood in the gut.

AXIOM

SERUM CREATININE IS A FAR BETTER TEST
THAN THE BUN WHEN LOOKING FOR RENAL
DYSFUNCTION.

X-RAYS. X-rays are the most diagnostic
and accurate means for evaluating urologic
injuries. The techniques used include: plain
x-rays of the abdomen, excretory urography,
urethral cystograms, retrograde pyelograms
and renal angiography.

Plain X-rays of the Abdomen. The so-
called kidney-ureter-bladder (K.U.B.) views
may provide important information concerning the retroperitoneal area and the
status of the kidneys. Displacement or abnormal size of the renal shadows may indicate a previous abnormality or disease process. Loss of the psoas shadow and scolio-
sis may suggest fluid, especially blood or
urine, in the retroperitoneum. X-rays may
also show fractures of the lower ribs, lum-

bar spine or pelvis which suggest adjacent urinary tract injury. The localization of foreign bodies or bullets in or near the urinary tract is also very helpful. With penetrating wounds, particularly those caused by bullets, radiopaque markers should be placed over the entrance and exit wounds.

AXIOM

IF THERE IS ANY SUSPICION OF RENAL DAMAGE, EXCRETORY UROGRAPHY SHOULD BE PERFORMED.

Drip-infusion Pyelography. The use of drip-infusion urography is highly recommended. Information obtained from a drip-infusion urogram generally produces a much higher incidence of excellent delineation of the urinary tract than the usual dehydration type of intravenous urogram. If there is any history of iodine sensitivity, a slow 1-ml intravenous injection of the radiopaque material can be given and the patient observed carefully for at least ten minutes. If there is a serious question of iodide sensitivity, possible reactions can usually be blocked by giving 250 mg of Solu-Medrol intravenously. The use of 50 mg of Benadryl intravenously, following the Solu-Medrol, is also often helpful. It should be noted, however, that intravenous Benadryl may cause central respiratory depression in some patients; therefore, if the time is available to wait 15 to 20 minutes, it may be preferable to give it intramuscularly. The intravenous Solu-Medrol, however, usually blocks any immune reaction.

If the patient has a systolic blood pressure of 90 mm Hg or higher, the standard intravenous pyelogram using direct intravenous injection of 60% iodide radiopaque material should provide films of diagnostic quality in about 50% of acutely injured patients. With the high-dose drip-infusion technique, the films are usually much better and are of diagnostic quality in about 80% of patients. When available, tomography combined with the excretory urog-

raphy may provide more detail and allow visualization of lacerations that would not otherwise be seen.[1]

The drip-infusion pyelogram provides 4 to 6 times the usual amount of contrast material in a rapid injection over 5 to 7 minutes, and also produces an increased osmotic load to the kidney. Because of the osmotic load, the urine output is greater and the renal collecting systems are more easily seen. The solution recommended for drip-infusion urography consists of 1 ml of 60% iodide radiopaque material for each pound of body weight up to 150 pounds. This is mixed with an equal quantity of saline and is given intravenously over 5 to 7 minutes. If the infusion is begun as the patient is being transported to the radiology unit, the films can usually be taken as soon as the patient has been positioned on the x-ray table.

Some of the changes that may be seen on excretory urography of an injured kidney include:

1. Delayed or decreased excretion of the contrast material on one side.
2. Extravasation of contrast material beneath the renal capsule.
3. Extravasation of contrast material outside the renal capsule in the perirenal space.
4. Enlargement or loss of the renal outline.
5. Perirenal mass.
6. Filling defects, such as clots, in the collecting system of the kidney.
7. Distortion of the calyceal system by a mass such as a hematoma.
8. Nonvisualization of a segment or total renal collecting unit.
9. Nonvisualization of the kidney.

PITFALL

FAILURE TO OBTAIN AN EXCRETORY UROGRAM BEFORE EXPLORING AN INJURED KIDNEY MAY PUT THE SURGEON IN THE PREDICAMENT OF BEING FORCED TO REMOVE AN INJURED KIDNEY WITHOUT KNOWING WHETHER OR NOT THE OTHER KIDNEY IS ADEQUATE TO SUPPORT LIFE.

In addition to delineating the status of the injured kidney, the drip-infusion urogram also serves to demonstrate the position and function of the normal kidney. Although the changes found in the injured kidney are extremely important, the functional status of the uninjured kidney may be much more critical. Since one out of every 2,000 patients has a single kidney, the surgeon must be absolutely certain that the other kidney is present and can support life by itself before performing an emergency nephrectomy. Since 25 to 60% of patients with a solitary kidney have no vas deferens on the side of the missing kidney, careful examination of the scrotum may occasionally provide a clue to this anomaly.[2]

Although the intravenous urogram does not provide visualization of the vascular pedicle, strong suspicions of a major renal vascular injury would be aroused if there is nonvisualization of the kidney following trauma, or if there is evidence of excessive extravasation of contrast material. In cases of nonvisualization, the patient should have renal angiography if at all possible.

The drip-infusion pyelogram, although not as accurate as retrograde cystography, may also provide some information on the size and configuration of the bladder if the Foley catheter is clamped during the pyelogram. The drip-infusion pyelogram, furthermore, provides a better chance of diagnosing ureteral injury which may be manifested by excretion of contrast material through a partially or completely transected ureter. Marked displacement of the ureters, which show much better on drip-infusion urography, may indicate the presence of a large retroperitoneal hematoma.

Retrograde Pyelography. In the past, retrograde pyelography was a much-used diagnostic tool, but with the advent of drip-infusion urography and renal arteriography it has become much less important. It provides information important to the management of the patient only in cases where there is a suspicion of a dismembered or transected ureter.

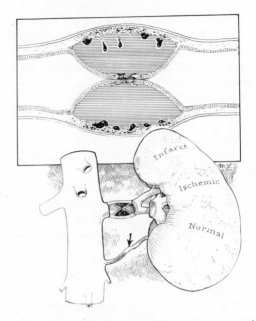

FIG. 1. Severe blunt trauma to the kidney may result in subintimal hemorrhage in the renal artery which may completely occlude the vascular lumen. In this instance, the blood supply to the inferior pole of the kidney is maintained by an accessory renal artery. (From Ross, R., Ackerman, E., and Pierce, J. M.[16])

Renal Arteriography. If an acutely injured kidney is not visualized on drip-infusion pyelography in a normotensive patient, renal arteriography should be performed immediately.[3] The kidney, especially during blunt trauma, can be subjected to a severe whiplash injury in which the renal artery and vein and sometimes the ureteropelvic junction may be torn as they are stretched across the vertebral bodies. The renal artery can sustain a medial subintimal hemorrhage, usually beginning about 1 cm from its takeoff from the aorta (Fig. 1). This may cause just a small localized narrowing or a severe dissection with occlusion of the renal artery, resulting in nonvisualization on drip-infusion urography.[4] A more severe degree of this injury is complete laceration of the renal artery near its origin from the aorta. With such an injury, the presence of a bruit and a rapidly expanding mass may be noted.

In young patients, completely dismembered renal arteries may stop bleeding almost instantly due to occlusion by constriction of the musculature. Since such renal arterial injuries are operative emergencies if any renal salvage is to take place, the arteriogram has to be done relatively soon after the injury.

PITFALL

FAILURE TO OBTAIN A RENAL ARTERIOGRAM WHEN THERE IS ANY SUGGESTION OF RENAL VASCULAR INJURY MAY DELAY OPERATIVE INTERVENTION WHICH MAY BE URGENTLY NEEDED TO MAINTAIN THE VIABILITY OF THE KIDNEY.

The method of renal arteriography most commonly used is percutaneous retrograde catheterization of the femoral artery using the Seldinger technique. A central aortic injection above the renal arteries is important to outline the contralateral kidney and any aberrant arteries or duplications. Sometimes selective injections of the renal artery or arteries may also be quite useful. If indicated, the celiac artery may be catheterized at the same time to evaluate for possible splenic or hepatic injuries.

Renal Scan. Because of their ease, safety and accuracy, renal scans may also be helpful in delineating areas of moderate parenchymal damage in stable patients with renal trauma.[5] At the present time, however, this technique is not readily available in most emergency rooms, particularly at night or on weekends. Furthermore, renal arteriography is much more important to the operating surgeon because it gives him a better anatomic understanding of the problem, especially if the major vessels are injured or abnormal.

Types of Renal Injuries

Renal injuries may be classified into six groups, depending upon their severity and location:

1. Contusions.
2. Renal cortical contusions with renal subcapsular extravasation.
3. Lacerations of renal cortex through renal capsule, but with bleeding confined to the perirenal space defined by Gerota's fascia.
4. Multiple lacerations of the kidney with bleeding not confined by Gerota's fascia.
5. Injuries to main renal vessels.
6. Ureteropelvic junction dismemberment and renal pelvic injuries.

Treatment

GENERAL APPROACH

PITFALL

AN EARLY AGGRESSIVE SURGICAL APPROACH TO ALL RENAL INJURIES WILL INCREASE THE MORTALITY RATE AND THE NUMBER OF NEPHRECTOMIES DONE FOR TRAUMA.[6]

Contusions and lacerations of the kidney not extending through the renal capsule, which make up the majority of renal injuries, usually heal very well without surgical intervention (Fig. 2). The more extensive lacerations extending through the renal capsule into the perirenal space also generally heal satisfactorily with conservative management, as long as the perirenal fascia remains intact. Multiple severe renal lacerations, however, almost always require nephrectomy. Sometimes a severely lacerated kidney may be treated with a partial nephrectomy, and rarely, under ideal circumstances, repair is possible so that all or most of the kidney can be saved.

Most urologists resort to early operative intervention only when there is evidence of severe, persistent hemorrhage or gross extravasation of urine beyond the renal capsule. Later surgery may be necessary if uncontrollable sepsis develops or if the involved kidney becomes functionless. When the patient has only one kidney, treatment should be even more conservative, and every effort should be made to salvage the solitary kidney, even when it is severely damaged or bleeding.

Bleeding from a damaged kidney may

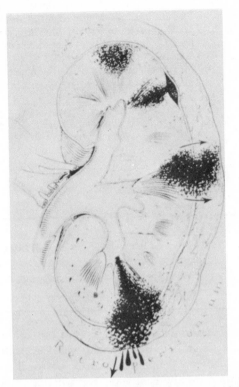

FIG. 2. Some of the more common injuries to the kidney include (starting at the top of the kidney) contusion, contusion with subcapsular hematoma, contusion with laceration of the capsule and hemorrhage into the perirenal fat, and (at the bottom of the kidney) contusion with hemorrhage through Gerota's fascia into the retroperitoneal space.

cause severe shock, but this is unusual and blood loss from other structures must be carefully considered. The perirenal fascia, if not torn, usually provides an excellent tamponading effect, and most hemorrhaging subsides very rapidly as the perirenal space fills. Therefore, if the hemoglobin and blood pressure continue to fall, the patient must be carefully checked for other possible sites of blood loss.

PITFALL

TRAUMA OFTEN INVOLVES MULTIPLE ORGANS. IF IT IS ASSUMED THAT PERSISTENT HYPOTENSION IN AN INJURED PATIENT IS DUE TO BLEEDING FROM A DAMAGED KIDNEY, MORE LIFE-THREATENING INJURIES ARE APT TO BE MISSED.

Hypotension associated with blunt trauma to the left or right kidneys is often due to splenic or liver injuries. Tearing of the mesenteric vessels may occur with blunt trauma to either side. Exploration is indicated if there is evidence of an enlarging abdominal-flank mass, or when the patient continues to deteriorate without other apparent injuries including hypotension from spinal trauma.

AXIOM

IF THE TIME IS AVAILABLE, ALL PATIENTS TO BE EXPLORED FOR RENAL TRAUMA SHOULD HAVE A RENAL ARTERIOGRAM PRIOR TO SURGERY.

The renal arteriogram may give the surgeon an excellent concept of the anatomy of the injury. If there are multiple renal vessels, and if certain segments of the kidney are involved where others are normal, it allows him to plan a much safer and effective operative intervention.

If a devascularized kidney is to be saved, its blood supply must be restored within a few hours of the injury. The decision as to whether or not a devascularized kidney can be salvaged usually depends on the appearance of the kidney at the time of exploration and control of the bleeding. If the kidney seems infarcted and dark, nephrectomy may be necessary.

Dismemberment of the ureteropelvic junction occasionally occurs, and, interestingly enough, the low-dose I.V.P. under such circumstances is often normal except that the contrast material is never seen in the ureter. If high-dose drip-infusion urography is used, however, the extravasation of contrast material in the retroperitoneal space is often seen.

Patients with this injury require emergency exploration and reestablishment of the continuity of the ureter. Rarely, in doubtful cases, a retrograde pyelogram will help delineate this injury.

Rupture of the renal pelvis from blunt

trauma is rare when the tissue in that area is normal; however, in patients with pre-existing disease, such as hydronephrosis, this type of injury is not uncommon. Early repair of such damage is indicated if the kidney is functional and viable. Failure to recognize a rupture of a part of the urinary collecting system, particularly the renal pelvis or ureter, may lead to the development of a urinoma. This pseudoencapsulated enlarging sac of urine usually develops inferior and medial to the kidney and pushes the kidney superiorly and laterally. Urinomas can become quite large and sometimes are not identified until 4 to 6 weeks after the injury. If the ureterogram has shown that the ureteropelvic junction is intact, simple incision and drainage are generally the easiest and most effective method of management.

Examination at the time of operation can be extremely difficult and deceiving. If there is evidence that the kidney has been damaged, a drip-infusion pyelogram should be performed preoperatively. This is particularly important if there is any thought that a nephrectomy might have to be performed. Sometimes, however, the patient is bleeding internally so rapidly that there is no time for intravenous drip-infusion urography and arteriography. Under these circumstances, once the bleeding is controlled, it is imperative that excretory urography be done in the operating room before the kidney is removed.

AXIOM

THE FUNCTION OF A KIDNEY CANNOT BE EVALUATED BY INSPECTION OF ITS SIZE OR APPEARANCE OR BY THE WAY IT FEELS ON PALPATION.

If a retroperitoneal hematoma is overlying the kidney, but the kidney has been demonstrated to be intact on the excretory urogram, it is usually better not to open the posterior peritoneum unless significant vascular damage or duodenal injury is suspected. When the retroperitoneal space around the kidney is opened, the tamponading effect of the perirenal fascia is lost, and the severe bleeding which may develop often forces the surgeon to perform a nephrectomy that might otherwise have been avoided.

AXIOM

A PERIRENAL HEMATOMA SHOULD NOT BE OPENED UNTIL THE RENAL VESSELS HAVE BEEN IDENTIFIED AND CONTROLLED.

APPROACH TO THE RENAL VESSELS. All explorations of a traumatized kidney should be carried out through a midline abdominal incision which can be extended as necessary to handle the various associated intra-abdominal injuries. Sometimes the hematomas are so large that great difficulty is encountered in making the usual approach to control the renal vessels. If the right kidney is involved, a Kocher maneuver followed by dissection and retraction of the right transverse colon to the left may expose the renal artery between the vena cava and the aorta. If there is severe bleeding from the kidney, it may be safer to get control of the right renal artery by incising the peritoneum over the aorta just inferior to, and at the base of, the transverse mesocolon and then dissecting along the aorta until the right renal artery is found. After the renal vessels are controlled, the peritoneum and perirenal fascia over the kidney can be opened, the hematoma evacuated, the kidney inspected and repair or nephrectomy performed. The left renal artery can be picked up in a similar manner or by entering the lesser sac and incising the posterior peritoneum over the aorta. If the bleeding is too great to be controlled by any of these techniques, a left thoracotomy and occlusion of the aorta just superior to the diaphragm should be seriously considered.

IN SOME INSTANCES, CONTROL OF THE RENAL VASCULAR SUPPLY MAY REVEAL THAT THE MAIN SOURCE OF BLEEDING IS NOT RENAL IN ORIGIN.

If the patient goes into shock while the renal vessels are being secured, pressure over the pedicle area, with sterile packs, will usually control the bleeding until the blood volume can be restored to a safe level. Following this, attempts to expose and control the renal artery can be begun again.

LACERATIONS. Unless the vascular injury to the kidney is so great that no repair can be done and the bleeding cannot be stopped, a nephrectomy should not be done unless it is certain that the contralateral kidney is adequate to support life. If the renal vein cannot be repaired on the right side, the kidney should be removed. On the left, however, the vein can be ligated near the inferior vena cava and an adequate venous return will be maintained by its rich collateral drainage.

If the kidney has severe injuries and is in three or four fragments, it is usually very difficult to repair and a nephrectomy is almost invariably required. However, if preservation of that kidney is important because of absence or poor function of the opposite kidney, in certain rare instances, a surgeon with special skill and facilities can remove the kidney from the patient and repair it while it is cooled with an ice-cold physiologic salt solution. This is similar to the technique used for renal transplantation. This so-called bench surgery requires a considerable amount of experience and optical magnification, either with a loupe or operating microscope, is usually also necessary. The kidney can then be returned to the patient as an autotransplant, usually into · the contralateral iliac fossa. Since these patients often go into renal failure, at least temporarily, and since they are not

candidates for peritoneal dialysis, hemodialysis must be readily available.

If the upper or lower pole of the kidney has been so badly torn from the rest of the kidney that it is no longer viable, but the rest of the kidney appears normal, a partial nephrectomy may be performed. The decision to perform this procedure is much easier to make if the patient had had a preoperative renal arteriogram. Less severe tears should be repaired to control the hemorrhage and to restore the continuity of the pelvicalyceal system. Horizontal mattress sutures tied over pieces of fat or Teflon pledgets, to reduce the chance of tearing the capsule, may be very useful for this purpose.

Following any surgery on the kidney for trauma, the perirenal space should be adequately drained, with the drains brought out through a stab wound in the flank.

Complications of Renal Injury

Although conservative management should be the general rule, the severely injured or ruptured kidney is subject to a number of complications. Some of the more immediate problems that may develop include hemorrhage, renal infection and nonfunction. Some of the delayed problems include perirenal infection, urinoma, urinary fistula, hydronephrosis (resulting from obstruction of the ureteropelvic junction), calculi, and renovascular hypertension. To facilitate early diagnosis of these complications, all patients with suspected or proven trauma should have frequent serial evaluations of their vital signs and daily blood counts, urinalyses and serum creatinine determinations. Later, after the patient appears to have recovered from the acute injury, a follow-up intravenous urogram should also be performed, usually before the patient leaves the hospital. Since late complications are not infrequent, follow-up after serious renal injuries, including urinalysis, blood pressure, and I.V.P., should be continued for at least two years.

INJURIES TO THE URETER

Etiology

Injuries to ureters from penetrating trauma were formerly quite rare, but with the rising incidence of gunshot wounds they are not at all infrequent in large city hospital emergency rooms.[17] The nature, location and direction of the penetrating trauma must be noted carefully, and a high index of suspicion by the surgeon must be maintained in order to discover these injuries. Early operative repair is essential to prevent serious complications and possible loss of the associated kidney.

The site of damage caused by stab or gunshot wounds is extremely variable. Although the track of the stab wound can often be followed rather accurately, bullets may ricochet off bone to produce injuries far from the path of the assumed trajectory. Ureteral injuries due to blunt trauma are rare and usually represent lacerations at the ureteropelvic junction from whiplash of the renal pedicle against the adjacent vertebral bodies. Not infrequently there is associated injury to the renal vascular pedicle.

Diagnosis

The diagnosis of ureteral damage is most frequently made on the basis of extravasation of contrast material on the drip-infusion urogram; however, this injury should also be suspected if there is nonfunction of one of the kidneys due to concomitant injury to the main renal vessels. On rare occasions, when ureteral injury is suspected and the drip-infusion urogram is nondiagnostic, it may be necessary to confirm the diagnosis by retrograde ureterogram on the suspected side (Fig. 3).

Treatment

The treatment of an injured ureter will vary with its location and severity. If at

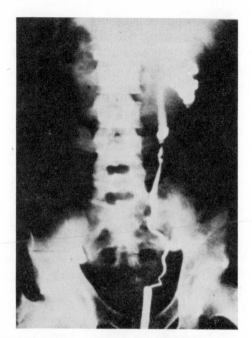

FIG. 3. Retrograde ureterogram demonstrating obstruction of the ureter and some hydronephrosis caused by a .38-caliber bullet that eroded from its original position in the renal cortex into the renal pelvis and then into the ureter over a 6-month interval.

all possible, with injuries involving its upper two thirds, the ends of the ureter should be freshened until they bleed properly, spatulated for about 1 cm and then sutured end to end.

PITFALL

EXCESSIVE MOBILIZATION OF THE URETER MAY RESULT IN NECROSIS OR POOR HEALING BY INTERFERING WITH THE BLOOD SUPPLY.

The ureter obtains its blood supply from the renal artery and from segmental vessels from the aorta, common iliac and hypogastric vessels. The segmental vessels can be sacrificed as long as the longitudinal vessels in the adventitia coming from either the lower or upper ureter are intact. If the adventitia is disturbed during the dissection or trauma, a segment of the ureter may necrose and form a ureteral fistula. Great care must be taken, therefore, to handle the ureter very gently.

The ureteral repair may be performed with two running 5-0 chromic catgut sutures so as to obtain a watertight anastomosis. No tension on the suture line is allowable because this almost inevitably leads to a breakdown of the anastomosis. If there has been no contamination of the ureter from an external penetrating injury or bowel leakage in the area, no stenting of the ureter is necessary. However, if there is any question of contamination, a stent should be utilized.[17] The stent should be small enough so that it will not cause pressure on the ureteral walls and should extend at least 3 to 4 cm above the anastomosis. The other end should be brought out through a cystotomy incision or through the urethra beside the Foley catheter. Silastic stents are generally used, but a red rubber Robinson catheter (8 to 10 French) is also perfectly satisfactory. With all ureteral injuries, a Penrose drain should be left in the periureteral area and brought out through a stab wound to remove any urine or blood that may leak in that area.

Although the lacerated end of the middle and upper third of the ureters can generally be reanastomosed directly, such repairs are generally not adequate in the lower third. If the ureter is damaged just above or near the bladder, it usually has to be reimplanted in the bladder, preferably employing an antireflux type of insertion. If the ureter is injured somewhat higher, near the pelvic rim, it may be necessary to use a pedicle flap of bladder known as a Boari or Ockerblad flap.[8]

Occasionally, it may be possible to obviate the need for a bladder flap by mobilizing the bladder and fixing it to the psoas muscles and the pelvic rim. The ureter can then be reimplanted into the mobilized bladder. This operation is known as a psoas-hitch type of ureteral reimplantation. The use of a transureteroureterostomy when the lower ureter is severely injured may also be considered in selected instances.[9]

Cutaneous ureterostomy may be utilized if it is difficult or impossible to provide ureterobladder continuity and especially if the functional status of the other kidney is in question. If it is certain that the contralateral urinary tract is normal, removal of the kidney on the side of the lesion is generally preferred to a cutaneous ureterostomy. Autotransplantation of the kidney from the lumbar fossa to the iliac fossa, on rare occasions, may be another method of handling the short ureter.[10]

INJURIES TO THE BLADDER

Etiology

When the bladder is empty, it is extremely well-protected against most types of trauma. When it is distended with urine, however, not only is it much more likely to be ruptured by blunt trauma or torn by spicules of bone from a pelvic fracture but it also presents a bigger target for a penetrating wound. Occasionally, a full bladder may be ruptured by a minor fall such as a slip on the ice.

Diagnosis

Bladder injuries should be suspected with any penetrating injury or blunt trauma to the lower abdomen or pelvis, especially if there is a fracture of the pelvic rami or separation of the symphysis pubis.[11,12] Symptoms and signs of bladder injury include gross hematuria and the inability to void. If the bladder rupture is intraperitoneal, the patient will also often have signs and symptoms of peritonitis, including pain, tenderness and rigidity. Careful rectal and vaginal examinations should be done in search of an enlarging pelvic mass or injury extending into the vagina or rectum.

Although examination of a voided urine specimen is an important part of the initial workup, if there is a high index of suspicion of bladder injury and the patient is unable to void, catheterization must be done.

X-ray examination of the bladder while it is filled with contrast material is the most accurate method for diagnosing rupture of

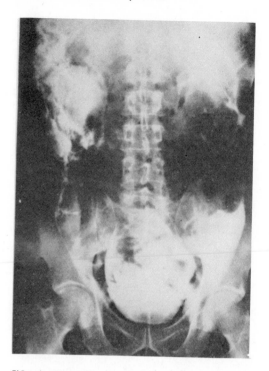

FIG. 4. Cystogram showing extravasation outside the bladder through a rupture into the peritoneal cavity with contrast material running up along the lateral gutters of the abdomen. (From Pierce, J. M.[19])

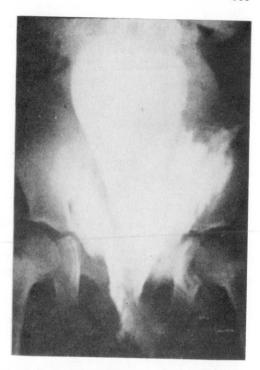

FIG. 5. Urethrogram showing a rupture of the prostatic urethra with extravasation around the bladder producing the so-called parachute bladder characteristic of this lesion. The bladder was filled by an intravenous urogram. (From Pierce, J. M.[19])

the bladder. In the male, this should be done with a retrograde urethrocystogram, and in the female with a cystogram (Fig. 4). The upper urinary tract should also be evaluated with a drip-infusion intravenous urogram. Sometimes the extravasation of contrast material from a ruptured bladder can be seen on the urogram, but there are many false-negatives.[13]

Retrograde cystograms are obtained by emptying the bladder with a catheter and then filling it by gravity with 200 to 300 ml of a 10 to 20% solution of contrast material made by diluting 100 ml of 60% organic iodide urography solution with 200 ml of saline. The technique of instilling a measured amount of water or normal saline into the bladder, and then emptying the bladder and measuring the recovered volume in lieu of a cystogram, is to be condemned.

The x-rays for the cystogram should include films taken in the AP and both posterior oblique projections and a postdrainage film of the bladder. If none of these studies shows any evidence of extravasation of the contrast material but there is gross hematuria and evidence of a pelvic hematoma, as manifested by a so-called parachute type of bladder, with the bladder elevated, narrowed and elongated (Fig. 5), the chances are excellent that the patient does have a ruptured bladder with tamponade of the tear by blood clot.

In penetrating wounds to the bladder, it is very common not to see extravasation on the cystogram because the hematoma in the wall of the bladder tamponades and closes off the hole. In some instances, tears up to 2 to 4 cm in length may be sealed by the hematoma. In 25 patients with proven ruptured bladder following blunt trauma, the diagnosis was made on cystogram in 23 of these; in two other cases, the cystogram looked normal, in spite of a ruptured bladder found at the time of surgery. Perivesical hematomas apparently prevented extravasation of the contrast material. Of three patients with penetrating wounds to the bladder, only one had an abnormal cystogram.[14]

In penetrating wounds of the urinary bladder, if the injury is incurred near a ureteral orifice, the ureteral insertion into the bladder may be severely damaged or blown off. Treatment of the bladder damage alone without proper attention to an associated ureteral injury will cause considerable morbidity and pelvic infection and may result in loss of the associated kidney.

Treatment

If there is extravasation of contrast material on the cystogram beyond the confines of the urinary bladder, or if there is severe hematuria with a perivesical hematoma, the patient should be explored through a vertical midline lower abdominal incision. The peritoneum is always opened before repairing the bladder to inspect for blood or injury to the bowel or other intraperitoneal organs.

If the vesical rupture is intraperitoneal, the rest of the bladder is inspected and then the mucosa and muscle are closed with a running 5-0 chromic catgut suture, followed by a second layer closing the muscle and serosa over this to further seal the bladder.

If the bladder rupture is extraperitoneal, the injury is best handled from within the bladder. After opening the peritoneum and inspecting its contents, it is closed. The bladder is then entered anteriorly through a midline incision and the area of rupture located. The muscularis is closed with either an interrupted or running 3-0 chromic catgut suture and the mucosa with a running 5-0 chromic catgut suture.

If the patient is a male, a Pezzar cystostomy tube is placed into the bladder through a stab wound away from the incision through the abdominal wall, halfway between the umbilicus and symphysis pubis, at least 2 to 3 cm from the incision. If the bladder injury is small and there has been minimal adjacent injury or contamination, or if the patient is a female, an 18 F. Foley catheter can be left indwelling without a cystostomy tube. However, if purulent urethritis and sepsis develop before it is safe to remove the Foley catheter, severe difficulties may arise.

The midline incision in the bladder is closed in three layers. A 4-0 or 5-0 chromic running catgut suture is used on the mucosal lining of the bladder; the muscularis and serosa are then closed as a second layer with a running 3-0 chromic catgut suture, and a third layer, consisting of a serosa-muscular suture of running 3-0 chromic catgut, is used to further seal the bladder cystotomy site.

Following all bladder surgery, a Penrose drain is left in the perivesical space and brought out through a stab wound separate from the incision. If healing is proceeding satisfactorily, this drain can usually be removed in 4 or 5 days. If a cystostomy tube has been utilized, this should be left in place for at least 8 to 10 days and then clamped. If there are no complications after it has been clamped for 24 hours and the patient can empty his bladder well, the tube can be removed.

INJURIES TO THE MALE URETHRA

The urethra is divided anatomically by the urogenital diaphragm into three parts (Fig. 6): (1) the prostatic urethra between the bladder and the superior leaf of the urogenital diaphragm, (2) the membranous urethra which traverses the urogenital diaphragm, and (3) the anterior urethra distal to the inferior leaf of the urogenital diaphragm. The anterior urethra may be further subdivided into the bulbous or perineal urethra (extending to the penoscrotal junc-

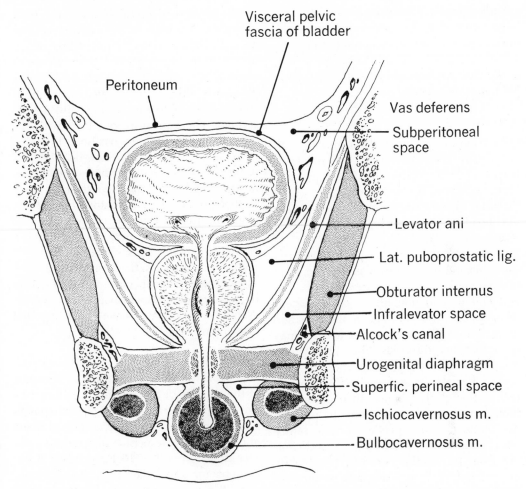

FIG. 6. The anatomy of the proximal urethra on a coronal section through the pelvis and urogenital diaphragm. (From Pierce, J. M.[19])

tion) and the distal penile or pendulous urethra.

Etiology

Penetrating wounds may damage any portion of the urethra. Blunt trauma, however, causes certain characteristic lesions. The classical straddle injury is one in which the male patient falls astride a bar such as a crossbar on a bicycle or a fence and sustains a severe blow to his perineum. In this injury, the bulbous urethra, just below the urogenital diaphragm, is crushed against the ischial rami and may rupture.

Severe blunt trauma to the lower abdomen and pelvis causing fractures of the pubic rami characteristically injures the prostatic, and occasionally the membranous, portion of the urethra. Classically, this type of trauma partially or completely severs the prostatic urethra just above the superior leaf of the urogenital diaphragm. Sometimes the urogenital diaphragm itself is torn as it is avulsed off an ischial ramus, and rarely the tear may extend into the membranous urethra itself.

AXIOM

MANIPULATIONS IN AND AROUND THE IN-JURED URETHRA MUST BE PERFORMED VERY GENTLY.

Unfortunately, excessively zealous attempts to catheterize or reapproximate the urethra may injure the membranous urethra, and this greatly compounds the problems, particularly with straddle injuries and prostatic urethral separations.

Diagnosis

Urethral injury should be suspected with any severe blunt trauma to the pelvis or perineum. If the patient has had a perineal blow and there is blood coming out of his urethral meatus, there is a very strong likelihood of rupture of the bulbous urethra with an associated perineal hematoma. If the patient has voided since the injury, there may also be extravasated urine in the perineum.

Rectal examination of the male patient who has had a separation of the prostatic urethra from the membranous urethra may show that the prostate is riding higher than usual. Sometimes a periprostatic and perivesical hematoma may make the prostate feel as though it is higher than normal although no separation is actually present. Any patient with a pelvic crushing injury who is unable to void, who has blood coming from the urethra, or who has bloody urine should have a retrograde urethrocystogram.

PITFALL

IF A FOLEY CATHETER IS INSERTED INTO A PATIENT WITH PELVIC TRAUMA BEFORE A URETHROGRAM IS PERFORMED, A URETHRAL INJURY MAY BE COMPLETELY MISSED.

If there is any suspicion of a urethral injury, a Foley catheter should not be inserted until a urethrogram has been performed. If there has been a partial urethral laceration with an incomplete separation and a Foley catheter is passed into the bladder, the injury may be completely missed and the catheter is apt to be removed long before healing is adequate.[18]

The retrograde urethrogram is the most important method for evaluating a suspected urethral injury. The urethrogram is obtained by injection of 10 to 25 cc of sterile 60% organic iodide contrast material, previously diluted with equal amounts of sterile saline, into the urethra with a bulb syringe. The x-rays are obtained with the patient in the oblique position. In many individuals, the bladder can be filled by using the same bulb syringe and gently instilling 200 to 300 ml of contrast material. If there is any resistance to filling of the bladder directly through the urethra, the cystogram should be performed through a catheter, if it can be inserted gently.

Areas of extravasation from the urethra should be noted. Special attention should be paid to determine whether the extravasation is below or above the urogenital diaphragm (Fig. 7).

Treatment

RUPTURE OF ANTERIOR OR DISTAL URETHRA. If the rupture of the urethra is confined by the fascial covering of the corpus spongiosum, and there is no extravasation of blood and urine into the perineum, urethral catheter drainage with a 16 F. 5-cc bag Foley catheter for 5 to 7 days is all that is necessary. If there is evidence of extravasation, the involved areas should be opened widely and drained for at least 5 to 7 days.

PITFALL

PERSISTENT ATTEMPTS TO PASS A URETHRAL CATHETER, ESPECIALLY AFTER A PELVIC INJURY, MAY CAUSE SEVERE COMPLICATIONS.

If, for some reason, a urethral catheter cannot be passed, a suprapubic cystostomy using a 30 F. Pezzar cystostomy tube is indicated. If the patient is on urethral catheter drainage, the catheter should be taped onto the anterior abdominal wall or medial thigh and cleansed frequently at the point where it enters the urethra. This cleansing is extremely important because

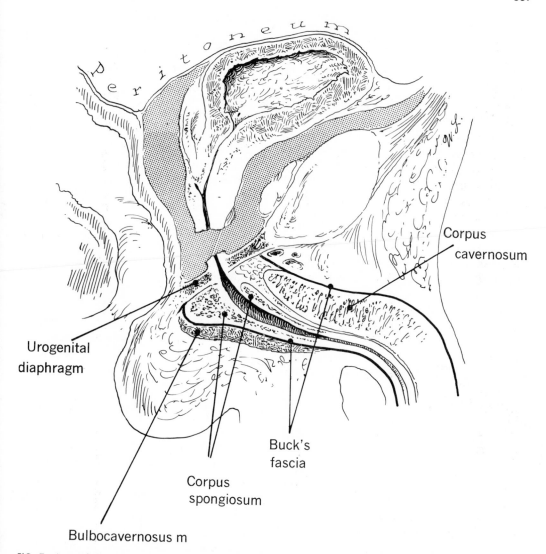

FIG. 7. A complete rupture of the prostatic urethra just above the urogenital diaphragm with a large pelvic hematoma. On rectal examination, the prostate would be noted to be much higher than normal. (From Pierce, J. M.[19])

one of the complications of urethral catheter drainage is purulent urethritis, which on occasion can lead to septic shock. Mechanical cleansing of the catheter at this point with soap and water five or six times a day is very effective. Use of a Betadine ointment around the catheter is also advantageous. The drainage system should be completely closed to reduce the chance of contamination.

If the urethra is ruptured completely through the corpus spongiosum, a suprapubic cystostomy with a 30 F. Pezzar catheter must be performed. If Buck's fascia is also torn, urine and blood may spread into the perineum and up the anterior abdominal wall. If the extravasated blood and urine become infected, the resultant sepsis has an extremely poor prognosis.

If a urethral catheter can be passed through the urethra up into the bladder, it may help by serving as a stent. The tip of the urethral catheter is then sutured to the tip of the cystostomy tube to keep it from falling out.

The use of interlocking sounds to try to reestablish urethral continuity, unless by a very experienced urologist, can lead to further damage to the urethra, especially in its membranous portion. If such iatrogenic damage occurs, the incidence and severity of later complications are greatly increased.

If there has been a complete rupture of the bulbous or distal urethra, the patient should be kept on cystostomy and Foley catheter drainage for at least three or four weeks. If urethritis develops, the Foley catheter must be removed sooner. At the end of this time, the urethral catheter, if still present, is removed by removing the cystostomy tube, cutting the tie that is holding it to the urethral catheter, and removing both the urethral and Pezzar catheters. The Pezzar catheter is then replaced with a 22 F. Foley catheter with a 5-cc bag as a cystostomy tube. This catheter can then be clamped and the patient given a trial of voiding. If the patient voids well for 24 hours, the cystostomy tube is removed. It is imperative that these patients are followed for at least a year to make sure that they are not developing a urethral stricture.

INJURIES OF THE MEMBRANOUS AND PROSTATIC URETHRA. These injuries are usually a result of severe blunt trauma to the pelvis with fractures of the pubic and/or ischial rami. These injuries carry a very high incidence of complications, including stricture of the urethra (which is often obliterative), sexual impotence, and chronic urinary infection (from prolonged drainage with tubes). The treatment of this group of injuries has been discussed extensively in recent years.

These patients should all have a suprapubic cystostomy and, if possible, an attempt should be made to pass a catheter in an antegrade fashion from the bladder into the urethra. If this is successful, then a urethral catheter can be sutured to its end and pulled into the bladder in a retrograde manner, to function as a urethral stent. Although this stent is very helpful, excessive attempts to insert the catheter should not be undertaken. If it cannot be passed easily in an antegrade manner, a suprapubic cystostomy, using a 30 Pezzar catheter, should be performed. A Penrose drain should be left in the perivesical area.

If a urethral catheter is easily passed in an antegrade manner and a retrograde catheter pulled through into the bladder, sometimes the prostate can be held down close to the urogenital diaphragm by passing nonabsorbable sutures through the prostatic capsule and out through the perineum and tying them over small packs. These are often referred to as vest sutures.

If the transection of the urethra is incomplete, it is important not to increase the injury by excessive operative manipulation; if one side of the urethra is intact, the autonomic nerves to the penis which pass through the urogenital diaphragm from the pelvis along the course of the urethra may be intact, and, if they are not damaged by further manipulation, the patient may not be rendered impotent.[15] In the past, it is certain that some people were made impotent by excessive operative attempts to reestablish continuity of the urethra. Occasionally, especially in young boys, approximation of the defect over a catheter can be carried out and the edges of the urethra sewn together. Attempts to do this, however, should not be pursued except by a surgeon with extensive experience in this area.

INJURIES TO THE PENIS AND SCROTUM

Most injuries to the penis and scrotum are due to direct trauma and are readily diagnosed. Penile injuries can occur under the most bizarre circumstances. If the injury is caused by blunt trauma when the penis is erect, the fascial covering of the corpora cavernosa may occasionally rupture without damage to the urethra. If this occurs, it should be treated by operative intervention with closure of the torn corpora cavernosum. Occasionally, the scrotal and penile skin is caught in mechanical belt-driven equipment and avulsed. This is treated by cleansing and minimal debridement so that as much viable skin as possible is left behind to reduce the amount of skin grafting that will be necessary. The penis can be temporarily protected with moist sterile dressings until it can be covered definitively with skin grafts. If the testes are exposed, they sometimes can be buried in subcutaneous pockets in the adjacent thigh.

Although there have been reported attempts to reanastomose a completely amputated portion of the penis to the remainder of the structure, the results have usually not been satisfactory. The initial treatment of an amputated penis after hemostasis is obtained consists of oversewing the ends of the corporal bodies and then spatulating the urethra to cover the end of the remaining penis.

INJURIES TO THE TESTES

Injuries to the testes may occasionally result from penetrating trauma, such as gunshots, but damage due to blunt trauma is much more common. The swelling and intracapsular testicular edema may cause severe pain. If the tunica albuginea is not ruptured, the initial treatment should consist of bed rest, scrotal support, analgesics and cold applications for 48 hours. If there is any suggestion that the tunica albuginea may be ruptured, the testicle should be explored, the area debrided, and the tunica albuginea reapproximated with sutures.

Lacerations of the testes by external trauma should be treated in the usual manner with debridement and surgical approximation of the separated tissues.

SUMMARY

Injury to the urinary tract should be suspected with any blunt or penetrating trauma to the lower chest, abdomen or pelvis. Any patient with hematuria, difficulty in voiding or severe pain or swelling in the flank should have his urinary tract completely investigated. Unless the mechanism of the injury is absolutely known to be localized either to the kidney or bladder, both drip-infusion urography and retrograde urethrocystography should be performed. The great majority of renal injuries are best treated nonoperatively initially, unless there is severe continued bleeding or urine extravasation.

Lower urinary tract injuries, involving the ureters or bladder, are generally best treated by early operation. The management of severe prostatomembranous urethral injury, however, is controversial. At this time, it is strongly advised that the general or urologic surgeon who sees these problems only occasionally use suprapubic cystostomy and perivesical drainage only. Subsequent urethral stricture, which is likely to occur, can be treated by those with expertise in this area at a later date.

TABLE 1. TEN FREQUENT ERRORS IN THE MANAGEMENT OF TRAUMA TO THE URINARY TRACT

1. Neglect of the patient's general condition and other injuries while investigating the urinary tract.
2. Failure to give a patient who is injured but whose condition is stable an opportunity to void spontaneously before a Foley catheter is inserted.
3. Failure to obtain early, high-dose drip-infusion excretion urography in patients who might have a renal injury.
4. Failure to obtain a renal arteriogram promptly if one of the kidneys is not visualized on the excretory urogram.
5. An aggressive surgical approach to renal injuries.
6. A conservative surgical approach to lower urinary tract injuries.
7. The assumption that a kidney is normal because it looks and feels normal.
8. Failure to obtain control of the renal vessels before opening a perirenal hematoma.
9. Excessive mobilization of the ureter while examining or repairing it.
10. Vigorous attempts to pass a Foley catheter in a patient who may have a urethral or bladder injury.

In the past, these injuries were often compounded by overzealous surgeons attempting primary repairs; primary repairs of these injuries can be performed successfully only on rare occasions. In treating gunshot wounds involving the urinary bladder, care must be taken not to miss a dismembered lower ureter or an associated rectal injury.

Frequent errors in management of trauma to the urinary tract are listed in Table 1.

REFERENCES

1. Mahoney, S. A., and Persky, L.: Intravenous drip nephrotomography as an adjunct in the evaluation of renal injury. J. Urol., 99:513, 1968.
2. Peters, P. C.: Trauma to the genitourinary tract. In: *Care of the Trauma Patient* (Shires, G. T., Ed.). New York, McGraw-Hill, 1966.
3. Elkin, M., et al.: Correlation of intravenous urography and renal angiography in kidney injury. Radiology, 86:496, 1966.
4. Morse, T. S., and Harris, B. H.: Nonpentrating renal vascular injuries. J. Trauma, 13:497, 1973.
5. Samuels, L. D., and Smith, J. P.: Kidney scanning in pediatric renal trauma. J. Trauma, 8:583, 1968.
6. Lucey, D. T., et al.: A plea for the conservative treatment of renal injuries. J. Trauma, 11:306, 1971.
7. Hinman, F., Jr.: Ureteral repair and the splint. J. Urol., 78:376, 1957.
8. Ockerblad, N. F.: Reimplantation of the ureter into the bladder by a flap technique. J. Urol., 57:845, 1947.
9. Anderson, H. V., et al.: Transureteroureterostomy experimental and clinical experiences. J. Urol., 57:845, 1947.
10. Hardy, J. D.: High ureteral injuries. JAMA, 184:97, 1963.
11. Reynolds, B. M., et al.: Pelvic fractures. J. Trauma, 13:1011, 1973.
12. Brosman, S. A., and Fay, R.: Diagnosis and management of bladder trauma. J. Trauma, 13:687, 1973.
13. Holland, M. E., et al.: Traumatic lesions of the urinary tract. Radiol. Clin. N. Amer., 4:433, 1966.
14. Wilson, R. F., and Birks, R.: Genitourinary injuries at Detroit General Hospital, 1960-1965. Unpublished data.
15. Seitzman, D.: Repair of the severed membranous urethra by the combined approach. J. Urol., 89:433, 1963.
16. Ross, R. R., Ackerman, E., and Pierce, J. M.: Traumatic subintimal hemorrhage of the renal artery. J. Urol., 104:11, 1970.
17. Fisher, S., Young, D. A., Molin, J. M., and Pierce, J. M.: Ureteral gunshot wounds. J. Urol., 108:238, 1972.
18. Pierce, J. M.: Management of dismemberment of prostatic-membranous urethra and ensuing structure disease. J. Urol., 107:259, 1972.
19. Pierce, J. M.: Trauma to the lower urinary system and genitalia. In: *The Practice of Surgery*. New York, Harper and Row, 1973.

Suggested Reading

1. Committee on Trauma, American College of Surgeons: Genitourinary tract (Chap. 14) in *Early Care of the Injured Patient*. Philadelphia, W. B. Saunders, 1972.

25 GYNECOLOGIC AND OBSTETRIC TRAUMA

T. N. EVANS
J. TESHIMA

GYNECOLOGIC INJURIES IN THE NONPREGNANT FEMALE (Table 1)

PITFALL

EXCESSIVE RELIANCE ON THE HISTORY AND CONCESSIONS TO MODESTY IN THE PHYSICAL EXAMINATION MAKE ACCURATE DIAGNOSIS OF GYNECOLOGIC TRAUMA EXTREMELY DIFFICULT.

Gynecologic injuries are important and yet are apt to be ignored or missed because of the patient's modesty or the doctor's reluctance to examine the perineum unless there is severe pain, bleeding or obvious wounds. In addition to the usual early complications of these injuries, such as pain, infection, or hemorrhage, certain more delayed sequelae may be extremely impor-

TABLE 1.   GYNECOLOGIC INJURIES AT DETROIT GENERAL HOSPITAL, 1960-69

TOTAL ADMISSIONS TO GYNECOLOGIC SERVICE—16,223

14 Vulvovaginal Injuries
   2 Rectal perforations by vaginal foreign bodies
38 Uterine Perforations
  20 During currettage
  10 During criminal abortions
   6 By gunshot wounds
   2 By intrauterine contraceptive devices

tant. These include infertility and pelvic contraction or distortion necessitating abdominal fetal delivery, rectovaginal or vesicovaginal fistulae, and vaginal and uterine synechiae.

Vulvovaginal Injuries

Because the history is often inaccurate or frankly deceptive, accurate diagnosis of vulvovaginal injuries depends primarily on careful complete examination.

PITFALL

IF GENERAL ANESTHESIA IS NOT USED IN THE UNCOOPERATIVE PATIENT TO OBTAIN A COMPLETE PELVIC EXAMINATION, SEVERE GYNECOLOGIC INJURIES MAY BE MISSED.

If there is any difficulty about obtaining patient cooperation, there should be no hesitancy in using general anesthesia; severe injuries of the urethra, bladder, rectum, and peritoneal cavity can be easily overlooked during the initial examination of a struggling, anxious patient. This is especially important with children, who are more likely to have serious associated injuries and are less likely to cooperate than adults.

The vulva and vagina, which are considered contaminated areas, and all associated wounds must be carefully cleansed prior to the examination. Since the bladder, if partially distended, can interfere with a proper pelvic examination, it should be emptied with a sterile catheter prior to the examination, and the urine submitted for analysis. In the adult, digital and speculum examination of the vagina and rectum is mandatory; in the child, vaginal endoscopy will usually suffice. If there is a possibility of high rectal damage, sigmoidoscopy is also indicated.

Additional information may be obtained by flat and upright x-rays of the abdomen. Free air, foreign bodies, and displaced loops of bowel all may have diagnostic value. If there is any suspicion of lower urinary tract injury, urethrograms and cystograms should also be performed.

HEMATOMAS. Before menopause, the vulva and vagina have a copious blood supply, and this rich plexus of veins is easily torn by any injury. Furthermore, there is little resistance in this area to the expansion of hematomas, and they may dissect deep into the perineum and ischiorectal fossa. Nevertheless, a nonpregnant woman with a large pelvic hematoma after only minimal trauma should be investigated for a blood dyscrasia, such as thrombocytopenia.

PITFALL

FAILURE TO OBTAIN IMMEDIATE COMPLETE COAGULATION STUDIES ON ANY PATIENT WITH EXCESSIVE BLEEDING MAY DELAY ACCURATE THERAPY AND SURGERY MAY BE UNDERTAKEN IN A PATIENT IN WHOM REASONABLE HEMOSTASIS IS IMPOSSIBLE.

Pain, the most common symptom of a pelvic hematoma, is usually directly proportional to the distension and disruption of the tissues. Ecchymoses about the perineum may be the only direct evidence of severe concealed hemorrhage into the ischiorectal fossa. Occasionally, excessive distension of a vulvar hematoma may either obliterate the vagina or cause a rupture of the overlying skin with external bleeding; rarely, the hematoma will continue to expand in spite of conservative treatment and cause hypovolemic shock. Although the presence of a vulvar hematoma is usually obvious, outlining its extent requires careful vaginal and rectal examination.

Most vulvar hematomas are less than 5 cm in diameter and resolve spontaneously without surgical intervention. However, progressively enlarging hematomas or hematomas greater than 5 cm in diameter require incision of the overlying mucosa or skin and evacuation of the clots. If the bleeding vessels are not found, and they usually are not, the hemorrhage may be controlled by multiple figure-of-eight sutures around the periphery of the hematoma followed by tight packing of the hematoma cavity over multiple Penrose drains. Concomitant packing of the vagina may also facilitate hemostasis. After removal of the pack in 24 to 48 hours, the hematoma cavity gradually disappears with subsequent restoration of normal anatomic landmarks. In rare instances a progressively enlarging subperitoneal hematoma may require laparotomy to achieve control of the bleeding.

LACERATIONS. Basic surgical principles in the management of vulvovaginal injuries are similar to those applied to any contaminated injury of the skin and subcutaneous tissues. Thorough cleansing, debridement and generous irrigation of all vulvovaginal wounds are essential. Additional treatment depends on the duration of the injury, the amount of inflammation and necrosis present and the presence of associated injuries to the urethra, bladder, rectum or peritoneal cavity. If the injuries are of less than 12 hours' duration and there is minimal tissue reaction, rectovaginal and vesicovaginal fistulae should be closed and any injuries to the anal sphincter carefully repaired. In many instances, a proximal colostomy will be needed if a large rectovaginal fistula is to heal properly.

RAPE AND COITUS

PITFALL

FAILURE TO PERFORM A COMPLETE INITIAL EXAMINATION ON AN ALLEGED RAPE VICTIM INCREASES NOT ONLY THE RISK OF COMPLICATIONS BUT ALSO THE POSSIBILITY OF GROSS INJUSTICE.

Rape is not always easily confirmed. The examining physician can only describe specific areas of obvious trauma and the presence or absence of spermatozoa. Any material in the vagina obtained during the speculum examination should be studied microscopically as a wet-mount. If the vagina is empty, it can be irrigated with saline which can then be removed and examined.

Coital trauma usually results in lacerations rather than hematoma formation. If the vagina is atrophic or the assault occurs in women with vaginismus, the lacerations are likely to be longitudinal. If the victim is a virgin, the rape or coitus may cause multiple hymenal and vaginal lacerations with severe bleeding. Occasionally the arterial bleeding following this initial coitus is so severe that ligation of the vessel and blood replacement are required. In addition to the pelvic evaluation, all rape victims should have a thorough general physical examination in search of extrapelvic injury; levels of consciousness and sobriety should be noted.

All suspected or proved victims of rape should be protected from pregnancy by the oral administration of estrogen, e.g. 25 mg of diethylstilbestrol twice daily for ten days.

FOREIGN BODIES

AXIOM

VAGINAL DRAINAGE IN A CHILD IS CAUSED BY A FOREIGN BODY UNTIL PROVEN OTHERWISE.

Trauma to the vulva or vagina from foreign bodies is most common in young children. Hemorrhage may occur immediately after insertion of the foreign body if it is sharp and causes a penetrating injury. Not infrequently, there is a delay of days or weeks before the child is brought to the physician because of a purulent vaginal discharge. Rectal examination with simultaneous insertion of a uterine sound into the vagina may detect a metallic foreign body. Because of the associated pain, anesthesia is often necessary to perform an adequate examination and to remove the foreign body.

If the foreign body is removed early, before there is severe infection, no additional therapy may be required. In all other instances, packing of the vagina with Vaseline gauze is important to prevent adhesive vaginitis and later vaginal atresia, dyspareunia, or infertility.

Pelvic Fractures

The rising number of high-speed automobile accidents has resulted in a marked increase in the incidence of severe pelvic fractures in females. Since the pelvis is a rigid, bony ring, great force is required to cause bony displacement, which will occur only if the ring is disrupted in at least two places. Such fractures may cause severe bleeding and extensive gynecologic and urologic injuries.[1] Not infrequently over 2000 ml of blood may be lost into the resulting retroperitoneal hematomas. Torn branches of the internal iliac vessels are the most likely source of bleeding under these circumstances.

PITFALL

SURGICAL ATTEMPTS TO CONTROL HEMORRHAGE FROM PELVIC FRACTURES USUALLY RESULT IN FURTHER BLEEDING AND SEVERE COMPLICATIONS.

If at all possible, pelvic hematomas due to fractures should not be opened; once the tamponading effect of the posterior peritoneum is lost, the bleeding may be almost impossible to control. Sutures, coagulation and other methods of direct hemostasis are frequently unsatisfactory in this area. If the hematoma is progressively expanding and the bleeding cannot be controlled, the area should be packed. Ligation of both internal iliac arteries occasionally also helps to control the bleeding. The pack should then be slowly withdrawn over 5 to 10 days, beginning on the fifth or sixth day.

Simultaneous injury to the lower urinary and genital tracts is a common complication of pelvic fractures. With the patient in a lateral position and using a Sims speculum, the physician can quickly gain some impression of the extent of injury to the base of the bladder, the vesical neck and the urethra. Injection of 2 ml of methylene blue into the bladder will often identify traumatic fistulae into the vagina. Use of radiopaque material may also be used to demonstrate openings into the peritoneal cavity.

Under most circumstances lower urinary tract injuries should be repaired immediately, especially if rupture of the bladder has been confirmed on cystography. Definitive treatment may have to be deferred if the patient's general condition is very poor at the time of the examination (Chap. 24).

Uterine Injuries

PENETRATING WOUNDS. *Iatrogenic Injuries.* Perforation of the myometrium from within the endometrial cavity with a curette, ovum forceps or uterine sound occurs about once in every 350 cases. Similarly, the uterine wall may be perforated during insertion of radioactive sources in the treatment of endometrial cancer.

When recognized immediately, uterine perforation of the nonpregnant uterus in the operating room can usually be managed conservatively by careful observation of the patient for evidence of occult hemorrhage and infection. Whenever uterine perforation is suspected, further attempts at curettage should be abandoned, except in cases of suspected malignancy, when they can be continued if care is taken to avoid the site of perforation. Similarly, curettage for incomplete abortion may be continued carefully with removal of large fragments of placental tissue if the perforation was caused by a uterine sound or small curette. When perforation occurs, culdocentesis may also be performed to rule out occult intraperitoneal hemorrhage.

In contrast, any evidence of omentum or bowel within the perforated uterus demands immediate laparotomy. When laparotomy is carried out, the bowel, omentum and all adjacent intraperitoneal structures must be carefully examined for injury. Parametrial bleeding may occur and sometimes will require hypogastric artery ligation. In general, an extensive laceration involving a grossly infected gravid uterus is best managed by hysterectomy.

Contraceptive Devices. Intrauterine contraceptive devices such as the "coil" may be pushed or migrate through the uterine wall. Such devices in the peritoneal cavity can result in bowel obstruction, especially when the device contains a closed loop.[2] Hysterography in such instances confirms the extrauterine location of the device which should then be removed.

Criminal Abortions

AXIOM

ATTEMPTED ABORTION MUST BE SUSPECTED IN ALL INSTANCES OF SEPTIC SHOCK IN YOUNG WOMEN OF CHILDBEARING AGE.

Perforation of the uterine wall commonly occurs as a result of attempts to induce abortion. A catheter inserted over a part of a coat hanger is commonly used. Repeated insertions of such instruments may result in multiple uterine wounds. These patients often delay in reporting to a physician for 7 to 10 days or until signs and symptoms of severe infection appear. Most of these patients will deny having attempted to cause the abortion. Vaginal bleeding, fever, tachycardia, and a tender uterus with or without hypotension should lead the physician to suspect instrumentation and the need for vigorous emergency measures.

Prompt treatment to combat shock and infection must be initiated (Chap. 5). After proper cultures have been obtained, massive amounts of antibiotics have been started, hypovolemia has been corrected, and the patient's condition is stabilized, the uterus should be evacuated.

Administration of the correct antibiotics to these patients is vital. The organisms most frequently involved are of the E. coli-Aerobacter category; however, anaerobic streptococci, staphylococci and Proteus vulgaris are often also present. Clostridium welchii infection is rare but often fatal when it occurs. Pelvic abscesses bulging into the cul-de-sac of Douglas should be confirmed by culdocentesis and then drained from below. Unless bleeding is active, oxytocic drugs are contraindicated in patients with septic abortions because the severe vasoconstriction they produce impairs circulation and the natural defenses to dissemination of infection.

All patients suspected of having a criminal abortion should have radiologic studies in search of an extrauterine foreign body. However, x-rays do not always rule out foreign bodies because some plastic instruments and tubes are not radiopaque.

When uterine perforation or rupture is suspected, exploratory celiotomy is indicated. If the uterus is found to be perforated and infected, a hysterectomy should be performed. In those patients who develop septic thrombophlebitis with septic pulmonary emboli, inferior vena caval and high bilateral ovarian vein ligation should be performed.

Stabs and Gunshot Wounds. Treatment of extensive uterine injury in young women depends on whether or not the uterus can be reconstructed well enough to make a future pregnancy reasonably safe. If this cannot be accomplished, hysterectomy is the treatment of choice. In the critically ill patient, it is unwise to insist on total hysterectomy unless the origin of bleeding is from the cervix and unless it can be accomplished as rapidly as a subtotal hysterectomy.

BLUNT TRAUMA TO THE UTERUS. Blunt injury to the uterus may result not only from direct trauma but also from seat belts following sudden deceleration. Signs of seat belt injuries include lower abdominal contusions, abrasions, and ecchymoses which may be associated internally with mesenteric lacerations, transection of the rectus muscles and bowel, and traumatic thrombosis of iliac vessels.[3] The nonpregnant uterus is usually well protected by the bony pelvis but may occasionally be so damaged by major pelvic trauma that hysterectomy may be necessary, especially in a woman of high parity whose uterus may be less able to contract and control bleeding.

CHEMICAL INJURIES TO THE UTERUS. Severe chemical injury to the uterus resulting in vaginal ulceration and bleeding may occur when agents such as potassium permanganate are used for criminal abortions. This initial chemical damage may be followed by fistula formation, extensive scarring and vaginal atresia. Treatment consists of careful irrigation with large quantities of saline, control of infection, and, in some instances, loose packing with Vaseline gauze to prevent vaginal synechiae.

Adnexal Injuries

Injury to the adnexa may be associated with extensive hemorrhage, usually resulting from disruption of the ovarian or ascending uterine arteries. The extent of deprivation of ovarian blood supply will determine the amount of ovarian tissue which can be preserved.

Minimal trauma may lead to torsion or rupture of adnexal structures, especially when ovarian cysts are present. The patient may have so much pain and tenderness that diagnosis can be accomplished only by examination under anesthesia. Rarely, a ruptured ovarian cyst may be fatal because of severe hemorrhage or severe chemical peritonitis resulting from rupture of a dermoid cyst or tubo-ovarian abscess.

OBSTETRIC TRAUMA

General Considerations

Trauma is an increasing cause of maternal death and deserves special attention because two lives are involved.[4] Knowledge of certain fundamental intrinsic changes which occur during pregnancy is essential to the management of these patients.

In assessing the status of the gravid female, the physician must be aware of the normal physiologic changes and alterations in laboratory values during pregnancy.[5,6] For example, the normal expansion of the extracellular fluid space during pregnancy may result in a significant dilutional hyponatremia.[7] During late pregnancy, this hyponatremia may be made even worse by restriction in sodium intake. Since fibrinogen levels in late pregnancy are generally two to three times those found in the nonpregnant patient, fibrinogen levels which would be normal in a nonpregnant female reflect a serious deficit in a patient near term. Traumatic abruption of the placenta may be caused by direct injury or indirectly as the result of shock and may produce disseminated intravascular coagulation with lethal hemorrhage unless the clotting defect is corrected.[8]

Problems correlating coagulation studies with therapy involving the use of fresh blood, fibrinogen, heparin, and epsilon amino caproic acid are discussed in Chapter 34.

PITFALL

IF A WOMAN INJURED DURING LATE PREGNANCY IS NOT KEPT ON HER SIDE, SEVERE HYPOTENSION UNRELATED TO THE TRAUMA MAY DEVELOP; IF THE CAUSE OF THIS HYPOTENSION IS MISINTERPRETED, EXCESSIVE QUANTITIES OF FLUIDS AND BLOOD MAY BE ADMINISTERED.

About 10% of women in late pregnancy develop hypotension in the supine position as a result of vena caval compression by the gravid uterus.[9] Hypotension from this supine vena caval syndrome following trauma may falsely suggest extensive internal damage, and the physician may dangerously overload the patient with fluid or blood. Turning the patient on her side, elevating the lower extremities, or displacing the uterus to the right will usually restore a normal pressure promptly. The vena caval compression which occurs in the supine position also increases venous pressure in the lower part of the body and may increase bleeding from injuries to the pelvis and lower extremities.

Distension of the spleen and liver with blood during gestation, as well as displacement and compression by the gravid uterus, makes them much more susceptible to rupture by minor trauma during the later stages of pregnancy.[10] Occasionally, there is catastrophic hemorrhage due to rupture of the liver when no history of trauma can be obtained.

PITFALL

IF TRANSFUSION TO A MODERATELY HYPOVOLEMIC BUT NORMOTENSIVE PREGNANT WOMAN IS DELAYED FOLLOWING TRAUMA, SEVERE FETAL DISTRESS MAY DEVELOP.

After trauma, both maternal and fetal homeostasis should be restored as soon as possible by replacing deficits in volume and red cell mass with whole blood transfusions. Dextran and lactated Ringer's solution may restore the circulatory blood volume but are not as effective as whole blood or packed cells because they do not improve fetal arterial oxygenation.[11,12] Vasopressors should be avoided, if at all possible, since these drugs further decrease uterine blood flow and increase fetal hypoxia.

Special Preoperative Preparations in Pregnant Women

In addition to the standard preoperative preparations of any patient, certain special safeguards must be taken with pregnant women. Because of the reduced gastrointestinal motility, early emptying of the stomach with a nasogastric tube is extremely important. Although insertion of a Foley catheter should always be done under sterile conditions, extra precautions should be taken in these women because of the high risk of bladder and renal infection during pregnancy. The gravid uterus must be shielded as much as possible during any diagnostic radiography, and only the most necessary x-rays should be taken.[13]

Specific Injuries

UTERINE DAMAGE. *Penetrating Trauma.* Paradoxically, the prognosis following pelvic wounds during pregnancy is surprisingly good. Gunshot wounds of the abdomen in the nongravid female have a mortality rate four times greater than that found during pregnancy. The enlarging uterus displaces other viscera and serves as a protective shield.[14,15] The uterine wall and amniotic fluid provide a cushioning effect, diminishing the force of any penetrating missile. In addition, force applied to the uterus, in contrast to a solid organ, is distributed equally in all directions.

With penetrating abdominal wounds during pregnancy, exploratory laparotomy should be performed as soon as the patient's condition permits. Speed is particularly important when there is a chance of salvaging the fetus. In such instances exploration of other viscera should be deferred until the infant is delivered.

Superficial uterine wounds may be closed primarily. If the penetration extends through the uterine wall and the gestation is greater than 32 weeks, prompt delivery by cesarean section is generally indicated. Removal of a premature infant by cesarean section is not warranted when the uterus appears to be intact. If uterine damage is extensive or if there has been gross contamination of the uterus, hysterectomy should be performed.

Blunt Trauma. Auto accidents are an increasingly frequent cause of severe pelvic trauma and are now the most common cause of nonobstetric uterine rupture. Although the seat belt may prevent some severe injuries, it is not entirely harmless and has been increasingly incriminated as a cause of severe abdominal damage.[16,17]

It may occasionally be extremely difficult to make the diagnosis of uterine rupture following blunt abdominal trauma. Vaginal bleeding is not always present and abdominal tenderness and guarding may be minimal and easily confused with damage to the anterior muscles of the abdominal wall.

AXIOM

UTERINE RUPTURE MUST BE RULED OUT WHENEVER LABOR SEEMS TO BE PRECIPITATED BY TRAUMA.

In some instances, the pain of uterine rupture may closely resemble the pain of parturition. When faced with this dilemma, it is important to follow the fetal heart tones closely. If they slow or become inaudible, severe uterine damage or blood loss must be suspected. The clinical distinction between labor and uterine rupture is critical. If one tries to induce labor with oxytocic drugs in a patient wth uterine rupture, one may increase uterine damage and cause fatal bleeding.

FETAL INJURY. *Penetrating Trauma.* Damage to the placenta or umbilical cord from penetrating wounds may result in severe hemorrhage into the amniotic sac.[18] Although the maternal prognosis is usually good following bullet and stab wounds of the pregnant uterus, the fetus has only about one chance out of four of surviving. The high associated perinatal mortality is due to premature delivery as well as direct injury to the fetus, placenta and umbilical cord. Assessment of the extent of fetal injury is not easy. Obtaining blood by amniocentesis is diagnostic and is a grave prognostic sign.

Although the fetus will occasionally survive after the death of the mother, he is much more likely to die than the mother as a result of shock and decreased uteroplacental perfusion.[19] Even relatively mild injuries to the mother may cause severe fetal hypoxia and alter the subsequent course of the pregnancy or delivery.

The treatment of a viable injured fetus should be approached much as that of any newborn infant. After rapid delivery of the fetus by cesarean section, a second team of physicians should immediately begin treatment. The umbilical vein provides rapid access to the fetal circulation, but great care must be taken not to overload the cardiovascular system with excessive fluids.

Some rather bizarre fetal injuries have been reported following penetrating trauma. In one instance an infant died shortly after birth as a result of severe hemorrhage from a gunshot wound of the femoral artery.[20] In another instance the fetus swallowed the bullet and, following birth, developed an intestinal obstruction which was cured spontaneously by passage of the bullet in the stool.[21]

Blunt Trauma. Severe fetal injury can result from blunt trauma with minimal uterine damage.[22] Although the severity of the external force is extremely important, the duration of gestation is also a critical factor. During early gestation, the uterus is shielded by the bony pelvis. Later, as the uterus enlarges up and out of the pelvis, the protective effect of the amniotic fluid is all that remains.

Although the total volume of amniotic fluid continues to increase until about the 38th week of pregnancy, the amount present in relation to the size of the uterus falls as the pregnancy progresses. Thus, the risk of fetal injury also increases and is particularly great after the fetal head has become

fixed in the maternal pelvis. This fixation of the fetal head may explain the high incidence of skull fractures and intracranial hemorrhage resulting from blunt trauma.[23] Many of these injuries, including multiple fractures, may heal partially or completely by the time of birth.

Postmortem Cesarean Section

PITFALL

IF A POSTMORTEM CESAREAN SECTION IS NOT PERFORMED IMMEDIATELY ON A PREGNANT WOMAN WHO DIES SUDDENLY, AN OPPORTUNITY TO SAVE A VIABLE FETUS MAY BE MISSED.

Although a successful postmortem cesarean section is seldom performed, almost 150 cases of fetal survival under such circumstances have been reported.[24] The more mature the fetus, the better the chances for survival, especially if the mother dies suddenly rather than after a prolonged illness. Chances for fetal survival are greatly diminished if cesarean section is delayed longer than five minutes after maternal death. To improve the chances of fetal survival, resuscitation efforts should be vigorous, and facilities for opening the abdomen rapidly should be immediately available. If need for a postmortem cesarean section is suspected, it is advantageous to attempt resuscitation of the patient in the operating room.

Medicolegal Aspects of Trauma in Pregnancy

The medicolegal implications of injuries during pregnancy are protean. If pregnancy continues normally for several weeks following trauma, subsequent abortion or premature labor is probably not due to the injury. Traumatic abortions of normal pregnancies are rare.[25] Hertig[26] suggests that a prima facie case for traumatic abortion must include evidence that the abortus was anatomically normal up to the time of trauma.

SUMMARY

Accurate diagnosis of gynecologic and obstetric injuries requires careful pelvic examination, often using general anesthesia when the patient cannot cooperate. Injuries due to blunt trauma, especially retroperitoneal hematomas, should usually be treated conservatively whereas most penetrating wounds should have early surgical exploration. Criminal abortions, which should be suspected in any young woman with severe sepsis and lower abdominal tenderness, must be treated aggressively with antibiotics, fluid, and early evacuation or removal of the uterus.

Since even mild hypovolemia in the pregnant woman may greatly reduce uterine blood flow, any delay in administering needed fluid or blood may cause severe fetal distress. If a penetrating injury to the pregnant uterus cannot be repaired well enough to make subsequent delivery safe, hysterectomy should be performed after delivering the mature fetus by cesarean section. If vaginal bleeding or labor pains develop after blunt trauma, uterine rupture should be suspected and oxytocic drugs are contraindicated. If a pregnant woman with a mature fetus dies suddenly, immediate postmortem cesarean section should be considered.

REFERENCES

1. Miller, W. E.: Massive hemorrhage in fractures of the pelvis. Southern Med. J., 56:933, 1963.
2. Shimkin, P. M., Siegel, H. A., and Seaman, W. B.: Radiographic aspects of perforated intrauterine contraceptive devices. Radiology, 92:353, 1969.
3. Doersch, K. B., and Dozier, W. E.: The seat belt syndrome. The seat belt sign, intestinal and mesenteric injuries. Amer. J. Surg., 116:831, 1968.
4. Committee on Trauma and Committee on Shock: *Accidental Death and Disability: The Neglected Diseases of Society.* Washington, National Academy of Sciences, National Research Council, 1966.
5. Peckham, C. H., and King, R. W.: A study of intercurrent conditions observed during pregnancy. Amer. J. Obstet. Gynec., 87:609, 1963.
6. Fine, J.: Glycosuria of pregnancy. Brit. Med. J., 1:205, 1967.
7. Rhodes, P.: The volume of liquor amnii in early pregnancy. J. Obstet. Gynec. Brit. Comm., 73:23, 1966.
8. Beller, F. K.: Hemorrhagic disorders in pregnancy. Clin. Obstet. Gynec., 7:269, 1964.
9. Marx, G. F.: Shock in the obstetric patient. Anesthesiology, 26:423, 1965.
10. Buchsbaum, J. H.: Splenic rupture in pregnancy. Report of a case and review of the literature. Obstet. Gynec. Survey, 22:381, 1967.
11. Boba, A., Linkie, D. M., and Plotz, E. J.: Effects of vasopressor administration and fluid replacement on fetal bradycardia and hypoxia induced by maternal hemorrhage. Obstet. Gynec., 27:408, 1966.
12. Greiss, F. C., Jr.: Uterine vascular response to hemorrhage during pregnancy, with observations on therapy. Obstet. Gynec., 27:549, 1966.
13. Whitehouse, W. M., Simons, C. S., and Evans, T. N.: Reduction of radiation hazard in obstetric roentgenography. Roentgenology, 80:690, 1958.
14. Buchsbaum, H. J.: Accidental injury complicating pregnancy. Amer. J. Obstet. Gynec., 102:752, 1968.
15. Beatie, J. F., and Daly, R. F.: Gunshot wound of the pregnant uterus. Amer. J. Obstet. Gynec., 80:772, 1960.
16. Fish, J., and Wright, R. H.: The seat belt syndrome . . . does it exist? J. Trauma, 5:746, 1965.
17. Rubovits, F. E.: Traumatic rupture of the pregnant uterus from "seat belt" injury. Amer. J. Obstet. Gynec., 90:828, 1964.
18. Wright, C. H., Posner, A. C., and Gilchrist, J.: Penetrating wounds of the gravid uterus. Amer. J. Obstet. Gynec., 67:1085, 1954.
19. Romney, S. L., Gabel, P. V., and Takeda, Y.: Experimental hemorrhage in late pregnancy. Effects on maternal and fetal hemodynamics. Amer. J. Obstet. Gynec., 87:636, 1963.
20. Bryant, J. F., and Moore, M. D.: Gunshot wound of gravid uterus with simultaneous exploration of mother and fetus: Report of a case. Amer. Surg., 30:207, 1964.
21. Buchsbaum, H. J., and Caruso, P. A.: Gunshot wound of the pregnant uterus. Case report of fetal injury deglutition of missile and survival. Obstet. Gynec., 33:673, 1969.
22. Theurer, D. E., and Kaiser, I. H.: Traumatic fetal death without uterine injury. Report of a case. Obstet. Gynec., 21:477, 1963.
23. Dyer, I., and Barclay, D. L.: Accidental trauma complicating pregnancy and delivery. Amer. J. Obstet. Gynec., 83:907, 1962.
24. Breen, J. L., and Peraglie, B. R.: Postmortem Cesarean section. Report of a case. Pacific Med. Surg., 74:102, 1966.
25. Javert, C. T.: Role of the patient's activities in the occurrence of spontaneous abortion. Fertil. Steril., 11:550, 1960.

26. Hertig, A. T.: Symposium on problems re-
lating to law and surgery: minimal criteria
required to prove prima facie case of traumatic abortion or miscarriage; analysis of 1000
spontaneous abortions. Ann. Surg., 117:596,
1943.

Suggested Readings

1. Barnes, A. C., and Holzman, G. B.: Gyneco-
logic injuries. In: *The Management of Trauma*
(Ballinger, W. F., Ed.). Philadelphia, W. B.
Saunders, 1968.

2. Fort, A. T.: Prenatal intrusion into the amnion.
Amer. J. Obstet. Gynec., 110:432, 1971.
3. Fleming, W. H., and Bowen, J. C.: Control of
hemorrhage in pelvic crush injuries. J.
Trauma, 13:567, 1973.
4. Olcott, C., et al.: Amniotic fluid embolism
and disseminated intravascular coagulation
after blunt abdominal trauma. J. Trauma,
13:737, 1973.
5. McNabney, W. K., and Smith, E. I.: Penetrating wounds of the gravid uterus. J.
Trauma, 13:1024, 1973.

26 PERIPHERAL VASCULAR INJURIES

J. YAO
J. PLANT
R. F. WILSON

Technical advances, particularly the increased use of arteriography, autogenous grafts and intra-arterial balloon catheters, have revolutionized the management of peripheral vascular injuries. Unfortunately, clinical acumen has not always kept pace; too many limbs are still lost or crippled through failure to appreciate the need for vigorous investigation of all limb injuries where there exists even a remote possibility of vascular damage.

PITFALL

ANY DELAY IN DEFINITIVE REPAIR OF AN ARTERIAL INJURY EXCEEDING 4 TO 6 HOURS GREATLY INCREASES THE INCIDENCE AND SEVERITY OF COMPLICATIONS.

Prolonged ischemia in a limb may result in irreversible tissue damage with subsequent loss of the limb or severe contractures due to replacement of muscle by fibrous tissue. In addition, hypotension combined with toxemia due to tissue necrosis may cause or aggravate renal, respiratory, and cardiac failure.

ETIOLOGY

Penetrating Injuries

An understanding of the forces involved in the various types of injuries is essential in the management of arterial trauma. The explosive force of high-velocity (2,000 to 3,000 feet/sec) missiles, such as high-power rifle bullets, creates a cavitational effect in the limb with massive destruction of soft tissues and any vessels in that area. Thus, the artery may not only be torn by the missile but may also be severely contused for several centimeters proximal and distal to the laceration.[1] Deep contamination of such wounds from clothing, dirt and debris is common. In contrast, low-velocity missiles (500 to 1,000 feet/sec), generally due to gunshot wounds from pistols, usually push the blood vessel ahead, stretching it slightly before penetration, and cause only minimal adjacent soft-tissue injury.

With close-range shotgun blasts, the multiple pellets can cause extensive soft-tissue damage. Furthermore, the wad and plastic caps used to separate the powder charge from the shot may also penetrate deeply into the wound and, if not recovered, can lead to severe infections later. Since these objects are not radiopaque, their presence may not be recognized unless a thorough exploration of the wound is performed.

Blunt Trauma

Damage to arteries is being increasingly recognized following automobile accidents and athletic injuries. In most instances, the arterial injury is associated with a fracture of a long bone or a severe dislocation. The vessel may be directly contused by the displaced bone or it may be torn or perforated by the sharp edges of the fracture fragments. However, vascular damage can also occur from simple prolonged compression without a fracture or dislocation, as when a leg is pinned between two bumpers or a bumper and a wall.

Some of the more common sites of vascular trauma with orthopedic injuries include: (1) fractured clavicle—subclavian artery and vein, (2) dislocated shoulder—axillary artery, (3) supracondylar fracture of the humerus—brachial artery, and (4) knee dislocation or fracture of the proximal tibia—popliteal artery. Another example of arterial injury following orthopedic trauma is thrombosis or aneurysm of the axillary artery from an improperly adjusted crutch impinging upon the axillary contents.

Damage or compression of the brachial artery by supracondylar fractures of the humerus, which occurs almost exclusively in children, is especially dangerous. Frequent and careful examination of the radial pulse and the circulation to the hand is essential following such an injury, particularly after reduction of the fracture. Any prolonged ischemia to the forearm may result in fibrosis of the muscle with later development of Volkmann's ischemic contracture.

TYPES OF VASCULAR INJURY

Compression

Compression of a vessel by an external force may occlude the lumen without apparent vascular damage. If mild to moderate pressure on the vessel persists for several hours, a firm clot may develop in the proximal lumen and cause continued obstruction of the vessel after the compression is relieved. If the compression force is severe, it may cause contusion with local thrombosis or development of a distally hinged intimal flap that may also result in occlusion.

Spasm

On rare occasions, severe sustained contraction of vascular smooth muscle, associated with little or no apparent external damage to the vessel, may partially or completely obliterate the lumen. Such a spasm is usually self-limiting and generally disappears within a few minutes following relief or removal of the local compression.

PITFALL

IF DISTAL ISCHEMIA PERSISTS AFTER REDUCTION OF A FRACTURE OR DISLOCATION, IT SHOULD BE ASSUMED THAT THE VASCULAR OCCLUSION IS DUE TO VESSEL DAMAGE OR THROMBOSIS RATHER THAN SPASM.

Unfortunately some physicians still attempt to correct vascular occlusion following trauma with proximal nerve blocks, such as lumbar, epidural, or stellate ganglion blocks. Attempts to relieve "spasm" with these indirect methods generally only cause dangerous delays in the exploration and repair of the affected vessel.

AXIOM

NERVE BLOCKS TO CORRECT SPASM FOLLOWING TRAUMA TO A VESSEL ARE TO BE STRONGLY CONDEMNED BECAUSE THE TIME LOST WITH SUCH PROCEDURES MAY RESULT IN IRREVERSIBLE TISSUE DAMAGE.

At the time of surgery after the injured artery has been repaired, some degree of spasm may persist at the site of injury. Under these circumstances, local stripping of the adventitia for 1 to 2 cm above and below the repair, together with the local application of papaverine or Xylocaine, may improve the flow. If the flow still remains inadequate, an arteriogram should be performed in the operating room. If the radiographs show any evidence of partial or complete block, the anastomosis should be excised and the vessel repaired with a new end-to-end anastomosis or insertion of an autologous vein graft.

AXIOM

THE GREAT MAJORITY OF VESSELS THAT AP-PEAR TO BE IN SPASM ACTUALLY HAVE SIG-NIFICANT INTERNAL DAMAGE WHICH MUST BE CORRECTED SURGICALLY.

Contusion

Direct trauma may cause hemorrhage or edema in the intima and media of the vessel, producing narrowing or partial occlusion of the lumen. Vessels suffering significant contusion usually have a mottled external appearance because of subadventitial hemorrhage. As with severe compression, obstruction may also occur if an intimal flap develops from a crack in the vessel or if a thrombosis develops on the injured intima.

Lacerations and Perforations

Lacerations and perforations of blood vessels are most frequently encountered following penetrating wounds but may also be caused by sharp fracture fragments produced by blunt trauma. With complete transection, distal blood flow will cease and constriction and retraction of the vessel ends will often keep bleeding to a minimum. In contrast, with a partial laceration or perforation, the vessel cannot retract adequately and, although some distal blood flow may continue, the local bleeding is apt to be severe and persistent.

False Aneurysm

If the wound in a partially lacerated artery does not become occluded, the associated hematoma will develop a cavity in continuity with the arterial lumen and become a "pulsating hematoma." Later, when this cavity becomes lined with endothelial cells, it may have the appearance of an aneurysm. Since this "aneurysm" does not have all the normal layers of the vessel wall, it is called a "false" aneurysm. Although distal blood flow usually continues, severe symptoms may result from pressure on adjacent structures by the aneurysmal mass.

Recently, there has been a great increase in the incidence of septic false aneurysms following arterial injury by drug addicts using unsterile needles. These aneurysms, unless treated by proximal and distal ligation away from the infected site, may rupture and rapidly cause death from exsanguination. Fortunately, the collaterals which develop around such aneurysms are often adequate to maintain tissue viability distally after the vessel is ligated.

Arteriovenous (AV) Fistulae

A traumatic arteriovenous fistula develops when a penetrating injury causes laceration in an artery and its adjacent vein. The high arterial pressure allows blood to flow continuously into the adjacent hematoma and then into the vein, or directly into the vein itself. Later, as the hematoma wall becomes fibrotic and retracts, the holes in the artery and vein are often brought into direct continuity.

A large AV fistula can produce a significant increase in pulse rate, pulse pressure and cardiac output;[2,3] if large enough, it can cause a high-output cardiac failure and may be associated with an increased incidence of bacterial endocarditis. Compression of the fistula often causes a characteristic decrease in the pulse rate (Nicolodani-Branham sign).

DIAGNOSIS OF VASCULAR INJURIES

AXIOM

ANY LONG BONE FRACTURE, MAJOR DISLO-CATION, OR PENETRATING WOUND SHOULD BE CONSIDERED TO HAVE CAUSED A VASCULAR INJURY UNTIL PROVEN OTHERWISE.

A high index of suspicion plus careful complete clinical examination and angiography, where necessary, should result in an accurate diagnosis of most vascular injuries.

Clinical Examination

Massive external bleeding, especially if it is bright red and pulsating, is an obvious sign of a major arterial injury. Although not as readily apparent, a large hematoma, especially if it is expanding, is also strongly suggestive of this diagnosis.

The acutely ischemic limb is classically described by the six Ps: pulselessness, pallor, poikilothermia, pain, paresthesia, and paralysis. Although these symptoms and signs are extremely helpful in diagnosing major arterial injury, many of them may be caused by hypovolemia, shock, or severe cold when no vascular injury is present.

Although the distal pulses usually disappear following a major arterial injury, they will occasionally persist, especially if the injury involves only a small portion of the wall. Pallor may never develop in the ischemic limb, or it may be present only transiently; it can also be difficult to appreciate in dark-skinned patients. Furthermore, if there is any obstruction to venous return, the limb will appear cyanotic rather than pale.

Poikilothermia or reduction in the temperature of the skin to that of the environment may be very helpful. However, if there is significant collateral blood flow, if the superficial vessels in the skin are dilated, or if the temperature of the environment exceeds 80 to 85 F, the limb may not become cool until tissue death has occurred.

Initially, the pain or paresthesia due to an inadequate blood flow may be quite severe; however, if the ischemia is severe and persists, the limb may quickly become anesthetic. Direct trauma to nerves may be extremely painful, but it can also cause complete anesthesia to the involved area.

PITFALL

IF THE DIAGNOSIS OF AN ARTERIAL INJURY IS NOT MADE UNTIL MOTOR FUNCTION IS IMPAIRED, THE DELAY IN TREATMENT MAY BE DISASTROUS.

Loss of distal motor function is a late sign of ischemia to the muscles or nerves and, therefore, of relatively little value to diagnosing vascular injuries early, when repair is most apt to be successful.

Occasionally a bruit or thrill over a pulsating hematoma or a continuous murmur over an arteriovenous fistula may be the only evidence of a major vascular injury. Consequently, careful auscultation over the area of trauma is an important part of the physical examination.

Arteriograms

Arteriography, if properly performed, is the single most accurate ancillary method for diganosing the site and extent of a vascular injury. It has particular value if an arterial injury is suspected but the clinical findings are equivocal. The arteriogram may reveal extravasation of contrast material, occlusion or narrowing of the vessel, an arteriovenous fistula, a false aneurysm or an intimal tear.

The vessels that particularly lend themselves to arteriography include the femoral, popliteal, subclavian, axillary, brachial and carotid arteries. Arteriograms may be obtained by direct needle puncture or through a catheter inserted by the percutaneous Seldinger technique.[4] This technique allows an arterial site to be selectively examined, and is of particular value in the diagnosis of proximal arterial and aortic injuries.

Although arteriograms are generally accurate and extremely informative, they are not without problems. In addition to complications of bleeding, hematoma formation or occlusion at the puncture site, the arteriogram may also cause undue delay in treatment, especially if performed at night or on weekends when the regular personnel and equipment are not readily available. If arteriography causes delay of needed surgery, it is certainly not to the patient's advantage. Successful relief of ischemia is time dependent, and in some instances even minutes may be precious.

AXIOM

ARTERIOGRAPHY IS GENERALLY UNNECESSARY IF THE NEED FOR EXPLORATION IS OBVIOUS.

One of the most frequent errors in the interpretation of arteriograms following trauma is the overlooking of an area of slight narrowing or "spasm" due to significant intimal injury. Reports of misinterpretation of arteriograms both in clinical[5,6] and in animal studies[7] have raised some questions about the need or value of performing these studies routinely before emergency vascular surgery. All factors should be considered carefully before ordering an emergency arteriogram and delaying surgery. Much will depend upon the availability of the personnel and equipment to perform the studies. If a good result is to be obtained, no more than 4 to 6 hours should elapse between the time of injury and the time of repair and reestablishment of an adequate distal blood flow.

TREATMENT

The first successful end-to-end arterial anastomosis in a human was performed by J. B. Murphy in 1896;[8] however, because of the high rate of thrombosis or infection following attempts at direct reconstruction, ligation was still the usual treatment for major arterial injuries until the latter part of World War II.

The inadequacy of ligation was well demonstrated by DeBakey and Simeone,[9] who reviewed 2,470 major arterial injuries treated in this manner and reported a 49% amputation rate (30% for brachial artery damage and 75% for femoral-popliteal injuries). As a result, during the Korean War a greatly increased effort was made to perform primary arterial repairs and the superiority of vascular repair was clearly demonstrated. In 1958, Hughes[10] reported 304 cases of major arterial injuries with an amputation rate of 50% when ligation was used and 13% when arterial reconstruction was performed.

Since then, the results of primary vascular repair have continued to improve, primarily as a result of increased use of emergency arteriography, autologous vein grafts (rather than end-to-end anastomosis under tension) and more complete distal thrombectomies using balloon-tipped and irrigating (Fogarty) catheters.

Initial Management

Active external bleeding is best controlled by direct digital compression over a sterile dressing. The use of a tourniquet is seldom necessary and can be extremely dangerous because it impedes blood flow through the collateral vessels and may cause severe pressure damage to the underlying muscle and nerves. Conversely, if the tourniquet loosens so that it allows arterial inflow but retards venous return, the external bleeding may be greatly increased.

Depending upon the extent of the injury and the amount of blood loss, two or three large intravenous catheters should be inserted. After the initial blood samples are drawn for a blood count and type and cross-matching, fluid and blood should be infused rapidly until the vital signs are restored to normal. Monitoring of central venous pressure is essential if the patient requires massive transfusions or remains hypotensive in spite of rapid volume replacement (Chap. 5).

When an obvious severe fracture or dislocation is present, the physician must decide whether to attempt reduction immediately in the emergency room or to splint the limb and delay manipulation until x-rays have been obtained. If the portion of the limb distal to the injury is obviously ischemic or if there is evidence of loss of sensation or motor nerve function, immediate reduction is warranted. If the circulation improves with the reduction, the limb should be splinted in that position while awaiting further studies or treatment. If the circulation does not improve with attempts at reduction, immediate arteriography and surgery are necessary. If the distal limb is not ischemic when first seen, splints should be applied and all manipulation should be avoided until x-rays are obtained.

AXIOM

IF A FRACTURED EXTREMITY IS NOT SPLINTED ADEQUATELY, ADDITIONAL VASCULAR AND OTHER TISSUE DAMAGE IS APT TO OCCUR.

In addition to the control of hemorrhage and restoration of blood volume, administration of tetanus toxoid or immune globulin and antibiotics should be begun in the emergency room (Chaps. 12 and 29).

Operative Treatment

AXIOM

PREPARE FOR ALL EVENTUALITIES AHEAD OF TIME. IN PARTICULAR THE POSITION AND DRAPING SHOULD ALLOW FOR RAPID SECURING OF PROXIMAL AND DISTAL CONTROL OF THE INJURED VESSELS AND, IF NECESSARY, THE OBTAINING OF AN AUTOLOGOUS VEIN.

In the operating room, the entire extremity and adjacent trunk should be prepared and draped so that the surgeon can readily secure proximal and distal control of the injured vessels and also evaluate the blood flow and pulses distally without risking contamination of the wound. Provision should always be made for obtaining an autologous vein graft in any patient with a possible major arterial injury. If the trauma involves one leg, the opposite groin, thigh,

and lower leg should be prepared and draped so that a saphenous vein graft can be readily obtained if needed. If there is a chance that the saphenous veins will not be suitable or available, one arm and shoulder should be prepared and draped so that the cephalic vein can be used. Whenever a vascular patch or graft is needed, especially after trauma, the patient's own veins provide the most suitable material.

GENERAL PRINCIPLES. The general principles that should be followed in the management or repair of any major arterial injury include:

1. proximal and distal control prior to exposing the site of vessel injury,
2. reduction and fixation of fractures or dislocations before repairing the vessel,
3. debridement of the vessel before repairing it,
4. heparinization of the vessel proximally and distally while it is occluded, and
5. thrombectomy or removal of clots from the proximal and distal portions of the vessel before completing the repair.

Proximal and Distal Control. In order to reduce hemorrhage and to improve the exposure of the area of injury, proximal and distal control of the involved vessel should generally be obtained at least several centimeters away from the damaged site. In some instances there may be a strong temptation to approach the injured vessel directly; although this is successful occasionally and may save a lot of time, it invites the risk of restarting massive hemorrhage before the surgeon is prepared to handle it.

AXIOM

FAILURE TO OBTAIN PROXIMAL AND DISTAL CONTROL BEFORE EXPOSING THE SITE OF INJURY OF A LARGE VESSEL MAY CONVERT A CAREFUL ANATOMIC DISSECTION AND REPAIR INTO A FRANTIC ATTEMPT TO STOP MASSIVE HEMORRHAGE.

During the dissection to obtain proximal and distal control, no collateral vessels or veins should be sacrificed unless absolutely necessary. The involved vessel should also be disturbed as little as possible until it is separated from the surrounding tissue and is looped with an umbilical tape or rubber band. If the artery is actively bleeding, it should be occluded with direct digital pressure or with special noncrushing vascular clamps as close as possible to the injury, so as to cause minimal interference with collateral blood flow.

Once proximal control has been obtained, there is less need for a separate incision to obtain distal control, especially if the vessels involved are relatively small. With the larger arteries and veins, however, back-bleeding can be severe, and distal control should be obtained either through the wound itself or, when necessary, through a separate distal incision.

Bone Fixation. When an arterial injury has occurred in association with a dislocation or fracture, the bone or fracture should generally be reduced and stabilized before any attempt is made to repair the vessel. It is, however, extremely important to have good proximal and distal control of the vessel prior to any attempts at reduction because the manipulation will often cause the bleeding to recur or increase. Whenever possible, the reduction should be performed with the artery under direct vision so that the sharp bone ends do not cause additional injury to the vessel.

If contamination is minimal, internal fixation of the bone fragments is the preferred method of stabilization. Bone plates may be needed in some instances, but the additional soft-tissue dissection required to apply them properly may not be desirable. If the wound is grossly contaminated, internal fixation is not advised and external traction or casts incorporating pins proximal and distal to the fracture are preferred. After the reduction has been accomplished, muscle or other tissue should be interposed between the fracture site and involved artery to prevent the fracture callus from involving the vascular repair and causing later occlusion.

Debridement. Prior to the vascular repair, the damaged tissue in the vessel should be excised. The extent to which an injured artery should be debrided prior to definitive repair is controversial. Vietnam War experience has found a lack of correlation between the amount of normal artery resected adjacent to the grossly traumatized segment and the ultimate success of the repair.[11,12] Recent experiments suggest that microscopic changes in the normal artery immediately above or below a grossly damaged segment do not affect the ultimate outcome of the vascular repair, and arbitrary removal of large amounts of normal vessel may not be warranted.[13] Debridement can probably be limited to the grossly damaged segment and 3 to 4 mm of normal vessel.

If the integrity of an apparently intact artery or its blood flow is in doubt at the time of surgery, an arteriotomy should be performed to evaluate the intima. In some instances the vessel damage may appear to be mild, but the blood flow may be impaired because of what appears to be spasm. Under such circumstances, the involved portion of the vessel should generally be excised. Even if there is no obstruction at the time of surgery, intimal damage may result in complete occlusion later.

When the ends of the artery are cut off to remove damaged tissue and to provide a smooth vessel edge, both ends should be cut obliquely to cause less narrowing when the artery is repaired.

Heparinization. As a general rule, heparin should be given intravenously during any arterial repair to reduce the tendency for clots to form proximal and distal to the vascular clamps. This is especially important when repairing vessels such as the popliteal artery, which has a relatively poor collateral blood supply.

The heparin can be given either systemically or locally. Systemic heparinization can generally be obtained by giving 40 to

80 mg (4,000 to 8,000 units) of heparin intravenously. Within 2 to 5 minutes the heparin will have circulated throughout the body, producing anticoagulation in virtually all vessels. Local heparinization can be obtained by injecting 5 to 10 ml of a dilute heparin solution (1 mg or 100 units of heparin per ml) into the proximal arterial lumen and 10 to 25 ml distal to the vascular clamps using a small-caliber bent needle; an irrigating catheter may also be used to inject the heparin distally. The term "local heparinization" is somewhat deceptive, in that some or all of the heparin eventually enters the general circulation producing some systemic heparinization. However, if the amount of heparin used locally is small, the general anticoagulant effect will usually be mild.

Systemic heparinization has the advantage of producing a more complete and effective anticoagulation; however, if there is little or no distal blood flow, some additional heparin may have to be injected beyond the injury to prevent distal thrombosis. Local heparinization is safer if the patient may potentially bleed elsewhere, especially intracranially or in the retroperitoneal space from possible associated injuries. When the vascular anastomosis is completed, the heparin can be allowed to wear off by itself. Giving protamine to counteract the remaining heparin effect is unnecessary and probably unwise because it may cause a rebound hypercoagulability.

Thrombectomy

AXIOM

IT SHOULD BE ASSUMED THAT SIGNIFICANT CLOTS HAVE DEVELOPED DISTAL TO ANY VASCULAR INJURY, EVEN IF PROFUSE BACK-BLEEDING IS PRESENT.

Formation of thrombi at and distal to the site of arterial injury prior to surgery is a frequent occurrence, especially if the vessel is occluded for a prolonged period and there is little or no collateral circula-tion. Profuse back-bleeding from the distal end of the cut vessel is deceptive; it tends to create the impression that the distal runoff is good and that there are no major distal thrombi. However, extensive back-bleeding may occur from collaterals entering the artery just distal to the injury while, beyond the collaterals, the vessel may be completely occluded with thrombi. Fogarty balloon and irrigating catheters are very effective for removing such clots. After the deflated balloon catheter is passed far down the distal vessel, the balloon is inflated and pulled back slowly, bringing any clots that may be ahead of it into the wound. The irrigating catheter can then be used to flush out the distal arterial tree with a dilute heparin solution.

SURGICAL TECHNIQUES

AXIOM

AMPLE EXPOSURE OF THE INJURED VESSEL IS A PREREQUISITE FOR A SUCCESSFUL REPAIR.

Repair in Continuity. This type of repair is often possible if the vessel has a tangential wound which involves only part of the circumference and has clean sharp edges. If it is anticipated that this direct lateral closure will cause a significant compromise of the lumen of the artery, the vascular wound should be patched with a piece of autogenous vein.

End-to-end Anastomosis. If the vessel is completely severed, repair must be accomplished by an end-to-end anastomosis with or without interposed graft. After the damaged ends of the vessel have been debrided, at least 1 to 2 cm of vessel should be freed proximal and distal to the injury. The assistant must gently pull the ends of the vessels together with the clamps to prevent any tension on the suture line while the repair is being performed. Such tension may not only cause the suture to pull through the ends of the vessel at the time of repair but later may also lead to thrombosis or narrowing at the anastomosis.

Two corner sutures are inserted and tied and then the posterior anastomosis is completed first by rotating the clamps 180°. Care should be taken to prevent any adventitia from projecting into the lumen after the repair is completed. The intimal layers should be closely approximated to prevent development of a distal intimal flap. After completion of the posterior suture line, the clamps are then returned to their original position and the anterior portion is completed. Anastomosing the posterior layer first allows the inspection of the suture line internally. Everting sutures have the advantage of creating a smoother internal surface at the site of anastomosis. Cutting the ends of the vessel in an oblique fashion prior to suture helps to reduce the narrowing at the anastomotic site. In children, at least half of the suture line should be performed with interrupted sutures to allow growth of the vessel at the site of the anastomosis.

Just prior to the completion of the anastomosis, the distal and then the proximal clamps must be alternately removed to flush out any clots which may have formed distal and proximal to the vascular clamps. When the proximal clamp is removed, the distal clamp must be in place to prevent any clots from the proximal end being flushed into the distal vascular bed.

At the completion of the anastomosis, the distal vascular clamp is removed and the suture line examined. Any large leak present at this time should be sutured. The proximal clamp can then be removed. Unless a large leak is present, oozing from the anastomosis can generally be controlled by pressure applied carefully over the bleeding points for 5 to 10 minutes. If significant leaks are still present after this period, the bleeding points should be oversewn. It should be emphasized that additional sutures are rarely needed if the initial repair is adequate.

Although direct repair or reanastomosis of the artery is generally preferred, vascular grafts are occasionally necessary. This is most likely to occur if more than 2 to 3 cm of artery are resected and the ends cannot be approximated without excessive tension. For graft replacement, every attempt should be made to use autogenous tissues such as the patient's own saphenous or cephalic vein. If no vein is available and an autologous graft is absolutely necessary, the internal iliac artery may be used. The use of prosthetic material in the presence of gross contamination is contraindicated because of the high risk of infection and the dire consequences of such infection. In Rich's[14] report on war wounds in Vietnam, it was noted that there was a high incidence of infection when prosthetic materials were used. If a synthetic graft is absolutely necessary, however, local and systemic antibiotics may reduce the risk of local sepsis which can cause later occlusion of the graft or leak at the anastomotic site.

Vascular Spasm. Arterial spasm is extremely rare and is often mistakenly diagnosed when intimal damage or mechanical obstruction is present. If true spasm persists following an adequate repair, however, several techniques to relieve it may be attempted. One of the preferred methods is to overexpand the vessel by an injection of saline. Other alternative measures include the application of a solution of 2.5% papaverine hydrochloride, stripping of the adventitia, or bathing the artery in a procaine or lidocaine solution. If spasm persists after these maneuvers, the anastomotic site should generally be excised or opened and another repair performed.

Vein Repair. Simple or minor injuries of large vital veins should be repaired if at all possible. This is especially true of the superior vena cava, the right renal vein, the inferior vena cava above the renals and the portal vein. It is particularly important that the portal vein be repaired. If the two ends of the portal vein cannot be sutured together, a portacaval shunt should be performed. Injudicious attempts to repair small veins in the presence of multiple injuries should be discouraged. Nonvital veins with long or large through-and-through lacerations should also be ligated because thrombi may form at the suture lines and act as sources for large pulmonary emboli.

Debridement of the Wound. Debridement of tissue adjacent to the injured vessel is generally left until the artery is repaired. The resultant improved local blood flow may greatly alter the appearance of the muscle distal to the injured vessel.

If the wound is caused by a high-velocity missile, the entrance and exit wounds are excised, debriding as little skin as possible. If there is much underlying tissue damage, the skin should be incised longitudinally to allow adequate drainage and repeated debridement. All muscle which appears to be devitalized because of loss of contractility or abnormal color and consistency should be excised. The entrance and exit wounds in the skin are left open at least 4 to 5 days for secondary closure later. Since questionable areas of viability may improve after adequate circulation is established, the final debridement of muscle and skin is best left until after flow to the area has been reestablished.

Wound Closure. The decision as to whether to leave the skin and subcutaneous tissue open will depend upon the amount of contamination and the availability of viable skin or skin flaps. Contaminated wounds are best left open. Nevertheless, vascular repairs and grafts should be covered if at all possible. Occasionally, muscle flaps may be used if they are readily available. With groin wounds, the sartorius muscle is ideal for the coverage of the femoral artery. If the contamination is severe and the risk of infection is very high, the exposed vessel may be covered with a porcine skin graft. The wound should then be debrided and a new porcine skin graft applied daily until healthy granulation tissue grows over the vessel.[15]

Adjunctive Measures

INTRAOPERATIVE ARTERIOGRAM. If there is any question about the adequacy of blood flow distal to a vascular injury after the repair has been completed, an intraoperative arteriogram should be performed. If the arteriogram is abnormal or shows an occlusion distally, appropriate corrective surgery should be carried out immediately.

FASCIOTOMY

AXIOM

THE NEED FOR FASCIOTOMY SHOULD BE ANTICIPATED WHENEVER THERE HAS BEEN ISCHEMIA FOR MANY HOURS FOLLOWING A VASCULAR INJURY, ESPECIALLY IF A MAJOR VEIN HAS BEEN OCCLUDED OR LIGATED.

Adequate and early fasciotomy is an important adjunctive procedure to improve the survival of ischemic limbs. The main indications for fasciotomy are (1) signs of muscular ischemia manifested by the loss of muscle function, and (2) massive swelling of soft tissue, impairing distal blood flow. Fasciotomy also has a definite place in the wringer type of injuries where extensive deep soft-tissue damage is present. After repair of injuries to the popliteal artery and vein, such a procedure is often especially rewarding.

Proper fasciotomy of the lower leg requires a detailed knowledge of the fascial compartments of the lower leg. Anatomically, the lower leg has four muscle compartments, bounded by the intermuscular and interosseous fascial structures: (1) anterior, (2) lateral, (3) superficial posterior, and (4) deep posterior. The anterior and the deep posterior are of special surgical significance because they contain the anterior tibial artery and posterior tibial and peroneal arteries respectively.

The main types of fasciotomy currently performed include: (1) limited skin incision with blind incision of the fascia, (2) extensive skin incision with open incision of the fascia, and (3) fasciotomy with resection of a portion of the fibula.

Since the skin is not usually the constrictive layer, blind division of the fascia between multiple skin incisions will often be adequate. This can be done both in the anterior and superficial posterior compartment of the lower leg. Extensive skin incision and open incision of the fascia are indicated when decompression by the multiple smaller skin incisions is not adequate. An extensive skin incision, however, often results in exposure of tendons and poor healing. An important point in the incision of the fascia is to be sure that it extends from the head of the fibula to the ankle retinaculum.

Since access to the deep posterior compartment is possible only at the junction of the middle and distal third of the leg, excision of the fibula to facilitate the decompression has been advocated.[16] The middle two quarters of the fibula are excised and only the head of the fibula is preserved proximally so that the lateral deep peroneal nerve will not be damaged. The lower end is preserved to maintain the mortise of the ankle joint. This fibulectomy-fasciotomy is of great value in the decompression of the deep compartments which contain the peroneal and posterior tibial arteries and veins.

Regardless of the type of fasciotomy performed, avoidance of the use of circular dressings after the operation is essential. An application of a tight pressure dressing following a decompression procedure defeats the purpose of fasciotomy.

Postoperative Care

PITFALL

IF A LOW CARDIAC OUTPUT OR HYPOTENSION IS ALLOWED TO DEVELOP AFTER VASCULAR REPAIR, THE DANGER OF THROMBOSIS AT THE ANASTOMOSIS IS GREATLY INCREASED.

One of the most important factors in keeping a vascular repair functioning is the maintenance of an adequate systemic blood pressure and cardiac output. This is especially important when the patient has multiple other injuries. Use of adequate quantities of blood and fluid is the best method for maintaining an adequate distal flow.

Repeated examination of the distal pulses and temperature postoperatively is extremely important. Recent development of the Doppler ultrasound instrument has made the determination of the patency of a reconstructed vessel a simple procedure.[17] This technique is of particular value when ankle edema makes palpation of the pedal pulses difficult. Various types of ultrasonic Dopplers are available; these include Park's Electronic Laboratory and Parke-Davis Portable pocket-size Doppler (Hemosone). These instruments operate on the Doppler effect and detect blood flow velocity through intact skin by the frequency shift of the reflected sound. Both audible and written signals are available for study. By using the flow probe as a stethoscope over the posterior tibial or dorsalis pedis arteries, systolic pressure of the lower limb can be recorded by applying a blood pressure cuff around the ankle (Fig. 1). Failure to obtain a normal systolic pressure and flow pattern when compared with the noninjured limb indicates the operation has not been successful (Fig. 2).

If the distal pulses are lost or if the distal blood flow becomes impaired, reoperation may be required. If the skin temperature is only slightly reduced and motor and nerve functions are adequate, the limb may be carefully observed while attempting to improve blood flow by infusing additional fluids, blood or L.M.W.D. If the limb is edematous, its circulation may be improved by elevating it. If the limb is not swollen, there may be some advantage to lowering it periodically slightly below the level of the bed. If the limb muscles become tense, a fasciotomy should be performed. If all these methods fail to provide an adequate distal blood flow, arteriograms should be performed. If any obstruction or

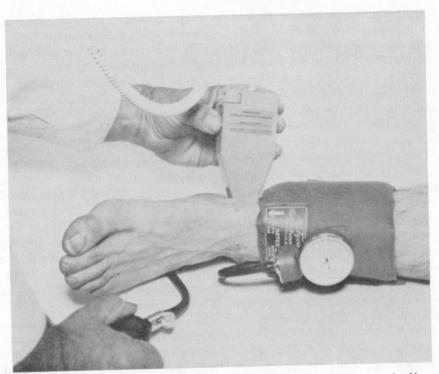

FIG. 1. Method of transcutaneous flow detection over the posterior tibial artery and recording of ankle systolic pressure by placing a pressure-cuff around the ankle.

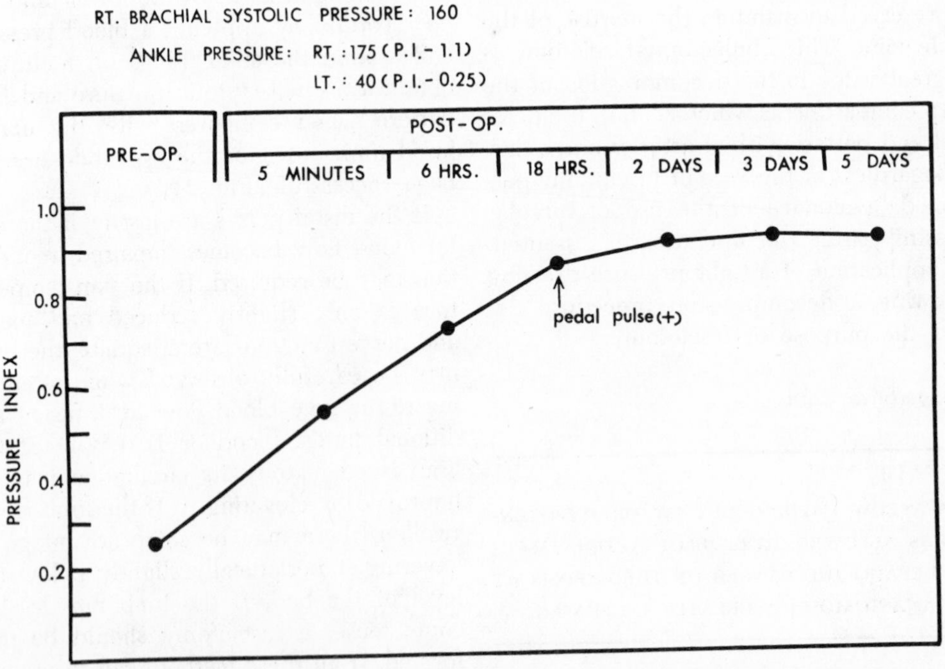

RT. BRACHIAL SYSTOLIC PRESSURE: 160

ANKLE PRESSURE: RT. : 175 (P.I. – 1.1)

LT. : 40 (P.I. – 0.25)

FIG. 2. Increased ankle systolic pressure is seen five minutes after repair of a transected superficial femoral artery in a patient with a gunshot wound of the thigh. The pedal pulse became palpable 18 hours after completion of the operation, at which time there was a marked increase in the ankle systolic pressure.

significant narrowing is noted on the arteriogram, reoperation is indicated.

AXIOM

IF THE SURVIVAL OF THE LIMB BEGINS TO APPEAR DOUBTFUL AT ANY TIME FOLLOWING A VASCULAR REPAIR, IMMEDIATE REOPERATION SHOULD BE PERFORMED WITH CORRECTION OF ANY ANASTOMOTIC PROBLEM AND CAREFUL COMPLETE DISTAL THROMBECTOMY WITH FOGARTY CATHETERS.

Antibiotics are administered just before, during and for at least 48 hours after any vascular repair, particularly if there has been any contamination (Chap. 29).

SPECIAL CONSIDERATIONS

Arterial Injuries Following Percutaneous Catheterization

The increasing use of percutaneous catheterization for the diagnosis of cardiac and vascular disease has resulted in a large number of iatrogenic vascular injuries. Femoral artery thrombosis is the most frequent complication of retrograde aortic catheterization by the percutaneous technique. The reported incidence varies from 1.2% to 7%.[18] Mechanical factors and altered blood flow are of primary importance in the development of these lesions. A low cardiac output, such as can occur in patients with mitral valve disease and other cardiac problems, may be an important contributing factor.

A cold, pale, pulseless, painful extremity strongly suggests the development of thrombosis following the catheterization. Persistent signs of ischemia during a short period (4 to 6 hours) of observation is a definite indication for arterial exploration. Arteriotomy and thrombectomy using the Fogarty catheter technique[19] usually result in prompt restoration of arterial patency. When thrombectomy is not carried out early, gangrene or claudication may develop later.

Arterial Injuries Associated with Drug Abuse or Addiction

Drug abuse or addiction has become an increasing problem in modern society. Apart from the systemic effects of the drugs and damage to the pulmonary vascular bed, local injury is also a serious problem. Methamphetamine, alone or in combination with heroin, can cause a necrotizing angiitis.[20] There has also been a report of arteritis leading to progressive arterial occlusion of the lower extremities in young Moroccans who were heavy smokers of cannabis extracts.[21]

Most addicts eventually resort to using the intravenous route (mainlining) for administering the narcotic. Thrombosed veins are thus a common sequela. In his search for usable veins, the addict often attempts to find femoral, axillary or even jugular veins. Lack of anatomic knowledge may lead to damage to the adjacent artery. The continuous use of unsterile needles makes infection a commonly associated feature; consequently, infected false aneurysms may result. Starch and other foreign materials, often added to the injected drugs, in addition to the local toxicity or occlusion they may produce when injected into a peripheral vein may also damage the pulmonary circulation. Digital artery thrombosis and gangrene of portions of the hand can also result from inadvertent injection of material into the brachial artery.[22]

The use of arteriograms is often necessary to delineate the exact site extent of an infected aneurysm. Unless bleeding makes immediate operation mandatory, the administration of large doses of systemic antibiotics for three days prior to surgical intervention is highly desirable. The most common site of infected aneurysms is the common femoral artery. If primary resection with graft replacement is carried out in an infected area, there is a very strong chance that the graft will also be infected. An infected common femoral artery aneurysm should, therefore, generally be treated either by using an obturator bypass graft,[22] thereby completely avoiding the infected area, or by performing proximal ligation of the external iliac artery, relying on the collateral channels to maintain the viability of the limb. The viability of the limb can be determined conveniently by using the Doppler ultrasound method. If flow is absent 4 to 6 hours after the ligation and the viability of the limb is in question, a graft passed through the obturator foramen down to the distal femoral artery becomes the form of treatment most likely to save the limb.

Arterial Injuries Associated with Massive Tissue Loss

If a major arterial injury is associated with severe tissue loss, as following close-range shotgun blasts, the treatment is greatly complicated and the chances of eventual loss of the limb are high. Repeated debridement of the involved tissue may be required every 24 hours for several days. If a viable muscle flap cannot be easily rotated over the involved artery after the area is clean, it should be covered with a porcine skin graft, which is then changed every 24 to 48 hours until the wound is clean. Autologous skin grafts can be applied after healthy granulation tissue grows over the area of repair. Any later bleeding from the repair sites is a warning that massive arterial disruption is imminent and should be treated by ligation of the normal artery proximal and distal to the involved area. If possible, reestablishment of distal blood flow may be attempted by insertion of a graft through an uninjured area of the same limb.

Blunt Trauma to the Carotid Artery

Soft-tissue injury to the side of the head and neck may rarely be the cause of intimal damage to the common carotid or internal carotid arteries. The symptoms and signs of carotid artery occlusion in most patients are delayed for hours or days after the time of injury. This problem should also be kept in mind with those patients who have neck injuries due to malplaced safety straps.

Examination of the affected vessel often shows an intimal tear with gradual propagation of a thrombus antegrade and retrograde. Early operation is essential if severe brain damage or death is to be prevented. The diagnosis depends upon eliciting the history of neck trauma, which may occasionally be quite mild, and an associated gradual onset of carotid artery ischemic symptoms, combined with prompt angiography to demonstrate the intimal tear. The usual local physical signs of vascular injury, such as bruit or decreased pulses, appear to be rare in this condition.

Once complete occlusion has occurred, reestablishment of blood flow may be difficult or only transient; furthermore, once the brain has infarcted, reestablishment of the flow may cause hemorrhage into the softened brain tissue with further extension of the damage.

Upper Extremity

In the upper extremity, a serious arterial injury may easily be overlooked because the excellent collateral circulation may keep the hand adequately perfused. In addition, in a small but significant number of patients, the brachial artery divides into the ulnar and radial arteries several inches above the elbow, higher than the usual position in the antecubital fossa. Following fracture dislocation of the shoulder, special efforts must be made to rule out damage to the adjacent axillary artery.

Lower Extremity

In the lower extremity, lesser trochanter and peritrochanteric fractures may involve the deep femoral artery. In elderly individuals, this vessel may have been the major arterial supply to the limb and severe ischemia may result.

In penetrating and blunt injuries around the knee joint, the usual rule of ligating the injured veins is not always applicable. If the popliteal vein can be repaired, it may remain open for 1 to 2 days postoperatively to help reduce the edema which may contribute to the poor results often seen with injuries of this area. Additionally, it is important to ligate as few venous and arterial collaterals as possible while dissecting the popliteal fossa to obtain exposure of the injured vessels.

Pulmonary Embolism

ETIOLOGY. Three factors are generally felt to play a role in the development of thrombi: (1) a slow blood flow, (2) increased coagulability of the blood, and (3) damage to or abnormalities of the intima of the blood vessel. Thus, the patient in shock or congestive heart failure who is confined to bed and has had trauma to his lower extremities or previous venous disease in the legs is a perfect candidate for the development of venous thrombi. There are more patients with pulmonary emboli on medical wards than on surgical wards. Apparently many of these thrombi can similarly form in the operating room, particularly if the surgery is prolonged.

DIAGNOSIS. Diagnosis depends upon a high index of suspicion and often cannot be confirmed even by pulmonary angiogram unless the emboli are quite large and occlude at least a lobar branch.

Most pulmonary emboli are not detected during life. Of 124 patients with gross evidence of pulmonary emboli at autopsy, the diagnosis was suspected in less than 10% before death. Less than one sixth of these patients had any of the classic signs of pulmonary emboli often described in the literature, such as sharp or pleuritic chest pain or hemoptysis. EKG signs of right heart strain were either absent or missed in virtually all patients. The chest x-ray often demonstrated nonspecific scattered infiltrates which were usually interpreted as plate-like atelectasis, congestion or mild pneumonitis. The largest emboli often had no x-ray abnormalities.

Four important clinical signs may be indicative of pulmonary embolus in the injured patient: sudden appearance of tachypnea, tachycardia, fever, and anxiousness or restlessness.

Virtually all these patients were noted to have tachypnea which seemed to increase at the time the embolism probably occurred. Tachycardia was also frequent, but seemed to be less reliable. In some instances the pulmonary emboli seemed to either cause some congestive heart failure or aggravate C.H.F. that was already present.

Fever of a low grade was present in many of these patients and this, with a few rales and nonspecific pulmonic infiltrates, was generally interpreted as a mild pneumonitis and/or atelectasis. The routine chest x-ray is of little or no value in the diagnosis of the condition and a normal x-ray never rules out pulmonary emboli.

If blood gases are available, a rise in the alveolar-arterial carbon dioxide difference to more than 5 mm Hg may indicate interference with perfusion in the lung.

A rise in the central venous pressure may indicate a pulmonary embolus, but this may also occur with a myocardial infarct or acute heart failure without an embolus. However, if the pulmonary wedge pressure (obtained with a Swan-Ganz catheter) is found to be low in the presence of a high CVP, this suggests a pulmonary embolus fairly strongly.

TREATMENT. Pulmonary emboli should be divided or classified into three major categories: those that kill immediately, those that cause persistent shock with survival for at least 4 to 6 hours, and those with no hemodynamic abnormality. If the patient with pulmonary embolic shock is in a hospital which does not have facilities for emergency pulmonary angiography and embolectomy, he should be immediately transferred to an institution with such facilities if at all possible.

Administration of 100 mg heparin rapidly I.V. may occasionally cause dramatic relief of hemodynamic and respiratory symptoms caused by pulmonary emboli. Under such circumstances, this response may be almost diagnostic. Heparin should then be administered subsequently by a continuous I.V. infusion of 10 to 15 mg/hour to keep the clotting time at 2½ to 3 times control values.

Oxygen should be given as needed to maintain the arterial Po_2 above 60 mm Hg and preferably at 80 to 100 mm Hg. If high concentrations of oxygen are required or if ventilation is inadequate, the patient should be put on a respirator.

If there is any bronchospasm, bronchodilators should be given. If the patient is hypotensive, ephedrine may be given. If the BP is normal or high, aminophylline may be given. With severe anxiety when the blood pressure is adequate, sedatives may occasionally be warranted.

If the blood pressure is low, a vasopressor such as norepinephrine (Levophed, 4 ampules in 500 ml glucose in water) is recommended. The addition of 2 ampules or 10 mg of phenotolamine (Regitine) to this mixture reduces the severe vasoconstriction that the norepinephrine causes when given by itself. Isoproterenol should not be given to raise the BP. Inotropic agents, particularly digoxin or Cedilanid, may also help to improve the BP and cardiac output.

If severe shock persists in spite of all efforts at correction, surgical removal of the emboli under cardiopulmonary bypass may be required. Such surgery, however, can be very dangerous and should not be undertaken unless the diagnosis is proven clinically by the circumstances of the case or by pulmonary arteriogram. Not infrequently in the past, patients were mistakenly operated on for a pulmonary embolus when they actually had an acute myocardial infarction.

Thrombolytic or fibrinolytic agents to remove pulmonary emboli are still experimental and may be of value.

Implantation and Amputations

See Chapter 18 for discussion.

SUMMARY

Success in the management of vascular injuries depends on an early accurate diagnosis, using arteriography whenever the clinical signs or symptoms are equivocal, followed by immediate repair and restoration of blood flow, whenever possible, within 4 to 6 hours. Ischemia distal to a vascular injury is virtually never due to "spasm"; attempts to correct spasm nonsurgically generally cause delays which greatly jeopardize the patient's life and limb. Continued ischemia after repair is generally due to an unsatisfactory vascular repair or distal thrombosis and early reoperation is usually indicated. The increased use of arteriography, autogenous vein grafts, Fogarty catheters to remove distal thrombi, and early complete fasci-

TABLE 1. TEN FREQUENT ERRORS IN THE MANAGEMENT OF PERIPHERAL VASCULAR INJURIES

1. Failing to rule out a vascular injury in patients with trauma near major vessels, particularly following penetrating wounds, fractures, or dislocations.

2. Assuming that inadequate circulation following trauma or vascular catheterization is due to "spasm" rather than mechanical occlusion of the vessel.

3. Delaying definitive diagnosis and treatment of a suspected vascular injury.

4. Delaying definitive repair to obtain when the need for vascular exploration is obvious.

5. Failing to prepare and drape the entire involved extremity and to make provisions for obtaining an autologous vein for grafting if needed.

6. Failing to obtain adequate proximal and distal control before exposing the site of vascular injury.

7. Failing to open an artery with "spasm" or a suspected intimal injury.

8. Failing to heparinize adequately above and below the sites of occlusion during vascular surgery.

9. Failing to perform an adequate thrombectomy following a vascular repair.

10. Delaying to perform an adequate fasciectomy in patients with prolonged ischemia or excessive swelling distal to a vascular injury.

otomy if tissue ischemia has been prolonged has greatly improved the prognosis for most arterial injuries.

REFERENCES

1. Amato, J. J., et al.: High velocity arterial injury: A study of the mechanism of injury. J. Trauma, 11:412, 1971.
2. Elkin, D. C., and Warren, J. V.: Arteriovenous fistulas, their effect on the circulation. JAMA, 134:1524, 1947.
3. Holman, E.: The anatomic and physiologic effects of arteriovenous fistula. Surgery, 8:362, 1940.
4. Seldinger, S. I.: Catheter replacement of needle in percutaneous arteriography. Acta Radiol., 39:368, 1953.
5. Mufti, M. A., et al.: Diagnostic value of hematoma in penetrating arterial wounds of the extremities. Arch. Surg., 101:562, 1970.
6. Dillard, B. M., Nelson, D. L., and Norman, H. G., Jr.: Review of 85 major traumatic arterial injuries. Surgery, 63:391, 1968.
7. Lain, K. C., and Williams, G. R.: Arteriography in acute peripheral arterial injuries: An experimental study. Surg. Forum, 21:179, 1970.
8. Murphy, J. B.: Resection of arteries and veins injured in continuity. End-to-end suture. Exp. Clin. Res. Med. Rec., 51:73, 1897.
9. DeBakey, M. E., and Simeone, F. A.: Battle injuries of the arteries in World War II. Ann. Surg., 123:534, 1946.
10. Hughes, C. W.: Arterial repair during the Korean War. Ann. Surg., 147:555, 1958.
11. Rich, N. M., Manion, W. C., and Hughes, C. W.: Surgical and pathological evaluation of vascular injuries in Vietnam. J. Trauma, 9:279, 1969.
12. Rich, N. M.: Vascular trauma in Vietnam. J. Cardiov. Surg., 11:368, 1970.
13. Amato, J. J., et al.: Vascular injuries, an experimental study of high and low velocity missile wounds. Arch. Surg., 101:167, 1970.
14. Rich, N., Baugh, J., and Hughes, C.: Significance of complications associated with vascular repairs performed in Vietnam. Arch. Surg., 100:646, 1970.
15. Ledgerwood, A. M., and Lucas, C. E.: Massive thigh injuries with vascular disruption: Role of porcine skin grafting of exposed arterial vein grafts. Arch. Surg., 107:201, 1973.
16. Patman, R. D., and Thompson, J. E.: Fasciotomy in peripheral vascular surgery: Report of 164 patients. Arch. Surg., 101:663, 1970.
17. Yao, S. T.: Experience with the Doppler ultrasound flow velocity meter in peripheral vascular disease. In: *Modern Trends in Vascular Surgery*. London, Butterworths, 1970.
18. Kloster, F. E., Bristow, J. D., and Griswold, H. E.: Femoral artery occlusion following percutaneous catheterization. Amer. Hosp. J., 79:175, 1970.
19. Fogarty, T. J., et al.: A method for extraction of arterial thrombi. Surg. Gynec. Obstet., 116:241, 1963.
20. Citron, B. P., et al.: Necrotizing angiitis associated with drug abuse. New Eng. J. Med., 283:1003, 1970.
21. Nahas, G. G.: Cannabis arteritis. New Eng. J. Med., 284:113, 1971.
22. Gasper, M. R., and Hare, R. R.: Gangrene due to intra-arterial injection of drugs by drug addicts. Surgery, 72:573, 1972.
23. Fromm, S. H., and Lucas, C. E.: Obturator bypass for mycotic aneurysm in the drug addict. Arch. Surg., 100:82, 1970.

Suggested Reading

1. Carrel, A., and Guthrie, C. C.: Uniterminal and biterminal venous transplantation. Surg. Gynec. Obstet., 2:266, 1906.
2. Steenberg, R. W., and Ravitch, M. M.: Cervicothoracic approach for subclavian vessel injury from compound fracture of the clavicle; considerations of subclavian-axillary exposures. Ann. Surg., 157:839, 1963.
3. Conn, J., Jr., Trippel, D. H., and Bergan, J. J.: A new atraumatic aortic occluder. Surgery, 64:1158, 1968.
4. Amato, J. J., et al.: Emergency approach to the subclavian and innominate vessels. Ann. Thorac. Surg., 8:537, 1969.
5. Motsay, G. J., Manlove, C., and Perry, J. F.: Major venous injury with pelvic fracture. J. Trauma, 9:343, 1969.
6. Levin, P., Rich, N., and Hutton, J.: Collateral circulation in arterial injuries. Arch. Surg., 102:392, 1971.
7. Reynolds, B. M., and Balsano, N. A.: Venography in pelvic fractures: A clinical evaluation. Ann. Surg., 137:104, 1971.
8. Margolies, M. M., et al.: Arteriography in the management of hemorrhage from pelvic fractures. New Eng. J. Med., 287:317, 1972.
9. Piyachon, C., and Arthachinta, S.: Arteriography in trauma of the extremities. Amer. J. Roentgen., 119:580, 1973.
10. McNamara, J. J., et al.: Management of fractures with associated arterial injury in combat casualties. J. Trauma, 13:17, 1973.
11. Rich, N. M., et al.: Subclavian artery trauma. J. Trauma, 13:485, 1973.
12. Yellin, A. E., and Shore, E. H.: Surgical management of arterial occlusion following percutaneous femoral angiography. Surgery, 73:772, 1973.
13. Volma, F. J.: Management of infected arterial grafts. Amer. J. Surg., 126:798, 1973.

27   INJURIES OF THE HAND

R. D. LARSEN

Physicians often remark with wonderment at the intricate mechanism and exquisitely engineered precision of the hand. Relatively few, however, have the opportunity to acquire the detailed knowledge which is essential for definitive care of injuries and infections of this unique organ. The surgeon treating badly injured hands must have a wide variety of skills; he must be capable of performing skin grafting and pedicle flap procedures, of caring for the skeletal injuries within the hand, and of repairing the injured nerves, tendons and vessels.

Since most injured patients must be cared for in the local community, it is important that physicians have a basic knowledge of the initial management of trauma to the hand. After this initial treatment, the more complex injuries can be referred to surgeons who have made a special study of the hand.

INITIAL MANAGEMENT OF HAND INJURIES

PITFALL

IF THE PRIMARY CARE OF THE SEVERELY INJURED HAND IS POOR, EVEN THE MOST EXPERIENCED HAND SURGEON MAY BE UNABLE TO RESTORE ADEQUATE FUNCTION LATER.

In few anatomic areas is an acute sense of priorities in initial care more essential to eventual function than in the hand. The margin of error allowed to the physician who first sees the patient is small. Moreover, technical surgical excellence is not enough; clinical judgment is also essential.

AXIOM

DON'T SACRIFICE THE PATIENT TO SAVE A HAND: DON'T SACRIFICE THE HAND TO SAVE A FINGER.

In patients with multiple injuries, treatment of the hand may have to be subordinated to other lifesaving measures such as maintenance of adequate ventilation and restoration of blood volume. In such circumstances, bleeding from the hand is best controlled by gentle compression over sterile dressings with elevation of the extremity. After the patient has been resuscitated and his condition stabilized, the hand can be examined properly.

Examination

Careful examination of the entire hand is mandatory before any intelligent decisions concerning therapy can be made. This is best accomplished under good light, and with sufficient analgesia to elicit patient cooperation. Desultory probing of the wound is highly undesirable; much more can be learned, and with safety, by a careful external inspection and a thorough assessment of motion and sensation. X-rays are taken if there is any possibility of fracture, dislocation, or foreign bodies. A negative pictorial record is better than no record at all. Since this must be done without moving the hand unduly, plastic radiolucent splints may be very helpful in this regard.

PITFALL

NERVE INJURIES MAY BE OVERLOOKED VERY EASILY UNLESS THE OVERLAP OF SENSORY IN-NERVATION AND THE FREQUENCY OF ANOMA-LOUS MUSCLE INNERVATION ARE CONSIDERED.

Sensory defects are relatively easy to detect unless the patient is uncooperative, a not infrequent problem in inebriated individuals and small children. Sensory function of the major nerves to the hand is best checked in the following areas (Fig. 1): ulnar nerve—center of the tactile pad of the little finger, radial nerve—first dorsal interosseous space, medial nerve—tactile pad of the index finger.

Motor function of the median nerve is best checked by having the patient bring the thumb into abduction. With the dorsal surface of the hand on a flat surface, the patient is asked to point his thumb toward the ceiling (Fig. 2). This motion is performed by the abductor pollicis brevis muscle which is almost constantly innervated by the median nerve only. For the ulnar nerve, abduction and adduction of the ex-

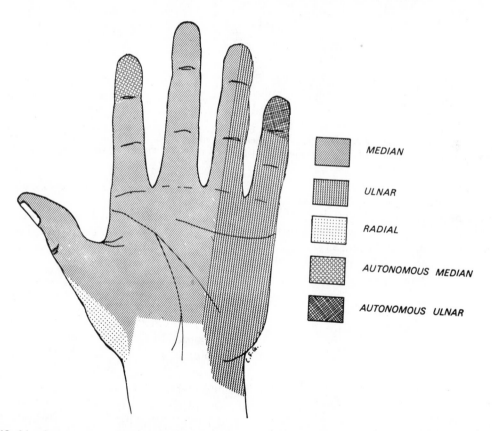

MEDIAN

ULNAR

RADIAL

AUTONOMOUS MEDIAN

AUTONOMOUS ULNAR

FIG. 1A: Sensory nerve supply—palm. Although the little finger and half of the ring finger are supplied by the ulnar nerve and the rest of the volar surface is supplied primarily by the median nerve, there is much overlap of the nerve supply. Only the volar surface of the distal phalanx of the index finger (supplied by the median nerve) and the volar surface of the distal phalanx of the little finger (supplied by the ulnar nerve) have an autonomous nerve supply with no overlap from adjacent nerves.

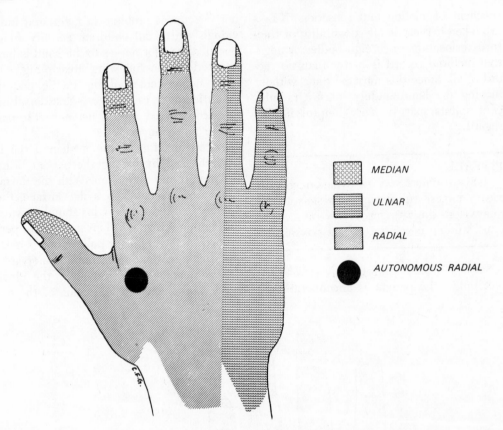

MEDIAN

ULNAR

RADIAL

AUTONOMOUS RADIAL

FIG. 1B: Sensory nerve supply—dorsal. On the dorsal surface of the hand, supplied primarily by the radial and median nerves, the only area with an autonomous nerve supply is the center of the first dorsal interosseous space which is supplied by the radial nerve.

tended fingers are the usual tests. Care must be taken that this test be performed with all finger joints fully extended; if the fingers are allowed to flex, false abduction and adduction may be performed by the extrinsic flexor and extensor tendons (Fig. 3).

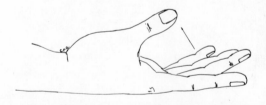

FIG. 2. The test for motor function of the median nerve is performed by asking the patient to place the back of his hand on a flat surface and then point his thumb toward the ceiling.

AXIOM

ABSENCE OF MOTION DOES NOT ALWAYS MEAN TENDON INJURY, WHEREAS SOME MOTION MAY PERSIST IN SPITE OF COMPLETE LACERATION.

Physiologic splinting, because of the local pain, may be extremely misleading and must always be considered when examining for tendon injuries. Inability to flex the distal interphalangeal joint of any finger implies damage to the profundus tendon; laceration of the sublimis tendon with an intact profundus tendon, however, may be extremely difficult to detect. Flexion of all joints should be checked with the proximal joints extended; otherwise, intrinsic hand muscles may be able to produce

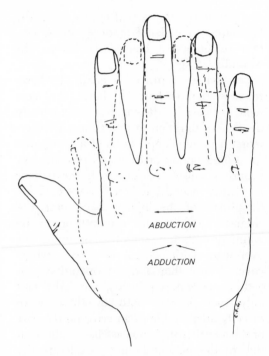

ABDUCTION

ADDUCTION

FIG. 3.   The test for motor function of the ulnar nerve is abduction and adduction of the fully extended fingers.

some flexion or extension, even when the extrinsic tendons are injured.

Initial Treatment

After resuscitation of the patient has been accomplished and the injured hand examined, the initial surgeon must make certain major decisions:

1. The extent of debridement required, keeping this to a minimum.
2. The extent of repair that is urgent and essential.
3. The extent of future reconstruction required to obtain ultimate maximum function.

AXIOM

THE LESS EXPERIENCED THE SURGEON, THE LESS HE SHOULD ATTEMPT WITH A BADLY INJURED HAND.

Whenever possible, the patient with a significant hand injury should be transferred to the care of a hand surgeon within 4 to 6 hours. Prior to the transfer, however,

bleeding should be controlled and the hand should be wrapped in sterile dressings, splinted and elevated. When appropriate, tetanus prophylaxis and antibiotics should also be given. If rapid transfer to a hand surgeon is impossible or impractical, the initial surgeon must then take certain steps to keep the hand in optimal condition until definitive care can be given.

If the surgeon can provide simple closure, an excellent beginning can be effected by cleaning the area, removing foreign bodies, controlling all bleeding points and conservatively debriding obviously devitalized tissue. In his zeal for tidiness the surgeon should not remove any more skin than he absolutely must; even if the skin appears to be in shreds, it may be a valuable source of coverage.

Control or prevention of infection is best accomplished by good surgical technique; however, tetanus toxoid and/or globulin should be given to all patients. Antibiotics should be begun if the wound is grossly contaminated or more than 6 to 8 hours old before it is closed or treated.

GENERAL CONSIDERATIONS IN THE DEFINITIVE MANAGEMENT OF HAND INJURIES

Two of the most important considerations in the surgical management of hand injuries are: (1) adequate anesthesia to prevent pain and inadvertent movement of the hand, and (2) proper application of a tourniquet so that the surgeon can operate with maximum visibility in a bloodless field.

Anesthesia

LOCAL INFILTRATION.   Adequate anesthesia for care of minor wounds can usually be obtained with simple local infiltration of the wound with 1% lidocaine or 1% procaine. Local anesthetics with epinephrine are avoided because they might cause irreversible spasm of the digital arteries with resultant necrosis of a finger. Digital block anesthesia is usually satisfactory only for the care of minor lacerations or superficial infections confined to a digit. Wrist block anesthesia is usually satisfactory only for the treatment of more minor wounds or infections. Direct local infiltration of a local anesthetic agent into a fracture will often produce sufficient anesthesia for a closed manipulation and reduction, but it will not usually be adequate for any type of open fracture surgery.

Local anesthesia within the hand itself, whether by direct infiltration or by a digital or wrist block, has the further disadvantage that a tourniquet cannot usually be inflated on the upper arm for more than a few minutes. Cut tendons, particularly if they have retracted, are also much more difficult to repair under local anesthesia since the motor nerve supply to the muscle which moves the tendon has not been paralyzed.

AXILLARY AND SUPRACLAVICULAR NERVE BLOCKS. Regional block anesthesia of the brachial plexus in the axilla or supraclavicular area, when properly performed, gives satisfactory anesthesia for the repair of most injuries of the hand and forearm; however, since an axillary block does not usually give adequate anesthesia for using a tourniquet on the upper arm, a ring of local anesthetic in the subcutaneous tissues just above and under the tourniquet is often also necessary. With supraclavicular blocks, pain from the tourniquet is not usually a problem. This technique has its greatest value in the patient in whom general anesthesia is undesirable because of various medical problems such as recent myocardial infarction.

INTRAVENOUS REGIONAL BLOCK ANESTHESIA. In recent years regional block anesthesia of the upper extremity by means of the intravenous infusion of a local anesthetic while a tourniquet is applied above the area to be anesthetized has been popularized. Although this technique seems to be satisfactory for minor procedures of fairly short duration, the quality and duration of the anesthesia obtained, in our limited experience, has been somewhat uncertain. An obvious disadvantage of this technique is

the loss of anesthesia that occurs when the tourniquet is deflated in order to be certain of complete hemostasis before the wound is closed.

GENERAL ANESTHESIA. General anesthesia remains the method of choice for most hand surgery as it ensures an adequate depth and duration of anesthesia. Furthermore, it permits application of a tourniquet for a long period of time and provides appropriate muscle relaxation. If the patient has eaten recently, it is necessary to delay the repair of the injured hand until the stomach has had time to empty or can be emptied with a nasogastric tube. In our experience with general anesthesia, which covers many thousands of operative procedures on injured hands, we have had only two deaths. Both of these were directly attributable to an error on the part of the anesthetist. In no case has death been due to the patient failing to tolerate the general anesthetic. Based upon this experience we definitely favor a general anesthetic for the management of hand injuries of any significance.

The Use and Abuse of the Tourniquet

PITFALL

IF HAND SURGERY IS ATTEMPTED WITHOUT A TOURNIQUET, IT MAY BE EXTREMELY DIFFICULT OR IMPOSSIBLE ACCURATELY TO IDENTIFY AND REPAIR INJURED TENDONS AND NERVES.

It is always more difficult, and at times it is impossible, to perform a satisfactory operation upon a hand without a bloodless field. Many small structures, such as the digital nerves and vessels, may be accidentally damaged or impossible to identify if the wound is oozing.

A standard blood-pressure cuff which does not leak makes an acceptable tourniquet. The tubing which leads to the bladder should be clamped in order to maintain the pressure at the desired level. Special tourniquets which are inflated by some type of compressed gas, with the pressure being maintained at a constant level by a regulating valve, are most satisfactory. The valve must be accurately calibrated, however. Since the pressure in some of these devices has a tendency to "creep," the pressure gauge must be examined frequently during the operation to be sure that an excessively high pressure is not applied accidentally.

The most feared complication of the use of the tourniquet is a tourniquet paralysis; however, the cases of tourniquet paralysis which we have seen have all been directly related either to too long an application of the tourniquet or to application of a pressure greater than 300 mm Hg.

PITFALL

IF THE TOURNIQUET IS NOT CHECKED CAREFULLY, EXCESSIVE PRESSURE MAY CAUSE SEVERE UNDERLYING DAMAGE.

Several layers of sheet wadding should be wrapped about the arm before the tourniquet is smoothly applied and taped in place. The tourniquet is elevated to a pressure between 280 and 300 mm Hg. If, at the end of 1½ hours, the surgeon is certain that the operation can be completed in another half hour, the tourniquet can be left inflated for the additional period. If the operation is going to extend beyond these limits, however, the tourniquet should be deflated for a period of 20 minutes. This 20 minutes of operating time can generally be usefully employed in obtaining hemostasis or in performing some stages of the procedure where a bloodless field is not absolutely essential. After the extremity has had 20 minutes of circulation, the tourniquet can then be safely inflated for an additional 1½ hours.

MANAGEMENT OF SPECIFIC HAND INJURIES

In descending order of priority, care of the injured hand is directed to restoration of blood supply, prevention or reduction of infection, provision of skin coverage where feasible, stabilization of fractures, and, in selected appropriate cases, repair of the nerves and tendons. There is, for example, little use in placing a good tendon graft in a finger which has permanently stiffened joints or no sensation.

Vascular Injuries of the Hand

Lacerations of the arteries and veins in the hand or wrist are usually managed by ligation. This must, however, be done carefully under direct vision, preferably in a bloodless field, because of the ease of injuring adjacent nerves and tendons. Under rare circumstances, if viability of the hand seems impaired, vascular repair of larger vessels may be attempted. Such repairs, however, usually require microvascular techniques. Repair of digital arteries and veins may reconstitute the blood supply of a damaged finger which would otherwise not survive. In general, however, if a single digit must have its blood supply reconstituted, it is usually so badly injured that worthwhile recovery of function is doubtful. Often, such fingers should be amputated. This does not apply to severe trauma to the thumb or to multiple fingers in which case every effort must be made to save the injured digits.

Reimplantation

This subject is discussed fully in Chapter 18.

Mechanical Injuries of the Skin of the Hand

DIRECT CLOSURE

PITFALL

AGGRESSIVE DEBRIDEMENT OF RAGGED HAND WOUNDS MAY MAKE WOUND CLOSURE EXTREMELY DIFFICULT.

Closure of skin wounds is desirable wherever possible and is the procedure of choice if locally available viable skin is

present. Ragged and irregular skin margins
are debrided economically to ensure a minimum of tension at the time of closure.
Wounds produced by machinery, explosions
or severe crushing often cause a bursting
type of irregular laceration with skin edges
which are badly contused and irregular
but which are generally still viable. Despite the extensive damage, such a wound
can often be closed with locally available
skin and soft tissue if the debridement of
the skin edges is appropriately conservative.

AXIOM

SKIN IS PRECIOUS IN THE HAND, AND IT IS
OFTEN HELPFUL TO MINIMIZE THE DEBRIDE-
MENT OF THE WOUND'S EDGES IN ORDER TO
OBTAIN DIRECT CLOSURE WITHOUT SKIN GRAFT-
ING.

CONVERSION OF FLAPS TO FULL-THICKNESS
GRAFTS. Long flaps of skin and subcutaneous tissue which have a very narrow
base are generally not viable, particularly
when the base of the flap is distal. If a flap
of skin and subcutaneous tissue is in good
condition but has an inadequate blood supply, the subcutaneous fat and the deeper
layers of the dermis can be removed, converting the flap into a full-thickness graft
which may then be sutured back into its
original position. If the skin of an obviously nonviable flap has been severely damaged, it is generally better to remove the
nonviable flap and resurface the defect
with a full-thickness or thick split-thickness skin graft, a rotation flap, or a pedicle
flap.

ROTATION FLAPS. Rotation flaps to close
skin defects of the hand are especially useful in wounds which have large skin defects with exposed tendon or bone; such
wounds do not make a good bed for a free
skin graft. If a local flap can be rotated to
cover the exposed tendon or bone, the area
from which the flap has been obtained can
generally be covered with a free skin graft.

The loose dorsal skin of the hands lends
itself to the construction of rotation flaps
much more readily than does the palmar
skin.

FREE SKIN GRAFTS

AXIOM

IN GENERAL, THE THINNER THE SKIN GRAFT,
THE BETTER IT TAKES; THE THICKER THE SKIN
GRAFT, THE BETTER IT FUNCTIONS.

Although full-thickness free skin grafts
are very effective for covering defects created during certain types of elective surgery, such as the correction of a scar or
burn contracture, they often do not heal
well when applied to an acutely injured
hand. Very thin grafts, 0.008 to 0.010 inch,
heal well but have a rather pronounced
tendency to contracture. Grafts of this
thickness are generally not used in the
closure of acutely injured hands unless the
amount of donor skin available is limited
and the donor area must be reused.

A suitable compromise can usually be
obtained with a medium-thickness graft of
approximately 0.015 inch; this will usually
provide rapid and satisfactory closure of
an acute hand wound which cannot be
closed by direct repair. If the split graft
proves to be too thin, it may be electively
replaced later with a full-thickness graft or
a pedicle flap. It is often surprising, however, to note how well a medium-thickness
graft will do permanently.

PEDICLE FLAPS. Although pedicle flaps of
skin and subcutaneous tissue are used most
commonly in elective reconstruction operations, they are also occasionally used to
resurface defects in the acutely injured
hand. A degloving injury of a digit, and
particularly the thumb, will frequently require the application of an immediate
pedicle flap in order to preserve length.
This can be done either as a wraparound
flap or a tubed pedicle to be placed over
the denuded digit. Defects on the hand
with exposed bones or tendons do much

better with a pedicle flap than with a free skin graft, and the flap can usually be applied at the time of the injury without fear of infection.

A useful rule in the construction of a pedicle flap is that the ratio of the length of the flap to the width of the base of the flap should not exceed 3 to 1. A flap of these dimensions will almost always survive unless it has been placed under undue tension. Although pedicle flaps provide good viable skin coverage, they have poor sensation and permanently retain the quality of the skin and hair of the areas from which they are obtained.

Burns of the Hand (see also Chap. 28)

FIRST-, SECOND- AND THIRD-DEGREE THERMAL BURNS. Thermal burns of the hand are best managed initially by a bulky occlusive dressing with a splint which maintains the hand in the position of function. We favor a layer of Vaseline gauze directly over the burn followed by multiple layers of fluff gauze. Although silver nitrate solution or paste minimizes the amount of infection which develops in a burned hand, the staining of the normal skin has the disadvantage of causing a delay in the accurate evaluation of the depth of the burn.

PITFALL

ANY DELAY IN RESURFACING THE BURNED HAND MAY GREATLY REDUCE ITS ULTIMATE FUNCTION.

In general, the aim should be to have the burned hand completely resurfaced by the end of the third week. It is usually possible to determine, within 7 to 10 days, those areas which have sustained a full-thickness loss and those which can be expected to heal spontaneously. Once this decision has been made, the area of obvious full-thickness loss should be excised. Since the raw area left behind is usually not acceptable for immediate skin grafting, a few days of warm hand baths and daily dress-ing changes are often needed to put the wound in good condition for grafting.

Sharply circumscribed areas of obvious full-thickness burn can be immediately excised and replaced with a free skin graft. This method of management of a rather localized burn which is definitely full thickness will hasten recovery of function, lessen the chance of infection, and decrease the total time of immobilization of the hand.

"FOURTH-DEGREE" THERMAL BURNS. Burns are generally classified according to their depth as first-, second- and third-degree burns. Some authors, however, recognize a fourth-degree burn, which involves structures deeper than the skin and immediate subcutaneous tissues. Such a burn is not uncommon in the hand, especially on the dorsal surface. Tendons, joint capsules and even bone may be burned to the point of complete necrosis. Residual disability is inevitable in burns of this severity. The surgeon should try, however, to preserve the maximal degree of residual function. This can be best accomplished during the early stages of management by maintenance of the hand in the position of function. The wrist should be maintained in a position of 30° extension and 10° ulnar deviation. The digital joints and the thumb should be maintained in about 30° flexion (Fig. 4).

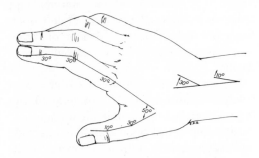

FIG. 4. The "position-of-function" of the hand (i.e. the position which preserves the maximal degree of function in an injured or disabled hand) consists of 30° extension and 10° ulnar deviation at the wrist, 30° flexion of the joints of the fingers and metacarpophalangeal joint of the thumb, a 50° angle between the first and second metacarpals, and 10° flexion of the interphalangeal joint of the thumb.

If this position cannot be maintained by splinting, temporary fixation of the joints with Kirschner wires may be indicated. Final coverage of burns of "fourth-degree" severity may involve pedicle flap transfer to the involved areas of the hand.

ELECTRICAL BURNS

PITFALL

FAILURE TO APPRECIATE THE SEVERE UNDERLYING INJURY IN AN ELECTRICAL BURN GREATLY REDUCES THE CHANCES OF RESTORING FUNCTION TO THE HAND.

Electrical burns of the hand are often deceptive. While the external wound may appear to be quite minor, the degree of deeper coagulation may involve almost any structure within the hand. Management includes splinting in the position of function and debridement of devitalized tissue, which often must be staged, followed by appropriate resurfacing. Restoration of deeper structures, such as nerves and tendons, may involve very complicated reconstructive surgery.

Amputations

In general, fresh amputations of fingers or the hand can be closed without fear of infection. Contaminated amputations and those from human bites are best left open for a few days, until the danger of infection has passed, and then closed secondarily.

In selecting the method of closure, consideration must be given not only to the injury itself, but to the individual's age, sex, usual occupation, hobbies, athletic interests, and eagerness to return to work. Individuals who prefer to return to their regular activities as rapidly as possible are usually not interested in going through a prolonged two- or three-stage flap procedure in order to preserve the full remaining length of the injured portion of the hand.

The cost to the patient in terms of lost time from work and in terms of the hospitalization and medical care must also be considered when selecting a method for closing an amputation.

Since the thumb provides about 50% of the function of the hand, an attempt is made to preserve as much of its length as possible regardless of the complexity of the method chosen. Similarly, when there have been injuries or amputations of multiple digits, more complicated and time-consuming procedures might be elected than for an injury which has involved only a single digit. In severe complex or crushing injuries of multiple parts of the hand, an attempt should be made to preserve all viable digits, even those which are so severely damaged that they would ordinarily be amputated.

DIRECT CLOSURE. When possible, direct closure of an amputation stump without the sacrifice of additional length, using locally available skin and soft tissue, is the procedure of choice. Small sharp spikes of bone are removed with a small ronguer or bone cutter, and the end of the bone is then smoothed off with a fine bone rasp. If possible, a pad of volar skin and subcutaneous tissue should be turned over the end of the bone; however, a great deal of additional bone should not be resected to effect such a closure.

Amputation stumps which are closed with equal anterior and posterior flaps are also usually acceptable and serviceable. Closure with a long dorsal flap is somewhat less acceptable because the scar on the volar surface may be tender and exposed to frequent trauma. When the level of amputation is so proximal that the digital nerves are recognizable structures, the nerves should be trimmed well back proximal to the actual level of amputation and ligated with fine silk suture to reduce the tendency toward formation of painful troublesome neuromas later.

PITFALL

FREE SKIN GRAFTS. Free skin grafts applied directly over exposed bone do not
provide satisfactory coverage; however, in
some amputations it is possible to draw fat
over the end of the bone and then apply
the free graft to the fat with a satisfactory
result.

PEDICLE FLAPS. Advancement of local
pedicle flaps or flaps from a distance are
generally indicated in those amputations in
which it is desirable to preserve all possible
length of the injured part. Such procedures
generally provide a much better functional
and cosmetic stump than skin grafts.

Advancement of Local Flaps. The two
most frequently used techniques for advancement of local flaps are the Kutler procedure[1] and the Moberg slide procedure.[2]
In the Kutler procedure, small triangular
flaps of skin and subcutaneous tissue in
which the neurovascular supply has been
retained are advanced over the end of the
amputation stump and sutured together.
The donor area of the triangular flap is
then closed in a V-Y manner. This procedure is quite useful in fingertip amputations where the level of bone amputation
is equal to, or slightly greater than, the level
of skin and soft-tissue amputation.

The volar V-Y flap advancement operation is a modification of the Kutler procedure which has been described by Klein-
ert.[3] In this modification a single triangular
flap of skin and soft tissue, constructed on
the volar surface of the finger immediately
proximal to the stump, is advanced over the
bone end and the resulting defect closed
in a V-Y fashion. This method should be
reserved for those amputations which are
either cut straight across or sloped dorsally,
and is not applicable to those amputations

in which the length of bone to be preserved
is longer than the volar skin.

The Moberg slide procedure, usually applied to amputations of the thumb, involves mobilization of the volar skin and
subcutaneous tissue together with the
neurovascular bundles over a sufficient
length of the digit so that the normal volar
skin and subcutaneous tissue can be drawn
over the end of the amputated bone.

Flaps from a Distance. THE PALMAR
PEDICLE FLAP. In this procedure, a flap of
skin and a small portion of subcutaneous
fat are elevated from the palm, the finger
is flexed to the palm and the flap of skin
and subcutaneous fat is sutured over the
amputation stump. This technique is usually indicated only in amputations through
the distal phalanx. The defect created by
the elevation of the palmar flap is covered
by a free skin graft. The finger then remains
in this position for 2 to 3 weeks. After circulation from the injured digit to the flap
has developed, the base of the flap is divided from the palm.

This procedure has the disadvantage of
requiring the involved finger to be maintained in acute flexion for a period of at
least 2 to 3 weeks. Adults, especially those
over 50 years of age, will frequently develop a considerable degree of joint stiffness if immobilized in this position for this
length of time. It is safer, therefore, to limit
this procedure to children.

THE CROSS FINGER PEDICLE FLAP. The raw
amputation surface is covered by a flap of
skin and subcutaneous tissue elevated from
the dorsal surface of the digit adjacent to
the one which has been amputated. It is
important that the plane of the dissection
of the flap be between the subcutaneous
fat and paratenon. The donor finger is then
covered with a full-thickness graft obtained
from as nearly hairless an area of the body
as possible. The flap of skin and subcutaneous tissue is then sutured over the open
amputation stump. After three weeks, the
base of the flap can be severed from the

donor finger and the amputated digit completely closed. These flaps usually develop a fairly satisfactory quality of sensation over a period of several months.

FLAPS FROM OTHER PARTS OF THE BODY. Large or multiple amputations of the hand will occasionally require resurfacing with pedicled skin from other areas of the body, especially the anterior abdominal wall. Such procedures, however, require two or more operations and the decision to resurface the hand with a pedicle flap from a distance should be made only when no other method of closure is possible without sacrificing remaining hand tissue. Although abdominal flaps have the disadvantages of other pedicle flaps, they are occasionally the only method available for the closure of very extensive injuries or large multiple amputations of the hand.

Infraclavicular skin is less hairy and of better quality than abdominal skin but is less able to cover large hand injuries. Cross-arm and cross-forearm flaps to resurface an amputated or denuded digit are also possible; however, they are rarely used because they limit the use of both extremities.

In all pedicle flap procedures, it is important that a completely closed wound be obtained. The donor area for the pedicle must either be closed primarily or skin grafted at the time of the application of the flap. The skin graft should extend across the base of the flap and for a short distance along the flap so that it can be sutured to the hand wound where the edges of the flap cannot be sutured.

Fractures

Once it is certain that the vascular supply is adequate and the wound can be closed with a reasonable chance of primary healing, the skeleton of the hand can be considered. The original surgeon is frequently the only one who has a good chance at complete restoration of normal skeletal anatomy; therefore, if he does not feel capable of accomplishing this with a particular injury, he should immediately transfer the patient to a facility where this type of care is available.

PITFALL

IF A FRACTURE, DISLOCATION OR INTRA-ARTICULAR FRACTURE IS ALLOWED TO HEAL IN MALPOSITION, LATER ATTEMPTS AT REDUCTION MAY FRUSTRATE EVEN THE BEST EFFORTS OF THE RECONSTRUCTIVE SURGEON.

TECHNIQUES OF MANAGEMENT. *Closed Reduction.* Whenever possible, closed fractures should be treated by closed manipulation and reduction and simple splinting of the part which has been injured. Mild angulation at the fracture site may be acceptable; however, marked angulation requires reduction to as nearly normal a position as possible. Any significant degree of rotation must also be corrected or there will be a tendency for the finger which has been fractured to overlap the adjacent finger.

If an accurate reduction cannot be maintained by closed methods, a percutaneous fixation of the fracture with fine Kirschner wires may be attempted. If this method of treatment is used, closed reduction and percutaneous pinning are attempted in the operating room and then a portable x-ray is obtained. If closed reduction has not been successful, open reduction of the fracture is then performed. In most cases of open reduction, the accuracy of the reduction can be determined visually; however, if there is any doubt, a portable x-ray should be obtained.

Open Reduction. If satisfactory reduction cannot be obtained by closed methods, an open reduction is indicated, exposing as little tendon as possible. With the safety and efficiency of present-day anesthesia and antibiotics, we no longer hesitate to perform open reductions nor to place metal pins across fractures in fresh open wounds.

Traction. Traction is now generally limited to those hand fractures with severe loss of bone or severe comminution, where it may be the only method for maintaining bone length and restoring something approaching anatomic alignment. In fractures where a considerable portion of the shaft of the bone has been lost, traction may also serve as a method of preserving the length of the digit until the wound is cleanly healed and the soft tissues are ready to accept a bone graft.

PITFALL

SOFT-TISSUE TRACTION, PARTICULARLY THROUGH THE TACTILE PAD ON THE DISTAL PHALANX, OFTEN LEADS TO A CONSIDERABLE DEGREE OF TISSUE NECROSIS WITH PAINFUL AND COSMETICALLY UNACCEPTABLE SCARS.

When traction is indicated for the management of a fracture of the hand, it should be applied through bone and should pull across as few joints as possible.

SPECIFIC INJURIES. *Bennett's Fracture.* Bennett's fracture is a fracture of the base of the first metacarpal in which the small bony prominence on its ulnar side at the base loses its contact with the major portion of the bone, which becomes displaced in a radial direction. Previous methods of reduction and immobilization of this fracture have involved the use of strong traction through the neck of the metacarpal or the base of the proximal phalanx or immobilization in a molded plaster cast. Superior results in recent years, however, have been obtained by reduction of the fracture and immobilization with a metal pin which is placed across the base of the reduced metacarpal into adjacent bone.

PITFALL

FAILURE TO REDUCE A BENNETT'S FRACTURE ACCURATELY MAY LEAD TO THE DEVELOPMENT OF A PAINFUL AND PROGRESSIVE DEGENERATIVE ARTHRITIS WITH SEVERE LOSS OF THUMB FUNCTION.

If a malunion and arthropathy develop, secondary procedures such as arthrodesis or arthroplasty of the carpometacarpal joint of the thumb may become necessary.

Intra-articular Fractures. Although undisplaced and minor chip fractures of the joints can be managed by simple immobilization of the involved bone and joint, any intra-articular fracture with displacement of 25% or more of the articular surface will, in general, require an open reduction. It is seldom possible to reduce such articular fragments accurately enough by closed methods. Although closed immobilization may occasionally be satisfactory after the reduction is obtained, internal fixation with thin Kirschner wires is often needed to maintain the proper position of all fragments.

Skeletal Injuries in which a Significant Amount of Bone Has Been Lost

PITFALL

IF A FRACTURED HAND BONE IS ALLOWED TO COLLAPSE INTO A SHORTENED POSITION, RESTORATION OF THE ORIGINAL LENGTH DURING RECONSTRUCTIVE OPERATIONS IS SELDOM POSSIBLE.

If a hand injury results in loss of significant amounts of the shaft of the bone while the proximal and distal joints remain in good condition, it is often advisable to preserve the length of the injured bone so that the bone loss can be restored later by a bone graft. With metacarpal injuries the original length can often be restored by traction upon the finger; the length can be maintained by passing a rather heavy Kirschner wire transversely across the heads of the metacarpals. With mid-shaft loss in the phalanges, it is usually necessary to use traction to maintain the length of the digit until the soft tissues are in sufficiently good condition to accept a bone graft.

Dislocations. Most dislocations of the hand are due to closed injuries, and closed reduction should be attempted as soon as possible. Fresh interphalangeal joint dislocations can almost always be reduced by closed manipulation with little or no local anesthesia. More proximal dislocations, however, often require a regional block or general anesthetic.

PROXIMAL INTERPHALANGEAL JOINT. Although it is usually possible to reduce fresh dislocations of the distal interphalangeal joints easily with little or no residual problem, with the proximal interphalangeal joints the volar plate and the central slip of the extensor tendon apparatus must also be considered. Loss of the attachment of the volar plate to the proximal phalanx, or rupture of the central slip of the extensor tendon apparatus at its insertion on the base of the middle phalanx, may be very difficult to detect by clinical examination at the time of the injury. If these injuries can be diagnosed within a few days of the accident, open reattachment of the structure may be the procedure of choice. The boutonniere deformity, which results from uncorrected rupture of the central slip of the extensor tendon at the base of the middle phalanx, is one of the most difficult of all hand injuries to treat successfully.

METACARPOPHALANGEAL JOINT. Most dislocations of the metacarpophalangeal joints are hyperextension injuries in which the head of the metacarpal is forced through the volar capsular structures. Attempts immediately to replace the head of the metacarpal into the interior of the joint may be frustrated by a noose of volar capsule encircling the neck of the metacarpal. After a few days, edema and fibrosis of the capsular structures may make a successful closed reduction almost impossible. If attempts at a closed reduction under local anesthesia in the emergency room are unsuccessful, the patient should be taken to the operating room for another attempt under general anesthesia. Hyperextension of the dislocated joint, traction on the proximal phalanx of the digit and flexion of the joint, in that order, will usually result in reduction.

If a metacarpophalangeal joint cannot be reduced by closed manipulation, open reduction should be performed immediately. The rent in the joint capsule is enlarged, the metacarpal head is returned to the interior of the joint, the injury of the volar capsular structures of the joint is repaired, and the reduction is maintained by splinting with the joint in gentle flexion. If the sesamoid bone which may be present on the volar surface of the metacarpophalangeal becomes lodged between the head of the metacarpal and the base of the proximal phalanx, it may be necessary to excise it before a stable reduction can be obtained.

SPONTANEOUS REDUCTIONS OF DISLOCATED JOINTS. Patients often have reduced a dislocated joint within the hand by themselves. The degree of motion which these patients have retained in spite of lack of medical treatment and immobilization causes one to wonder whether or not a dislocated joint within the hand should ever be immobilized following reduction.

Since most dislocations of joints in the hand are hyperextension injuries, it is our practice to immobilize the reduced joint in 30° flexion with a small padded metal splint applied to the dorsal surface for 3 to 4 weeks. This splint is applied in a manner which allows the patient to remove the restraining tape for active flexion of the joint daily but prevents any possibility of a recurrence of the hyperextension.

Nerve Injuries Within the Hand

Nerve injuries present some of the most challenging of all problems in hand surgery. In each instance, the surgeon must decide whether the patient will achieve a better ultimate functional result with a primary or with a secondary repair. The crux of the problem is the condition of the wound itself. When peripheral nerves in the hand or wrist have been injured in a cleanly incised laceration, they should be repaired primarily following debridement of the proximal and distal ends of the lacerated nerve to the level of visible hemorrhage. A tension-free anastomosis is essential and may require a minor degree of mobilization of the proximal and distal ends of the nerve. Nonabsorbable suture of the smallest possible size, usually 6-0, 7-0, or 8-0, should be used. It is extremely important that the nerve ends be lined up accurately, that the suture include only the perineurium, and that the suture not encircle and strangulate any bundles of nerve fibers within the nerve. Magnification, either by an operating microscope or by a loupe, will make the nerve repair more accurate, particularly when dealing with digital nerves.

AXIOM

PRIMARY REPAIR OF PERIPHERAL NERVES SHOULD NOT BE ATTEMPTED IN ANY WOUND WHICH HAS ANY ELEMENT OF CRUSHING, TEARING, OR CONTAMINATION OR WHICH CANNOT BE CLOSED.

With any wound that is not a neat clean laceration, the patient is better served either by no surgery upon the nerve itself or by a temporary gross suturing of the nerve ends with the expectation of performing a secondary repair later. Other conditions which enter into the decision for or against a primary nerve repair include the availability of skilled personnel, anesthesia and operating facilities. If one or more of these conditions cannot be met, the patient is better served by a delayed repair of the nerve within six weeks to three months.

Tendon Injuries About the Hand and Wrist

INJURIES TO FLEXOR TENDONS. The technique of flexor tendon repair is not as important as the application of good general surgical principles, with gentle handling of tissues, absolute hemostasis in the wounds and appropriate postoperative splinting. The suture material used in flexor tendon repair should be nonabsorbable. The newer synthetic sutures of nylon, Dacron, Teflon and Mersilene, in our experience, seem to cause less foreign-body reactions and fewer adhesions about the tendon repair.

AXIOM

TO BE TRULY FUNCTIONAL, TENDONS MUST BE ABLE TO GLIDE.

Recent experience with synthetic absorbable suture (polyglyconic suture) indicates that this material is quite suitable for tendon repair. There have been no instances of tendon dehiscence nor have troublesome granulomas developed about these sutures. However, since experience with this material is still somewhat limited, a positive recommendation cannot be made at this time.

The Flexor Digitorum Profundus Tendon Injury Distal to the Insertion of the Flexor Digitorum Sublimis Tendon. Almost all injuries of the flexor digitorum profundus tendon distal to the insertion of the flexor digitorum sublimis tendon at the base of the middle phalanx should be repaired primarily. Even though the profundus tendon may be in somewhat less than ideal condition for primary repair, the worst that can happen is a tenodesis effect with the tendon repair badly bound down in surrounding scar.

The problems of attempting to restore flexion or stability to the distal joint of a finger which has lost its profundus tendon but still has an intact and functioning sublimis tendon are considerable. Many authorities would never attempt to restore the profundus tendon with a tendon graft through an intact sublimis tendon; others, including ourselves, will perform this procedure only under ideal circumstances. Often, it is preferable to resort to a stabilization procedure for the distal interphalangeal joint to prevent the distal joint from going into hyperextension. These procedures involve either a tenodesis of the portion of the profundus tendon distal to the level of the injury or an arthrodesis of the joint.

It is occasionally possible with this injury to avoid the problems of a tendon suture line, and the adhesions which always form about such a suture line, by advancement and reinsertion of the proximal cut end of the flexor digitorum profundus into a new insertion on the distal phalanx. No attempt should be made, however, to reinsert a profundus tendon which has been lacerated at a considerable distance from its original insertion. Although some authorities indicate that a tendon can be advanced a distance of 1 to 1½ inches, our own feeling is that this procedure should be limited to flexor digitorum profundus tendon lacerations which have occurred within 1.0 to 1.5 cm of the original insertion.

Tendon Injuries in "No-man's-land"

PITFALL

IF A SURGEON WITHOUT EXPERIENCE IN HAND SURGERY ATTEMPTS PRIMARY REPAIR OF TENDONS IN "NO-MAN'S-LAND," THE RESULTS MAY BE DISASTROUS

The so-called no-man's-land or critical area for flexor tendon injuries lies between the distal flexion crease of the palm and the insertion of the sublimis tendon at the base of the middle phalanx (Fig. 5). It is in this area that the poorest results of all of the flexor tendon repairs are obtained. Many authorities feel that primary tendon repair should never be performed here, even by thoroughly experienced hand surgeons and with cleanly incised wounds. Nevertheless, in our experience, primary repair of flexor tendon injuries in this area is a useful and successful procedure if the wound is fresh and cleanly incised and does not involve a joint, a fracture or more than one neurovascular bundle. Unless all the conditions are ideal, however, the patient with a flexor tendon injury in the critical area is better off with immediate closure of the wound and later secondary surgery.

If primary repair of a lacerated flexor tendon within the critical area is decided upon, the following rules apply:

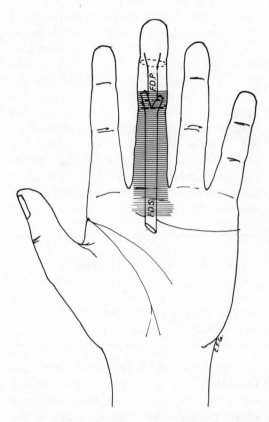

FIG. 5. "No-man's-land" or the critical area for flexor tendon injuries (which is shaded in) lies between the insertion of the flexor digitorum sublimis (F.D.S.) at the base of middle phalanx of each finger and the distal palmar crease. In this critical area, the flexor digitorum profundus (F.D.P.) and the F.D.S. are enclosed together within a rather tight tendon sheath.

1. When both the flexor digitorum profundus and the flexor digitorum sublimis tendons have been completely lacerated, the sublimis tendon is sacrificed and only the profundus tendon is repaired. However, an intact sublimis tendon should never be sacrificed in order to regain function of the profundus tendon.
2. If the profundus tendon is completely lacerated while the sublimis tendon sustains little or no damage, the sublimis tendon is not disturbed, and the profundus tendon is repaired.
3. If one slip of the sublimis tendon has been lacerated and the other has not, and there has also been a complete laceration of the profundus tendon, it is generally wise to resect the lacerated slip of the sublimis tendon, to leave the uninjured slip of the sublimis tendon

alone and to repair the profundus tendon. Small "nicks" in the sublimis insertions, with a complete laceration of the profundus tendon, are best managed by repair of the profundus tendon; nothing whatever is done to the sublimis tendon in this situation.

Flexor Tendon Injuries within the Palm. It is our practice to repair all lacerated flexor tendons within the mid-portion of the palm. The tendency for the formation of adhesions between the repair of a profundus and sublimis tendon of the same digit can be minimized by interposing the lumbrical muscle between the two tendon repairs. Since the nerves lie between and superficial to the tendons in the palm, patients who have flexor tendon lacerations of two digits in this area usually also have a laceration of the common digital nerve carrying sensation from the contiguous aspects of the two digits. Careful evaluation of sensation prior to surgery is, therefore, essential.

Flexor Tendon Injuries within the Carpal Tunnel. Nine flexor tendons and the median nerve pass through the carpal tunnel and the ulnar nerve lies against it. Since the tendency toward formation of adhesions within the area of the carpal tunnel is considerable, some authorities recommend that, with multiple flexor tendon injuries in this area, only the flexor pollicis longus and profundus tendons be repaired. Our own opinion is that the sublimis tendons are powerful and important and should not be sacrificed unless absolutely necessary. We, therefore, repair all structures which have been lacerated in the carpal tunnel even though a tendolysis may be necessary later.

Flexor Tendon Injuries between the Level of the Carpal Tunnel and the Musculotendinous Junctions. It is generally agreed that all lacerated tendons proximal to the carpal tunnel should be repaired. This includes the wrist flexors, the flexor pollicis longus and the profundus and sublimis tendons.

EXTENSOR TENDON INJURIES. Extensor tendon injuries usually demand a good primary repair, even with less than ideal conditions. Secondary surgery on extensor tendons is more difficult and less rewarding than secondary surgery upon flexor tendons. An end-to-end repair of an extensor tendon injury at 4 to 6 weeks is often impossible, and delayed extensor tendon injuries often require a tendon graft or tendon transfer procedure for proper results.

The Mallet Finger. The mallet finger is due to a loss of continuity of the extensor tendon apparatus over the dorsal surface of the distal interphalangeal joint. Although this may occur as an open laceration of the tendon, it more commonly is the result of a closed rupture of the extensor tendon or avulsion of a portion of the bone of the distal phalanx.

In the open laceration, it is our practice to extend the wound, as indicated, in order to repair the lacerated tendon directly with 6-0 silk sutures. The distal joint is then maintained in slight hyperextension by a Kirschner wire for a period of six weeks. Closed ruptures of the extensor tendon apparatus over the dorsum of the distal interphalangeal joint are immobilized with the distal joint in slight hyperextension for a period of six weeks. For an old mallet-finger deformity due to an untreated closed rupture, the scar between the tendon ends is resected, the distal joint is maintained in slight hyperextension with a Kirschner wire, and the tendon ends are reapproximated with 6-0 silk.

The mallet-finger deformity with avulsion of a bone fragment is somewhat more complex. This fracture, if left untreated, will heal with the formation of a rather prominent "beak" of bone on the dorsal aspect of the distal phalanx and irregularity of the articular surface of the distal interphalangeal joint. If the bone fragment has less than 25% of the articular surface of the distal phalanx, the injury is treated as if it were a closed rupture of the extensor tendon, the bone fragment is ignored, and the injury is treated by simple splinting for a period of six weeks. If the bone fragment contains 25% or more of the articular surface, it is our feeling that this injury is best managed by an open reduction and replacement of the avulsed bone fragment. This is accomplished by immobilization of the distal interphalangeal joint in slight hyperextension by a Kirschner wire and replacement of the bone fragment with a pull-out wire suture.

The Boutonniere Deformity. The boutonniere deformity is one of the most difficult of all tendon injuries to treat successfully. This deformity occurs when the central slip of the extensor tendon apparatus over the dorsal aspect of the proximal interphalangeal joint has been injured. The lateral bands of the extensor tendon apparatus then become dislocated into a position anterior to the flexion-extension axis of the proximal interphalangeal joint, and therefore become flexors of this joint rather than extensors.

Direct laceration of the central portion of the extensor tendon apparatus does quite well with either immediate repair of the lacerated portion of the extensor tendon over the dorsal aspect of the proximal interphalangeal joint or with excision of the scar and secondary repair. If it is a closed injury with avulsion of the insertion of the central slip of the extensor tendon from the middle phalanx, splinting of the proximal interphalangeal joint in extension for a period of six weeks will usually result in a satisfactory, if not normal, functional result. If this injury is not diagnosed and treated soon after injury, secondary repairs are extremely difficult and the results are relatively poor.

Extensor Tendon Injuries Proximal to the Proximal Interphalangeal Joint. Direct repair of extensor tendon injuries about the proximal phalanx, the metacarpophalangeal joint, the dorsum of the hand and the wrist and forearm are usually quite successful and are preferable to secondary surgical procedures. Rare exceptions may be pres-

ent when there has been actual avulsion of extensor tendons from the dorsal surface of the hand or wrist.

SUMMARY

AXIOM
THE SURGEON WHO INITIALLY CARES FOR A HAND INJURY MAY WELL DETERMINE THE ULTIMATE OUTCOME.

When the surgeon is confronted with an injury of the hand involving multiple structures, he should follow certain priorities. Restoration of vascularity, although rarely a problem, certainly has the first priority. Skin coverage is next, followed by restoration of the anatomic integrity of the skeleton. Restoration of sensation and motor function of peripheral nerves has the fourth priority, while restoration of tendon function has the lowest.

When only one or two structures have been injured, the question of priority may not arise and the individual structures are repaired immediately. This is particularly true of vascular, cutaneous and skeletal structures. The advisability of, and neces-

TABLE 1. TEN COMMON ERRORS IN THE MANAGEMENT OF HAND INJURIES

1. Failure to take an x-ray when there is a possibility of a fracture or foreign body.
2. Failure to use a tourniquet to obtain a bloodless operative field.
3. Incomplete cleansing and debridement of the wound.
4. Incomplete hemostasis or reliance on skin sutures to stop deeper bleeding.
5. Attempts to repair significant hand injuries under suboptimal conditions in an emergency room.
6. Failure to correct rotation or angulation of fractures.
7. Failure to recognize tendon injuries, particularly those to extensors, because of a cursory examination.
8. Failure to recognize nerve injuries because of an improper examination.
9. Closure of wounds under significant tension.
10. Application of a dressing that is too tight.

sity for, immediate repair of nerve or tendon injuries depend upon the nature of the wound and the skill of the surgeon.

Some of the common errors made in hand surgery are listed in Table 1.

If the principles outlined in this chapter are adhered to, most patients who have acutely injured hands will recover satisfactorily following initial care. In addition, those hands with the most severe and complicated injuries will have been placed in the best possible condition for later reconstructive surgery.

REFERENCES

1. Moberg, E.: Aspects of sensation in reconstructive surgery of the upper extremity. J. Bone Joint Surg., 46A:817, 1964.
2. Kutler, W.: A method for finger tip amputation. JAMA, 133:29, 1947.
3. Atasoy, E., et al.: Reconstruction of the amputated finger tip with a triangular volar flap. J. Bone Joint Surg., 52A:921, 1970.

28 THERMAL INJURIES

J. R. LLOYD
K. IMAMOGLU

BURNS

AXIOM
MOST BURNS ARE PREVENTABLE.

Over 2,000,000 burn injuries occur in the United States annually.[1] While many of these burns are minor, the resultant morbidity and economic loss can be very serious. The patients with the more severe burns occupy 11,000 hospital beds per day and 12,000 patients die of their burns each year. Any severe burn is a tragedy but the most regrettable aspect of the burn problem is the fact that 80% of all these injuries are avoidable accidents. In no other area of major trauma is education of the general public on prevention so severely lacking.

During the past three decades, major strides have been made in the management of burn injuries, with a dramatic improvement in the survival rates in patients with 30 to 50% burns. Burn shock, one of the major problems in the past, has been nearly eliminated as a cause of death. More sophisticated respiratory support has greatly improved the mortality rate of the victims of severe smoke inhalation. The use of topical antimicrobials has contributed significantly to the control of invasive burn wound sepsis in burns less than 50% and has made survival possible in some patients with burns in the 80 to 85% range. Malnutrition is still a formidable problem, but occlusive dressings, topical antimicrobial agents, better control of the ambient temperature and improved nutrition, especially by the intravenous route, have helped curtail the ravages of burn hypercatabolism.

In spite of these advances, however, patients with major burn injuries still die, often just short of the point where survival should be ensured. These late deaths are generally due to a combination of sepsis, negative nitrogen balance, suppressed immunity, and a general depletion of the patient's reserves.

Classification of Thermal Injuries

Burns are classified according to the depth and the extent of the injury. The depth of injury is expressed as the degree of burn; classically, three or four categories are recognized, progressing from first degree which is the mildest to third or fourth degree which is the most severe. The extent of injury is expressed in terms of the percentage of involvement of the body surface area. A further classification based on a combination of the depth and the extent of involvement can be used to subdivide thermal injuries into major and minor burns.

In general, all first-degree burns are considered minor. Second- and third-degree burns involving less than 10% of the body surface are also considered minor. Any combination of second- and third-degree burns that exceeds 20% of the body surface, however, is considered a major burn. Some authors refer to burns in excess of 40% of the body surface as "severe" burns.

DEPTH OF INJURY. *First-degree Burns.* The first-degree burn is characterized by erythema, moderate to severe pain and minimal to moderate edema. These changes are due to dilatation of the intradermal vascular bed and are exemplified by the common nonblistering sunburn. These wounds rarely, if ever, become infected. They heal without any scarring and do not require any surgical intervention. The amount of fluid lost into the injured areas can be significant but is rarely of sufficient magnitude to require intravenous fluid administration.

Second-degree Burns. Second-degree burns are characterized by vesiculation (blisters) and moderate to severe pain. If severe infection does not supervene, they generally heal with little or no scarring. In terms of their appearance, management and prognosis, second-degree burns are often subdivided into superficial, intermediate, and deep.

Superficial second-degree burns develop thin-walled vesicles from within a few minutes up to 18 hours after injury. The pain is moderate to severe, the edema is moderate, healing occurs within 7 to 10 days, and there is no scarring or contracture problem.

Intermediate second-degree burns are the classical variety of second-degree burn injury. Vesiculation including the basal layer of the epithelium occurs at the time of injury or within the first hour. The pain is severe. The edema and fluid loss are significant and extensive untreated burns of this type, in excess of 15% in children and over 20% in adults, can rapidly produce shock of life-threatening severity. Superficial infection may occur but invasive sepsis causing full-thickness skin loss is unusual. Healing or re-epithelialization is ac-

complished by spreading or migration of epithelium from hair follicles and sweat glands that have not been destroyed by the burn. This process is usually complete in 10 to 17 days. There is generally little or no scarring, and contractures are rare.

Deep second-degree burns extend through the epidermis into the dermal layer, destroying varying numbers of hair follicles and sweat glands depending on the depth to which the dermal destruction occurs. Vesiculation occurs at the time of injury, and many of the blisters rupture very soon after being formed. The surface of the wound has a blanched appearance and may be covered with remnants of ruptured blisters. The pain may be very severe but some areas may be anesthetized because of damage to the underlying superficial nerves.

The time required for re-epithelialization varies with the depth to which the dermis is involved, the number of hair follicles and sweat glands that have been destroyed, and the amount of burn which has been converted to a full-thickness injury by bacterial infection. Healing may occur as early as 15 to 20 days but not infrequently takes as long as 50 days. The scarring and contractures are often severe, particularly if more than 30 days are required for healing. Under such circumstances excision of the areas which are unhealed after 25 to 30 days, followed by skin grafting, provides a more satisfactory end-result and saves many hospital days.

Third-degree Burns. Third-degree thermal injuries result in full-thickness loss of the skin and its component parts, including the hair follicles and sweat glands. The appearance of third-degree burns can vary somewhat, and the inexperienced individual may occasionally not recognize that the area is burned. Classically the third-degree burn appears as an eschar through which thrombosed blood vessels can be seen; the eschar is anesthetic and will not bleed when incised. In some instances the skin may be so severely injured by thermal exposure that it is charred and the subcutaneous tissue will be exposed.

Fourth-degree Burns. Extremely severe burns that char or burn away the skin and extend into muscle, tendon, joint or bone have been referred to by some physicians as fourth-degree burns. The lethality of such wounds is equivalent to severe crush injuries. When an extremity is involved with a burn of this severity, early amputation is frequently the procedure of choice.

EXTENT OF INJURY

AXIOM

THE EXTENT OF A SEVERE BURN CANNOT BE ACCURATELY DETERMINED WITHOUT THE USE OF A DIAGRAM.

An accurate assessment of the extent of the burn is essential for proper treatment, particularly in estimating the initial fluid needs. Brief inspections often provide erroneous data which in turn may result in poor decisions concerning therapy. The extent of the burn should be traced on a human diagram, such as that devised by Lund and Browder[2] (Fig. 1), which takes into consideration changes in the percent of surface area of various parts of the body during growth.

The "rule of nines" may be employed when such a chart is not available. On the average, each upper extremity of the adult comprises about 9% of the total body surface area, each lower extremity 18%, the front and the back of the trunk 18% each, the head 9% and the perineum 1%. During infancy the head is relatively larger and constitutes about 18% of the surface area while each of the lower extremities may account for only 12% of the total.

Etiology

The causes of heat injuries, in the order of the frequency with which they occur, are: scald burns, flame burns, direct heat, friction or abrasion burns and electrical burns.

SCALD BURNS. Scald burns are for the most part first- and second-degree burns; however, third-degree burns can be incurred if the temperature of the scalding liquid or vapor is very high and the duration of exposure is prolonged. Clothing may offer some protection from this type of injury, but, on the other hand, clothing saturated with a scalding liquid can hold the excess heat in apposition to the skin and produce a more severe burn. Rapidly divesting the patient of clothing saturated with a scalding liquid may significantly reduce the depth of injury. Severe scalds in some instances may be due to chemicals such as alkalis or acids. In these cases the burn is apt to be much more severe and involve deeper structures.

FLAME BURNS. In general, flame burns produce a more serious injury than scalds, and there is almost always some element of third-degree burn. House fires account for a significant number of these burns, and the injury is usually much more severe if the patient's clothing ignites. Flames in the proximity of the individual may not actually make contact with the skin but the intense heat generated can by itself produce a severe burn injury.

Although considerable legislation is being instituted to require the textile industries to use fire retardants in the manufacture of cloth and clothing, some materials are still available that can ignite with explosive violence, almost always producing an extensive third-degree burn.

Burns due to flammable liquids may range from superficial flash burns to extensive, deep, life-threatening injuries. The telltale odor of gasoline or turpentine is often a clue to the cause of these burns.

DIRECT HEAT. The third most common cause of burns is direct contact with a heated object, e.g. a hot iron or the heating element of a kitchen range. While these burns are usually limited in extent, they are almost always third-degree in depth.

BURN SHEET

BURN RECORD. AGES — BIRTH - 7½

DATE OF OBSERVATION_____

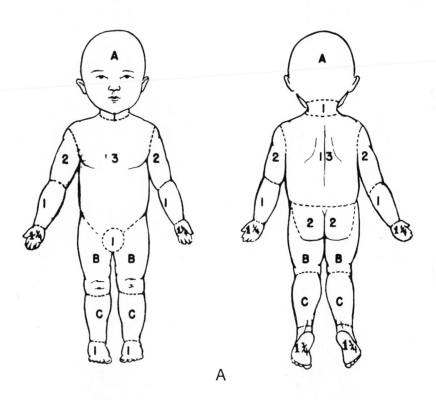

A

RELATIVE PERCENTAGES OF AREAS AFFECTED BY GROWTH

Area	Age 0	1	5
A = ½ of Head	9½	8½	6½
B = ½ of One Thigh	2¾	3¼	4
C = ½ of One Leg	2½	2½	2¾

% BURN BY AREAS

Probable 3rd° Burn	Head_____ Neck_____ Body_____ Up. Arm_____ Forearm_____ Hands_____
	Genitals_____ Buttocks_____ Thighs_____ Legs_____ Feet_____
Total Burn	Head_____ Neck_____ Body_____ Up. Arm_____ Forearm_____ Hands_____
	Genitals_____ Buttocks_____ Thighs_____ Legs_____ Feet_____
Sum of All Areas_____ Probably 3rd°_____ Total Burn_____

NUR-15

FIG. 1A. Burn sheet for infants and young children.

BURN SHEET

BURN RECORD. AGES 7 TO ADULT

DATE OF OBSERVATION _____

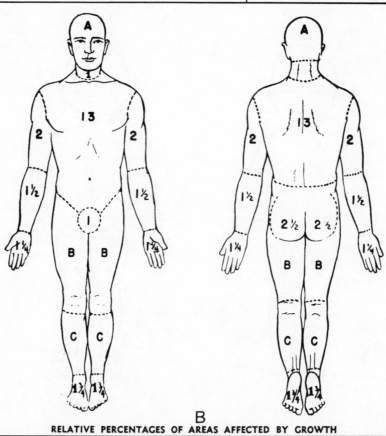

B

RELATIVE PERCENTAGES OF AREAS AFFECTED BY GROWTH

Area	Age 10	15	Adult
A = ½ of Head	5½	4½	3½
B = ½ of One Thigh	4¼	4½	4¼
C = ½ of One Leg	3	3¼	3½

% BURN BY AREAS

| Probable 3rd° Burn | Head___ Neck___ Body___ Up. Arm___ Forearm___ Hands___ |
| | Genitals___ Buttocks___ Thighs___ Legs___ Feet___ |

| Total Burn | Head___ Neck___ Body___ Up. Arm___ Forearm___ Hands___ |
| | Genitals___ Buttocks___ Thighs___ Legs___ Feet___ |

Sum of All Areas_____ Probably 3rd°_____ Total Burn_____

NUR-15

FIG. 1B.   Burn sheet for older children and adults.

ELECTRICAL BURNS. Electrical burns are particularly bad since they can cause severe thermal burns as well as coagulation necrosis of deep structures along the course of the electrical current. In high-voltage electric arc exposures, the individual may be engulfed in flames with temperatures to 4,000 to 5,000 F. Although the duration may only be fractions of a second, a very serious and extensive flame-like burn may result. With this type of contact there is little or no tissue coagulation related to the electrical current.

PITFALL

THE PHYSICIAN MAY FAIL TO APPRECIATE THE EXTENSIVE DEEP TISSUE DAMAGE THAT MAY OCCUR, IN SPITE OF MINIMAL SKIN DAMAGE, IN ELECTRICAL BURNS.

The other major type of electrical burn occurs when a patient comes in contact with a high-voltage wire or conduit. There may be relatively small skin burns at the points of contact, but the intervening tissues, through which the current is conducted, will frequently be severely coagulated by the intense heat generated in the tissues. The tissue necrosis is further compounded by thrombosis of major vessels in the area. Not infrequently, the external appearance may suggest that only a minor burn occurred, but extensive underlying damage to tendons, muscles and bone may occasionally require amputation or extensive debridement.

FRICTION BURNS AND ABRASIONS. Severe abrasions are the result of the scraping action of coarse substances or surfaces against the skin. The heat generated by the friction may cause additional damage. The severity of these injuries may vary from mild first-degree burns to extensive third-degree burns such as those that may occur when an individual is struck by an automobile and dragged along the pavement. The management of abrasions is roughly the same as other burns, but the removal of ground-in debris or dirt may present special problems. Failure to remove foreign bodies early in the management will result in lifelong tattooing that is almost impossible to remove as a secondary procedure. In some instances vigorous scrubbing with a brush under anesthesia is required.

Pathophysiology

The pathologic changes in the skin and underlying tissues will vary depending on the intensity of the heat and the length of time that it is applied. The epidermis is partially or completely destroyed by the heat, the capillaries in the area become dilated and capillary permeability is increased. Edema fluid accumulates rapidly in and around the damaged tissues during the first 18 to 24 hours after the burn. This fluid shift occurs at the expense of the intravascular volume and may cause hypovolemic shock if not replaced adequately. Loss of fluid from the vascular compartment gradually decreases during the second 24 hours as the capillaries recover their tone and their permeability is restored to normal.

In addition to the great losses of plasma that occur, there is often a decrease in the red cell mass. Initially this red cell loss may not be appreciated because of the severe hemoconcentration caused by the plasma loss. If large numbers of red cells are hemolyzed, the patient will develop severe hemoglobinemia which will be followed by hemoglobinuria within 1 to 4 hours.

The coagulation necrosis which occurs in a third-degree burn produces an ideal environment for infection. In addition, the patient's polymorphonuclear leukocytes may be damaged by the burn so that they are much less capable of phagocytizing and destroying the invading bacteria.

Treatment

The management of any individual who has suffered a severe burn has three major objectives: (1) to save life, (2) to close the wound, and (3) to minimize or correct deformities.

The major life-threatening problems encountered in the management of severely burned patients are shock, sepsis and malnutrition. Probably no other injury or illness demands greater physical and emotional endurance on the part of the patient and more patience and effort on the part of the physician. The multiple problems encountered require the expertise of numerous specialists, and, ideally, severely burned patients are managed by the team approach in a facility designed specifically for this purpose.

PITFALL

THE PHYSICIAN MAY FAIL TO OBTAIN ADEQUATE HELP IN THE MANAGEMENT OF A PATIENT WITH A SEVERE BURN.

INITIAL OR EMERGENCY TREATMENT. *Minor Burns.* Minor burns can usually be managed on an outpatient basis. If the burn is small and located in an area accessible to the patient, he may do his own treatments at home; if the patient is a child or unable to care for himself properly, instructions should be given to some responsible member of the family who can do the necessary dressings. These patients may then be followed at intervals in an outpatient department or in the physician's private office.

The following outline for the initial management of minor burns is suggested:

1. Administration of cool compresses or pain medication as indicated.
2. Cleansing with a mild detergent soap.
3. Debridement of all blisters and other devitalized tissue.
4. Application of a topical antimicrobial such as:
   Silvadene   Silver nitrate paste
   Betadine   Furacin gauze
   Sulfamylon   Vaseline gauze
5. Application of a bulky dressing which is then wrapped snugly with bias-cut stockinette.
6. Instructions to the patient or a member of his family to start soaks of the involved area after the third day.

7. Instructions on the availability and types of dressing materials to be used after each soak.
8. Instructions on the intervals between outpatient visits.

Some small third-degree burns that will eventually need grafting may be treated on an outpatient basis; the patient can be brought back later for grafting after debridement has been completed and a clean granulating bed is achieved.

Major Burns (Table 1). Criteria that generally indicate that admission to the hospital is necessary include a second-degree burn involving more than 15% of the body surface, a third-degree burn involving more than 10% of the body surface, or involvement of the hands, face, or genitalia. If the patient is younger than two years, older than 65 years, or has other injuries or illness, he may have to be admitted even if the burns are much less severe.

An initial rapid examination should be made to ascertain that the patient has an adequate airway and vital signs. If smoke inhalation is suspected, oxygen and mist should be started immediately. The time of the burn should be established and all subsequent treatment related to this time.

If the burn is very serious, it warrants the attention of several physicians. While one member of the team is evaluating the extent of injury and the patient's general status, another should be removing any remaining clothing and looking for an opportunity to obtain an accurate weight. The patient should then be covered with a sterile sheet and enough blankets to ensure warmth. A third member of the team should establish a reliable intravenous line to administer 5% dextrose in lactated Ringer's solution at the rate of 5 cc per pound per hour.

AXIOM

ANY DELAY IN THE ADMINISTRATION OF ADEQUATE INTRAVENOUS FLUIDS MAY CAUSE SEVERE HYPOVOLEMIA AND SHOCK.

TABLE 1. OUTLINE OF INITIAL TREATMENT OF PATIENTS WITH SERIOUS BURNS

1. Establish an airway and administer oxygen or assisted ventilation as indicated.
2. Remove all clothing.
3. Weigh the patient.
4. Make baseline CBC, electrolyte, BUN and glucose determinations.
5. Start IV of 5% D/L.R. and administer at the rate of 5 ml/lb/hr.
6. Relieve pain with:
   a. narcotic as indicated or
   b. cool compresses to burn areas or immersion of the injured part in cool (55 F) water or saline.
7. Debride all loose foreign material, blisters and blister debris.
8. Cleanse with cool saline—NO HEXACHLOROPHENE.
   a. If the wound is essentially clean, copious irrigations alone are adequate.
   b. If moderately contaminated or previously treated with a home remedy such as butter or ointments, gentle sponging of wound with mild detergent soap is indicated.
   c. To scrub out ground-in dirt, aggressive debridement is required, using sedation or anesthesia as indicated.
9. Make an accurate assessment of the extent of the burn wound (burn sheet—Fig. 1).
10. Apply dressings using Silvadene, Betadine, Sulfamylon, silver nitrate cream or silver nitrate soaks.
11. Calculate fluid requirements.
12. Insert indwelling Foley catheter for burns greater than 15% in children and geriatric patients, and for burns greater than 20% in young and middle-aged adults.
13. Start burn record data based on time of burn.
14. Consider CVP monitoring for patients in shock or with burns over 60%.
15. Observe for effects of smoke inhalation.

An indwelling urinary catheter should be inserted to follow the hourly urine output. The necessity for CVP monitoring should be evaluated. Tetanus immunization should be administered and blood should be drawn for CBC, electrolyte, BUN and glucose determinations. Serial blood gases should also be obtained if smoke inhalation is suspected.

Without any additional delay, the patient should be sent to the burn unit for further cleansing of the wound and dressings. When the hospital does not have a burn unit, the patient should be dispatched to an appropriate area where further treatment can be carried out, or he should be carefully observed in the emergency room and arrangements made to send him to the nearest facility where adequate burn care is available.

PITFALL

THE PHYSICIAN MAY FAIL TO NOTE THE PRESENCE OF OTHER INJURIES AND MAKE ARRANGEMENTS FOR THEIR APPROPRIATE MANAGEMENT.

Before any patient is transported from the E.D., any emergent associated injuries should have had appropriate first aid, including control of any bleeding, establishment of an airway and a reliable intravenous infusion line, application of an adequate temporary dressing, insertion of an indwelling urinary catheter, and administration of analgesics as indicated.

AIRWAY AND PULMONARY PROBLEMS

AXIOM

THE LUNGS ARE ALMOST NEVER DAMAGED BY HEAT FROM A FIRE.

Even when there is evidence of severe flame burns around the face, nose and perioral region, it is extremely unusual for the thermal injury to extend below the vocal cords. The pulmonary problems caused by burns are more commonly due to smoke inhalation with resultant chemical pneumonitis or to asphyxiation due to the formation of carboxyhemoglobin from the inhaled carbon monoxide. In some instances, a comparatively minor skin burn may be associated with severe damage to the lungs, particularly if the burn occurred in a closed space. Many patients may seem to improve rapidly when they are first removed from the site of the noxious fumes. The initial improvement, however, may be only transient and 8 to 12 hours later a severe chemical pneumonitis may become evident. Patients who cough up carbonaceous material should be observed with particular care since this is evidence of severe smoke inhalation. Large doses of steroids are helpful and blood gases should be monitored closely in these patients. If there is any evidence of inadequate oxygenation or ventilation, respiratory support should be given.

AXIOM

PERFORMANCE OF AN EMERGENCY TRACHE-OSTOMY ON A PATIENT WITH MODERATE TO SEVERE DYSPNEA FOLLOWING A SEVERE FLAME BURN IS CONTRAINDICATED.

Initially the severely burned patient with dyspnea may appear to have an airway problem, but he is much more likely to be suffering from carbon monoxide poisoning which can usually be treated with high concentrations of maximally humidified oxygen. In some instances ventilatory assistance through an endotracheal tube for 12 to 24 hours may be required.

AXIOM

TRACHEOSTOMY SHOULD BE AVOIDED, IF AT ALL POSSIBLE, IN BURNED PATIENTS, PARTICU-LARLY SMALL CHILDREN.

The acute management of severe respiratory distress is very adequately conducted with an endotracheal tube, but prolonged ventilatory support is better provided with a tracheostomy. If the severity of the skin burn is relatively minor and respiratory distress is a major problem, a tracheostomy is appropriate; however, in severe burns, a tracheostomy should be avoided because of

the high incidence of pneumonia and its poor prognosis in such critically ill patients. When it is obvious that several weeks of respiratory support will be needed, a tracheostomy is performed and precautions are carefully observed to minimize contamination of the airway and hopefully avoid severe pneumonia.

FLUIDS AND ELECTROLYTES

AXIOM

INTRAVENOUS FLUIDS SHOULD BE STARTED PROMPTLY IN ALL PATIENTS WITH SEVERE BURNS.

In the United States there has been a tendency to give large volumes of isotonic fluids during the initial resuscitation. Although this may correct or prevent the severe hypovolemia that might otherwise develop, it can greatly increase the edema at the burn site. Since the sodium appears to be the primary factor in effective resuscitation, several burn experts have begun to use hyperosmolar solutions to prevent the excessive formation of edema fluid. Fox et al. feel that the most effective solution for resuscitation of the burn patient is one that contains 225 mEq of sodium and 160 mEq of chloride per liter.[3] A portion of the sodium should be provided by sodium bicarbonate to combat the acidosis that is frequently present in the severely burned patient.

AXIOM

THE AMOUNT OF FLUID GIVEN TO A SE-VERELY BURNED PATIENT MUST BE INDIVID-UALIZED.

The classical Evans formula (Table 2) for calculating fluid requirements in burned patients, introduced over two decades ago,[4] is still an effective approach to the prevention of burn shock. The major deterrent to using the Evans formula at present is the

TABLE 2. FORMULAS FOR CALCULATING FLUID REQUIREMENTS

Evans formula

Day 1   % Burn $\times$ body weight (kg) $\times$ 1 = ml colloid
        % Burn $\times$ body weight (kg) $\times$ 1 = ml 5% D/N.S. $\Big\}$ 1/2 in first 8 hrs

        Plus maintenance fluids 2000 ml 5% D/W/day

Day 2   % Burn $\times$ body weight (kg) $\times$ .5 = ml colloid
        % Burn $\times$ body weight (kg) $\times$ .5 = ml 5% D/N.S.

        Plus maintenance fluids 2000 ml 5% D/W/day

Day 3 and thereafter—I.V. fluids as indicated
        (burns over 50% calculated as 50% burn)

Brooke Army formula

Day 1   % Burn $\times$ body weight (kg) $\times$ 1.5 = ml 5% D/N.S. $\Big\}$ 1/2 in first 8 hrs
        % Burn $\times$ body weight (kg) $\times$ .5 = ml   colloid*

        Plus maintenance fluids 2000 ml 5% D/W/day

Day 2   % Burn $\times$ body weight (kg) $\times$ .75 = ml 5% D/N.S.
        % Burn $\times$ body weight (kg) $\times$ .25 = ml colloid

        Plus maintenance fluids 2000 ml 5% D/W/day

* Because colloid is now considered ineffective during the first 24 hours after burn, some authors advocate eliminating colloid from the Brooke Formula.[4]

Children's Hospital of Michigan formula

Day 1   % Burn $\times$ body weight (kg) $\times$ 2 = ml 5% D/L.R. (2/3 in first 8 hrs)
        Plus maintenance fluids 1500 ml 5% D/L.R./m^2/day

        % Burn 40-60%, add 50 mEq NaHCO$_3$ to each liter of fluid and reduce rate by 10%

        % Burn over 60%, add $\Big\{$ 40 mEq NaHCO$_3$ to each liter of fluid
                          50 mEq NaCl (12.5 ml of 15% NaCl) to each liter of fluid.
                          Slow rate by 20%

Day 2   Same fluids—but for burns over 40% with hyperosmolar solutions in use, monitor electrolytes at 18-24-30-36 hours and q4 hours thereafter. Stop hyperosmolar solution when serum sodium rises to or above 150 mEq or serum osmolarity exceeds 350 millimoles. Resume 5% D/L.R. at original rate.

Day 3 and thereafter—5% D/L.R. at a rate sufficient to maintain urinary output of 40 ml/m^2/hr.

---

difficulty in obtaining adequate quantities of plasma and the risk of hepatitis even with carefully screened fresh plasma.

It is absolutely essential to maintain an awareness that formulas are only guides to therapy. In all severe burns, careful monitoring of the patient's vital signs, urine output, electrolytes, hemoglobin and hematocrit levels and weight are far more important guides to treatment.

Numerous modifications of the Evans formula have been introduced; the most popular is the Brooke Army formula[4] which uses less colloid and more saline than the Evans formula (Table 2). The Brooke Army formula demonstrated that burn patients could be resuscitated with less colloid and that, in the event of a major catastrophe, the locally available colloid stores could be stretched further in the management of a large number of patients.

Moyer et al. in St. Louis went even further and demonstrated that severely burned patients could be resuscitated without the use of any colloid, employing only a balanced electrolyte solution.[5] It is generally recommended that blood should never be given to the burn patient during the first 24 to 48 hours unless there is a significant preexisting anemia, in which case blood should be administered as packed cells through a separate intravenous line.

There are, however, many physicians who still believe strongly that colloids should be employed in the prevention or treatment of burn shock. If colloid is used, plasma is preferred. It has been shown that during the first 24 hours serum albumin is not retained in the vascular system of the burn patient, but is rapidly lost into the injured tissue. Sequestration of albumin in these tissues may then result in increased fibrosis and scarring as healing occurs.

In the department of surgery at Wayne State University there are two burn units—the pediatric burn unit at the Children's Hospital of Michigan and the adult burn unit at Detroit General Hospital—each having a different approach to initial fluid resuscitation.

At Detroit General Hospital the severely burned adult is given 1000 to 2000 ml of 5% glucose in saline or Ringer's lactate immediately. Subsequent fluid administration is based on the patient's hourly urine output, attempting to maintain a urine flow of 30 to 50 ml/hr if the urine is clear. If the patient has hemoglobinuria the output should be increased to 100 to 150 ml/hr until the urine is clear again.

The Children's Hospital resuscitation program using 5% D/L.R. has been effective in managing burns up to 35 to 40%. For burns over 40%, 50 mEq of sodium bicarbonate are added to each liter of fluid. For burns of 60% or greater, 40 mEq of sodium bicarbonate and 20 ml of a concentrated salt solution containing 2.5 mEq NaCl/ml are added to each liter of fluid which provides 220 mEq sodium and 158 mEq chloride, approximating the ideal resuscitation fluid advocated by Fox.[3]

The rapid shift of water and sodium from the vascular compartment to the interstitial space generally declines rather abruptly approximately 24 to 36 hours postburn. When using hyperosmolar solutions, it is essential to monitor serum electrolytes at 4- to 6-hour intervals to avoid a sudden severe hypernatremia. If an abrupt rise in the serum sodium level is noted, the concentrated salt solutions are discontinued, and the patient is maintained thereafter on 5% dextrose in lactated Ringer's solution.

Unlike the adult patient, an average output of X amount of urine per hour is not appropriate in children because of the wide range of weights of the patients. A convenient guide to urine output in children is 40 ml/m²/hr, a figure that incidentally is also appropriate for adults.

AXIOM

SEVERELY BURNED PATIENTS, PARTICULARLY CHILDREN, SHOULD NOT BE PERMITTED TO TAKE ORAL FLUIDS AS DESIRED DURING THE FIRST 24 TO 48 HOURS.

The severe hypovolemia that develops following extensive burn injuries often results in the patient being excessively thirsty and begging for water and other liquids to drink. In the ensuing hours when ileus develops, he is likely to vomit back all or most of the fluids taken. The hazard of aspiration in such patients, who are partially and sometimes completely immobilized, poses a serious threat to their lives. The incidence of nausea and vomiting following trauma is especially great in small children, and oral intake should be withheld until normal function of the gastrointestinal tract has been demonstrated. Furthermore, an excessive intake of water may result in a severe dilutional hyponatremia and water intoxication.

PAIN RELIEF

PITFALL

NARCOTICS ARE SOMETIMES ROUTINELY ADMINISTERED TO BURNED PATIENTS TO RELIEVE PAIN.

One of the primary duties of the physician is the relief of pain. He must be careful, however, not to administer excessive amounts of narcotic agents. There is a tendency to give narcotics immediately following a burn injury without first carefully evaluating the degree of suffering. In many burn injuries, especially third degree, the injured area is anesthetic; if the patient is not in obvious pain, such medication should be withheld. It is also important to inquire as to whether or not the patient received pain medication earlier at the site of the injury or at another institution. In some instances, the patient may have received an adequate dose of analgesic but, because of his failing circulation, the drug has not been absorbed from its intramuscular injection site; rather than an additional dose of narcotic, such a patient needs rapid expansion of his reduced blood volume.

In the burn patient there is frequently a strong element of apprehension in addition to the pain, and morphine is the most efficacious drug for relief of both pain and associated fear and anxiety. This is given in a dose of 0.1 mg/lb up to a maximal dose of 15 mg.

A simple and frequently overlooked method for relieving burn pain is the use of cold applications or cold immersion for burns of the extremities.

PITFALL

USING WATER OR SALINE THAT IS EXCESSIVELY COLD TO TRY TO RELIEVE BURN PAIN MAY CAUSE MORE DISCOMFORT THAN THE BURN ITSELF.

Since the patient's ability to maintain his normal body temperature is compromised by the burn injury, excessive cooling can do more harm than good. Water at approximately 55 F can effectively relieve pain, does not itself cause discomfort and is not apt to produce severe hypothermia. In general, cool applications can effectively relieve burn pain if started within one hour after injury, and continuous cool applications for a period of approximately one hour will usually result in pain relief even after the cool compresses are discontinued.

In some instances, several hours of cooling may be required.

DEBRIDEMENT. The main objective in the treatment of burns is the restoration of the integument in as little time as possible. In theory, the ideal approach to this problem would be to remove the devitalized tissue as soon as the patient's condition has stabilized and then cover the wound with skin grafts. If inadequate skin is available to cover the defect, even using a 6:1 mesh graft, the remainder of the defect can be covered with a skin substitute until the donor site is ready for reharvesting.[6]

PITFALL

EARLY DEBRIDEMENT OF BURNED SKIN MAY SACRIFICE AREAS THAT MAY STILL BE VIABLE.

At first glance, aggressive early debridement appears to be a fairly simple and direct approach. However, large volumes of blood must be transfused during the excision of extensive areas of eschar. Furthermore, it may be extremely difficult to differentiate second- and third-degree burns during the first 2 to 3 weeks. Many burns which were thought to be third degree during the first two weeks have proved later to be deep second-degree burns that epithelialized spontaneously. We have been reluctant to excise large areas of burned skin when there has been any possibility that we might be sacrificing areas that would eventually heal spontaneously. It appears wise to take advantage of all the spontaneous healing that can be achieved, especially if the burns approach 80% full-thickness loss.

Since the use of topical antibacterial agents may almost completely eradicate the bacterial breakdown and removal of dead tissue, the eschar tends to remain intact for long periods of time and must be mechanically debrided. Recently, enzymes that may assist in this debriding process have become available.[7] The major drawback to these enzymes is the absence of antibacterial properties and, although they may accomplish debridement rapidly, the patient may become severely septic. We have found that the use of the enzyme sutilains in combination with silver sulfadiazine decreases the debriding time by approximately 50% and at the same time avoids overt wound infection. A collagenase has recently become available which appears to work about as well as the sutilains. These debriding enzymes must be used very carefully because their inappropriate use may convert second-degree burns into third-degree burns.

ESCHAROTOMY

PITFALL

AN ESCHAROTOMY ON CIRCUMFERENTIAL BURNS MAY BE UNDULY DELAYED.

Circumferential third-degree burns of extremities are potentially hazardous because the inelastic eschar that forms may act as a tourniquet. As edema develops in the area of the burn, the increasing interstitial fluid pressure may occlude first venous return from and then arterial blood flow into the extremity. If this problem develops, escharotomies must immediately be made through the circumferential burn in three or four quadrants. Anesthesia is usually not necessary because most of the nerve endings will have been destroyed with the skin. The eschar is excised just deep enough to allow the edges to separate significantly. If the excision extends too deeply into the noninvolved subcutaneous tissue, troublesome bleeding may develop when the circulation is restored.

Circumferential burns of the thorax may be particularly dangerous because they cause progressively severe restriction of ventilation and tidal volume until respiratory failure develops. Escharotomies made longitudinally over the chest in at least four quarters will significantly relieve this problem. Occasionally a circumferential eschar over the abdomen may, in the presence of severe ileus, elevate the diaphragm and contribute to the development of respiratory distress.

CLEANSING, INITIAL DEBRIDEMENT AND DRESSING. For the most part burn wounds are comparatively clean when first seen. Overt contamination is seen only occasionally but may occur with an explosive flame burn or if the patient has been rolled on the ground to extinguish flames. In wounds with little or no contamination, irrigation with copious amounts of saline usually suffices to cleanse the surface. At the same time, all devitalized tissue should be debrided and blisters, even though intact, should be opened and the blister skin removed. This maneuver is essential if optimal results are to be obtained with topical agents.

If there is overt contamination and if irrigation alone does not effectively cleanse the surface, it may be gently sponged with a mild detergent soap. Since hexachlorophene is rapidly absorbed through the burned tissues in sufficient quantities to produce neurotoxic effects and convulsions,[8] preparations containing this agent should be avoided.

DRESSINGS AND TOPICAL AGENTS. There continue to be two schools of thought in regard to the manner in which burns should be dressed. Some institutions prefer the open method, in which topical ointments are applied without dressings. It has been our observation, however, that most patients, particularly children, are more comfortable with a dressing in place. The exposed burn wound is very sensitive, even to minor drafts, and patients treated in this manner are much less likely to move about properly.

For the initial dressing, any one of the commercially available topical creams or ointments may be applied directly to the wound. Burn pads consisting of 30 layers of single-ply cheesecloth are commercially available in sheets 18 × 36 inches in size. These may be readily cut to fit any particular wound and save a considerable amount of time in applying dressings. They are wrapped around extremities or layered over the trunk and held in place with snugly wrapped bias-cut stockinette.

By the fifth day after the burn, the colonization of the burn wound by coliforms, particularly Pseudomonas organisms, has usually taken place. During the early 1960s, Pseudomonas infection (which had previously been more of an annoyance than a threat) became the major cause of death in burn patients. In the middle 1960s the introduction of topical anti-infectives proved to be a valuable weapon against Pseudomonas and other organisms responsible for invasive burn wound sepsis.

The first two topical agents successfully employed were Sulfamylon, introduced by Lindberg,[9] and ½% silver nitrate soaks, introduced by Moyer.[5] Since then, additional agents have been made available, e.g. Garamycin cream, Silvadene and more recently Betadine ointment. An additional agent that can be made up in most pharmacies is ½% silver nitrate paste. Success with the various topical agents is similar; however, the enthusiasm with which the agent is used and the attention given the patient significantly influence the outcome.

Although these topical agents have greatly reduced the incidence and severity of burn sepsis, there are significant drawbacks to each. The problems associated with ½% silver nitrate soaks are primarily those of severe fluid and electrolyte disturbances and failure of the agent to penetrate to tissues below the eschar.

The main disadvantage of Sulfamylon, which is effective against Pseudomonas and a wide spectrum of bacteria, is the severe pain it causes upon application. In addition, Sulfamylon is a carbonic anhydrase inhibitor and can cause severe alkalosis.[10] Further, it has little or no effect against Candida albicans or Providencia species, an organism that has recently developed a virulent strain that has become a significant factor in burn mortality.[11]

The major drawback to Betadine is its cost and a significant amount of discomfort upon application to the burn wound. It also has an inhibiting effect on any enzymes used to debride the wound.

Garamycin cream, when originally introduced, was very effective and good results were reported. However, resistant strains of Pseudomonas have developed in patients while it was being used. Consequently, if a virulent strain should arise and the patient become septic, the use of gentamicin parenterally might be totally ineffective.

Experience with treating over 500 burn patients with silver sulfadiazine at the Children's Hospital of Michigan has led us to believe that this is the most effective topical agent available at the present time. The major advantages of silver sulfadiazine are, in addition to its excellent antibacterial properties, an almost total lack of pain and in some instances a soothing effect upon application to the burn wound, relative ease of dressing changes, a remarkable ability to prepare donor sites for reuse within 9 to 10 days following skin grafts,[12] a total lack of fluid and electrolyte problems, the ability to suppress Candida albicans, and a prolonged effectiveness which permits 24 to 36 hours between dressing changes. The cream may be applied directly to the patient or impregnated in gauze strips which may then be layered on the wound. Hypersensitivity reactions to silver sulfadiazine have not been encountered.

ANTIBIOTICS. While antibiotics may be a great help in managing many burn infections, adequate nutrition and good local wound care, with the adjunctive support of biological dressings, either homografts or xenografts, are essential to minimize the incidence and severity of sepsis.

With the use of topical ointments, it is often possible to carry a patient with fairly extensive burns through his course of therapy without resorting to the use of antibiotics. On the other hand, streptococcal invasion of the burn wound by endogenous organisms can occur rapidly in an acute burn, producing a severe streptococcal sepsis. To avoid this complication almost all patients with severe burn injuries are given intravenous penicillin or ampicillin during the first 4 to 5 days after the burn. Beyond the fifth day, the burn wound will generally be colonized by staphylococcal organisms, and by the seventh to tenth day by coliforms. Cultures should be obtained from the wound when first seen and at intervals of approximately every three days thereafter. After the fifth or sixth day, antibiotics, if used, are chosen on the basis of the cultures and sensitivity studies.

When facilities are available to quantitate bacterial populations, valuable information is made available. Bacterial counts in excess of 100,000 (10^5) organisms per square cm of burn surface or per gm of burn tissue are recognized as the level at which invasive sepsis occurs.[13,14] When such sophisticated techniques are not available, it is necessary to rely on the bacteriologist's interpretation of the severity of infection in terms of light, moderate or heavy growth. In general, heavy growth should be considered a forewarning that invasive wound sepsis is imminent and that more vigorous local care of the wound is indicated.

Blood cultures should be obtained at intervals of one week and any time that septicemia is suspected. In burn patients, a high spiking temperature or a sudden episode of hypothermia in the range of 95 to 96 F is often an indication that severe sepsis is developing. Other signs may include ileus, lethargy, coma, oliguria, polyuria, bradycardia, arrhythmias, cyanosis and shock. The septic burn patient is a major problem in management. He generally requires intensive therapy which may include fresh blood, massive steroids, cooling or warming to bring the patient's temperature back to normal, massive antibiotics and, not infrequently, respiratory support.

Pseudomonas sepsis continues to be the major problem on many burn units, but the incidence of candidiasis is increasing and overlooking or treating a Candida sepsis as a bacterial sepsis only makes matters worse. Gentamicin and carbenicillin are the most effective agents for treating Pseudomonas sepsis. The antifungal agent Fungizone (amphotericin B) has been effectively employed against yeast sepsis but must be used with great caution because of its toxicity. The most serious problem of amphotericin is permanent renal damage, if recommended doses are exceeded.

NUTRITION AND HYPERALIMENTATION (Chap. 4)

PITFALL

EXTRA PROTEIN AND CALORIES MAY NOT BE SUPPLIED TO SEVERELY BURNED PATIENTS.

It has been demonstrated that normal skin permits water to evaporate at the rate of 3 ml per square meter per hour, while water evaporates from burn-injured skin at the rate of 300 ml or more.[5] Some authors believe that the major cause of burn cachexia is a direct result of an increased caloric expenditure on the part of the body in an attempt to keep up with evaporative heat loss. However, it has also been shown that the hypermetabolic rate continues to some degree even when evaporative water loss is completely blocked.[15] Thus, burn hypercatabolism may be an overshoot of a normal physiologic response.

Due to the marked heat loss and increased metabolic rate of the severely burned patient, it is frequently necessary to administer two or three times the normal requirements of calories and proteins. Patients with less than 40% burns who are treated with closed dressings, which curtail evaporative heat losses, and are kept in a warm environment with an ambient temperature of 80 to 84, should theoretically be able to maintain adequate nutrition by oral intake alone after the fifth day. In more extensively burned patients, additional sources of nutrition are often required.

As soon as the patient's gastrointestinal tract is functioning properly, he is advanced as rapidly as tolerated to a high-protein, high-caloric diet. In most instances the use of an elemental diet administered by mouth or through a feeding tube may provide the necessary supplemental nutrition.

The psychologic aspects of the injury interfere with the appetite in many patients, and they will frequently have little or no desire to eat. Such patients, however, will ordinarily tolerate nasogastric feedings well and, even though psychologically depressed, their nutrition can be maintained with well-balanced tube feeding.

In the severely burned patient who cannot maintain adequate nutrition through his gastrointestinal tract, parenteral nutrition has made it possible to supply an additional 2,000 calories per square meter of body surface area per day. When added to the high-protein, high-caloric diets that most of these patients are able to take, these additional calories can generally maintain body weight and plasma protein concentrations quite well.

Extensive burns over 60% involving all four extremities often present serious problems in establishing a central venous catheter for parenteral nutrition. In our experience, the most crucial factor in avoiding infection with the catheter is to provide a 3-inch tunnel through the subcutaneous tissue between the site where the catheter enters the skin and the point where it enters the vein. Cutdowns on veins have been performed safely, and with little or no later infection, through burned tissue if the cathether is tunneled through 3 to 4 inches of subcutaneous tissue and then brought out and anchored. If possible, it is desirable to have the catheter exit through even a small patch of unburned skin so that it can be firmly anchored with a nylon suture. If there is no skin, the catheter is anchored with a nylon suture which is passed through the deep fascia. Several satisfactory parenteral nutrition formulas are available (Chap. 4).

PITFALL

THE BURN PATIENT'S HEMOGLOBIN SHOULD BE MAINTAINED ABOVE 12.0 GM/100 ML AND HIS PLASMA PROTEINS ABOVE 5.0 GM/100 ML.

In general if the patient's hemoglobin is maintained at 12 gm/100 ml or higher, the plasma proteins will also usually remain at relatively normal levels. Maintaining a satisfactory hemoglobin is directly related to providing adequate nutrition, including iron and vitamin supplements. With more severe burns, however, small transfusions of packed cells are often necessary to maintain a hemoglobin of at least 12 gm/100 ml. Even in the most severe burns, the circulating red cell mass is rarely decreased by more than 10% due to the thermal injury. There is, however, an increased fragility of many of the circulating red cells and within as few as 5 or 6 days there will be an accelerated rate of hemolysis, resulting in a drop of hemoglobin that can be corrected only with transfusions.

In a few severely burned patients, in spite of a maximal oral intake, good parenteral nutrition and a hemoglobin above 12 gm/100 ml, the plasma protein concentrations may fall and persist in the range of 3.5 to 4 gm/100 ml. These low protein levels are associated with poor wound healing and poor tolerance of infection. In such instances, a 50-cc ampule of 25% serum albumin is given for each 20 pounds of body weight per day up to a maximum 5 ampules per day. It has been observed that this adjunctive protein load maintains the plasma proteins and healing at satisfactory levels.

CLOSURE OF THE WOUND. Rapid permanent closure of the burn wound is the primary goal in burn therapy. When less than 20% of the body surface is available for skin grafting, permanent closure of a major full-thickness defect is a long-drawn-out process. Surgeons for years have sought a skin substitute or method to close the burn wound temporarily. Homografts partially solved this problem and, even though they were rejected, they helped buy valuable time for the severely burned patient. More recently, porcine xenografts have been demonstrated to be nearly as effective as homografts for biologic dressing.[16]

As the eschar is debrided and granulation tissue begins to take its place, homografts or xenografts protect the wound, reduce the bacterial colonization and decrease fluid and protein loss from the injured tissues. Currently, it is recommended that such grafts be employed as a temporary biologic dressing, that they be changed every 1 to 5 days, depending on their appearance, and that they not be permitted to remain on the wound beyond six days. This is particularly important with homografts, which become vascularized at about this time and subsequent removal is attended with brisk, troublesome bleeding.

With burns that are unequivocally third degree and involve less than 15% of the body surface, primary excision by the second to fourth day and immediate skin grafting give good results and save many days of hospital or outpatient treatment. Partial excision of more extensive burn may be managed in this manner when there is an adequate amount of donor skin available. MacMillin at Cincinnati Shriner's Burn Unit reports success with early radical excision of major burns and use of 6:1 mesh autografts as far as they will go. Porcine xenografts can then be used to close the remainder of the defect temporarily until the sparse autogenous donor sites have healed sufficiently to provide skin for definitive closure of the wound.

These heroic measures must not be approached lightly and the surgeon should be prepared to transfuse massive amounts of blood during the debridement. The blood loss can be roughly estimated at one unit per each square foot of eschar excised.

AXIOM

LOCAL ANESTHESIA SHOULD BE USED FOR DEBRIDEMENT OR GRAFTING WHENEVER POSSIBLE.

General anesthesia is poorly tolerated by severely burned patients and, in those patients who have very small donor areas available, it does not seem justifiable to harvest 35 to 40 square inches of skin. We have found that infiltrating these areas with 1/5% Xylocaine in saline produces adequate anesthesia and, over bony prominences such as the rib cage, elevates the skin so that excellent grafts may be obtained. The Castroviejo dermatome is a very valuable tool in harvesting skin from small donor sites and, in some instances, the scalp, if it has not been burned, provides an excellent donor site that will permit as many as 8 to 10 grafts without causing significant damage to the patient's hair follicles.

AXIOM

IN THE EXTENSIVE BURN, RESTORATION OF AN INTACT INTEGUMENT IS LIFE-SAVING AND MUST BE THE PRIMARY CONCERN.

Appearance and function are only secondary considerations in patients with severe burns. Once the skin has been replaced, problems related to sepsis are significantly diminished and reconstructive work can be accomplished electively after the scar has matured. Extensive surgery on contractures during the hypertrophic scarring phase before they have matured is a relatively useless procedure.

ASSOCIATED INJURIES. The patient with multiple trauma and severe burns continues to be a major problem in management and will almost always require a team approach. Under these circumstances, blood loss should be replaced as accurately as possible while, at the same time, the additional fluids and electrolytes needed to compensate for the losses due to the burn itself are administered. In these instances, separate I.V. lines are often necessary to keep up with both the hemorrhage and burn edema. Although the problem is much more complicated in these patients, the details of good burn care must be followed carefully. A cooperative effort on the part of all persons concerned can achieve a favorable outcome in the face of what often appears to be a hopeless situation.

Complications

The most frequent complications of burns include carbon monoxide poisoning, sepsis (which is the most important cause of death), pulmonary edema, heart failure, renal failure, gastrointestinal erosions or ulcerations, acute gastric dilatation, ileus, urinary tract infection, contractures and disfigurations. Therapy must be directed toward minimizing the problems associated with each of the potential complications, most of which may be lethal in themselves.

TABLE 3. FREQUENT ERRORS IN THE MAN-AGEMENT OF BURNS

1. Estimating rather than accurately evaluating the depth and extent of a severe burn.
2. Underestimating the extent of underlying tissue necrosis after an electrical burn.
3. Delay in administering fluids to a severely burned patient.
4. Failing to individualize fluid therapy to maintain optimal tissue perfusion and urine output.
5. Precipitously performing a tracheostomy on a burn patient if and when oxygen with mist or ventilation through an endotracheal tube would be just as effective.
6. Allowing severely burned patients, particularly children, to drink excessive amounts of fluid during the first 24 to 48 hours.
7. Using narcotics or ice-cold solutions excessively to relieve pain from large burns.
8. Delaying to perform an escharotomy on a circumferential third-degree burn.
9. Failing to provide adequate calories and protein and to maintain an adequate hemoglobin concentration in severely burned patients.
10. Excising early and unnecessarily partial-thickness burn and excising excessively late full-thickness burn.

Any of the above complications may cause death. Most common causes of death are sepsis, renal failure, heart failure, respiratory failure and other infections.

COLD INJURIES

In many instances the damage caused by excessive cold may be as devastating as that caused by severe heat. Although attention is generally focused on the injuries caused by local cooling, the effects of generalized cooling may be much more important and are more apt to be lethal.

Local Cooling

A number of conditions caused by local cooling have been described. These include chilblain, immersion foot, trench foot and frostbite.

CHILBLAIN (PERNIO). Chilblain refers to the swelling and reddish or violaceous plaques that may develop on fingers, toes or ears following repeated chronic exposure to damp cold with temperatures just above freezing. Burning, itching and tingling are prominent symptoms as the involved part warms. In some instances, the erythema and edema may go on to vesiculation and ulceration. Any underlying metabolic or vascular disorder may contribute to this problem.

Local treatment is nonspecific and consists of careful rewarming of the involved part and protection from further cold or trauma. Correction of any underlying problem such as anemia, malnutrition or hypothyroidism may accelerate healing and reduce the likelihood of injury if further exposure cannot be avoided.

IMMERSION FOOT AND TRENCH FOOT. Immersion foot refers to the inflammation and occasional gangrenous changes that occur because of prolonged immersion of the feet in water at a temperature below 50 F. Trench foot is very similar and refers to the changes that occur when the feet are wet (but not immersed) and are exposed for prolonged periods to temperatures from just above freezing to 50 F.

Treatment consists of warming the feet in water of 100 to 105 F and then carefully drying. Any ulcerations or gangrenous areas should be given local care and protected from any further cold or trauma.

FROSTBITE. The term frostbite refers to the damage caused by crystallization of tissue fluids in the skin or subcutaneous tissue by exposure to temperatures of freezing or below.

Etiology. In most instances, the individual exposed to excessive cold may not be aware of the fact that he is in danger of suffering cold injury. Failure to provide adequate protection to the face, ears and extremities is a common factor. The wind chill factor may be entirely ignored and the individual, aware that the outside temperature is only a few degrees below the freezing point, fails to take into consideration the fact that a 30-mph wind may reduce the effective temperature to well below zero. Being engaged in some variety of winter sport may be a distracting influence and the danger of impending frostbite is not recognized until a significant injury has been incurred.

Pathogenesis. There are two main theories on the pathogenesis of frostbite. (1) The vascular theory postulates that the tissue injury is indirectly caused by the cold which initially causes vasoconstriction and then later vasodilatation, edema, red cell sludging, thrombosis and then necrosis. (2) The cold theory postulates that the tissue damage is caused directly by the cold itself. It is likely, however, that both factors play a role and that the initial vasoconstriction and resultant decreased blood flow to the surface makes it much more susceptible to the direct cold injury.

Signs and Symptoms. Sudden blanching or an unusual whiteness of the skin, with a pale-glassy appearance, may be the first indication of cold injury. There is generally also an uncomfortable sensation of coldness followed by numbness which, as rewarming occurs, may be followed by tingling, stinging, burning or an aching sensation.

The severity of frostbite may be divided into degrees: first degree (frost nip), which is characterized by hyperemia and edema; second degree, which is characterized by hyperemia and blisters; third degree, involving necrosis of the skin and subcutaneous tissue; and fourth degree, involving necrosis of underlying fascia and muscle.

FIRST-DEGREE FROSTBITE (FROST NIP). At this stage, the skin following rewarming becomes mottled blue or purple and then red and swollen. The edema may persist for a week or longer and is followed by skin peeling, which may persist for many weeks or months.

SECOND-DEGREE FROSTBITE. With this degree of damage, the first-degree changes are followed by formation of multiple tiny vesicles or a single large vesicle within 12 to 24 hours of rewarming. The blisters dry and form black eschars in 1 to 3 weeks; these gradually peel away revealing underlying intact but easily injured skin. Initially the area may be anesthetic, but with rewarming tingling and burning are followed within 1 to 5 days by throbbing and aching which may be quite severe.

THIRD-DEGREE FROSTBITE. This injury involves the full thickness of the skin. The edema of the entire involved hand or foot may be very severe and blisters may be present at the periphery of the damaged tissue. In addition to the pale white waxy appearance, the areas become firm and there is no "give" to the underlying tissues with compression. The involvement is now equivalent to a third-degree burn. The thick black eschar that subsequently develops peels away very slowly over the next several weeks and reveals granulating tissue which slowly epithelializes, usually from the surrounding intact skin. Severe aching or throbbing may persist for several weeks.

FOURTH-DEGREE FROSTBITE. The destruction of tissue with this injury may extend down to and involve bone. The very edematous damaged tissue gradually develops the appearance of dry gangrene. Severe paresthesias may be present at the line of demarcation which develops between the gangrenous tissue and that which will survive. This demarcation may not be apparent for at least several weeks.

Treatment. FROST NIP. The damage is usually minor and prompt warming and subsequent protection from further exposure generally completely reverses the process. If artificial heat is not available, the area should be warmed by covering it with hands or by breathing on it.

AXIOM

AN AREA OF COLD INJURY SHOULD NEVER BE RUBBED AND MOST PARTICULARLY IT SHOULD NEVER BE RUBBED WITH SNOW OR COLD WATER.

SUPERFICIAL FROSTBITE. First-aid measures are directed toward rapid rewarming of the affected area. The involved surface should never be rubbed or massaged. Small areas may be warmed by the hands or by blowing warm breath over them. If artificial heat is available, steady warming should be carried out. Warm compresses with a temperature between 100 F and 105 F are applied until the warming has been achieved.

AXIOM

A PATIENT WITH A COLD INJURY MUST NOT SMOKE A CIGARETTE.

Smoking can cause severe vasoconstriction in the skin, causing a slower rewarming and additional tissue damage.

The blisters may be unroofed and treated with a topical burn ointment. Healing, in the absence of additional insult, occurs within 5 to 7 days. If the patient is still out of doors and further cold must be endured, the area should be padded with a soft material and further exposure carefully prevented.

DEEP FROSTBITE. Warming should be continuous with warm compresses, and large areas may benefit from the use of intravenous heparin. Rubbing or massaging the injured part is to be avoided. On warming, the skin will remain blanched if full-thickness destruction has occurred. Little or no pain is experienced and the presence of pain, purplish mottling or the occurrence of vesiculation suggests that there may be patchy survival of tissues.

The eschar that forms should be managed much as a third-degree burn. If there is no evidence of viability, the eschar and involved subcutaneous tissues may be mechanically debrided after 36 to 48 hours and split-thickness skin grafts applied. If blistering has occurred, even though sparsely, the area may be treated expectantly as a deep second-degree burn, from which re-epithelialization may occur from remnants of hair follicles and sweat glands.

The residual damage from severe frostbite or generalized cooling may result in extensive areas of gangrene or loss of fingers, toes, parts of ears and sometimes destruction of the nose. Additionally, severe persisting paresthesias or causalgia may intervene, which in some instances may be benefited by sympathectomy.

Generalized Cooling
(Total Body Hypothermia)

There are progressions of signs and symptoms and physiologic changes caused by generalized cooling. As chilling occurs, there is intense shivering which gradually abates as the individual lapses into an apathetic state. From this point on, cooling is rapid. The apathy and lethargy deepen until unconsciousness occurs. There is a glassy stare, little or no response to external stimuli and the pulse and respiration become progressively weakened and slower. The extremities become frozen and death soon follows.

If the individual is brought to aid before the extremities become frozen, active warming may permit survival. The problem is frequently complicated by cardiac irregularities and continuous monitoring is advisable.

The individual in a hypothermic state who has lost the shivering response has no mechanism for increasing the metabolic rate; he must be warmed externally since he is unable to generate any internal body heat. Warm compresses, a warming mattress or, better still, immersion in warm water at 100 to 105 F should be employed. While there has been some controversy as to the best way of warming these patients, it appears to be generally agreed that warming as rapidly as possible by the direct application of heat in the 100 to 105 range is the best therapeutic measure. Slow warming may only permit additional ischemic damage and cold applications should never be used. Smoking should not be permitted.

AXIOM

VASOCONSTRICTORS SHOULD NOT BE USED IN PATIENTS WITH HYPOTENSION DUE TO COLD.

Vasoconstrictors will interfere with rewarming and may cause severe additional tissue damage. As the temperature rises, the myocardial function will improve and the blood pressure will rise.

Other measures that may help in the treatment of the severely hypothermic patient include intravenous heparin, vasodilators and correction of severe anemias. Prolonged anticoagulation with coumadin may help to prevent thromboses in healing areas.

Summary

The essential therapeutic measures with any cold injury include rapid warming, good local wound care, use of heparin and vasodilators as needed, appropriate pain medication and correction of underlying metabolic, nutritional or vascular disorders. Trauma to the tissue or repeated exposure to the cold (particularly after rewarming) must be prevented. Smoking and other agents or drugs which may cause vasoconstriction should be strictly prohibited.

TABLE 4. FREQUENT ERRORS IN THE MANAGEMENT OF COLD INJURIES

1. Causing additional injury to frozen tissue by rubbing it or immersing it in excessively hot water in an effort to warm it rapidly.
2. Failing to adequately protect tissue which has been frozen from repeated cold or physical trauma after it has been rewarmed.
3. Allowing a patient with a cold injury to smoke or be given a vasoconstrictor drug.
4. Giving inadequate attention to the generalized or systemic effects of cooling.
5. Failing to detect and treat underlying systemic diseases such as hypothyroidism or vascular insufficiencies.

REFERENCES

1. Arts, C. P.: Therapy for burns. Drug Therapy, January 1973.
2. Lund, C. L., and Browder, N. C.: The estimation of areas of burns. Surg. Gynec. Obstet., 79:352, 1944.
3. Fox, C. L., and Stanford, J. W.: Comparative efficacy of hypo-, iso-, and hypertonic sodium solutions in experimental burn shock. Surgery, 75:71, 1974.
4. Hutcher, N., and Haynes, B. W.: The Evans formula revisited. J. Trauma, 12:453, 1972.
5. Moyer, C. A., et al.: Treatment of large burns with 0.5% silver nitrate solution. Arch. Surg., 90:812, 1965.
6. Law, E. J., and MacMillan, B. G.: Excision of acute burns with immediate meshed autografting. Proceedings American Burn Association, Fifth Annual Meeting, Dallas, 1973.
7. Mandi, I.: Collagenase. New York, Gordon and Breach, 1972.
8. Lockhart, Jean D.: How toxic is Hexachlorophene? Pediatrics, 50:229, 1972.
9. Lindberg, R. B., et al.: The successful control of burn wound sepsis. J. Trauma, 5:601, 1965.
10. Schaner, P. J., et al.: A possible ventilatory effect of carbonic anhydrase inhibition following topical sulfamylon in burned patients. Anesthesiology, 29:207, 1968.
11. Zawacki, B. E., and Pearson, H. E.: Epidemic nosocomial infection by antibiotic proof Providencia. Proceedings American Burn Association, Fifth Annual Meeting, Dallas, 1973.
12. Lloyd, J. R.: Improved management of skin graft donor sites with silver sulfadiazine dressings. Arch. Surg., 108:561, 1974.

13. Georgiade, N. G., et al.: A comparison of methods for the quantitation of bacteria in burn wounds. I. Experimental evaluation. Amer. J. Clin. Path., 53:35, 1970.
14. Georgiade, N. G., et al.: Clinical evaluation. Amer. J. Clin. Path., 53:40, 1970.
15. Zawacki, B. E., et al.: Does increased evaporative water loss cause hypermetabolism in burned patients? Ann. Surg., 171:236, 1970.
16. Rappaport, I., et al.: Early use of xenografts as a biologic dressing in burn trauma. Amer. J. Surg., 120:144, 1970.

Part 5
COMPLICATIONS OF TRAUMA

29 SEPSIS IN TRAUMA

R. F. WILSON
R. CUSHING

As surgeons have become increasingly successful in their resuscitation of severely injured patients, the incidence of sepsis and related complications has risen sharply. Currently infection, directly or indirectly, is the most frequent cause of morbidity and mortality in patients surviving for at least 48 hours after major trauma.

It is the purpose of this chapter briefly to discuss infections in injured patients from the following points: (1) factors increasing the risk of infection, (2) methods for preventing infection, (3) methods for diagnosing infection, (4) the types of treatment available, with particular attention to antibiotics, and (5) the clinical characteristics of and suggested treatment for some specific infections.

FACTORS INCREASING THE CHANCES OF INFECTION

Much of the sepsis following trauma can be prevented by careful attention to the wound, particularly during the first 4 to 6 hours after injury. Even with optimal care, however, certain factors greatly increase the likelihood of infection.[1]

Bacterial Factors

Several bacterial properties may increase their virulence or their chances of causing infection. For example, the capsule of Klebsiella and the M protein of streptococci in-hibit phagocytosis, and Escherichia coli and other gram-negative aerobic bacilli release endotoxins from their cell walls when they die. Other bacteria, such as the staphylococci, produce powerful exotoxins while living and multiplying.

The amount of wound contamination is also important; the greater the number of organisms present, the more likely is infection. Even in so-called clean wounds, positive cultures can be obtained in up to 68% of cases.[2] The infection rate in clean wounds with positive cultures was five times greater than that found in clean wounds with sterile cultures (5.4% versus 1.0%), and wounds contaminated with coagulase-positive staphylococci were infected seven times more frequently than those contaminated with other organisms.

PITFALL

FAILURE TO OBTAIN SMEARS AND CULTURES FROM CONTAMINATED WOUNDS DELAYS IDENTIFICATION OF THE INVOLVED ORGANISMS.

Impaired Host Defenses[3]

Some of the factors that may reduce the patient's resistance to infection include reduced blood flow, a decreased or abnormal phagocytosis, abnormal formation of antibody or complement, and impaired intracellular digestion.

AXIOM

BLOOD FLOW TO AN AREA OF TRAUMA
SHOULD BE MAINTAINED AT NORMAL OR
HIGHER LEVELS.

REDUCED BLOOD FLOW. Blood flow to an
injured tissue may be reduced by the
trauma itself or by previous cardiovascular
disease. Direct vascular damage may inter-
rupt or occlude blood vessels within or
leading to the damaged area. Devitalized
tissue, foreign bodies, hematomas, and
seromas not only produce an ideal culture
medium for bacteria but may also compress or occlude adjacent capillaries and
veins. Mild to moderate hypovolemia can
greatly reduce blood flow, especially to the
skin and subcutaneous tissue, long before
any drop in blood pressure is noted. If
hypotension develops blood flow is further
impaired, and if vasopressors are used effective circulation to these areas may cease.
Even without the injury, however, preexisting cardiac disease or arteriosclerosis,
particularly in diabetics, may have already
greatly reduced nutrient blood flow to
these tissues.

DECREASED INFLAMMATORY RESPONSE. The
inflammatory response, an essential part of
man's defense against bacterial invasion,
depends upon vascular and cellular changes
which may be elicited by the bacteria, their
products or the tissue injury. There is a
greatly increased blood flow to the inflamed
area and large numbers of leukocytes accumulate in the surrounding capillaries and
migrate into the involved tissue through
intercellular spaces in the capillaries and
venules. A decreased vascular inflammatory
response, unrelated to blood flow, may be
found in uremia and in patients receiving
steroids.

DECREASED OR ABNORMAL PHAGOCYTOSIS.
Both monocytes and neutrophils are capable of phagocytosis and intracellular destruction of bacteria, but it is the neutro-
phil that plays the dominant role, especially
in acute suppurative infections. Any condi-

tion which decreases the delivery of phagocytes to an area of bacterial contamination
will promote the development of infection.
Factors decreasing the delivery of phagocytes to a wound include reduced blood
flow, depressed inflammatory response, or
a decreased production of phagocytes. Decreased phagocyte production in the bone
marrow may occur in patients with neo-
plasms involving bone marrow and in those
receiving irradiation or antineoplastic drugs.
Defects in the ingestion of bacteria by
phagocytes have been found in uremia, diabetes mellitus, and certain malignancies,
especially the leukemias.

ABNORMAL ANTIBODY FORMATION OR COM-
PLEMENT. Virtually all antibodies are developed as a result of previous contact with
foreign substances or organisms referred to
as antigens. Antibodies enable the body to
eliminate the antigen more rapidly and effectively upon repeated contact.

Specific antibody directed against a mi-
croorganism can combine with its surface
antigens, resulting in a specific activation
site for complement. Complement, a col-
lective term for eleven chemically distinct
serum constituents, serves as a biologic
amplification system for the interaction between antigen and antibody. Neither complement nor specific antibody has bactericidal capabilities, but acting together they
may kill many species of gram-negative
bacteria and a few species of gram-positive
bacteria.

If the host has had no prior experience
with the organism, he will have no specific
antibody, and the rate of phagocytosis by
competent leukocytes will be considerably
reduced. In rare individuals who produce
minimal or abnormal gamma globulin, little
or no antibody is produced in response to
an antigenic stimulus, and as a consequence
phagocytosis is also impaired.

IMPAIRED INTRACELLULAR DIGESTION. After
bacteria are ingested, they usually become
confined to intracellular vacuoles called
lysosomes, which contain large numbers of
powerful hydrolytic enzymes. Although

most bacteria are destroyed by these enzymes, certain bacteria such as mycobacteria, salmonella, and Brucella often successfully resist this intracellular digestion and may remain viable for long periods of time. Recently, it was demonstrated that the leukocytes of patients with severe burns may have normal phagocytosis, but the intracellular killing is reduced.[4]

PREVENTION OF INFECTION

AXIOM

MANY WOUND INFECTIONS FOLLOWING TRAUMA CAN BE PREVENTED BY GOOD SURGICAL TECHNIQUE, EARLY THOROUGH DEBRIDEMENT OF ALL CONTAMINATED OR NECROTIC TISSUE, AND COMPLETE DRAINAGE OF ANY COLLECTIONS OF BLOOD OR OTHER FLUID.

Although much attention has been given to antibiotics, strict adherence to the surgical principles of good wound care, maintenance of optimal tissue perfusion and proper immunization against tetanus are by far the most effective means for preventing infection following trauma.

PITFALL

TOO MUCH RELIANCE ON PROPHYLACTIC ANTIBIOTICS TO PREVENT INFECTION MAY PRODUCE AN OPPOSITE RESULT.

One of the most frequently employed and yet least well understood efforts to prevent infection is the administration of so-called prophylactic antibiotics. By this we mean the use of antimicrobial drugs in patients who have no apparent infection and in whom there is little or no contamination at the site of surgery or injury. Although prophylactic antibiotics are frequently used, they have greater potential for harm than benefit in otherwise healthy patients in whom the risk of infection is small and the consequences of infection are not grave.

In spite of several well-controlled double-blind prospective studies on the value of prophylactic antibiotics in certain types of elective surgery,[5,6,7] relatively little is known of their value in injured patients. It might be suspected, however, that antibiotics might be even more beneficial following trauma; these patients are generally much more susceptible to infection than the general hospital population, particularly if they have suffered prolonged hypotension.

AXIOM

ANTIBIOTIC THERAPY SHOULD NOT BE DELAYED WHEN ITS USE IS CLINICALLY INDICATED.

In injured patients, particularly those with intra-abdominal wounds, the amount of contamination present may not be apparent for at least several hours. Yet it is clear that the sooner antibiotics are started, the more effective they are apt to be. For example, Altemeier has shown that, if antibiotics are to be given for abdominal injuries, they are more effective when begun preoperatively than intraoperatively or postoperatively.[8]

For most surgeons, the use of antibiotics soon after injury seems reasonable in patients with open fractures, serious burns, wounds which are heavily contaminated or have a poor blood supply, and injuries which require insertion of a large prosthesis. Although a sterile nonreactive prosthesis, e.g. a vascular graft or intramedullary nail, may not greatly increase the likelihood of infection, if it does become infected the results may be disastrous. Some physicians feel that prophylactic antibiotics may also be justified following serious injuries in certain infection-prone individuals, e.g. those taking steroids or immunosuppressive drugs and those with severe malnutrition, uremia, diabetes, anemia, or malignancies. However, broad antibacterial coverage may lead to overgrowth of relatively antibiotic-resistant organisms which are potential pathogens.

DIAGNOSIS OF ESTABLISHED INFECTIONS

Diagnosis involves finding the source and extent of the sepsis and determining the organisms involved. Although the diagnosis of most surgical infections is usually relatively easy, deep-seated wound sepsis and abscesses of the liver or retroperitoneal or subphrenic spaces may be extremely difficult to identify.

AXIOM

SEVERE INFECTIONS MAY SOMETIMES DEVELOP WITHOUT PAIN, FEVER OR LEUKOCYTOSIS.

When steroids or antineoplastic drugs are used, large abscesses may be present with little or no fever, tenderness, or leukocytosis. In overwhelming infections developing in the face of antibiotic therapy, particularly in debilitated patients, the only evidence of infection may be a shift in the differential white blood count to the left (i.e. more band or immature forms) with little or no change in the total white blood count.

History

The most frequent symptoms of infection include chills and fever, pain, cough, dysuria, and night sweats. The past history may be very helpful, particularly if it includes infections which tend to recur or illnesses which might reduce the patient host defenses.

CHILLS AND FEVER. Although fever is one of the classic signs or symptoms of infection, significant sepsis can occur without fever; indeed, some of the worst infections, especially those caused by gram-negative organisms, may be associated with hypothermia. Severe tooth-chattering chills are of some diagnostic help because they are often associated with lobar pneumonia, acute pyelonephritis, cholangitis, or large abscesses. Temperatures above 105 or 106

F often indicate a neurologic or metabolic problem in addition to or complicating the sepsis.

AXIOM

TEMPERATURES SHOULD BE TAKEN FREQUENTLY, PARTICULARLY IN THE EARLY EVENING, IN PATIENTS WHO MAY DEVELOP INFECTIONS.

Initially many infections, particularly if the patient is receiving antibiotics, may cause only mild temporary temperature elevations which may be missed unless the temperature is taken at least every four hours. If the patient has any fever it is most apt to be present in the late afternoon and early evening, and special efforts should be made to take the temperature at least once or twice during that time. In patients who are stuporous or mouth breathers, the temperature must be obtained rectally.

PAIN. Pain is usually well localized to the site of the infection if somatic nerves are involved. Pain sensation from intra-abdominal infection, however, often is carried by splanchnic nerves, which tend to produce only vague, poorly localized "visceral" symptoms that are not infrequently referred to another area. The tenderness from intra-abdominal collections of pus is usually better localized than the pain and may be of great diagnostic value.

COUGH. A new or increased cough in a septic patient generally indicates a tracheobronchial or pulmonary infection of some type, particularly if it is productive of copious or purulent sputum. Copious amounts of foul sputum are usually associated with lung abscess or bronchiectasis. If the cough is associated with sharp chest pain, this generally indicates some pleuritic inflammation.

DYSURIA. Acute cystitis is characterized by frequency of urination, dysuria, and urgency. Such symptoms are not uncommon in injured patients who have had a urinary catheter for more than two or three days.

NIGHT SWEATS. Excessive or unusual sweating at night may be the only or earliest sign of mild, deep-seated or chronic infection. Unfortunately, this sign is non-specific and frequently occurs in patients without sepsis.

Physical Examination

The classic signs of inflammation are pain, redness, heat, and swelling. If, in addition, the involved area is indurated with softness or fluctuation in its center, this is strongly indicative of an abscess. Swelling of the lower leg, especially at the calf, may indicate thrombophlebitis or phlebothrombosis. Rales in the lung may be associated with pneumonia, atelectasis, or congestion. Flank tenderness may indicate infection in the kidney or subphrenic space. A pelvic abscess is often first noted as an area of tenderness and induration on rectal examination.

PITFALL

IF DAILY RECTAL EXAMINATIONS ARE NOT PERFORMED ON PATIENTS WHO MAY DEVELOP A PELVIC ABSCESS, SEVERE SYSTEMIC TOXICITY MAY DEVELOP BEFORE THE DIAGNOSIS IS MADE.

The anatomic location of a lesion may provide valuable clues concerning the probable etiologic agent. For example, most wound infections are caused by staphylococci or a mixed bacterial flora and rapidly spreading subcutaneous cellulitis and lymphagitis often result from infection by Streptococcus pyogenes. Recently, increasing numbers of anaerobic and gram-negative aerobic bacteria have been cultured from infections following trauma, particularly when the abdomen is involved. If the colon is injured, Bacteroides species are usually involved; however, since these are anaerobic organisms, they are difficult to culture and frequently missed.

X-rays

Increased space or free air behind the trachea in the neck is strongly suggestive of upper mediastinal sepsis. The plain chest x-ray is the most accurate method for diagnosing virtually all intrathoracic infections except bronchitis and bronchiectasis. An elevated diaphragm, especially with an abnormal air-fluid level beneath it, is almost diagnostic of a subphrenic abscess. Loss of the psoas shadow on one side may indicate retroperitoneal infection or irritation on that side. Air in the fascial planes of an extremity or the abdominal wall may indicate infection with Clostridia or other gas-forming organisms.

Radioisotopes may be used to detect collections larger than 2 cm in diameter in intra-abdominal organs. This technique may be especially valuable when a liver abscess is suspected; a filling defect in the liver under such circumstances may be virtually diagnostic. Gallium-labeled citrate may also be useful in localizing abscesses.[9]

Laboratory Studies

The presence of a bacterial infection is often reflected by an elevated white blood cell (W.B.C.) count with an increased percentage of polymorphonuclear leukocytes (P.M.N.), especially if there is a "shift to the left" (an increased number of the immature band or stab forms).

PITFALL

IF SMEARS AND CULTURES ARE NOT OBTAINED BEFORE ANTIBIOTIC THERAPY IS STARTED, A PRECISE BACTERIOLOGIC DIAGNOSIS MAY BE DELAYED OR IMPOSSIBLE.

Whenever possible, pus or exudate from an infected or contaminated area should be smeared and cultured prior to beginning antibiotic therapy. The earlier the smears and cultures are obtained, the sooner the physician will have accurate information as to the antibiotics to use. All too often the simple approach of obtaining and reading a gram-stained smear of pus or exudate is ignored, thereby losing potentially invaluable information regarding the etiologic agent. Not infrequently, moreover, various factors or technical errors may cause either no organisms or the wrong organisms to grow out on culture; under such circumstances, the information obtained from examination of the initial smear may be especially valuable.

Whenever possible, both aerobic and anaerobic cultures should be made of all infected or contaminated material. Anaerobic cultures must be taken with the same precautions as arterial blood gases and then placed immediately into tubes containing carbon dioxide and no oxygen. The material should then be placed into appropriate media and incubated as soon as possible. Culture tubes or swabs that are allowed to dry out or are kept at room temperature for more than a few hours often yield inconclusive or deceptive results, particularly when mixed infections are present. When rapid information is desired, a direct smear of the infected material onto blood agar plates will often yield characteristic colonies within a few hours.

In patients with septicemia and chills, several blood cultures should be obtained at intervals of at least 20 to 30 minutes because one or more cultures are often negative, and a single positive blood culture may be due to a contaminant. Diurnal variations in temperature are probably related primarily to steroid production by the body rather than to organisms in the blood. Chills, however, are often due to a bacteremia and thus blood cultures drawn while they are occurring are more likely to be positive.

If the patient has been receiving antibiotics but continues to have evidence of sepsis and the cultures keep showing "no growth" or "normal flora," a special effort should be made to culture out anaerobic organisms.

AXIOM

THE LOCATION AND EXTENT OF AN INFECTION AND THE BACTERIA INVOLVED MAY BE MASKED WHILE THE PATIENT IS RECEIVING ANTIBIOTICS.

In some instances antibiotics cannot control the infection but they will mask its signs and make it extremely difficult to locate the infection or culture out the responsible organisms. If the infection is not controlled after one or more changes of antibiotics or if the location of the sepsis cannot be definitely determined, it may be advisable to stop the antibiotics. After 24 to 48 hours of discontinuing these agents, cultures are more apt to be positive and the abscess or site of infection may declare itself. The decision to stop antibiotics under these circumstances must be individualized, however, because the patient's infection may get considerably worse if the antibiotics are discontinued. In some instances, the fever will disappear after the antibiotics have been discontinued. If the fever does not reappear in 48 to 72 hours, it can generally be assumed that the patient had antibiotic or drug fever.

Biopsy of the lesion in granulomatous infections may provide valuable information in establishing the definitive diagnosis. Utilization of the fluorescent antibody technique for identifying organisms in tissue sections has also added significantly to the value of biopsy. Culture of biopsy material for fungi and acid-fast organisms is necessary and must be done on nonformalinized tissue.

TREATMENT OF INFECTIONS

Surgical

AXIOM

MOST INFECTIONS FOLLOWING TRAUMA CAN BE TREATED SUCCESSFULLY BY THOROUGH DEBRIDEMENT OF ALL CONTAMINATED OR NECROTIC TISSUE AND COMPLETE DRAINAGE OR REMOVAL OF ALL COLLECTIONS OF PUS, BLOOD, AND OTHER FLUID.

The optimal treatment of infections varies with the location of the infection, the amount of cellulitis, the duration of the infection, and the presence of complicating diseases. The most effective method of treating established localized collections of pus is incision and complete drainage. Surgical drainage not only removes bacteria, dead leukocytes, and necrotic tissue, it also permits access of new phagocytes, antibodies, complement, and antibiotics to the remaining bacteria.

The incision into an abscess should be located so that the drainage is as dependent as possible. If the abscess is deep seated, it is important to keep the drainage tract open with soft rubber (Penrose) drains, sumps, or catheters. The abscess cavity may also be irrigated periodically with saline or antibiotic solutions to improve drainage and help control the local infection.

AXIOM

AN ABSCESS CAVITY WHICH CONTINUES TO DRAIN LARGE QUANTITIES OF PUS OR FLUID FOR SEVERAL DAYS AFTER SURGICAL INCISION IS INADEQUATELY DRAINED.

If the amount of drainage from an abdominal abscess exceeds 100 to 200 ml/day for several days, it can usually be assumed either that the abscess is inadequately drained or that a fistula from the gastrointestinal or urinary tract is emptying into the abscess. If an abscess is adequately incised, it should drain only a small amount of serous fluid produced as a reaction to the drains or catheters. If the initial drainage fluid is extremely malodorous there is a strong possibility that anaerobic organisms are present, and if the drainage continues to be malodorous the incision was probably inadequate.

Abdominal incisions to drain intra-abdominal abscesses or resect contaminated or necrotic tissue should be only partially closed. The peritoneum and fascia may be sutured together but the skin and subcutaneous tissue should be left open for four or more days until a good granulating

base is obtained and there is no longer a threat of infection.

Chemotherapy and Antibiotic Therapy

Most infections in injured patients are prevented or managed best by good surgical technique and early drainage or debridement of all pus or necrotic tissue; antibiotics, under such circumstances, are usually of only secondary importance. However, if a diffuse cellulitis develops, antibiotics may be extremely important.

AXIOM

ONCE TREATMENT IS BEGUN WITH A CAREFULLY SELECTED ANTIBIOTIC, IT SHOULD BE CONTINUED FOR AT LEAST 48 TO 72 HOURS BEFORE EMPIRICALLY ADDING OR CHANGING TO ANOTHER AGENT.

If the systemic signs and symptoms of infection fail to recede within this period of time, this usually indicates a resistant organism or the development of an abscess or metastatic infection. Notable exceptions are staphylococcal and Pseudomonas endocarditis which may show no clinical response for more than 7 to 10 days in spite of treatment with appropriate agents.

SELECTION OF ANTIBIOTIC AGENT

PITFALL

IF A BROAD-SPECTRUM ANTIBIOTIC IS USED WHEN ONE OF A LIMITED SPECTRUM MIGHT BE ADEQUATE, THE RISK OF SUPERINFECTION IS INCREASED.

Whenever possible, only one or, at the most, two antibiotics should be used at a time. In addition, the antibiotic should not have a spectrum extending beyond that necessary to control the organisms involved. "Shotgun" therapy with three or more broad-spectrum antibiotics is to be discouraged, except rarely in the presence of unusual life-threatening infections in which the involved microorganisms and their sensitivities are unknown.

Some of the factors that may help in deciding on the proper choice of antibiotics include the location of the infection, the culture and sensitivity reports, the severity of the infection, the status of the organ systems that may be damaged by antibiotics, and the toxicity and side effects of the available antibiotics.

Location of the Infection. WOUND INFECTIONS. Many wound infections developing outside the hospital in patients who have had no antibiotic therapy are caused by penicillin-sensitive staphylococci and streptococci. The staphylococci causing wound infections in the hospital, however, are generally coagulase-positive penicillinase-producing organisms which are resistant to penicillin but may be responsive to methicillin, oxacillin, and other synthetic penicillins. If the patient is allergic to penicillin, drugs such as erythromycin, lincomycin, or clindamycin, which are relatively nontoxic, may be used effectively. The drug of choice for life-threatening staphylococcal infection in the patient with anaphylactic penicillin allergy is vancomycin.[10]

Recently more and more of the wound infections developing in the hospital, particularly in patients who have intraabdominal injury or have been receiving broad-spectrum antibiotics, are caused by one or more gram-negative bacilli. For life-threatening gram-negative infections or those caused by Pseudomonas, gentamicin is the drug of choice. For less severe infections caused by E. coli, Enterobacter or Klebsiella, drugs such as kanamycin, cephalothin, or tetracycline are often effective.

PULMONARY INFECTIONS. A wide variety of organisms may cause pulmonary infections after trauma, and a gram stain of the sputum is essential. If the patient has not been receiving antibiotics, gram-positive diplococci (pneumococci) and gram-positive cocci in chains (streptococci) are usually sensitive to penicillin. Gram-positive cocci in clusters (staphylococci) may be

treated with cephalosporins or penicillinase-resistant synthetic penicillins such as methicillin. Gram-negative cocci associated with mild to moderate acute infections may be treated with kanamycin, cephalosporins or tetracycline. For severe gram-negative infections developing after antibiotic therapy and those caused by Pseudomonas, a frequent invader in patients requiring prolonged respirator assistance, gentamicin with or without carbenicillin is the drug of choice.

Pulmonary abscesses due to aspiration are generally caused initially by aerobic gram-positive cocci and mouth anaerobes, including the fusospirochetes, which are usually quite sensitive to penicillin. The few which do not respond to penicillin will often improve with clindamycin. Gram-negative organisms may also become involved and therapy with gentamicin, kanamycin, or tetracycline is often required to effect an adequate clinical response.

PERITONITIS. The organisms most likely to cause intraperitoneal infections are the family of Enterobacteriaceae (including Escherichia, Klebsiella, Enterobacter and Proteus species), Pseudomonas species, streptococci and anaerobic organisms, particularly Bacteroides species. Although Bacteroides species are involved in most infections following trauma to the colon, this may not be reflected in the culture reports because these anaerobic organisms are so difficult to culture. For mild peritoneal contamination not involving the lower gastrointestinal tract, we prefer penicillin and tetracycline. For severe peritoneal contamination, especially if it involves the colon or distal small bowel, we prefer gentamicin and clindamycin. With lesions of the small bowel, particularly those involving jejunum or proximal ileum, it might be wise to add penicillin to cover the enterococci that are also present in significant quantity.

URINARY-TRACT INFECTIONS. Although sulfa preparations are the most frequently used drugs for mild to moderate urinary-tract infections in ambulatory patients, they are seldom used in patients with severe infections and are of no value if the patient is unable to take oral medications. Ampicillin, tetracycline, and colistin may be effective against the gram-negative organisms that are usually involved, but gentamicin is the antibiotic of choice for the most severe kidney infections; this drug is especially effective if the urine is alkaline.

Bacterial cystitis may often be prevented by irrigating the bladder with dilute Neosporin solutions containing 40 mg neomycin and 20 mg polymyxin B per liter of fluid with an infusion rate of 40 ml/hr. Some physicians, however, feel that irrigation with antibiotic solutions should be avoided and that a closed urinary drainage system is the only effective method for preventing catheter cystitis. If fungal infection in the bladder is present, 20 mg of amphotericin B may be added to each liter of sterile water for use as an irrigating fluid. Since this agent is broken down by light, the I.V. bottle should be covered with a brown paper bag.

Culture and Sensitivity Reports. Although clinical experience and a sound knowledge of bacteriology may be invaluable in predicting the organisms likely to be involved in a particular infection, culture and sensitivity reports still form the foundation upon which most antibiotic therapy is based. However, the initial organisms cultured might not be those responsible for the patient's sepsis, or superinfection with other organisms may have developed.

AXIOM

ALTHOUGH CULTURE AND SENSITIVITY REPORTS ARE USUALLY IMPORTANT GUIDES TO ANTIBIOTIC THERAPY, THE INFORMATION THEY PROVIDE IS OCCASIONALLY DECEPTIVE OR FALSE.

Culture and sensitivity reports cannot be completely relied upon. It is not uncommon for the organisms that are causing the infection either not to grow in culture or else to be overgrown by less important but faster-growing bacteria; this is especially true for some of the gram-negative organisms, particularly if the patient has already had antibiotic therapy.

Severity of the Infections. The milder the infection, the more important and safer it is to use single and less toxic antibiotics, preferably by the oral route. In more severe infections, larger doses of parenteral antibiotics are likely to be needed. For the worst infections, these antibiotics should usually be given intravenously to get the highest possible blood and tissue levels. It must also be remembered that many of the most severe infections, especially those acquired in the hospital, are caused by organisms which are often quite resistant to the usual antibiotics.

Status of Various Organ Systems. The main organ systems to be evaluated before giving antibiotics are the kidneys, liver and bone marrow. Some of the laboratory tests that should be done before starting antibiotic therapy include a CBC, platelet count, BUN, creatinine, urinalysis, SGOT, and serum protein determinations. If antibiotics known to be damaging to these systems must be given to the patient, the appropriate laboratory tests must be repeated frequently, usually at least once or twice a week.

The antimicrobial drugs that should be avoided where possible with various types of organ impairment include chloramphenicol if there is bone marrow disease and aminoglycosides if there is renal disease.

If agents such as the aminoglycosides (kanamycin, gentamicin or streptomycin), which are excreted by the kidneys, must be used in spite of renal dysfunction, the interval between doses has to be increased substantially to prevent the serum levels of the antibiotics from rising to toxic levels. As a general rule of thumb, a third of the usual daily dose can be given at intervals equal to eight times the serum creatinine levels. Thus an average-sized adult male with a normal serum creatinine of 1.0 mg/100 ml may be given 80 mg of gentamicin every 8 hours; however, if his serum creatinine were 6.0 mg/100 ml, that same dose should only be given at 48-hour intervals.

Toxicity of the Antibiotics. The least toxic drug that may be effective should be used. Chloromycetin, for example, because of its possible effects on the bone marrow, should never be given to infants and young children, except in life-threatening situations where no other effective antibiotic is available. Polymyxin, although quite effective against a number of gram-negative bacilli, including Pseudomonas, is rarely used now because of its severe toxicity, especially to the kidneys.

ADMINISTRATION OF ANTIBIOTIC AGENTS. Although oral antibiotics are often used to treat infections, especially in patients who are not hospitalized, absorption by the intestine is often unreliable or may result in relatively low blood levels of the agent. Intramuscular injections are much more effective but may be very painful, limiting the frequency and dose that a patient will tolerate.

The highest serum and tissue levels are generally achieved if the antibiotic is given intravenously. When the intravenous route is used, intermittent injection by I.V. piggyback is often preferred to continuous infusion, because it can provide much higher peak levels in the blood and tissue. Antibiotics which are very stable in solution can be given by continuous I.V. infusion; however, agents which deteriorate rapidly after being placed in solution are best mixed fresh and infused every 4 to 6 hours by I.V. piggy-back.

MOST FREQUENTLY USED ANTIBIOTICS. The main groups of antibiotics used in acutely injured patients include: (1) penicillins, (2) cephalosporins, (3) aminoglycosides, (4) tetracyclines, (5) erythromycin, (6) lincomycins, (7) chloramphenicol, (8) polymyxins and (9) amphotericin B. The mechanisms of action, spectrum, toxicities,

and dosages of these agents should be familiar to all physicians treating injured patients and using these drugs.

Penicillins. The penicillins are bactericidal agents which act by inhibiting cell wall synthesis in growing cells, thus forming protoplasts. Without the protection of the cell wall the hyperosmotic bacteria absorb so much water that they burst. The main groups of penicillins used in injured patients include penicillin G, phenoxymethyl penicillin, ampicillin, carbenicillin and the penicillinase-resistant penicillins.

PENICILLIN G. Penicillin G is bactericidal against gram-positive cocci, gram-negative cocci, gram-positive bacilli, fusiform bacilli, and some gram-negative anaerobic bacilli. In high doses it may also be effective against E. coli and Proteus mirabilis. It is ineffective against penicillinase (beta-lactamase) producing staphylococci.

Crystalline aqueous penicillin G, 600,000 units I.M. every four hours, is painful but effective in treating many pyogenic infections, especially those caused by pneumococci and aerobic streptococci. Procaine penicillin is less painful but more apt to cause allergic reactions.

Intravenous aqueous penicillin in doses of 2 to 8 million units per day is usually very effective for treating severe infections caused by sensitive organisms. Some physicians have used up to 20 to 40 million units per day; such doses, however, are rarely needed unless bacterial endocarditis supervenes. In addition, doses of penicillin exceeding 3 million units per day may greatly increase the incidence of superinfection by other organisms.[11] In the rare instances when very high sustained blood levels of penicillin may be required, probenecid (Benemid) 500 mg every 6 hours may, by reducing the renal excretion of penicillin, more than double the blood levels of penicillin and its duration of action.

Allergic reactions such as drug fever, rashes and urticaria are not infrequent and a number of fatal anaphylactic reactions have been reported. As a consequence, all patients given an I.M. injection should be watched closely for 15 minutes for any evidence of a reaction and this drug should be avoided in patients who have had an allergic reaction to it in the past.

PITFALL

IF A LARGE AMOUNT OF AQUEOUS PENICIL-LIN IS GIVEN RAPIDLY I.V., ESPECIALLY TO A CHILD, THE PATIENT MAY DEVELOP SEVERE ARRHYTHMIAS OR A CARDIAC ARREST.

When using large quantities of penicillin G, it is important to remember that it contains 1.6 mEq of potassium in each million units. In patients with renal failure, it may be wise to use sodium penicillin to decrease the chances of a dangerous hyperkalemia.

PENICILLIN V. The alpha-phenoxy penicillins, such as penicillin V, Pen-Vee, and V-Cillin, are acid stable and thus may be given orally, in doses of 250 to 500 mg every 6 hours.

AMPICILLIN. Ampicillin has a spectrum quite similar to that of penicillin G against gram-positive cocci; however, it is more effective against many strains of enterococci, most strains of Proteus mirabilis, and occasional strains of other Proteus species. It also may have some activity against H. influenzae, salmonella, shigella and E. coli. The oral dose is 0.25 to 1.0 gm every 4 to 6 hours.

CARBENICILLIN. Carbenicillin has antibacterial activity against many strains of Escherichia coli, Proteus species and Pseudomonas aeruginosa. This agent has been used with urinary-tract infections and lacks the nephrotoxicity of the aminoglycosides. It may also be effective with pneumonia, peritonitis, or wound infections; however, we use it only in combination with gentamicin for treating severe Pseudomonas infections. Since this antibiotic contains about 5 mEq of sodium per gram of drug, patients receiving high doses may have a significant load of extra sodium to handle.

For adults with urinary-tract infections, the usual dose of carbenicillin is 1 to 2 gm every 6 to 8 hours I.M. or I.V. For infections outside the urinary tract in adults without azotemia, up to 4 to 6 gm may be given I.V. every 4 to 6 hours; with oliguria, only about a quarter of this dose is given.

BETA-LACTAMASE RESISTANT PENICILLINS. Staphylococci that produce penicillinase (beta-lactamase) are resistant to penicillin G, penicillin V, ampicillin and carbenicillin. A number of synthetic penicillins which are beta-lactamase resistant, however, have been developed. These include methicillin, oxacillin, cloxacillin, dicloxacillin, and nafcillin. The usual intramuscular dose of methicillin is 1 gm every 3 to 6 hours, and the intravenous dose is 1 to 2 gm every 4 to 6 hours, depending on the severity of the infection. Since these drugs are relatively unstable, especially in an acid pH, they should be made up just prior to use and given via I.V. piggy-back.

Cephalosporins. The cephalosporins are similar to the penicillins in structure and action, and an occasional patient who is allergic to penicillin is also allergic to cephalosporins.

The cephalosporins have a moderately broad spectrum and are effective against many gram-positive cocci including the penicillin-resistant Staphylococcus aureus; they are, however, usually not active against the enterococci. These antibiotics are also effective against many gram-negative bacilli.

CEPHALOTHIN. Since cephalothin injections intramuscularly are very painful and since this drug is inactive orally, it is virtually always given by I.V. infusion. The usual dose is 0.5 to 2.0 gm by I.V. piggy-back every 4 to 6 hours. Its main side effects are allergic reactions.

CEPHALORIDINE. Cephaloridine must be given intramuscularly but is much less painful than cephalothin. Its spectrum is similar to that of cephalothin except that it is more active against susceptible anaerobic organisms. It is nephrotoxic in doses exceeding 4 gm per day and should be avoided in severely injured patients if there has been any hypotension, oliguria or renal damage.

CEPHALEXIN. Cephalexin may be given orally in doses of 1 to 4 gm per day. This allows the physician to continue cephalosporins painlessly after the I.V. infusions have been discontinued.

CEFAZOLIN. Cefazolin is a new cephalosporin which produces excellent blood levels, is not as nephrotoxic as cephaloridine, and is not painful. It probably should be used instead of cephaloridine.

Aminoglycosides. The aminoglycosides are bactericidal agents which act on the bacterial ribosomes to inhibit protein synthesis. These drugs are effective against many bacteria, particularly gram-negative bacilli; however, they all tend to have some ototoxicity and nephrotoxicity, especially if large doses are given for prolonged periods.

AXIOM

THE FREQUENCY OF AMINOGLYCOSIDE ADMINISTRATION MUST BE REDUCED IN PATIENTS WITH IMPAIRED RENAL FUNCTION.

The aminoglycosides are excreted primarily through the kidneys and, if there is any interference with renal function, the concentration of these agents in the blood may rise rapidly to levels which are toxic to the kidneys and ears. The urine output must be watched very closely, but the serum creatinine levels and the creatinine clearance are much more accurate guides.

STREPTOMYCIN. For many years, the combination of penicillin and streptomycin was popular in the treatment of injured patients, particularly after abdominal trauma. However, now streptomycin is used rather infrequently except in the treatment of tuberculosis. It is effective against only about a third of the gram-negative bacilli, susceptible bacteria rapidly develop resistance to it, and it has many side effects including vestibular nerve damage, nephro-

toxicity, drug fever, and dermatitis. If given I.V. or into a body cavity during anesthesia, it may have a curare-like effect.

Because of these problems and because there are many more effective drugs available for treating infections caused by gram-negative bacilli, streptomycin should be used almost never now unless indicated by specific sensitivity tests. The usual dosage is 0.5 gm I.M. every 6 to 12 hours.

KANAMYCIN. Kanamycin is very effective against a number of gram-negative aerobes and has been a valuable addition to our therapeutic armamentarium. It is, however, relatively ineffective against Pseudomonas, streptococci, pneumococci and anaerobes. Its main disadvantages are its potential nephrotoxicity and ototoxicity, especially in patients with renal failure. Kanamycin should generally be avoided in older patients, as they are more susceptible to these side effects, and during general anesthesia because it may occasionally cause a curare-like effect with respiratory paralysis.

Although kanamycin injections are usually quite painful, the preferred route of administration is deep intramuscular injection in doses of 10 to 15 mg/kg/day divided into 2 or 4 equal doses. Since it is dangerous to exceed a total dose of 10 to 12 gm, kanamycin is seldom given for more than 10 to 12 days. Oral kanamycin is poorly absorbed from the gastrointestinal tract and, therefore, may be used to reduce the bacterial count in preparation for bowel surgery.

GENTAMICIN. At the present time gentamicin is the most effective antibiotic against gram-negative aerobes, including Pseudomonas and Proteus species. Its greatest value is its effectiveness against serious Pseudomonas infections, especially when combined with carbenicillin. It is ineffective against most streptococci, pneumococci and anaerobes but may act against staphylococci.

The toxicity of gentamicin is similar to that of kanamycin, and both branches of the eighth cranial nerve may be involved.

However, in contrast to kanamycin, the vestibular involvement with gentamicin is generally greater. It is given intramuscularly in doses of 0.6 to 1.0 mg/kg every 8 hours, with appropriate adjustments for any renal impairment. If there is any possibility of renal damage or disease, we are careful to maintain a urine output of at least 50 ml/hr. In serious infections, doses as high as 1.0 to 1.5 mg/kg every 8 hours have been used for limited periods of time.

Tetracyclines. The tetracyclines are bacteriostatic agents which inhibit protein synthesis by blocking the transfer of amino acids from the aminoacyl RNA to polypeptides. These antimicrobials are effective against many gram-positive and gram-negative aerobic and anaerobic bacteria and for some time they were considered the drug of choice against Bacteroides species. However, some staphylococci and some pneumococci and group A beta-hemolytic streptococci are resistant. The combination of I.V. penicillin and tetracycline has for some time been a popular choice in patients with abdominal wounds. Recently, however, we have found many gram-negative bacilli and Bacteroides that are resistant to tetracycline.

These agents are relatively safe, but hepatotoxicity has been reported, particularly in pregnant women, if more than 2 gm was given I.V. daily. The dosage causing hepatotoxicity is much lower if there is impaired renal function. Other problems with the tetracyclines include an occasional rise in BUN due to their catabolic effect and permanent staining of the teeth in children.

Erythromycin. Erythromycin is a bacteriostatic agent which acts by selectively inhibiting protein synthesis. It is effective against most streptococci and many S. aureus strains. It is a relatively safe drug and its greatest usefulness lies in treating infections caused by gram-positive organisms in patients who are allergic to penicillin. However, since I.M. injections of this drug are painful, it is generally administered orally.

Lincomycin and Clindamycin. Lincomycin, which is bacteriostatic, and clindamycin, which is frequently bactericidal, inhibit protein synthesis by binding to 50s subunits of ribosomes and preventing peptide bond formation. Lincomycin and clindamycin are active against many gram-positive cocci, including most strains of S. aureus. Although lincomycin is effective against many anaerobes, clindamycin is particularly valuable, especially against Bacteroides fragilis, and is now the drug of choice for intra-abdominal anaerobic infections.

Because lincomycin tends to develop higher concentrations in the bone than most other antibiotics, it may be of special value in patients with open fractures.

Although both drugs are generally considered very safe, there have been occasional reports of mild neutropenia and slight elevations of the SGOT during or following their use. Recent reports of serious colitis following the use of these drugs must be evaluated.[12] The drugs should be discontinued immediately if diarrhea develops during their use.

Chloramphenicol. Chloramphenicol is a bacteriostatic agent which inhibits protein synthesis by interfering with assembly of amino acids in peptide synthesis. This antimicrobial is effective against many gram-positive and gram-negative aerobes, and is one of the most effective drugs against the intestinal anaerobes, including Bacteroides. Unfortunately, it may cause severe bone marrow depression. It should probably never be given to children and should seldom be used in adults except in difficult situations when no safer drug is apt to be effective.

AXIOM

CHLORAMPHENICOL SHOULD NOT BE USED IN CHILDREN BUT SHOULD BE USED IN ADULTS WITH SERIOUS INFECTIONS WHEN SENSITIVITY STUDIES SHOW THAT IT IS THE MOST EFFECTIVE DRUG.

Polymyxin B and Colistimethate. Polymyxin B and colistimethate are bactericidal agents which act as cationic detergents to increase cell membrane permeability. They also interfere with cellular oxidative phosphorylation. Unlike many other antimicrobials, the bacteria do not have to be growing or multiplying for these agents to be effective. In spite of their action against most gram-negative bacilli, except Proteus, they are so toxic that they are rarely used in acutely injured patients. They both cause severe pain at I.M. injection sites and cause frequent nephrotoxic reactions and occasional neurotoxicity.

AXIOM

POLYMYXIN B AND COLISTIMETHATE SHOULD NEVER BE GIVEN TO ACUTELY INJURED PATIENTS AND SHOULD NOT BE GIVEN LATER UNLESS ALL OTHER ANTIBIOTICS HAVE BEEN SHOWN TO BE INEFFECTIVE.

They should be avoided during general anesthesia, particularly if muscle relaxants are used, because they can cause neuromuscular blockade with respiratory paralysis if administered intraperitoneally, intrapleurally, or intravenously. Colistin is seldom used now by us except in the treatment of urinary-tract infections caused by antibiotic-resistant organisms, particularly Pseudomonas aeruginosa. Polymyxin B is used very rarely, and then only as a last resort to control Pseudomonas organisms that have become resistant to all other antibiotics.

Amphotericin B. Amphotericin B is effective against a wide variety of fungi including Histoplasma and Candida. The increasing incidence of Candida infections (moniliasis) in patients who have received multiple antibiotics or I.V. hyperalimentation over long periods of time makes this drug increasingly important. Unfortunately, this is an extremely toxic drug with many side effects including nephrotoxicity, an-

emia, fever, hepatotoxicity and phlebitis. It should be used only if the patient has a life-threatening infection which cannot be treated in any other way.

Amphotericin B must be given very cautiously, beginning with a daily dose of 5 mg and increasing by 5 mg per day until a dosage of 25 to 40 mg per day is reached. The dosage throughout is regulated according to the BUN, blood count, and liver function tests. This drug must be administered in 5% glucose in water, using 100 to 150 ml of solution to each 10 mg of drug, and the infusion should be slow (taking at least six hours). The total dosage should only rarely exceed 2 to 3 gm.

COMPLICATIONS AND SIDE EFFECTS OF ANTIBIOTIC THERAPY. The most important complications and side effects of antibiotic therapy include (1) hypersensitivity and idiosyncratic reactions, (2) toxic effects, (3) irritative effects, and (4) superinfection.

Hypersensitivity. The most frequent hypersensitivity reactions caused by various antibiotics, especially the penicillins, include skin rashes, angioneurotic edema, serum sickness, anaphylaxis.

When an alternative antibiotic agent may be equally effective, the penicillins should probably be avoided in patients who have histories of severe allergic reactions to any drugs or foods. Certainly penicillin should not be given if the patient has a history of penicillin allergy, particularly if the allergic reaction was manifested as anaphylactic shock or angioneurotic edema. In an occasional patient who has a history of mild skin rash or itching following penicillin and who has a severe life-threatening infection which is not apt to respond to other drugs, careful scratch testing with a dilute penicillin solution may be attempted. Prior to such testing, however, the physician should review the pertinent literature.[13] The testing must be done with personnel, drugs, and equipment immediately available to handle any possible reaction, including anaphylactic shock or cardiac arrest. In some instances, simultaneous administration of antihistamines may prevent or reduce mild reactions.

Whenever penicillin is given parenterally, the patient must be watched for any reaction for at least 15 to 30 minutes. If an immediate penicillin reaction occurs, the administration of any further drug must be stopped at once and, if possible, a tourniquet should be applied above the site of injection. Epinephrine, steroids, and Benadryl should then be given. The usual dose of Benadryl is 50 mg I.M., which can be repeated in 4 to 6 hours. Hydrocortisone can be given I.V. in doses of 100 to 200 mg and repeated as often as necessary. The use of penicillinase (Neutrapen) in doses of 800,000 units I.M. and repeated once or twice in the next 24 to 48 hours has been advocated by some physicians for treating reactions to injections of long-acting penicillins. However, it has no place in the management of an acute anaphylactic reaction and the resultant penicillin fragments may in themselves be antigenic. If there is evidence of anaphylaxis, 0.3 to 0.5 cc of 1:1000 epinephrine (Adrenalin) must be given subcutaneously or I.V. depending on the severity of the reaction. An I.V. should be started and measures for supporting ventilation and cardiovascular function must be immediately available at all times.

Chloramphenicol and the sulfonamides may, in addition, cause agranulocytosis or aplastic anemia. The aplastic anemia caused by chloramphenicol is especially severe and has sharply limited the use of this drug; if it is used, complete blood counts should be performed every 48 hours during treatment.

Toxic Effects. The penicillins have little or no specific organ toxicity; however, CNS effects manifested by convulsions have occurred when large doses were given to patients on cardiopulmonary bypass or in severe renal failure. Patients, especially pregnant women, given tetracycline in daily doses of 2.0 gm or more per day may develop jaundice and fatty degeneration of the liver.

In addition to the aplastic anemia which chloramphenicol can cause as an idiosyncratic effect, this drug can also produce a dose-related anemia which is manifested by a maturation arrest of erythroid precursors in bone marrow with development of cytoplasmic vacuoles. The cephalosporins have also been reported, rarely, to depress leukopoiesis.

Kanamycin, gentamicin, polymyxin, and colistin can produce renal damage, particularly in individuals with oliguria or preexisting renal disease. Streptomycin, kanamycin, and gentamicin may all produce ototoxicity when given in large doses or for a prolonged period.

Kanamycin and neomycin have a curarelike action on neuromuscular transmission and paralysis of respiration has been reported following intraperitoneal instillation of these drugs, particularly if the patient in under the influence of a general anesthetic or muscle relaxant.

Irritative Effects. The tetracyclines, chloramphenicol, erythromycin, polymyxins, and kanamycin may cause gastrointestinal irritation manifested by epigastric burning, nausea, emesis, and diarrhea, with occasional vaginitis or pruritus ani. Intravenous administration of tetracyclines and cephalosporins is frequently followed by thrombophlebitis. Photosensitivity of skin may occur with demethylchlortetracycline. Cephalothin, streptomycin, aqueous penicillins and polymyxins are very painful on I.M. injection and may cause sterile abscesses at the injection site.

Superinfection. The use of multiple antibiotics in critically ill patients for more than 1 to 2 weeks often results in superinfection by various gram-negative bacilli, particularly Pseudomonas organisms. The emergence of resistant organisms is particularly prone to occur when the patient is on a respirator or has lesions subject to continued external contaminations, such as open wounds, leg ulcers, or burns. Not infrequently vigorous antibiotic therapy may control the gram-negative superinfection only to have Candida organisms emerge and continue the sepsis.

Immunotherapy

At present, the usefulness of specific immune therapy in the practice of surgery is limited primarily to the administration of antitoxins against tetanus, rabies, and poisonous snakes (Chap. 8). Recently, there have been some reports of beneficial results from the use of anti-Pseudomonas vaccine in burned patients.[14] Polyvalent gas gangrene antitoxin is no longer used in the treatment of gas gangrene because its efficacy is questionable and it frequently causes severe allergic reactions.

Hyperbaric Oxygenation

PITFALL

EXCESSIVE RELIANCE ON HYPERBARIC OXYGENATION TO CONTROL ANAEROBIC INFECTIONS MAY REDUCE THE EFFORTS OF THE SURGEON TO PROVIDE OPTIMAL INCISION AND DRAINAGE.

Hyperbaric oxygenation should theoretically be extremely helpful in controlling infections caused by anaerobic organisms, particularly Clostridia. The clinical results, however, have often been inconclusive and, unless the facilities are readily available, the risks of moving critically ill patients probably outweigh the potential benefits. Furthermore, there may be a tendency to be less vigorous with the debridement and surgical drainage if the use of hyperbaric oxygenation is contemplated. Finally, hyperbaric oxygen may be dangerous in the hands of personnel who are not thoroughly trained and experienced.

SPECIFIC INFECTION

The signs, symptoms, and clinical course of the most frequent infections following trauma are characteristic and, in some instances, may be virtually diagnostic.

Staphylococcal Infections

The lesions produced by Staphylococcus aureus are characteristically well localized and consist of an indurated area of cellulitis which undergoes abscess formation with the development of a thick, creamy, odorless pus. Fever and leukocytosis are usually present if the infection is uncontrolled, spreading or causing septicemia. Bacteremia or septicemia may occur and can be very dangerous because of the frequency with which metastatic abscesses can develop. Treatment consists of complete surgical drainage with or without penicillinase-resistant penicillins.

Streptococcal Infection

A wide variety of streptococcal infections may be seen in surgical practice; however, since most of the infections caused by these organisms respond so well to penicillin, they are rarely a problem once they are recognized. Most of these infections are caused by Streptococcus pyogenes (group A, beta-hemolytic); however, other streptococci such as Streptococcus viridans (alpha-hemolytic), Peptostreptococcus, microaerophilic streptococcus and Streptococcus faecalis (group D enterococcus) may also be encountered.

STREPTOCOCCUS PYOGENES. The lesions caused by Streptococcus pyogenes are characterized by a rapid progression of cellulitis, lymphangitis, lymphadenitis, and extension of the inflammation along fascial planes. A thin watery pus may develop, but frank abscess formation rarely occurs. Bacteremia occurs frequently with chills, high fever, a rapid, thready pulse, and general signs of toxemia. Erysipelas, which classically appears as a superficial spreading cellulitis with indurated, raised and irregular margins, is most often caused by Streptococcus hemolyticus and is usually associated with high fever, chills, rapid pulse, and severe toxemia.

STREPTOCOCCAL GANGRENE. Streptococcal gangrene, usually caused by anaerobic streptococci, is a rapidly spreading, invasive, fascial and subcutaneous infection which may be associated with thrombosis of nutrient vessels resulting in necrosis and slough of the overlying skin. Occasionally, the patient may also develop clear, bullous lesions which may coalesce and become filled with hemorrhagic fluid. These infections usually occur in wounds of the lower extremities or abdomen. Treatment involves complete excision of the involved tissue and large doses of antibiotics, especially the penicillins.

MICROAEROPHILIC STREPTOCOCCI. Microaerophilic organisms grow best in an anaerobic environment but also can tolerate slightly aerobic conditions. Meleney's chronic burrowing ulcer, caused by microaerophilic streptococci, is characterized by chronic, slowly progressive, painful surface ulcerations and communicating subcutaneous sinus tracts with little or no systemic toxicity.

Chronic progressive cutaneous gangrene is caused by the synergistic action of microaerophilic nonhemolytic streptococci and aerobic hemolytic Staphylococcus aureus or other strains of bacteria such as Proteus. This infection is characterized by a bright-red cellulitis which widens and develops a purplish center which becomes gangrenous, followed by a progressively enlarging painful ulcer. Treatment of both infections requires radical excision of the involved tissue and systemic antibiotic therapy with penicillin or erythromycin.

Infections Caused by Gram-negative Bacilli

Gram-negative bacilli are almost invariably involved in any infection associated with injury to the gastrointestinal or genitourinary tracts. Most of these infections are polymicrobial and often involve both anaerobic and aerobic organisms. Infections caused by the gram-negative aerobes generally have a longer incubation period than those caused by staphylococci or streptococci, and tend to cause less systemic toxicity.

PITFALL

IF PHYSICIANS FAIL TO CHECK FREQUENTLY THE SENSITIVITIES OF THE BACTERIA FOUND WITHIN THEIR HOSPITALS, THEIR INITIAL ANTIBIOTIC CHOICES ARE LIKELY TO BE INCREASINGLY INCORRECT.

The gram-negative bacilli in many hospitals have become increasingly resistant to many of the most frequently used antibiotics. In a recent study at Detroit General Hospital, it was found that the antibiotic sensitivities of the E. coli, Enterobacter, and Klebsiella organisms tested were: gentamicin—84%, kanamycin—64%, cephalosporins—48%, tetracycline—45%, streptomycin—44%, Chloromycetin—34% and ampicillin—34%. Since we have tried to reserve gentamicin for severe life-threatening infections, particularly those due to Pseudomonas, we have tended to use kanamycin, cephalosporins or tetracycline for the mild to moderate infections. If there is any suspicion of renal impairment, we avoid gentamicin, kanamycin and streptomycin. Although we have rarely seen aplastic anemia in adults from the use of Chloromycetin, we avoid this drug unless it is specifically indicated because of the severity of the infections and the sensitivity of the organisms.

The antibiotic sensitivities of the Proteus species vary depending on whether they are indole-positive or indole-negative. Taken as a group, however, we found the following sensitivities on the organisms tested: gentamicin—82%, kanamycin—64%, cephalosporins—61%, ampicillin—59%, streptomycin—44%, Chloromycetin—24% and tetracycline—5%.

Pseudomonas organisms are different in several ways from other gram-negative enteric bacilli. For some time it was thought that Pseudomonas organisms were not responsible for production of any endotoxin; however, evidence to the contrary has recently been reported.[15] Since the Pseudomonas is also the only bacterium with elastase, and since it invades the small arterioles by way of the vasa vasorum, producing a homogeneous destruction of the arterioles, its infections can be diagnosed histologically. After several days or weeks of treatment with broad-spectrum antibiotics, highly resistant Pseudomonas organisms may be cultured from many parts of the body, particularly the tracheobronchial tree. In such cases it is difficult to be sure whether the Pseudomonas cultured is indeed the cause of the sepsis or whether it has only colonized the area.

Treatment of Pseudomonas infections may be extremely difficult. Any collections of pus or necrotic tissue should be drained or excised. If the lungs are involved, frequent thorough removal of pulmonary secretions with a flexible bronchoscope may be extremely helpful. Antibiotics are notoriously ineffective in obtaining complete control of well-established Pseudomonas infections. Even in vitro, these organisms are extremely resistant to most of the safer antibiotics. The sensitivities of the Pseudomonas organisms tested recently at Detroit General Hospital were: gentamicin—90%, carbenicillin—52%, streptomycin—19%, and tetracycline—4%. For the most severe Pseudomonas infections, we have had our greatest clinical success using a combination of gentamicin and large doses of carbenicillin. We have had no experience with Pseudomonas vaccines, but there have been some reports of success in patients with severe burns.[10]

Mixed Bacterial Infections
HUMAN BITE INFECTIONS

AXIOM
LACERATIONS CAUSED BY A HUMAN BITE SHOULD NOT BE SUTURED.

The human bite often causes severe mixed synergistic bacterial infections, involving oral spirochetes and other aerobic and anaerobic mouth bacteria. These infections are characterized by marked swelling and tenderness, a thick, foul-smelling purulent exudate, and necrosis of the underlying areolar and fibrous tissues. Such wounds should be thoroughly debrided and left open, hot soaks should be applied to the involved areas for 20 to 30 minutes at least 3 to 6 times a day, the part should be put at rest or immobilized with a dressing incorporating a splint, and antibiotic therapy should be instituted. If an infection develops, complete surgical drainage and debridement should be done, and continuous hot soaks and intensive antibiotic therapy should be instituted immediately.

NONCLOSTRIDIAL CREPITANT CELLULITIS. This mixed infection usually occurs in wounds contaminated by gastrointestinal or genitourinary contents and is characterized by necrosis of the areolar and fascial tissues with progressive gangrene in the skin from thrombosis of the local nutrient vessels. A wide variety of etiologic agents have been associated with this condition, including Bacteroides, the anaerobic streptococcus, and many strains of the coliform group. Crepitation in the wound caused by gas formation by the bacteria often causes the physician to make an incorrect diagnosis of a clostridial infection. Treatment includes early surgical decompression with extensive debridement of all involved tissue combined with high doses of antibiotics, such as clindamycin and gentamicin.

Infections Caused by Anaerobes

With improved techniques for culturing anaerobic bacteria, anaerobic organisms are being recognized increasingly as causes of infections following trauma or surgery. The anaerobic bacteria are divided into five main groups: (1) the gram-negative, nonsporulating rods such as the Bacteroides and Fusobacteria, (2) the gram-positive, nonsporulating rods including the Eubacterium. Catenabacterium and Bifidobacterium, (3) the clostridial organisms, (4) the gram-positive cocci, the Peptostreptococci, and (5) the gram-negative cocci, the Veillonella. The most frequently encountered anaerobes in surgical infections, particularly after colon injuries, are Bacteroides fragilis and other Bacteroides species, followed by Peptostreptococci and clostridial organisms.

BACTEROIDES INFECTIONS. Because these organisms may cause only minimal local inflammatory changes, Bacteroides infections are often extremely difficult to identify or localize. The presence of an infection by these organisms usually requires thorough drainage of any localized pus and debridement of associated necrotic tissue.

CLOSTRIDIAL INFECTIONS. The clostridial infections most apt to occur in injured patients include clostridial cellulitis, clostridial myositis and tetanus. The surgeon faced with a patient who has obvious gangrenous tissue must try to categorize the lesion accurately because the extent and urgency of the treatment required may differ markedly. All gangrene, even when associated with gas in the tissue, is obviously not always due to clostridial organisms, and all clostridial lesions are not of the same seriousness. For example, although clostridial cellulitis may be extremely painful and may look extremely serious, it is seldom fatal unless the patient is debilitated and treatment is inadequate. Clostridial myositis, on the other hand, causes severe prostration of the patient and may be rapidly fatal.

Clostridial Cellulitis. Clostridial cellulitis is caused by one or more of the Clostridia, most frequently Clostridium welchii. This infection of the skin, subcutaneous and connective tissues is a crepitant cellulitis which spreads rapidly along fascial planes and produces a gray or reddish-brown discharge. Eventually, necrosis and sloughing of the involved areolar tissues, fascia, and skin may occur as a result of thrombosis of local blood vessels. Pain in and around the wound is severe. Treatment includes surgical incision and decompression of all fascial planes together with radical debridement of all involved tissue and

the administration of systemic antibiotic agents, particularly penicillin and ampicillin or one of the tetracyclines.

Clostridial Myositis. Gas gangrene, usually caused by Clostridium welchii, C. novyi, C. septicum, and C. sordellii, is a dreaded complication of any injury. This lesion should be anticipated in any wound in which there is extensive destruction of muscle combined with severe contamination of the tissues, particularly if there is any delay in therapy or an associated vascular injury.

The infection is characterized by a rapidly spreading gangrene of muscle and profound toxemia. Gas formation with crepitation within the muscle and along fascial planes is usually found, but may be absent. Swelling and pain occur early, usually within the first 24 hours after injury. The infected muscle becomes soft, swollen, and dark red, and there is frequently a foul-smelling, brown, watery exudate. The prostration of the patient is often far out of proportion to his fever. Early diagnosis is facilitated by examination of the discharge which may contain many large gram-positive rods, usually without spores.

Surgical treatment should be prompt with extensive decompression of all involved muscle compartments and thorough debridement of all involved tissue. If irreversible gangrenous changes have developed in the extremity, amputation may be the only hope of cure. Speed is extremely important in the management of these patients because the infection may progress to shock and death within 24 to 48 hours. Very high doses of intravenous antibiotics, particularly penicillin in combination with cephalosporins, Chloromycetin, or clindamycin, should also be started immediately.

Tetanus. Tetanus, caused by Clostridium tetani, is an extremely serious anaerobic infection. It is much less common in the United States than in past decades because most citizens have had at least partial immunization. A few, however, particularly women, escape, and others often fail to obtain subsequent booster doses at the prescribed intervals (Chap. 8). Tetanus is a unique infection in that virtually all the symptoms are caused by a powerful exotoxin released by the growing bacteria. Although this infection is most apt to occur with deep and dirty wounds, it is occasionally seen in patients with small lacerations.

The latter stages of the incubation period, which averages 4 to 21 days, are characterized by restlessness, headache, stiffness of the jaw muscles, and intermittent tetanic muscle contractions near the wound. Tachycardia and excess sweating and salivation are also often present. Generalized tonic contractions may follow within 12 to 24 hours, producing the classic facial distortion (risus sardonicus), opisthotonos and rigidity. Clonic contractions may result from even the slightest stimulation, and death is most likely to result from a respiratory arrest occurring during one of these convulsive seizures. Since these patients are often remarkably alert, the disease may be agonizing.

The treatment of established tetanus is extremely difficult, often unsuccessful, and in no way has it replaced the ease and effectiveness of prior active immunization. Once the diagnosis is suspected, treatment must be intensive and proceed rapidly along multiple lines.

SEROTHERAPY. A single I.M. dose of 3,000 to 6,000 units of tetanus immune globulin should be given immediately. In the unusual circumstances in which tetanus immune globulin may not be available, equine or bovine antitoxin may be used if skin or eye sensitivity testing is negative. The immediate dose of equine and bovine antitoxin is 100,000 units consisting of 50,000 units I.V., 40,000 units I.M. and 10,000 units injected into the tissue around the site of injury prior to excision of the wound; 5,000 units are then given I.M. daily until the disease is controlled.

It must be emphasized that tetanus immune globulin is much safer and probably much more effective than equine or bovine antitoxin. No hospital caring for injured patients should be without adequate quantities of tetanus immune globulin.

SURGICAL DEBRIDEMENT. All necrotic tissue and as much of the involved wound as possible should be excised with wide incision of the adjacent tissue so that it is well exposed to the air. Careful reexamination of the wound every 12 to 24 hours is essential and will often reveal additional tissue that must be incised or debrided. Frequent irrigations with hydrogen peroxide or zinc peroxide may be beneficial. Oxygen should be added to the inhaled gas mixtures to keep the arterial Po_2 at 100 mm Hg or higher. All efforts must be made to produce an environment which is hostile to anaerobic growth.

SEDATION AND ANTICONVULSIVES. Adequate sedation is important and may require a continuous I.V. drip of 0.1% Pentothal. This may be supplemented with chloral hydrate through a feeding tube or by retention enemas. Valium 5 to 10 mg I.M. or I.V. every 4 to 6 hours may also be helpful. If seizures occur in spite of all these drugs, additional short-acting barbiturates or muscle paralyzers such as succinylcholine or curare may be required.

TRACHEOSTOMY AND RESPIRATORY ASSISTANCE

AXIOM

DEATH FROM TETANUS IS USUALLY RELATED TO RESPIRATORY ARREST DURING A SEIZURE.

If there is any difficulty in removing the tracheobronchial secretions or if respiratory assistance is needed, a tracheostomy should be performed over a previously placed endotracheal tube. In virtually all cases of any severity, a tracheostomy will be required to ensure adequate ventilation during the seizures.

NURSING CARE. Constant nursing care is

essential to immediately recognize and treat any seizures or respiratory arrest. The patient should be placed in a dark room and protected from as much auditory, visual and other stimuli as possible. Maintenance of adequate fluid and calories is essential, preferably I.V. so there is less risk of vomiting and aspiration.

ANTIBIOTICS. Antibiotics have no effect on the tetanus toxin already released but they should be given to control or prevent secondary infections of the wound or respiratory tract.

HYPERBARIC OXYGEN. The value of hyperbaric oxygen in established tetanus is not clear; however, if the facilities for such treatment are readily available they may be of some assistance.

ACTIVE IMMUNIZATION. Tetanus infection does not produce immunity; therefore any patient who survives tetanus must be given a full course of tetanus toxoid.

Fungal Infections

Within the past few years, the incidence of fungal infections, particularly by Candida species, has risen sharply, especially in patients on I.V. hyperalimentation and those with diminished host resistance from severe debilitation or prolonged therapy with steroids or antineoplastic agents. Candida superinfection is always a threat in severely injured patients who have been receiving broad-spectrum antibiotics for two weeks or longer. Candidiasis is a frequent problem during I.V. hyperalimentation; Candida is one of the few organisms that can live and multiply in hyperosmotic, concentrated glucose solutions.

PITFALL

THE PHYSICIAN MAY FAIL TO CONSIDER CANDIDIASIS WHEN BACTERIAL CULTURES IN A SEPTIC PATIENT ARE REPEATEDLY NEGATIVE.

Most fungal infections cause relatively few systemic symptoms. Their presence is often not suspected until a pulmonary lesion is seen on a chest x-ray or until the organisms are identified in pulmonary secretions or wound drainage. Systemic Candida infections, however, may cause severe toxicity and may closely resemble gram-negative septicemia. These infections should be suspected when cultures from patients with this clinical picture are repeatedly negative for aerobic and anaerobic bacteria. Even if Candida organisms cannot be cultured from the blood, their presence should be suspected if they are found in large quantities in the mouth, urine and feces.

In some instances, oral nystatin, by reducing the number of Candida organisms in the bowel, may decrease the likelihood of systemic candidiasis. Once the systemic infection is established, treatment is directed primarily toward removing all predisposing factors. If the patient is on I.V. hyperalimentation, the I.V. catheter should be removed and the infusion started at another site. If the patient is on antineoplastic drugs or steroids, they should be discontinued as soon as possible. If candidiasis persists in spite of all these measures, amphotericin B may have to be given.

SUMMARY

Infection is the most important cause of morbidity and mortality in the injured patient who survives more than 48 hours.

Sound surgical principles are the cornerstone of the prevention and treatment of post-traumatic sepsis. Persistent fever in an injured patient suggests undrained pus, and every effort should be made to locate an abscess rather than change antibiotics. The appropriate use of antibiotics, however, may be extremely helpful and is not infrequently lifesaving. It is rare for an organism to become resistant to an antibiotic during a course of therapy. The correct use of chemotherapeutic agents is based on the understanding of bacteria apt to be involved and the pharmacology of the drugs used (Table 1).

TABLE 1. TEN FREQUENT ERRORS IN MANAGEMENT OF INFECTION

1. Depending on prophylactic antibiotics instead of sound surgical principles.
2. Beginning antibiotics without cultures and smears.
3. Assuming that the cause of persistent fever is an antibiotic-resistant organism.
4. Mistaking colonization for superinfection.
5. Administering an agent with broad-spectrum coverage when specific therapy is indicated.
6. Failing to search for hidden abscesses.
7. Failing to think of unusual organisms when cultures are repeatedly negative.
8. Improper collecting and handling of material for cultures, particularly for anaerobic organisms.
9. Discontinuing antibiotics before the infecting organisms have been adequately controlled.
10. Failing to check antibiotic sensitivities in the hospital at frequent intervals.

It must be apparent to the reader that this short discussion of therapy cannot possibly mention all of the precautions and dangers with each drug. Before administering any of these agents, careful examination of package inserts and the current literature is advised. Furthermore, bacterial sensitivities may vary tremendously from place to place and time to time. Consequently each physician must keep abreast of the current cultures and sensitivity results in the areas in which he practices.

REFERENCES

1. Alexander, V. W., and Meakins, J. L.: Natural defense mechanisms and clinical sepsis. J. Surg. Res., 11:148, 1971.
2. Howe, C. W.: Bacterial flora of clean wounds and its relation to subsequent sepsis. Amer. J. Surg., 107:696, 1964.
3. Altemeier, W. A., and Alexander, J. W.: Surgical infections and choice of antibiotics. In Davis-Christopher Textbook of Surgery: The Biological Basis of Modern Surgical Practice, 10th ed. Philadelphia, W. B. Saunders, 1972.
4. Alexander, J. W., et al.: Periodic variation in the antibacterial function in human neutrophils and its relationships to sepsis. Ann Surg., 172:206, 1971.
5. Bernard, H. R., and Cole, W. R.: The prophylaxis of surgical infections: The effect of prophylactic antimicrobial drugs on the incidence of infection following potentially contaminated operations. Surgery, 56:151, 1964.
6. Campbell, P. C.: Large doses of penicillin in the prevention of surgical wound infection. Lancet, 2:805, 1965.
7. Feltis, J. M., and Hamit, H. F.: Use of prophylactic antimicrobial drugs to prevent postoperative wound infections. Amer. J. Surg., 114:867, 1967.
8. Fuller, W. D., et al.: Prophylactic antibiotics in penetrating wounds of the abdomen. J. Trauma, 12:282, 1972.
9. Balair, D. C., et al.: 67 Ga-citrate for scanning experimental staphylococcal abscesses. J. Nucl. Med., 14:99, 1973.
10. Kirby, W. M. M.: Vancomycin. New Eng. J. Med., 262:49, 1960.
11. Tillotson, J. R., and Finland, M.: Bacterial colonization and clinical superinfection of the respiratory tract complicating antibiotic treatment on pneumonia. J. Infect. Dis., 119:597, 1969.
12. Page, M. I.: Sounding board. Beware the anaerobe bandwagon. New Eng. J. Med., 290:338, 1974.
13. Howard, V., et al.: Clinical detection of the potential allergic reactor to penicillin by immunologic tests. JAMA, 196:679, 1966.
14. Alexander, J. W., et al.: Immunologic control of Pseudomonas infections in burn patients—A clinical evaluation. Arch. Surg., 102:31, 1971.
15. Sensakovic, J. W., and Bartell, P. F.: The slime of Pseudomonas aeruginosa. Biological characterization and possible role in experimental infection. J. Infect. Dis., 129:101, 1974.

Suggested Reading

1. Lucas, C., et al.: Altered renal homeostasis with acute sepsis. Arch. Surg., 106:444, 1973.
2. Gale, E. F., et al.: The Molecular Basis of Antibiotic Action. London, John Wiley and Sons, 1972.
3. Dubos, R. J., and Hirsch, J. G.: Bacterial and Mycotic Infections of Man, 4th ed. Philadelphia, J. B. Lippincott, 1965.
4. Finland, M.: Changing ecology of bacterial infections as related to antibacterial therapy. J. Infect. Dis., 120:419, 1970.

30 ACUTE VASOMOTOR NEPHROPATHY

I. K. ROSENBERG

"It is no exaggeration to say that the composition of the blood is determined, not by what the mouth takes in, but by what the kidneys keep."

HOMER W. SMITH, 1959

PITFALL

IF IT IS ASSUMED THAT AN INJURED PATIENT HAS GOOD RENAL FUNCTION BECAUSE HIS URINARY OUTPUT IS NORMAL OR HIGH, PROGRESSIVE RENAL FAILURE MAY NOT BE APPRECIATED UNTIL IT IS EXTREMELY DIFFICULT TO CORRECT.

AXIOM

IN THE USUAL CLINICAL SETTINGS, THE ROUTINE MEASURING OF SERUM CREATININE IN THE POSTOPERATIVE PERIOD IS THE BEST AND SIMPLEST METHOD FOR DETECTING EARLY CHANGES IN RENAL FUNCTION.

When a patient suffers a massive injury, the kidneys are usually given attention only if there is hematuria or if the urine flow rates fall below 25 to 50 ml per hour. If the rate of urinary flow can be restored to normal, however, further thought is seldom given to the kidney or its functional state unless laboratory tests are ordered and a rise in BUN, creatinine, or serum potassium is noted. Although the rate of urine flow is often monitored quite closely in critically injured patients, it has serious limitations as an index of the functional status of the kidney. It is becoming increasingly apparent that complex changes occur in the kidney following even minor trauma or sepsis; however, sophisticated studies are usually required to reveal the alterations in function.

In order to understand the effects of trauma and sepsis on renal function, and why acute insufficiency may develop in spite of a normal or high urine output, a brief review of some basic aspects of renal physiology is presented.

NORMAL RENAL FUNCTION

Glomerulus

The formation of urine begins in the coiled capillary tufts of the glomerulus. The hydrostatic force of the blood forces a portion of the plasma water and its crystalloids through the glomerular capillary membrane into Bowman's space. The rate at which this ultrafiltrate of plasma is formed is called the glomerular filtration rate. In a state of health this rate is constant, at about 125 ml/min in a normal

485

sized man, and is maintained by a system of autoregulation within the kidney despite wide fluctuations of hydration, blood pressure, and renal blood flow.[1]

If cardiac output falls, renal vascular resistance usually increases and renal blood flow declines. Under these circumstances, a relative rise in efferent arteriolar resistance and decline in afferent arteriolar resistance may serve to maintain the filtration rate and pressure. When renal vascular resistance rises and renal plasma flow falls, the ratio of glomerular filtration rate to renal plasma flow, known as the filtration fraction, rises above the normal value of 20%.

Proximal Tubule

The proximal tubule reabsorbs about 85% of the glomerular filtrate and is the major site of salt and water reabsorption in the kidney. Many of the constituents of the glomerular filtrate are actively resorbed in this area, and, since no osmotic gradient is established, it is assumed that water diffuses through the tubule wall passively with the absorbed solute.

Following injury, the glomerular filtration rate may decline precipitously. Since resorption in the proximal tubule is partially dependent on the length of time the filtrate is exposed to its cells, the resorption of electrolytes and water under these circumstances is increased. This reduces the volume of urine and its sodium content and helps to maintain the total body content of sodium and water. If the glomerular filtration rate rises as a result of fluid loading or an alteration of vascular dynamics, the rate of proximal tubular flow also increases and increased quantities of sodium and water are lost into the urine. Although the balance between the glomerulus and the proximal tubule provides the bulk of salt and water regulation, fine adjustments in this system are made by aldosterone, antidiuretic hormone (ADH), and several other factors.[2]

Loop of Henle

After the glomerular filtrate, much reduced in volume, leaves the proximal tubule, it enters the loop of Henle. In the ascending limb of the loop of Henle, sodium ion is pumped into the adjacent tissue, making the interstitium of the renal medulla adjacent to the loop of Henle and the collecting tubules hypertonic. As the urine passes through the collecting tubule, water moves from it into the interstitium of the renal medulla according to the osmotic gradient. If limited quantities of glomerular filtrate are presented to the loop of Henle, as may occur during dehydration, increased quantities of sodium may be pumped into the renal medulla, the urine volume will decrease, and its concentration of solutes will increase. During hypovolemic shock or general anesthesia, however, the quantity of sodium ion that can be pumped out by cells of the loop of Henle decreases; consequently the osmolar concentration of the renal medulla falls and the degree to which the urine can be concentrated is reduced.

This passive movement of water out of the collecting tubule, however, can take place only if the tubular epithelium is rendered permeable by the action of ADH from the posterior pituitary gland. The maximal osmolality of the urine in the acclimatized healthy male is about 1400 mOsm/L and is a direct reflection of the osmolality created in the medullary interstitium and the action of ADH.

Distal Tubule

The fluid in the distal convoluted tubule is hypotonic with respect to plasma as a result of the active pumping of the sodium ion out of the ascending limb of the loop of Henle into the interstitium of the renal medulla. Final adjustments in sodium content in the distal tubule are made by active sodium reabsorption, which is accelerated by aldosterone and matched by passive chloride reabsorption or by exchange for potassium and hydrogen.

The macula densa is a specialized portion of the distal convoluted tubule at the point where it is close to its own glomerulus. The afferent arteriole adjacent to the macula densa also has altered cellular elements in its media and adventitia which merge with a proliferation of the mesangium called the polkissen. The structure so constituted by these areas is called the juxtaglomerular apparatus and is responsible for the production of renin by the kidney. The control mechanisms for this area are not yet clearly elucidated, but may include the volume of fluid in the distal tubule, the sodium transport rates from the distal tubule, and the pressure and flow relationships in the afferent arteriole. It has been suggested that the juxtaglomerular apparatus may allow each individual nephron to control its filtration rate by a local feedback loop.[3]

Collecting Tubules

As the tubular fluid passes down the final segment of the nephron, it is exposed to progressively greater osmotic forces in the renal medulla tending to abstract water from the interior of the tubule. If sufficient ADH activity is present, the osmolality of the urine may then approach that of the renal interstitial tissue. If the patient is dehydrated, the osmoreceptors in the hypothalamus cause increased secretion of ADH, resulting in an increased absorption of solute-free water, a fall in urine volume, and an increase in urine osmolality. In this area of the nephron, potassium and hydrogen ions are actively excreted into the tubular lumen, generally in exchange for sodium ion. Ammonia is also secreted and is one of the mechanisms for excreting hydrogen ion.

THE EFFECTS OF TRAUMA

Renal Blood Flow

Studies on severely injured patients with burns and major trauma have consistently shown a marked decline in renal blood flow

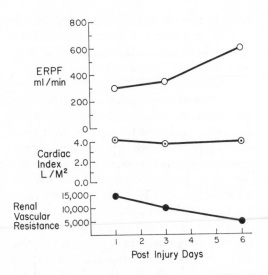

FIG. 1. Sequential changes in effective renal plasma flow (ERPF), cardiac index, and renal vascular resistance in a typical patient who suffered massive trauma.

as measured by PAH clearance techniques. This reduction may be even further aggravated by general anesthesia (Fig. 1). Following injury this patient's renal blood flow fell to 30% of normal and did not return to normal levels for several days. During the period that the renal blood flow was diminished, the cardiac output and total peripheral resistance were normal. The calculated renal vascular resistance was markedly elevated. This increased renal vascular resistance results in the kidney receiving less then the 20% of cardiac output with which it is usually perfused.

Calculation of renal plasma flow from para-aminohippuric acid (PAH) clearances is predicated on the assumption that the removal of PAH is virtually complete during one passage through the kidney. The extraction ratio, $\dfrac{A_{PAH} - V_{PAH}}{A_{PAH}}$ (where A_{PAH} represents arterial concentration of PAH and V_{PAH} represents renal vein concentration of PAH), under varying conditions and wide extremes of renal blood flow, has been shown to be quite constant in the dog unless renal blood flow falls to less than 3% of normal.[4] Although the PAH extraction ratios in humans have not been extensively studied, and then usually under conditions of health, it has been assumed that PAH extractions are 90% complete under most circumstances.[5]

Preliminary observations measuring PAH extraction directly, with a catheter in the right renal vein in patients with overwhelming sepsis and high cardiac outputs, have provided some interesting data. In a few septic patients studied in this fashion, we have found PAH extraction ratios to be less than 50%, with actual renal blood flows calculated to be 150 to 200% of normal.[6,7] The kidneys, therefore, appear to participate in the hyperdynamic circulatory changes of sepsis. Whether these reduced PAH extraction ratios are due to anatomic shunting, redistribution of blood flow, or a failure of cellular transport mechanisms cannot be determined by this method.

In a study of massively wounded individuals at our hospital, the reduction of renal plasma flow was found to vary directly with the extent of the injury and the number of blood transfusions.[6] The reduction in renal plasma flow may persist for several days after injury, but if recovery is uneventful it usually rises to normal by the sixth postinjury day. Since the reduction of blood flow is proportionally greater than that of the GFR, the filtration fraction is increased, producing a rise in oncotic pressure in the postglomerular capillary surrounding the tubule. This increases the gradient between the tubule and the surrounding plasma and encourages salt and water transport out of the tubule, aiding the retention of salt and water by the body.[8]

Glomerular Filtration Rate (GFR)

Although the GFR in severely injured patients requiring multiple transfusions may be considerably reduced, the urine output may be normal or increased. Unless renal failure develops, the GFR is maintained above 40 ml/min and is generally not affected as much as the renal plasma flow (Fig. 2).

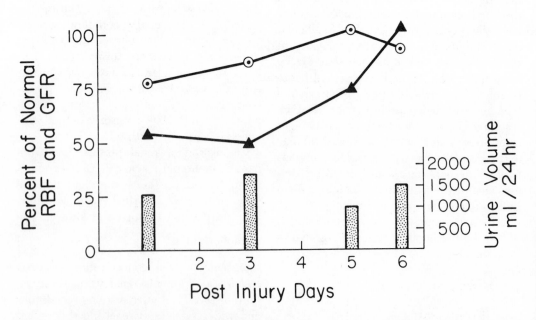

FIG. 2. Triangles represent renal blood flow (RBF), dotted circles represent glomerular filtration rate (GFR), and dotted bars represent urine volume in a typical patient after massive trauma. All vital signs were stable and urine volumes over 60 ml/hr. Note the marked depression in RBF and its lack of effect on urine volume. The early reduction of GFR is less striking.

AXIOM

As might be expected with a decline in the GFR and an increased endogenous protein breakdown, most of our patients with severe trauma and sepsis have had an increased BUN. As the GFR returns to normal, the serum levels of BUN and creatinine also begin to fall toward normal.

Under certain conditions, the glomeruli in various parts of the kidney may get widely differing blood flows.[10] If flow to the glomeruli in the outer cortex is reduced but blood flow to the juxtamedullary nephrons is maintained, a concentrated urine with low urinary sodium levels may result because these nephrons have long loops of Henle. On the other hand, if juxtamedullary blood flow is reduced while cortical blood flow is maintained, the urine will be relatively dilute and its sodium levels will be closer to those of the plasma. In addition, if blood flow is greatly increased to some glomeruli and greatly decreased or absent to others, the few functioning nephrons may be submitted to a higher osmotic load per nephron, resulting in a urine which is closer to pure glomerular filtrate than would ordinarily be found.[11] The urine in many patients with the nonoliguric variety of renal failure has a composition consistent with this thesis of altered renal hemodynamics.

Urinary Concentration

During major operations and for a variable period thereafter, the kidneys may be unable to concentrate the urine to more than 600 mOsm/L despite the administration of pharmacologic doses of ADH[12] (Fig. 3). In patients with severe trauma or sepsis, a large volume of urine is required to excrete the increased osmolar load. If an

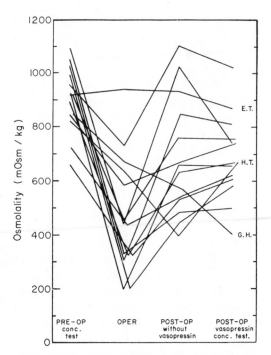

FIG. 3. Inability to concentrate urine during and immediately after operation even when vasopressin is infused at supramaximal levels. (From Gullick, H. D., and Raisz, L. G.[12] Used with permission.)

increased urine volume cannot be achieved because of a blood volume deficit or a decline in the GFR, azotemia will develop. Such a combination of events occurs frequently and the definition of oliguria, arbitrarily set at 400 ml/day, should be revised upward to 1000 ml/day in patients with severe trauma or sepsis.

Urinary Volume

Many factors combine to reduce urinary volume in the intraoperative and postoperative periods. Large fluid deficits may develop preoperatively, especially if the patient is kept N.P.O. for 12 to 18 hours and has suffered large fluid losses through use of laxatives, nasogastric suction, or multiple enemas. In patients with congestive heart failure, sodium restriction and potent diuretics may serve to further deplete total body sodium and water.

All these factors are potent stimuli to the secretion of aldosterone and ADH and may directly reduce GFR. The administration of a general anesthetic and the hypovolemia accompanying most severe injuries and major operative procedures, by depressing renal plasma flow and GFR, contribute to the reduced urinary flow and sodium content. Measurement of urinary sodium and osmolality can thus be extremely helpful in distinguishing post-traumatic or postsurgical oliguria from the oliguria of acute renal failure.

ACUTE VASOMOTOR NEPHROPATHY

Pathogenesis

What was formerly referred to as acute renal failure, lower nephron nephrosis, and shock kidney is now referred to as acute vasomotor nephropathy, reflecting a revised concept of pathogenesis. We now consider this syndrome to be related to altered distribution of blood flow within the kidney mediated by vasomotor changes. The mechanisms by which acute vasomotor nephropathy is produced following injury are still conjectural, despite many experimental animal models which can produce changes closely resembling the clinical entity. It appears fairly certain, however, that several concurrent factors contribute to the pathogenesis.[13]

A period of decreased rate of urine flow seems important in setting the stage for the development of acute vasomotor nephropathy.[14,15] This reduction in urinary flow rate may be due to hypovolemia, hypotension, or a maximal antidiuresis secondary to many other stimuli. The production of a relatively concentrated urine may allow the precipitation of casts[16,17] which can obstruct the tubules or produce high concentrations of circulating toxins in the tubules. Many observations of pigments appearing in the urine and in the tubules on histologic section have suggested that tubular plugging may cause this syndrome; however, such findings are inconstant and of such limited extent as to cast doubt on their causal relationship.[18] Although the casts

may be the end-results of low rates of urine flow associated with high pigment loads from transfusion reactions or muscle damage, they are probably not responsible for the development of renal insufficiency.[19] Certain antibiotics, anesthetic agents, and contrast media may contribute to the development of renal failure; however, the relationship of the syndrome to the administration of these drugs is inconstant enough to discount them as causative in more than a few cases.

Although the conditions that produce low rates of urine flow are often the same as those responsible for low renal blood flow, a reduction in renal perfusion may occur without hypotension and is part of the physiologic response to trauma.[6,20] The decline in blood flow may or may not be sufficient to produce renal ischemia, but it does seem to contribute to the production of vasomotor nephropathy. On the other hand, there are many situations in which there is prolonged ischemia of the kidneys but renal failure is a distinct rarity. For example, patients with bleeding duodenal ulcers, myocardial infarction, or diabetic acidosis all may have prolonged periods of renal ischemia but rarely develop acute renal failure. In contrast, the patient who suffers massive trauma or abruptio placentae has a significantly increased likelihood of developing renal failure.[21,22]

Krypton washout studies in patients with acute injury, and micropuncture studies in rats, indicate that the oliguric phase in shock or trauma results primarily because of increased vascular resistance in the renal cortex with redistribution of blood flow to the medullary and the juxtamedullary nephrons. Under these circumstances, total renal blood flow may be unchanged while cortical hypoperfusion is occurring. Some of the changes in urinary concentrating ability and sodium excretion in this syndrome may be explained by such a redistribution of blood flow. Preliminary studies by electron microscopy on some of these patients suggest that mechanical obstruction

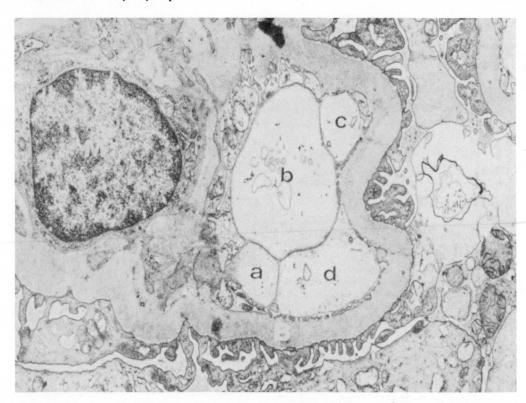

FIG. 4. Electron micrograph of part of a glomerular capillary from a patient with severe sepsis. Lumen is filled with membrane-bound cytoplasmic remnants (a-d). One of these (a) can be seen to arise from mesangial cell cytoplasm extruding through endothelial pore (arrows). Mesangial cell (M), basement membrane (B). (×15,940.) (From Rosenberg, I. K., et al.[6] Used with permission of the American Medical Association.)

of glomerular capillaries by the formed elements of blood and by extrusion of mesangial cells into the capillary lumen contributes to these changes[6] (Fig. 4).

Although measurements of glomerular filtration rates by classical clearance techniques in oliguric patients are unreliable, the GFR and RBF in nonoliguric patients with vasomotor nephropathy are consistently depressed to extremely low levels.[17] The histologic changes in renal biopsy material or at autopsy as seen on light microscopy, however, do not account for these alterations.[19] Nevertheless, a functional or mechanical alteration of the renal vasculature might well explain the disturbed parameters observed. A marked increase in tone of certain afferent arterioles may cause such reduced glomerular capillary pressures that filtration would cease in the involved neph-

rons. Such changes might be mediated via a local feedback loop involving tubular flow rates, the juxtaglomerular apparatus, and local renin release. This concept implies individual nephron control of filtration rate as determined by tubular fluid transport rates.[23] In some nephrons, filtration may continue but, because of high osmotic loads, the urine volume may be relatively high, with a high sodium content, and reabsorption of solute-free water may be reduced. The number of functional units would, in part, determine urine volume. If a large number of nephrons were open, endogenous osmotic effects could produce the high urine output of nonoliguric renal failure syndromes with urine/plasma (U/P) ratios of various solutes approaching unity (Fig. 5). The relatively large reduction of GFR would produce azotemia, and the os-

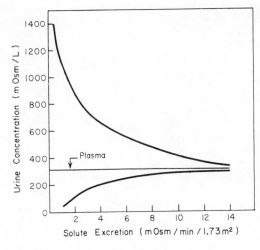

FIG. 5. Effect of osmotic diuresis on concentration and dilution of urine in normal subjects. (From Seldon, D. W., Carter, N. W., and Rector, F. C. In: *Diseases of the Kidney* [Strauss, M. B., and Welt, L. G., Eds.]. Boston, Little, Brown & Co., 1963. Used with permission.)

motic diuresis would account for isosthenuria. Such changes have been observed in some of our patients with trauma and sepsis.

In some patients suffering severe sepsis, we have observed exceptionally high rates of urine flow, more than 300 ml/hr, in the absence of excessive fluid loads. This phenomenon may be related to the generalized vasodilatation and increased blood flow often seen in sepsis.[6,7,24] Since the calculated renal blood flow in these patients often exceeded 2 L/min, it appears that the kidney

shares in the hyperdynamic state seen in many patients with sepsis. Vasodilatation of the intrarenal vessels with hydralazine or phenoxybenzamine causes similar high renal blood flows, high urine flow rates, and decreased PAH extraction (Table 1). If the high volumes of urine flow are not replaced, the patient may become hypovolemic, and oliguric renal failure may then supervene. To avoid this series of events, the patient's fluid intake and output, blood pressure, and pulse must be carefully monitored (Fig. 6). Diuretics should be used cautiously in patients with severe trauma or sepsis because surprisingly large fluid losses can occur before the extent of volume depletion is recognized by the physician.

In some septic patients the high rates of urine flow are inadequately replaced by intravenous fluids. Since sepsis often causes severe pulmonary congestion, the CVP in these patients may be high in spite of marked hypovolemia. A rising pulse rate and a falling urine output, however, suggest that the circulating blood volume is reduced and tissue perfusion may be failing. This is confirmed if the sodium content of the urine falls to less than 20 mEq/L. Unless aggressive fluid replacement is begun rapidly in such a patient, oliguria and acute vasomotor nephropathy are the usual sequelae. Fluid deficits may also result from excessive urine output if diuretics such as furosemide or ethacrynic acid are

TABLE 1. SUMMARY OF RENAL FUNCTIONAL PARAMETERS STUDIED
IN 25 SEPTIC PATIENTS*

	GFR	ERPF†	Cosm**	Clearance Na(ml/min)	ExPAH	TRBF†	TRBF/ CO(%)
Mean	85	75	3.25	1.2	43%	188	21
SD	±30	±29			4-62%	56-305	16-26

*From Rector, F., et al.: Renal hyperemia in association with clinical sepsis. Surg. Forum, 23:51, 1972. Used with permission.
†% of normal.
**% of GFR.
GFR = Glomerular filtration rate, ERPF = effective renal plasma flow, Cosm = osmolar clearance, ExPAH = extraction ratio of para-aminohippuric acid, TRBF = true renal blood flow, CO = cardiac output.

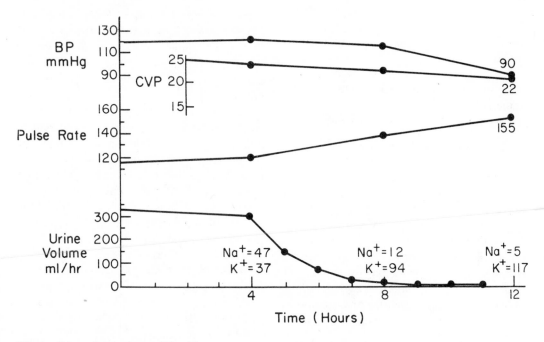

FIG. 6. Urine volumes of over 300 ml/hr in a young man with massive peritonitis. Aggressive fluid therapy might have prevented the oliguric renal failure which supervened. (From Lucas, C. E., et al.[7] Used with permission of the American Medical Association.)

used indiscriminately. Great care should be exercised to avoid depleting the circulating volume in a misguided attempt to prevent vasomotor nephropathy by producing high flows of urine with diuretics. The end-result of such efforts may be diminished circulating volume resulting finally in oliguric vasomotor nephropathy, which few severely injured or septic patients survive.

Prevention of Renal Failure

Situations which cause oliguria are associated with a high incidence of renal failure, especially if sepsis and trauma are also present. Prevention of renal failure in the injured patient, therefore, is directed primarily toward avoiding oliguria or quickly determining the cause and correcting it. Determining the cause of oliguria in an injured patient can sometimes be extremely difficult; however, the urgency of the situation demands an approach which is systematic and rapid.

RULE OUT MECHANICAL OBSTRUCTION

PITFALL

IF IT IS ASSUMED THAT COMPLETE ANURIA IS DUE TO ACUTE RENAL FAILURE, AN EASILY CORRECTABLE MECHANICAL OBSTRUCTION MAY BE OVERLOOKED.

If a Foley catheter is not already present in a patient who has a high risk of renal failure or is suspected of having oliguria, it should be inserted to assure that no obstruction of the bladder outlet is present and to measure the hourly urine output. If the presence of oliguria is confirmed, and the operative procedure or trauma was such that the ureter might have been occluded by ligatures or injured, retrograde pyelography is indicated. An alternative which may take less time, but is often nondiagnostic because of the poor contrast on the films, is a high-dose drip-infusion intravenous pyelogram with delayed films.

AXIOM

OLIGURIA FOLLOWING TRAUMA IS USUALLY DUE TO INADEQUATE ADMINISTRATION OF FLUIDS.

Even with no obvious blood loss, injured patients can develop severe hypovolemia and impaired tissue perfusion. These blood or fluid deficits may be even further aggravated by contusions, fractures, anesthesia and various drugs. Other factors, such as previous disease or direct trauma to the heart, lungs or kidneys, may occasionally cause inadequate renal perfusion and oliguria, but these should be considered seriously only if there is little or no response to rapid infusion of adequate quantities of fluid.

IMPROVE CARDIAC OUTPUT. If oliguria persists in spite of adequate fluids and there is evidence of cardiac disease or trauma, steps should be taken to improve myocardial function using digitalis or other inotropic agents. If the blood pressure and cardiac output can be improved, overall renal perfusion should increase, the vasoconstriction in the cortex should decrease and a normal renal cortical blood flow may be reestablished.

CORRECT ELECTROLYTE ABNORMALITIES. Serum concentration of electrolytes should be measured frequently in severely injured patients, especially those with hypotension or oliguria. In some patients, oliguria may be due to a severe hyponatremia. Although water restriction is generally the preferred method for treating dilutional hyponatremia, this method may not be appropriate or effective rapidly enough in the acutely injured patient, especially if his total body content of sodium is reduced. Under such circumstances, administration of hypertonic (3%) saline may produce a dramatic diuresis. The concentration of sodium in the urine of patients with salt deficiency and normal kidneys is generally less than 20 mEq/L. If the sodium concentration in the urine is greater than 40 mEq/L in the presence of severe hyponatremia, the syndrome of inappropriate secretion of ADH should be considered. Severe acidosis or hypoproteinemia also may occasionally cause oliguria.

REDUCE METABOLITE AND PIGMENT LOAD TO THE KIDNEY. A thorough debridement of nonviable or contaminated tissue must be performed as soon as possible to reduce the release of pigments and nitrogenous substances into the blood from infected or necrotic tissue. Blood should be carefully cross-matched for major and minor incompatibilities, especially if the patient has previously been given uncross-matched O- or type-specific blood. Whenever a patient receiving a blood transfusion develops oliguria, the possibility of a mismatch must be considered strongly and appropriate steps rapidly taken (Chap. 10).

ADMINISTER DIURETICS. If correction of existing volume deficits and hypotension fails to produce an adequate urine flow following massive trauma, it may be necessary to use diuretics.

Mannitol. Under these circumstances, 25 gm of mannitol in 250 cc of saline administered I.V. in 20 to 30 minutes may be useful. The mechanisms by which this osmotic diuretic may reverse impending renal insufficiency are not definitely known; however, it is felt that high rates of urine flow in the distal tubule may influence the juxtaglomerular apparatus and the distribution of blood flow within the kidney parenchyma. Thus the cortical ischemia that usually occurs under these circumstances may be prevented. Since mannitol may rapidly expand the blood volume prior to its diuretic effect, this drug should be used cautiously if there is evidence that the patient is overloaded with fluid or has heart disease.

Furosemide and Ethacrynic Acid. Potent diuretics such as ethacrynic acid and furosemide (Lasix) have been used extensively for the prevention of acute vasomotor nephropathy, with some success. The recommended dose of furosemide is 20 to 40 mg

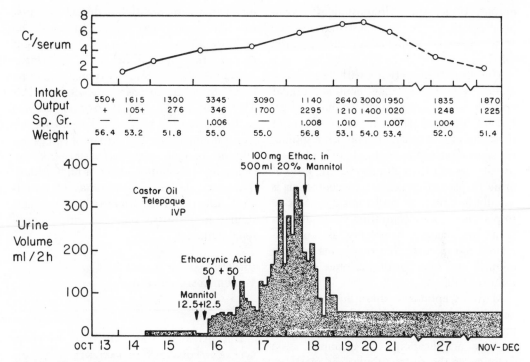

FIG. 7. This 82-year-old man became dehydrated (weight loss 5 kg) while being evaluated for abdominal pain. Urine output was restored after 2 doses of ethacrynic acid 32 hours after oliguria, and sustained by an infusion of ethacrynic acid and mannitol. The serum creatinine continued to rise for 4 days, but recovery followed. (From Kjellstrand, C. M. Nephron, 9:339, 1972. Used with permission.)

intravenously. If an adequate response is not obtained, the dose is doubled every half hour until a total of 2 gm has been administered. If no response is obtained by that time, efforts to force urine flow with diuretics are abandoned. In an occasional patient who is unresponsive to furosemide, 50 to 100 mg of ethacrynic acid I.V. have produced a significant diuresis. Since these agents are potent agents which eventually poison transport mechanisms, great care should govern their use. Adequate correction of electrolyte imbalances and restoration of volume deficits must precede their use (Fig. 7). In the patient with normal renal perfusion, there may be a detrimental effect on filtration rate.

PITFALL

FAILURE TO REPLACE THE FLUID AND ELECTROLYTE LOSSES ADEQUATELY FOLLOWING THE USE OF DIURETICS MAY HAVE DIRE RESULTS.

The patient's vital signs and intake and output must be watched very carefully whenever a diuretic is used. If a significant diuresis is obtained, the patient may rapidly develop hypovolemia or hypokalemia. If steps are not taken to prevent or rapidly treat such a problem, hypotension and irreversible oliguric renal failure may develop.

Diagnosis

If all volume deficits are replaced, hypotension is corrected, and serum electrolytes are restored to normal, and if urine flow still does not respond to osmotic or natriuretic diuretics, the diagnosis of renal failure is reasonably well established; however, complete anuria is distinctly unusual and should suggest either an obstruction of the outflow tract or a vascular lesion. It must also be remembered that acute vasomotor nephropathy may also occur in the presence of a normal or increased urine output. Under such circumstances a two-hour creatinine clearance test may provide early objective evidence of an impaired GFR.

The urine from patients with acute vasomotor nephropathy may contain tubular epithelial cells, casts, small amounts of albumin, and red cells; however, none of these findings is constant. The urine sodium concentration in the acute oliguric phase is usually greater than 50 mEq/L, the ratio of urine to plasma creatinine concentration is usually less than 20, and the ratio of urine to plasma urea concentration is usually less than 10. Urinary osmolality is approximately the same as that of plasma in both oliguric and nonoliguric varieties of renal failure (Table 2).

Many exceptions to these findings occur, and there is considerable evidence for varying degrees of persisting tubular function.[25] Urinary acidification, for example, is a function of the distal tubule, yet most patients have an acid urine even with severe oliguria. Potassium secretion is also a distal tubular function; however, the urinary concentration of potassium in oliguric patients is usually maintained at normal levels. The nonoliguric patient seldom has difficulty with potassium retention unless there is exogenous administration of this ion or extensive tissue breakdown.

The patient with nonoliguric vasomotor nephropathy is seldom recognized until uremia occurs. It is important, therefore, to measure serum creatinine during the first few days after any major trauma. The findings in the urine are somewhat different than in the oliguric variety. The urinary sodium is variable and occasionally may be low if there are extensive deficits of salt.[24] This is especially characteristic of patients with massive burns. Formed elements are less prominent in the urine of the nonoliguric patient, perhaps because of the cleansing and dilution effect of high urinary flow rates. Urine/plasma ratios of osmolality, urea, and creatinine, however, are similar to those in patients with oliguric renal failure.

Treatment

FLUID ADMINISTRATION

PITFALL

THE PHYSICIAN MAY FAIL TO LIMIT FLUID INTAKE ADEQUATELY IN PATIENTS WITH OLIGURIC RENAL FAILURE.

If the treatment of acute vasomotor nephropathy is to be successful, early recognition is mandatory. In the oliguric variety, the volume of fluid given to the patient is governed largely by changes in his body weight. This must, however, take into account that a negative nitrogen and caloric balance is expected, and the patient should lose about 0.5 kg to 1.5 kg per day, depending on the extent of the injury. The

TABLE 2.   COMPARISONS OF FINDINGS IN PATIENTS WITH INADEQUATE CIRCULATORY VOLUME AND ACUTE VASOMOTOR NEPHROPATHY

	Inadequate Circulating Volume	Acute Vasomotor Nephropathy
Cardiac index	Usually reduced	Normal
Mean arterial pressure	Normal or low	Normal or high
Urine sodium concentration	<20 mEq/L	>50 mEq/L
U/P osmolality	>1.2	about 1
U/P urea	>10	<10
U/P creatinine	>20	<20
Endogenous creatinine clearance	>40 ml/min	<40 ml/min
BUN/serum creatinine	>20	about 10

rate of rise of the BUN may be reduced and the feeling of well-being improved by the administration of a diet containing the essential amino acids in proper proportion with a nonprotein caloric source.[26,27] This is often given intravenously because many of these patients have an adynamic ileus.

With extensive trauma or sepsis, especially when accompanied by fever, even greater losses of body weight are expected. Attempts to prevent this weight loss by fluid administration can lead to overhydration, edema, and congestive heart failure. In the usual oliguric patient, administration of 400 to 500 cc of water per day added to the measured renal and gastrointestinal losses is generally sufficient to keep the patient in balance. This fluid may be supplied as 25% dextrose in water administered by continuous I.V. infusion through a caval catheter. A minimum of 100 gm of carbohydrate per day should be provided to keep nitrogen catabolism to a minimum.

PITFALL

FAILURE ADEQUATELY TO REPLACE FLUID AND ELECTROLYTE LOSSES IN PATIENTS WITH NONOLIGURIC RENAL FAILURE MAY LEAD TO HYPOVOLEMIA.

Patients with nonoliguric renal failure can rapidly develop hypovolemia if the vital signs and fluid intake and output are not watched carefully. The oliguric renal failure which might then develop is much more difficult to treat, especially if the patient becomes septic.

SODIUM BALANCE. Sodium balance in patients with oliguric vasomotor nephropathy is not usually a problem. Urinary sodium losses are minimal and, unless the patient is perspiring excessively, only the gastrointestinal losses require replacement. Hyponatremia is more often a result of hemodilution due to overzealous fluid administration than it is of total-body sodium deficits.

In patients with the nonoliguric variety of the syndrome, the sodium and potassium losses in the urine must be carefully monitored and replaced. Potassium loss has more often been a problem than hyperkalemia in these patients. Creatinine clearances can be measured in patients producing more than 50 to 60 ml of urine per hour and are useful in monitoring the recovery of renal function.

POTASSIUM BALANCE. After trauma or surgery, the blood potassium level not infrequently rises above 4.5 to 5.0 mEq/L, in spite of hemodilution. This is largely due to leakage of intracellular potassium across the cell membrane and will be worse if the patient becomes acidotic. This hyperkalemia would probably not occur if renal excretion could keep pace with endogenous production.[28]

AXIOM

IF OLIGURIC VASOMOTOR NEPHROPATHY DEVELOPS, THE BIGGEST THREAT TO THE PATIENT'S LIFE IS HYPERKALEMIA.

High concentrations of potassium cause conduction block in the atria, A–V node, and ventricles, with the heart eventually stopping in diastole. EKG monitoring is very important in patients with renal failure and is generally an earlier clue to potassium excess than are serum levels. Elevated levels of intracellular potassium are manifested electrocardiographically by high, peaked T waves followed by widening of the QRS complex and finally sine waves heralding an imminent cardiac arrest.

It should be remembered that the usual type of aqueous penicillin contains roughly 1.67 mEq of potassium in each million units. Sodium penicillins are available and should be used if potassium accumulations are a problem.

Blood samples for potassium determinations must be drawn carefully. Trauma to blood while it is being drawn can cause a false or misleading hyperkalemia in the blood sample because of release of potassium from damaged red blood cells.

The emergency management of hyperkalemia has been well outlined by Levinsky.[29] If cardiac toxicity is severe, calcium infusion is the most rapidly effective measure; 5 to 15 ml of 10% calcium chloride can be infused intravenously in less than an hour. Extreme caution, however, is necessary in the digitalized patient. Infusion of glucose solutions is also helpful; 200 to 500 ml of 10% glucose are given in the first half hour and the infusion is then maintained at a slower rate. It is customary to give 10 units of regular insulin subcutaneously or in the infusion to enhance cellular uptake of glucose, but this is probably required only in diabetic patients. Alkalinization of the plasma by I.V. infusion of sodium bicarbonate also rapidly lowers plasma potassium levels by causing potassium to shift into cells; 2 to 3 ampules of sodium bicarbonate, each containing 44.6 mEq, can be given slowly I.V. or added to one liter of the glucose solution. Hypertonic sodium infusions will counteract hyperkalemic toxicity, especially in hyponatremic or volume-depleted patients. The beneficial effect is due in part to dilution of plasma potassium by an expanded extracellular volume and may also be due to the opposing effects of plasma sodium and potassium levels on cardiac function.

Potassium can be removed from the body by the use of cation exchange resins such as sodium polystyrene sulfonate (Kayexalate). Up to 20 gm can be given by mouth 3 or 4 times a day. To potentiate the effect of the resin and to prevent fecal impaction, 20 ml of a 70% sorbitol solution may be administered with each dose of resin. In patients who cannot take medication by mouth, or when a more rapid effect is desired, the resin can be given as a retention enema; 50 gm of resin are suspended in a mixture of 50 ml of 70% sorbitol and 100 to 150 ml of tap water. The enema should be retained for at least half an hour and may be repeated 3 to 4 times a day.

PERITONEAL DIALYSIS. The use of peritoneal dialysis is simple and safe with modern closed techniques. It has been used without complication even following abdominal operations involving bowel resection or vascular grafting. It is less efficient than hemodialysis but may be adequate in patients with low to moderate rates of increasing azotemia. If a hypertonic dialysis fluid is employed, it can also be used to remove any excess water from the patient.

HEMODIALYSIS. The early use of hemodialysis in the treatment of post-traumatic renal insufficiency has become increasingly popular. If it is to be used, however, it should be begun before toxemia is apparent and should be performed at frequent intervals.[30] Indwelling arterial and venous catheters, such as the Scribner shunt, and disposable coils for the hemodialysis machine have greatly simplified the procedure. Urgent indications for dialysis are hyperkalemia, cerebral confusion, and increasing neuromuscular irritability. Hemodialysis may also be of value if there is concomitant respiratory insufficiency due to a fluid overload.[31] Under such circumstances, the CVP is often but not always elevated.

MANAGEMENT OF THE DIURETIC PHASE OF ACUTE RENAL FAILURE. The oliguric phase of renal failure is followed by a diuretic phase. The period of oliguria may be a few days or many weeks, with a median duration of about 10 to 12 days. During the phase of increasing urine volumes, the urine/plasma ratios of creatinine and urea differ little from those found during the oliguric phase. The urinary sodium content is variable. The losses of sodium, water, and potassium during the diuretic phase may be excessive and may quickly lead to extracellular fluid volume deficits if replacement is inadequate. Measurement of urine volume and electrolyte concentrations under these circumstances allows precise replacement. Slight underreplacement may be helpful because accumulations of excess water usually occur during the oliguric period, even with careful fluid restriction. During the diuretic phase, azotemia may continue to increase in spite of high urine outputs because the GFR is still depressed.

PITFALL

OVERCONFIDENCE AND NEGLECT OF FLUID AND ELECTROLYTE BALANCE DURING THE DI-URETIC PHASE OF RENAL FAILURE MAY LEAD TO DEATH.

Although recovery may seem obvious clinically, there may still be functional inadequacy of the kidney as measured by sensitive tests of renal function—maximal concentrating ability, tubular transport maximum for PAH, and inulin clearance. These deficits may persist for many weeks or months.

SUMMARY (Table 3)

Renal function is an exquisitely balanced mechanism for the regulation of the volume and composition of body fluids. Trauma and sepsis may cause a number of changes resulting in failure of the kidney to perform some or all of its functions. The presence of increased circulating pigments in the plasma and low rates of urine flow potentiate the tendency for redistribution of blood flow within the kidney parenchyma. The stage is then set for the development of acute vasomotor nephropathy. The maintenance of adequate renal blood flow and high urine output seems to protect the kidney from this syndrome.

Once renal failure is established, it is spontaneously reversible if an internal milieu consistent with life can be maintained. Restriction of fluids, reduction of catabolism, control of potassium accumulations, and avoidance of infection all contribute to the maintenance of homeostasis. Dialysis may be lifesaving and should be started early and employed frequently if the trauma is massive. Spontaneous return of renal function seems assured if complications can be averted.

REFERENCES

1. Smith, H. W.: *Principles of Renal Physiology.* New York, Oxford University Press, 1956.
2. Schrier, R. W., and de Wardener, H. E.: Tubular reabsorption of sodium ion: Influence of factors other than aldosterone and glomerular filtration rate (second of two parts). New Eng. J. Med., 285:1292, 1971.
3. Powers, S. R., Jr.: The maintenance of renal function following massive trauma. J. Trauma, 10:554, 1970.

TABLE 3. SOME OF THE MOST FREQUENT ERRORS MADE IN THE DIAGNOSIS AND TREATMENT OF RENAL FAILURE AFTER TRAUMA

1. To assume that oliguria is on the basis of renal failure without adequately ruling out mechanical obstruction.
2. To assume that oliguria is due to renal failure without ascertaining that adequate volume replacement and electrolyte balance have been restored.
3. To assume that an elevated central venous pressure assures an adequate blood volume.
4. To fail to appreciate that a large volume of urine does not necessarily mean volume overload.
5. To fail to recognize that polyuria may result in volume deficits and acute oliguric vasomotor nephropathy.
6. To restrict sodium excessively in patients who are already either volume or sodium depleted prior to injury or operation.
7. To administer loop diuretics without being careful to maintain an adequate circulating volume.
8. To administer blood during anesthesia (when reactions are easily missed) if the transfusion could have been delayed until later.
9. To fail to maintain high volume urine flow during extensive operative manipulations.
10. To fail to control sepsis by drainage, debridement and appropriate antibiotics in the severely injured patient.
11. To administer potassium-containing fluids before ascertaining that renal function is adequate.
12. To overload the oliguric patient with intravenous fluids in a vain attempt to stimulate urine flow.
13. To restrict fluids in the hopes of preventing pulmonary insufficiency to the detriment of the kidney.
14. To neglect fluid and electrolyte balance during the recovery diuretic phase of acute vasomotor nephropathy.

4. Phillips, R. A., et al.: Effects of acute hemorrhagic and traumatic shock on renal function of dogs. Amer. J. Physiol., 145:314, 1945.

5. Smith, H. W.: *The Kidney: Structure and Function in Health and Disease.* New York, Oxford University Press, 1951.

6. Rosenberg, I. K., et al.: Renal insufficiency after trauma and sepsis. A prospective functional and ultrastructural analysis. Arch. Surg., 103:175, 1971.

7. Lucas, C. E., et al.: Altered renal homeostasis with acute sepsis—Clinical significance. Arch. Surg., 106:444, 1973.

8. Windhager, E. E., Lewy, J. E., and Spitzer, A.: Intrarenal control of proximal tubular reabsorption of sodium and water. Nephron, 6:247, 1969.

9. O'Neill, J. A., Jr., et al.: Renal function during the early postburn period. Surg. Forum, 18:67, 1967.

10. Barger, A. C.: Renal hemodynamic factors in congestive heart failure. Ann. N.Y. Acad. Sci., 139:276, 1966.

11. Bricker, N.: On the meaning of the intact nephron hypothesis (editorial). Amer. J. Med., 46:1, 1969.

12. Gullick, H. D., and Raisz, L. G.: Changes in renal concentrating ability associated with major surgical procedures. New Eng. J. Med., 262:1309, 1960.

13. Teschan, P. E., and Mason, A. D.: Mechanism of renal lesions induced by shock: Hemodynamic data. Proc. 1st Int. Congr. Nephrol., Geneve/Evian 1960, Vol 1—56:303, 1961.

14. Teschan, P. E., and Lawson, N. L.: Studies in acute renal failure. Prevention by osmotic diuresis, and observations on the effect of plasma and extracellular volume expansion. Nephron, 3:1, 1966.

15. Welt, L. G., and Peters, J. P.: Acute renal failure. Lower nephron nephrosis. Yale J. Biol. Med., 24:220, 1951.

16. Myers, J. K., et al.: The role of renal tubular flow in the pathogenesis of traumatic renal failure. Surg. Gynec. Obstet. 123:1243, 1966.

17. Hollenberg, N. K., et al.: Acute oliguric renal failure in man; Evidence for preferential renal cortical ischemia. Medicine, 47:455, 1968.

18. Mason, A. D., Jr., Alexander, J. W., and Teschan, P. E.: Studies in acute renal failure. I. Development of a reproducible lesion in experimental animals. J. Surg. Res., 3:430, 1963.

19. Sevitt, S.: Pathogenesis of traumatic uraemia —A revised concept. Lancet, 2:135, 1959.

20. Cameron, J. S., and Miller-Jones, C. M. H.: Renal function and renal failure in badly burned children. Brit. J. Surg., 54:132, 1967.

21. Ladd, M.: *Renal Sequelae of War Wounds in Man. Studies of Surgical Research Team,* Vol. IV. Washington, Army Medical Service Graduate School, Government Printing Office, 1955.

22. Lauson, H. D., Bradley, S. E., and Cournand, A.: The renal circulation in shock. J. Clin. Invest., 23:381, 1944.

23. Britton, K. E.: Renin and autoregulation. Lancet, 2:329, 1968.

24. Hermreck, A. S., and Thal, A. P.: Mechanisms for the high circulatory requirements in sepsis and septic shock. Ann. Surg., 170:677, 1969.

25. Sevitt, S.: Renal function after burning. J. Clin. Path., 18:572, 1965.

26. Berlyne, G. M., et al.: The dietary treatment of acute renal failure. Quart. J. Med., 36:59, 1967.

27. Wilmore, D. W., and Dudrick, S. J.: Treatment of acute renal failure with intravenous essential L-amino acids. Arch. Surg., 99:669, 1969.

28. Moore, F. D.: *Metabolic Care of the Surgical Patient.* Philadelphia, W. B. Saunders, 1959.

29. Levinsky, N. G.: Management of emergencies. VI. Hyperkalemia. New Eng. J. Med., 274:1075, 1966.

30. Teschan, P. E., et al.: Prophylactic hemodialysis in the treatment of acute renal failure. Ann. Intern. Med., 53:992, 1960.

31. Zimmerman, J. E.: Respiratory failure complicating post-traumatic acute renal failure: Etiology, clinical features and management. Ann. Surg., 174:12, 1971.

32. Smith, H. W.: *From Fish to Philosopher: The Story of Our Internal Environment.* Summit, Ciba Pharmaceutical Products, 1959.

31 RESPIRATORY FAILURE IN TRAUMA

R. F. WILSON
M. L. NORTON

"And the Lord God formed man of the dust of the ground and breathed into his nostrils the breath of life."

Genesis 2:7

As the management of patients with severe trauma has improved, increasing numbers of patients have survived the initial period of shock only to die later of a severe progressive respiratory failure.[3,4] In many areas of Vietnam[5] respiratory failure was the most frequent cause of death in our wounded soldiers. In our own experience, it is second only to sepsis as a cause of postoperative death in patients with trauma.

We define acute respiratory failure in the adult as an acute pathophysiologic process due to pulmonary damage or disease resulting in impaired alveolar ventilation and gas exchange which is then inadequate to maintain an arterial Po_2 above 60 mm Hg and Pco_2 below 50 mm Hg.

Acute respiratory failure in the adult is a major part of the "post-resurrection syndrome" which we define as the multiple organ system failure which develops in patients who have had severe prolonged shock or cardiac arrest. In the past, most such patients would have died promptly of these cardiovascular problems; now, however, because of improved technology and treatment in our emergency rooms and intensive care units, a large number survive the initial insults. Unfortunately, within hours, many of these critically ill or injured patients begin to deteriorate again with evidence of progressive failure of the lungs, kidneys and liver.

During World War II, Burford and Burbank studied this problem extensively and used the term "wet-lung syndrome" to describe the vicious cycle of increased pulmonary exudation, secretions and atelectasis seen in many of their patients with chest trauma.[6] Burke has referred to the reduced oxygen extraction in spite of increased volume and work of ventilation in patients with trauma and peritonitis as characteristic of a "high-output respiratory failure syndrome."[7]

ETIOLOGY

The etiology of respiratory failure after trauma has been attributed by various authors to one or more of the following: hypoxic damage to the lung, fat emboli, platelet emboli, vasoactive substances, fluid overload, or aspiration. Pulmonary embolism is discussed in Chapter 26, and may also contribute to respiratory complications.

Hypoxic Damage to the Lungs

Inadequate blood flow to the lungs interferes with local cellular metabolism with a resultant decrease in mucociliary clearance and surfactant production.[8] Surfactant, a phospholipid produced in the lungs, is important in lowering surface tension in alveoli and preventing atelectasis.[9] It has a half-life of 14 to 18 hours which coincides with the usual lag period between trauma or shock and the onset of the respiratory failure. The work of Levin suggests that the ability of the lung to produce "surface-active alveolar lining material" may depend on adequate alveolar perfusion.[10] Henry et al. found that lung tissue from animals in shock had a decreased oxygen uptake and a reduced capacity to convert inorganic ^{32}P to phosphoprotein, suggesting that the shock lung has a reduced metabolism with impairment of the cells that produce surfactant.[8] Surfactant activity may also be reduced by fluid leaking into the alveoli through damaged or abnormal alveolar lining cells. This fluid contains a high concentration of proteins, including fibrinogen which markedly reduces the activity of the surface-active alveolar lining.

Complete isolation of one lung from the circulation during shock, however, protects it from many of the morphologic changes found in the opposite lung which continues to be perfused, suggesting that the pulmonary ischemia is of less importance than the substances brought to the lungs during and following shock and trauma.

Fat Emboli (see also Chap. 17)

"Fat embolism" is the name given to a fascinating, but poorly understood, clinical syndrome characterized by cerebral and respiratory dysfunction following long bone fractures or massive soft-tissue trauma. There is generally a relatively asymptomatic interval of 24 to 72 hours after injury, following which the patient begins to demonstrate increasing tachypnea, restlessness and confusion. If this progresses to the full-blown syndrome of severe hypoxemia, respiratory acidosis and coma, death may occur in 10 to 20% or more. Large numbers of platelets adhere to these fat emboli so that, characteristically, thrombocytopenia develops and petechiae may appear on the chest, axillae and conjunctivae.

The chest x-ray demonstrates diffuse fluffy infiltrates throughout both lung fields, and the EKG may reveal some right heart strain. Fat can usually be found in the urine and sputum; however, this may also occur occasionally in normal patients and is not thought to be of great diagnostic significance. Serum lipase levels are occasionally elevated after 4 to 6 days. There is considerable variation in the reported incidence of this syndrome; however, fat emboli have been found in the lungs of over 85% of patients dying of severe blunt trauma.[11]

In 1862 Gauss[12] postulated that fat from the marrow entered the vascular system through capillaries or veins torn by the fracture. In 1927, Lehman and Moore[13] challenged the mechanistic theory of Gauss, pointing out that fat emboli were also found in nontraumatic conditions such as infections and burns. They felt that fat emboli were the result of a biochemical derangement which altered the stability of fat and similar substances in the blood. In 1959, LeQuire[14] supported this theory by demonstrating that the concentration of cholesterol compounds in fat emboli is more than 10%, whereas fat from bone marrow contains less than 1%.

The time lag of 24 to 72 hours between injury and the development of respiratory and central nervous system symptoms has been the subject of much discussion. Peltier explained this delay as the time needed to convert neutral fats, which have little effect on the lungs, to fatty acids, which may be extremely irritating and damaging.[15] These fatty acids may cause a local tissue reaction with edema and inflammation progressing to congestion and hemorrhage. At autopsy, the lungs are heavy, congested and atelectatic, with many fat emboli 20 to 100 μ in size.

The relationship between platelets and fat emboli following trauma, stressed by Bergentz in 1961, appears to be extremely important.[16,17] McCarthy and Wilson have shown that a syndrome of "subclinical fat embolism" can be demonstrated after virtually all trauma.[18] Even in patients hospitalized with relatively uncomplicated extremity fractures, there are generally increased alveolar-arterial oxygen differences, decreased platelet counts, and increasing fibrinogen levels.[18,19] In patients with relatively mild nonthoracic trauma, the arterial P_{O_2} averaged 65 to 70 mm Hg, the P_{CO_2} averaged 30 to 35 mm Hg, and the A-aDO_2 averaged 40 mm Hg. Interestingly, virtually all patients with moderate to severe blood gas changes were essentially asymptomatic.

AXIOM

EVEN MILD NONTHORACIC TRAUMA MAY CAUSE SIGNIFICANT BLOOD GAS AND PLATELET ABNORMALITIES.

Platelet Emboli

Robb,[20] Blaisdell[21] and others have shown that a wide variety of physiologic changes can cause extensive platelet aggregation and embolization. In addition to the platelet emboli, many other particles found in stored blood or formed in the peripheral vascular bed during shock and trauma may be filtered out by the lung. Swank[22] has shown how severely these emboli may impede blood flow. These particles or the serotonin and other vasoactive substances which are released when they disintegrate may greatly alter or impair pulmonary blood flow and ventilation.

When pulmonary thromboembolism is negligible or when reticuloendothelial and fibrinolytic activity is normal, large amounts of procoagulants, products of coagulation and various particles may be cleared

from the microcirculation with minimal morbidity. If reticuloendothelial function has been overwhelmed by intravascular coagulation or microvascular debris or is deficient because of shock or trauma, the stage may be set for progressive pulmonary thromboembolic obstruction.

PITFALL

FAILURE TO USE ADEQUATE IN-LINE FILTERS WHEN GIVING MASSIVE BLOOD TRANSFUSIONS MAY CONTRIBUTE TO MORE RAPID AND MORE SEVERE DEVELOPMENT OF PULMONARY THROMBOEMBOLISM.

Vasoactive Substances

A number of vasoactive substances—including catecholamines, serotonin, histamine, and polypeptides—are released in shock, sepsis and trauma. Thal and Sukhnandan[23] and others have shown that these agents may have profound effects on pulmonary perfusion in experimental animals. Our later studies on isolated perfused dog lungs confirmed these findings and demonstrated that these substances, even in minute quantities, greatly accelerate the development of congestive atelectasis and pulmonary edema even when ventilation, blood flow and perfusion pressure are kept constant.[24]

In recent years much attention has been directed to the role of lysosomes in the development of organ failure following shock, sepsis or trauma. These intracellular vacuoles contain a number of very powerful enzymes which are important in intracellular digestion, particularly in polymorphonuclear leukocytes (P.M.N.). Even mild cellular damage due to trauma, ischemia, hypoxia or infection can cause the lysosomes to break down and liberate their enzymes into the cell, destroying the cell and any other tissue they may contact. James Wilson[25] has shown that leukocytes tend to stick to the pulmonary capillary endothelium after shock or trauma, and breakdown of their lysosomes may cause many of the lung changes that occur following these conditions.

Fluid Overload

Any increase in pulmonary venous or left atrial pressure, whether due to fluid overload or cardiac failure, greatly increases the rate at which respiratory failure develops. Unfortunately, the resuscitation of severely injured patients often requires such large quantities of blood and other fluids that it is extremely easy to administer excessive quantities, particularly during surgery to control massive hemorrhage. Use of large quantities of crystalloids, such as Ringer's lactate, rather than colloids or blood, may have been a major contributing factor to the high incidence of respiratory failure during the Vietnam conflict.

Most patients who die following severe prolonged shock will have extremely heavy, wet lungs at autopsy. This was often felt to be evidence that the physician had overloaded the patient with fluid. Interestingly, however, close examination of the intake and output records of these patients often revealed that excessive fluid had not been given. Furthermore, our studies using the isolated perfused dog lung showed that regardless of how low the pulmonary venous pressure was kept, the lungs eventually became heavy and wet with a microscopic appearance of congestive atelectasis and pulmonary edema.[24] Even after incision of all accessible pulmonary veins to get the pulmonary venous pressure as close to zero as possible, pulmonary edema would develop if the perfusion continued for a long enough period. However, if the pulmonary venous pressure was elevated even slightly, the rate of development of pulmonary edema was increased two- to three-fold. Use of a perfusate with a hematocrit less than 30%, perhaps due to simultaneous dilution of the plasma proteins, also accelerated the formation of the congestion and edema.

The Swan-Ganz catheter[26] for measurement of pulmonary capillary wedge pres-

sure (PWP) has proved to be a valuable monitoring aid in patients with acute respiratory failure, cirrhosis, acute myocardial infarction or failure, peritonitis and extensive trauma. Civetta[27] and Berger[28] have shown that there is often a poor correlation between central venous pressure and pulmonary capillary wedge pressure. However, over a range of 0 to 40 mm Hg, pulmonary capillary wedge pressure and left atrial pressure were essentially identical. There may be elevation of the pulmonary artery systolic and diastolic pressures in patients with respiratory failure, and the severity of the condition is related to the magnitude of the gradient between pulmonary artery end-diastolic pressure and the pulmonary capillary wedge pressure. This gradient, normally less than 3 mm Hg, decreases as the condition improves. These observations have demonstrated that previously unsuspected changes of great magnitude occur in the lesser circulation with great frequency.

AXIOM

FLUID OVERLOADING OR CONGESTIVE FAILURE MAY GREATLY INCREASE THE LIKELIHOOD OR SEVERITY OF RESPIRATORY FAILURE.

Aspiration

Aspiration of gastric contents occurs frequently following major trauma and can quickly cause severe damage to the lungs. Aspiration is most apt to occur either at the time of the trauma or during the induction of or emergence from anesthesia. It is good practice, therefore, to insert a nasogastric tube when a patient with severe trauma is first seen to remove as much gas or fluid as possible, especially if the patient is lethargic or may be given a general anesthetic. However, if great care is not taken to keep the stomach empty and the nasogastric tube functioning well, gastric contents may move up along the nasogastric tube into the pharynx and then into the larynx and lungs.

PITFALL

THE PHYSICIAN'S CONFIDENCE IN LEVIN OR SALEM-SUMP TUBE SUCTION OF THE STOMACH TO PREVENT ASPIRATION, PARTICULARLY IN PATIENTS WHO HAVE RECENTLY EATEN SOLID FOOD, MAY BE EXCESSIVE.

Pathology

The pathologic changes that occur in the lung during the development of respiratory failure following trauma tend to follow a sequence:

1. swelling and disruption of the pulmonary capillary endothelium,
2. interstitial edema,
3. congestive atelectasis,
4. pulmonary edema,
5. hyaline membrane formation, and
6. varying amounts of pneumonitis.

AXIOM

BY THE TIME THAT THE PULMONARY PROBLEM BECOMES APPARENT CLINICALLY, A RATHER ADVANCED DEGREE OF CONGESTIVE ATELECTASIS IS USUALLY PRESENT.

Very soon after shock or trauma, abnormal polymorphonuclear leukocytes accumulate and appear to fuse to the walls of capillaries.[25] As seen on electron photomicrography, the limiting membrane of these polymorphonuclear leukocytes became tightly opposed to the plasmalemma of the endothelium in arterioles, capillaries, and venules. As the abundant lysosomes in these leukocytes break down, the powerful hydrolytic enzymes that are released can cause severe damage to the capillary endothelium and adjacent tissue. Spaces between endothelial cells develop and allow increasing quantities of fluid to enter the interstitial spaces.

The increasing quantity of fluid in the interstitial spaces causes the lungs to stiffen and become heavy and interferes with the movement of oxygen from the alveoli into the capillaries. This process is accelerated if excessive quantities of fluid, especially crystalloids, are administered at this time. As a consequence, tidal volume tends to fall and the work of respiration increases. In spite of an increased minute ventilation due to an increased respiratory rate, the arterial Po_2 tends to fall. Since carbon dioxide diffuses so readily and since the patient is usually hyperventilating at this time, the excretion of carbon dioxide is generally increased and the arterial Pco_2 is often decreased by at least 5 to 10 mm Hg.

As the process continues, a progressive atelectasis develops. At the same time, perhaps because of fat or platelet emboli or the action of vasoactive substances, the capillaries may become so disrupted that interstitial hemorrhage may also occur. It is this congestive atelectasis that is so characteristic of the post-traumatic or shock lung syndrome.

If the process is not corrected, increasing quantities of fluid eventually begin to enter the alveoli. This pulmonary edema fluid is relatively high in protein and not only further interferes with ventilation and gas exchange directly but, by inactivating surfactant, also increases the tendency toward atelectasis. At this point the lungs are often at least two to three times their normal weight and so beefy-red with congestion that they appear to resemble liver on cut section. Many patients die during this phase, but if the patient lives long enough the protein in pulmonary edema fluid tends to precipitate out and forms hyaline membranes lining the alveoli.

The amount of pneumonitis present varies considerably; however, eventually all these patients develop a significant amount of superimposed pulmonary infection. This pneumonitis further compounds the problem by increasing the amount of bronchopulmonary secretions and atelectasis and by further destruction of the involved tissue. Sudden development of large areas of pneumonitis may be due to aspiration of gastric contents.

DIAGNOSIS

Clinical

PITFALL

IF VENTILATORY ASSISTANCE IN THE CRITI-
CALLY INJURED IS DELAYED UNTIL THERE IS
CLINICAL EVIDENCE OF RESPIRATORY FAILURE,
MANY PATIENTS WILL DIE.

If pulmonary insufficiency in critically
ill or injured patients is allowed to progress
to the point that respiratory distress is apparent clinically before intensive therapy is
begun, the mortality rate approaches 95%.[1]

On the other hand, when specific pulmonary changes are anticipated and prophylactically treated vigorously, the morbidity and mortality are substantially reduced.

SITUATIONS FREQUENTLY ASSOCIATED WITH
RESPIRATORY FAILURE. Some of the clinical
situations that are frequent precursors to
respiratory failure following trauma include shock, three or more organ injuries
or large bone fractures, sepsis, flail chest,
coma, previous pulmonary disease and age
greater than 65 years.[29] Although there is
much individual variation, the greater the
number of these situations or factors involved, the greater the chance that respiratory failure will develop. It is practically
certain that virtually all patients with shock
and sepsis, especially from severe peritonitis, will develop some degree of respiratory failure.

PHYSICAL EXAMINATION

AXIOM

THE FIRST AND OFTEN THE ONLY CLINICAL
EVIDENCE OF EARLY RESPIRATORY FAILURE IS
A MILD TO MODERATE TACHYPNEA.

In spite of a reduced tidal volume, the
tachypnea often increases minute ventilation by at least 25 to 50%. Examination of
the lungs at this time usually reveals nothing more than a few rales and perhaps a
slight decrease in the breath sounds at the
lung bases.

As the process continues, the work of
breathing subtly but progressively increases. Although this increased effort is
usually associated with an increased minute
ventilation until late in the process, the
effective alveolar ventilation progressively
decreases. These changes often occur so
slowly that they may not be noticed unless
looked for carefully.

PITFALL

IT IS SOMETIMES ASSUMED THAT A PA-
TIENT'S PULMONARY FUNCTION IS SATISFAC-
TORY BECAUSE "HIS COLOR IS GOOD."

Cyanosis is a late sign of respiratory failure and may not develop in anemic patients until or unless there is a very severe
impairment of blood flow to the skin. It
usually takes a minimum of 5.0 gm of reduced hemoglobin in the capillaries of the
skin before a patient appears cyanotic.

Use of the accessory muscles of respiration, flaring of the alae nasi and restlessness
are usually very late signs of respiratory
failure and generally indicate severe cerebral hypoxia. The restlessness due to the
discomfort caused by an injury, surgery or
an endotracheal tube is sometimes difficult
to differentiate from restlessness due to
hypoxia. Close examination of hypoxic patients, however, will reveal that their movements tend to be purposeless, abrupt and
irregular, whereas the actions of a patient
who is adequately oxygenated are generally directed to reducing a particular irritant and are slower and more repetitive.
If in doubt, it is best to assume that the
patient is hypoxic; if narcotics or sedatives
are given to a patient with a pulmonary
problem, ventilation will be further reduced.

PITFALL

IF A PATIENT WHO IS RESTLESS FOLLOWING
TRAUMA OR SURGERY IS SEDATED WITHOUT
CAREFUL ATTENTION TO HIS VENTILATION, HE
MAY DIE OF HYPOXIA OR HYPERCARBIA.

X-rays

AXIOM

IT CANNOT BE ASSUMED THAT PULMONARY FUNCTION IS SATISFACTORY IF THE LUNGS APPEAR RELATIVELY NORMAL ON THE CHEST X-RAY.

Acute respiratory failure following nonthoracic trauma may be associated with minimal changes on the chest x-ray until relatively late in the process. The earliest changes noted usually consist of scattered areas of mild plate-like atelectasis, particularly at the lung bases posteriorly, and increased prominence of the vascular markings. As the pulmonary function continues to deteriorate, the total lung volume often seems to diminish and there is evidence of increasing congestion, progressing to frank pulmonary edema. Simultaneously, many of these patients also develop scattered, fluffy, irregular areas of increased density, similar to those seen with interstitial pneumonitis. These may coalesce into larger areas often exceeding 2 to 3 inches in diameter. These larger areas of pneumonitis-like densities occasionally break down into lung abscesses; when this occurs, there is a possibility that aspiration may have occurred 24 to 96 hours earlier. In patients with thoracic trauma, pulmonary contusions may appear rapidly as large rounded irregular infiltrates, usually confined to one side of the chest. There may also be varying degrees of pleural changes and hemothorax or pneumothorax, intra-abdominal damage or infection causing elevation of the diaphragm, and occasionally a significant hydrothorax, which greatly increases the tendency to atelectasis.

Blood Gases

AXIOM

YOU CAN'T JUDGE A PATIENT'S BLOOD GASES BY LOOKING AT HIM—UNTIL IT IS TOO LATE.

Although arterial blood gases provide data which are invaluable for guiding therapy, they cannot be followed blindly and they must be carefully checked to ascertain that they correlate properly with the patient's clinical condition and other chemical studies. If there is any suspicion that a blood gas report may be in error, it should be repeated; if there is still any question concerning its reliability, the test should be repeated at the same time as a sample from an individual known to have normal gas values is tested.

P_{CO_2}. Carbon dioxide is so readily diffusible across the alveolar-capillary membrane that it is an excellent guide to the amount of alveolar ventilation. Proper transfer of oxygen, on the other hand, requires that ventilation, distribution, perfusion and diffusion all be relatively normal.

Traditionally the normal range for the arterial P_{CO_2} has been considered to be 35 to 45 mg. Following trauma, however, patients generally hyperventilate, lowering the average arterial P_{CO_2} by at least 5 to 10 mm Hg, so that the normal values in an injured patient should generally be considered 30 to 40 mm Hg. If the P_{CO_2} in an acutely injured patient who does not have a metabolic alkalosis exceeds 40 mm Hg, an airway, pulmonary, chest wall, diaphragm or central nervous system problem must be strongly suspected, and if the underlying cause cannot be corrected almost immediately ventilatory assistance with a respirator should be provided.

AXIOM

IF THE ACUTELY INJURED PATIENT IS NOT HYPERVENTILATING, DAMAGE TO THE BRAIN, AIRWAY, LUNGS OR CHEST WALL OR CEREBRAL DEPRESSION DUE TO DRUGS OR ALCOHOL MUST BE SUSPECTED.

CO_2 is so diffusible that it is excreted rapidly as long as there is reasonable alveolar ventilation. By the time that the pulmonary changes are so severe that the P_{CO_2} begins to rise above 45 mm Hg in the acutely injured patient, the respiratory failure is often irreversible.

If the Pco_2 is less than 20 to 25 mm Hg, excessive pain, inadequate tissue perfusion, sepsis or metabolic acidosis must be looked for. Severe hypocarbia should not be allowed to persist because it can interfere with proper cerebral blood flow. In rare instances, the cerebral vasoconstriction may be so severe that the respiratory center may become hypoxic and stimulate even more severe hyperventilation. Furthermore, if the patient is allowed to develop a severe combined metabolic and respiratory alkalosis, the prognosis is much poorer.[30]

When evaluating the arterial Pco_2, it is important to consider it in the light of the standard bicarbonate and pH. For example, an elevated Pco_2 in the presence of an elevated pH and metabolic alkalosis is a normal compensatory response and, although it does indicate hyperventilation, it does not indicate whether or not the lung is damaged. On the other hand, if the patient has a metabolic acidosis, an elevated Pco_2 is generally not found until severe, irreversible respiratory failure has developed.

Po_2. The arterial Po_2 is important because it reflects not only the function of the lungs but also the potential amount of oxygen available to the tissues. Hemoglobin saturation of 100% may be associated with a Po_2 exceeding 670 mm Hg, and a saturation of 97.7% is generally associated with a Po_2 of 100 mm Hg. In contrast, an oxygen saturation of 90% is usually found with a Po_2 of only 60 mm Hg, which is generally considered borderline respiratory failure and the minimal acceptable oxygenation for adequate tissue metabolism.

In order to properly interpret the arterial Po_2, it must be correlated with the clinical condition and other factors including ventilation, the Fio_2 (concentration of inspired oxygen), age, temperature and pH (Bohr effect), 2,3-diphosphoglycerate (2,3-DPG) and pulmonary disease or damage. The adequacy of ventilation is the first factor to consider whenever there is any decrease in the arterial Po_2. Even a mild reduction in ventilation, which may have relatively little effect on the Pco_2, can cause a moderate to severe decrease in arterial Po_2, particularly in severely injured patients.

The Fio_2 must always be considered when evaluating the blood gases in a patient breathing a mixture other than room air. Even mild increases in the inspired oxygen concentration can raise the arterial Po_2 to normal levels during early respiratory failure and can easily lead to the belief that only a minimal impairment of pulmonary function is present. A patient breathing 40% oxygen ($Fio_2 = 0.4$), for example, would be expected to have an arterial Po_2 of 190 to 240 mm Hg, and a patient breathing 100% oxygen ($Fio_2 = 1.0$) would be expected to have an arterial Po_2 of 550 to 670 mm Hg.

After the age of 30 years, the average arterial Po_2 in apparently healthy persons falls about 3 to 5 mm Hg for each additional decade. Whereas a young man might have an arterial Po_2 of 90 to 100 mm Hg while breathing normally, an apparently healthy patient of 70 years or older might be expected to have an arterial Po_2 as low as 60 to 70 mm Hg. Thus, while a low arterial Po_2 in an elderly individual may not be unusual, there may be some value to empirically giving some oxygen to older patients following trauma while maintaining adequate ventilation.

Increased temperature and acidosis shift the oxygen-hemoglobin dissociation curve to the right (Bohr effect) so that, at any particular oxygen saturation, the plasma Po_2 will be increased. In contrast, cold and alkalosis tend to shift the oxygen-hemoglobin dissociation curve to the left, thereby reducing the plasma Po_2. In general, an increase of 0.1 in the pH reduces the Po_2 by about 10%, while an increase in temperature 1 C tends to increase the Po_2 by about 5%. Thus, a patient with a 97.7% oxygen-hemoglobin saturation at a pH of

7.4 and temperature of 37 C would generally provide a P_{O_2} of 100 mm Hg, and, at a pH of 7.6 and temperature of 35 C, a P_{O_2} of about 72 mm Hg.

Blood storage and sepsis alter red blood cells so that their content of 2,3-diphosphoglycerate (2,3-DPG) falls, thereby reducing the ability of the red cells to release oxygen to the plasma. As a consequence, patients who are septic or who have received multiple transfusions will tend to have a low arterial P_{O_2} even if the oxygen saturation is relatively normal, and less oxygen will be available to the tissue. Thus, there appears to be some value to maintaining a hemoglobin concentration above 12.5 gm/100 ml, using the freshest blood possible, in acutely injured patients.

Previous pulmonary disease can cause hypoxemia or hypercarbia, but diagnosis from the history, physical examination and chest x-ray may be difficult. In the critically injured patient, however, if no other cause for a low P_{O_2} is evident, it must be assumed that pulmonary disease or damage is present and treatment planned accordingly. If the patient has a very low arterial P_{O_2} on room air, but an arterial P_{O_2} close to the expected range when breathing higher concentrations of oxygen, this may be a clue that the patient has pre-existing pulmonary disease.

ALVEOLAR-ARTERIAL OXYGEN DIFFERENCES (A-aDO_2). Although serial arterial P_{O_2} and P_{CO_2} determinations are far superior to physical examination for diagnosing early pulmonary insufficiency, when considered separately they can also be deceptive. With most injuries or illnesses, especially sepsis, patients generally are tachypneic and, in spite of a reduced tidal volume, often increase minute ventilation by at least 25 to 50%. As a consequence, the arterial and alveolar P_{CO_2} may fall to 20 to 30 mm Hg. Since there is normally an A-aDO_2 of only 10 to 20 mm Hg, the arterial P_{O_2} in a young, healthy hyperventilating patient with a low arterial P_{CO_2} (even

if the arterial P_{O_2} remains constant or falls only slightly) the A-aDO_2 will be increased significantly. Consequently, in patients who are hyperventilating the A-aDO_2 is a much better guide to pulmonary function than the arterial oxygen saturation, P_{O_2} or P_{CO_2} alone.

We have found that the A-aDO_2 while breathing room air in patients with previously normal pulmonary function can be estimated fairly accurately by subtracting the sum of the arterial P_{O_2} and P_{CO_2} from 145. Thus, if the arterial P_{O_2} is 70 mm Hg and the arterial P_{CO_2} is 20 mm Hg while breathing room air, the A-aDO_2 is about 55 mm Hg, indicating a rather advanced pulmonary problem. A more accurate indication of the degree of pulmonary damage is obtained if the arterial P_{O_2} is corrected to a pH of 7.40. Thus, an arterial P_{O_2} of 70 mm Hg at a pH of 7.50 would be approximately 10% higher (77 mm Hg) if the pH were 7.40 (see Bohr effect above). When evaluating the A-aDO_2 on room air, we generally consider 10 to 20 mm Hg as normal, 20 to 40 mm Hg as mild respiratory insufficiency, 40 to 55 mg as moderate respiratory insufficiency and 55 or more mm Hg as severe respiratory failure.

If the patient has had previous pulmonary disease, particularly an alveolar-capillary block, the A-aDO_2 on room air may be extremely high while the A-aDO_2 on 100% oxygen may be relatively normal. Interestingly, we found empirically that the A-aDO_2 on room air in mm Hg, on the average, is about 15 greater than the percentage of physiologic shunting in the lungs (Qs/Q). Thus, an acutely injured, previously healthy patient with an A-aDO_2 of 55 mm Hg on room air on the average has a physiologic shunt in his lungs of about 40%.

Some authors have stressed the value of the A-aDO_2 while the patient is breathing 100% oxygen, and they have suggested that significant respiratory failure is present if the value is greater than 300 mm Hg. We have found, however, that the A-aDO$_2$ on 100% oxygen often does not correlate with the Qs/Q as well as the A-aDO$_2$ on room air. Furthermore, many of our patients who have A-aDO$_2$ of 300 mm Hg or more on 100% oxygen have had only mild to moderate evidence of a respiratory problem.

PHYSIOLOGIC SHUNTING IN THE LUNG[1,2]

AXIOM

PHYSIOLOGIC SHUNTING IN THE LUNG IS THE MOST ACCURATE TEST FOR DIAGNOSING IMPENDING OR EARLY RESPIRATORY FAILURE.

Normally the amount of blood that is shunted through the lung without being completely oxygenated is about 3 to 8% of the cardiac output. Mild to moderate pulmonary damage may increase the shunt to 20 to 40%, which generally is well tolerated as long as reasonable respiratory care is provided and sepsis is prevented or controlled.

If the shunt exceeds 40%, however, most patients with severe trauma, sepsis or shock will die of respiratory failure unless the primary disease and the changes in the lung can be reversed with intensive treatment. Patients with shunts greater than 60% rarely survive regardless of the treatment given.

AXIOM

TRENDS ARE MUCH MORE IMPORTANT THAN ABSOLUTE NUMBERS WHEN EVALUATING BLOOD GASES OR PULMONARY FUNCTION TESTS.

One of the advantages of determining physiologic shunting of the lung is the relative ease with which it can be measured. All that is needed is an airtight system for giving 100% oxygen and apparatus for measuring hemoglobin-oxygen saturation and the Po$_2$. After the patient receives 100% oxygen for 15 to 30 minutes, arterial blood

and mixed venous blood are drawn from the right ventricle or pulmonary artery. Using the differences between the maximum possible (theoretical) arterial oxygen content, the actual arterial oxygen content and the actual venous oxygen content, the percentage of physiologic shunting may be calculated from Berggren's formula:[31]

$$\% \text{ Physiologic shunting} = \frac{{}^cA_{O^2} - {}^cC_{O^2}}{{}^cV_{O^2} - {}^cC_{O^2}} \times 100\%$$

${}^cA_{O^2} = $ Oxygen content of arterial blood

${}^cC_{O^2} = $ Theoretical maximal oxygen content of pulmonary venous blood (assuming 100% saturation and a Po$_2$ of 667 mm Hg)

${}^cV_{O^2} = $ Oxygen content of mixed venous blood

Thus, if the theoretical oxygen content of pulmonary venous blood is 20 vol %, the arterial content is 19 vol % and the mixed venous oxygen content is 15 vol %, the shunt is:

$$\frac{20 - 19}{20 - 15} \times 100 \text{ or } 20\%$$

The formula for calculating oxygen content is:

$$O_2 \text{ content (ml/100 ml)} = \frac{(O_2 \text{ satn})}{100}$$

$$\times (\text{Hb conc}) \times 1.34 + (Po_2) \times (0.003)$$

Thus, if the Hb is 10.0 gm/100 ml, the oxygen saturation is 90% and the Po$_2$ is 60 mm Hg. The oxygen content is $(10.0) \times (1.34) \times (0.9) + (60) \times (0.003) = 12.24$ ml/100 ml. If a Swan-Ganz catheter is in place, the mixed venous blood from the pulmonary artery is ideal for these calculations. However, if pulmonary artery or right ventricular blood is not available, blood drawn from the superior vena cava through a CVP line has an oxygen content which is normally relatively close to that of mixed venous blood. Calculations using a CVP sample, although not nearly as accurate as those using a mixed venous sample, can provide a useful estimate of the Qs/Q. In patients with severe sepsis or high cardiact output, the shunt calculated from the CVP blood may be 25 to 50% higher than the shunt calculated from pulmonary arterial blood.

Lung Compliance

It is rather easy to gain some impression of lung compliance if the patient is on a respirator. Passive ventilation of a "normal patient" with a tidal volume of 500 ml requires an inflation pressure of about 10 to 15 cm H_2O. Of this 10 to 15 cm H_2O pressure, 4 to 5 are usually needed to overcome airway resistance, 3 to 5 to overcome chest wall resistance, and 3 to 5 to overcome lung resistance. Most of the increase of inflation pressure needed as acute respiratory failure develops is due to increased stiffness or resistance of the lung itself. For example, if it takes 30 cm H_2O pressure to inflate the lungs with a tidal volume of 500 ml, it probably took about 20 cm H_2O pressure to inflate the lungs themselves. Thus, the stiffness or resistance of the lungs in this individual is probably about four times greater than normal and, as a corollary, lung compliance is only one fourth of normal.

AXIOM

IF THE INFLATION PRESSURES ON A VENTILATOR SUDDENLY RISE, A PNEUMOTHORAX OR MAJOR AIRWAY OBSTRUCTION MAY HAVE DEVELOPED.

Oxygen Consumption

Although oxygen consumption might be expected to suffer very quickly and severely when the patient develops respiratory failure, it often remains relatively normal until very late, even with advanced pulmonary insufficiency.[32] Measurements of oxygen consumption are, therefore, of little value in the diagnosis of impending or early respiratory failure.

TREATMENT

Our best results in the prevention and treatment of respiratory failure have been obtained when the problem was anticipated and intensive care was provided before there was clinical or blood gas evidence that pulmonary insufficiency was developing.

AXIOM

PULMONARY INSUFFICIENCY IN CRITICALLY ILL OR INJURED PATIENTS IS USUALLY EXTREMELY DIFFICULT TO REVERSE WHEN IT HAS REACHED THE STAGE WHERE ITS DIAGNOSIS IS OBVIOUS CLINICALLY.

The prevention or treatment of respiratory failure may be divided into the following categories: nursing care, general supportive measures, careful regulation of fluids, drugs, inhalation therapy, correction of airway problems and ventilators.

Nursing Care

Various aspects of nursing care can greatly reduce the incidence and severity of respiratory failure. These include encouraging the patient to cough and take deep breaths, frequent position changes, elevation of the head and chest, and chest physiotherapy. Such care should be almost routine in any nursing unit caring for critically ill or injured patients.

COUGH

AXIOM

THE SIMPLEST AND MOST EFFECTIVE WAY TO PREVENT ATELECTASIS AND RESPIRATORY FAILURE IS A GOOD COUGH.

The mechanism of coughing may be divided into two phases. During the first phase, the glottis is closed, the abdominal muscles are tensed and the intrathoracic pressure is increased. This "tussive squeeze" may literally push or squeeze secretions out of the alveoli and smaller bronchioles into the larger bronchioles. During the second phase of the cough, the glottis is opened and the air rushes out of the alveoli as a "bechic blast" carrying the secretions from the larger bronchioles and bronchi into the pharynx.

If the patient has excessive chest and abdominal pain after surgery or trauma, he will be unable to bear down effectively to build up the intrathoracic pressure needed for a good cough, and his efforts to cough will sound as if he is only trying to clear his throat. It is important to give just enough pain medication to reduce the pain so that he can cough and take deep breaths, but not enough to depress his ventilation.

If the patient has a tracheostomy, it will also be impossible for him to bear down properly unless the tracheostomy is temporarily occluded. It is important to stress that a tracheostomy allows the nurse and physician to remove excess secretions from the large bronchi but reduces the effectiveness of deep coughing which is needed to remove secretions from the alveoli and smaller bronchioles.

DEEP BREATHS. Although the tidal volume in a healthy individual is usually about 6 to 10 ml/kg, he unconsciously takes a deep breath or "sighs" at least several times an hour. This tends to open alveoli that are not inflated by the normal tidal volumes. Prolonged ventilation of the lung with a low fixed tidal volume tends to result in atelectasis in the poorly ventilated portions of the lung. This atelectasis, in turn, causes increased production of secretions, and thus a vicious cycle of increased secretions and atelectasis may begin.

Stimulating the patient and encouraging him to breathe deeply, cough and move must be done frequently, but with proper allowance for resting between these efforts. Several techniques have been used to encourage an improved ventilation; these include "blow-bottles" (in which the patient blows into a tube forcing colored fluid from one bottle into another), various gadgets which increase the patient's external dead space (the resultant increase in the arterial P_{CO_2} should increase the patient's efforts to breathe), and incentive spirometers (in which a light goes on if the patient inhales to a predetermined volume on pressure). All of these are valuable if used conscientiously and intelligently as part of a comprehensive approach to improving ventilation.

FREQUENT POSITION CHANGES. Gravity is an important factor in regulating regional blood flow in the lungs. Thus, the dependent portions of the lung tend to contain more blood, are stiffer and more difficult to ventilate. As a consequence, patients who lie flat on their backs for prolonged periods tend to develop atelectasis and pneumonia in the posterior and inferior portions of their lungs.

To prevent these changes in the dependent portions of the lungs, the patient's position should be changed frequently, both up and down and from side to side. Critically ill patients, particularly those who are elderly or have congestive heart failure, must not be kept flat on their backs for more than an hour or two at a time. Nurses may be reluctant to move or turn severely injured patients because it is difficult and may require the combined effort of several people, and there may be tubes or I.V.s that might become disarranged when the position is changed.

If the patient has pulmonary disease or damage confined primarily to one lung, that lung should be kept elevated as much as possible. In other words, the patient with a contusion of the right lung should lie on his left side much more than on his right.

Early ambulation is generally the optimal type of position change. The erect position is ideal for coughing and ventilating deeply and the walking improves the venous return from the legs and may reduce the incidence of pulmonary emboli.

ELEVATION OF THE HEAD AND CHEST. The head and chest should be kept as high as possible for as long as possible unless the patient is hypovolemic. This tends to relieve some of the intra-abdominal pressure on the diaphragm and allows the diaphragm to move further with less effort, thereby increasing tidal volume and reducing the work of respiration. Elevation greater than 30° may be difficult to accomplish in some individuals, but padded foot supports may be of great help in this regard.

Position is particularly important if the patient is obese or pregnant or has severe distension of the abdomen from ascites or ileus. The obese patient particularly should be nursed on his side or with his head elevated. If the patient has atelectasis, pneumonitis, or pulmonary contusion confined to one lung, that lung should be kept superior to the uninvolved lung as much as possible; otherwise, the weight of the chest and the elevation of the diaphragm by the adipose tissue in and on the abdomen will greatly reduce intrathoracic volume and increase the effort and pressure required to maintain adequate ventilation.

CHEST PHYSIOTHERAPY. Chest physiotherapy can be an important part of respiratory care, but is almost completely ignored in many hospitals. Breathing exercises may improve the patient's ability to take deep breaths and to cough. When done properly with the patient in various positions, almost all portions of both lungs may be systematically inflated. Other techniques— use of vibrators and gentle thumping or pounding on the patient's chest or back, particularly with the basilar or injured portions of the lung in an elevated position —may help loosen and remove secretions that the patient might otherwise be unable to mobilize.

General Measures

There are several general supportive measures that may be performed by the physician to decrease the factors which can cause respiratory failure or to increase the ability of the patient to ventilate and cough properly. These include control of infection, reduction of abdominal distension, control of pain, reduction of oxygen demands and, in an occasional case, thoracentesis.

CONTROL OF INFECTION

AXIOM

PROGRESSIVE RESPIRATORY FAILURE IS ALMOST IMPOSSIBLE TO REVERSE IF THE PATIENT HAS SEVERE UNCONTROLLED SEPSIS.

Sepsis, especially when due to pneumonia or peritonitis, causes an early, severe deterioration of pulmonary function which may not be apparent clinically or on casual examination of blood gases until quite late. All sites of infection must be rapidly and completely drained, removed, or controlled. Early and complete debridement of any necrotic tissue is extremely important; such tissue not only increases the likelihood of infection but also is a source of vasoactive substances and other material which may damage the lungs. The use of specific antibiotics, on the basis of appropriate cultures, forms an important second line of defense. If culture reports are not available, antibiotics directed toward the most likely organisms must be started after cultures of all possible infected material are taken (Chap. 29).

REDUCTION OF ABDOMINAL DISTENSION. Distended bowel and increased ascitic fluid may elevate the diaphragm markedly, reducing tidal volume and increasing the work of respiration. This should be prevented or corrected with early nasogastric suction or paracentesis as needed. To function properly, the nasogastric tube must be positioned properly and checked frequently for patency. Irrigation with 10 to 20 cc of saline every one to two hours may be very helpful in this regard. If the small bowel is already severely distended, a long intestinal tube can occasionally be manipulated past the ligament of Treitz to deflate this area.

Patients who may develop respiratory difficulty and require prolonged gastrointestinal intubation may benefit by having such tubes passed through a gastrostomy or jejunostomy rather than the nose or mouth. Tubes in the pharynx tend to increase upper respiratory secretions and the incidence and severity of atelectasis. The irritation of the upper respiratory passages by these tubes may also increase the pain of coughing and reduce its effectiveness.

Severe ascites, usually due to previous liver or cardiac disease, should be relieved carefully. Rapid paracentesis may improve ventilation but may also cause sudden severe hypotension. Sudden release of the pressure of the ascitic fluid against the inferior vena cava and other intra-abdominal veins may cause a rapid expansion of the intra-abdominal vascular capacity, resulting in a sudden decrease in the venous return to the heart.

REDUCTION OF PAIN. One of the greatest deterrents to effective ventilation and coughing following trauma is pain from an injury or surgery involving the chest or upper abdomen. In most patients, mild to moderate pain from chest wall contusions or one or two fractured ribs can be controlled fairly well with codeine, using ½ to 1 grain every 4 to 6 hours. Morphine or meperidine may be more effective for relieving pain, but can also depress the cough reflex and ventilation quite markedly. For patients with severe pain from multiple fractured ribs or a thoracotomy incision, an intercostal nerve block may produce dramatic benefit for many hours (Chap. 20).

REDUCTION OF OXYGEN DEMAND. If the patient has a high fever or is severely agitated, his oxygen requirements may be greatly increased. Under such circumstances, the patient's temperature should be reduced to normal with drugs, sponging, or induced hypothermia and sedatives may be used with caution.

The accurate diagnosis of the cause of restlessness in an injured or postoperative patient is often difficult to make and yet is extremely important. If the restlessness is due to pain, analgesics may be indicated; however, if the restlessness is due to hypoxia, such agents may be lethal.

THORACENTESIS. A restricted tidal volume, especially in patients with chest trauma or peritonitis, may be due to increased pleural fluid in one or both sides of the chest. Although 300 to 500 ml of fluid often cannot be detected on routine physical or x-ray examination of the chest, it may be important to remove it in patients with marginal respiratory function. The thoracentesis should be performed relatively high to avoid injury to the diaphragm or subdiaphragmatic organs. Use of a plastic catheter to aspirate the fluid may help reduce the incidence of puncture of the lung. A chest x-ray should be obtained at the termination of the procedure to detect any pneumothorax that may have been caused by the procedure. It should also be remembered that rapid removal of large amounts of pleural fluid may occasionally cause hypotension or pulmonary edema in the lung which is suddenly expanded.

AXIOM

A SUDDEN RISE IN INFLATION PRESSURE FOLLOWING THORACENTESIS OR INSERTION OF A SUBCLAVIAN VEIN CATHETER IS DUE TO A PNEUMOTHORAX UNTIL PROVEN OTHERWISE.

Fluid Therapy

"KEEP THE PATIENT DRY." During the initial resuscitation of critically injured patients, large amounts of blood and other fluids may be required to restore adequate vital signs and tissue perfusion. Unfortunately, in such patients there is often a fine line between the quantity of fluid needed to correct hypovolemia and the amount which may overload the circulation and increase pulmonary congestion. Although rapid restoration of the blood volume is important to survival, the administration of fluid must be done carefully, with close attention to vital signs, CVP or PWP, urine output and tissue perfusion and frequent auscultation of the lung bases. Proper regulation of the fluids may be particularly difficult during surgery to control massive hemorrhage from larger veins or arteries in the chest or abdomen. Since anesthesia, respiratory failure, and positive pressure ventilation may all raise the CVP, these must be considered when regulating the fluid intake.

Once the patient has been resuscitated, it is extremely important to limit fluid intake while at the same time maintaining an adequate tissue perfusion and urine output.

Hill,[33] for example, attempts to dehydrate the patient until the serum osmolarity rises from a normal of 270 to 290 mOsm/L to 350 mOsm/L. In our own experience, it has been difficult to dehydrate patients above 310 to 320 mOsm/L without compromising tissue perfusion.

In patients likely to develop respiratory failure, the hourly fluid intake should be carefully correlated with the hourly vital signs, CVP and urine output, the hematocrit and blood gases every 8 to 24 hours, the body weight and serum electrolyte determinations daily. If the serum proteins are low, they should also be measured every 48 to 72 hours. Urine sodium determinations may also be helpful. In some patients, the earliest evidence of inadequate tissue perfusion and hypovolemia is a urine sodium concentration less than 20 mEq/L.

In the patient with renal insufficiency and frank or impending respiratory failure, a severe dilemma exists. If inadequate fluid is given, the renal problem may become more severe; if enough fluid is given to maintain a good urine output, the respiratory problem may be greatly aggravated. In such patients careful use of small doses of diuretics, for example 5 mg of furosemide every 1 to 2 hours as needed, may allow slow dehydration without causing hypovolemia due to a sudden severe diuresis.

USE MORE COLLOIDS AND LESS CRYSTALLOIDS. Experimentally, hemodilution with excessive amounts of crystalloids greatly accelerates the movement of fluids into the interstitial spaces and alveoli and causes rapid deterioration of isolated lung preparations. Maintenance of relatively normal plasma protein levels and colloid osmotic pressure may temporarily help to reduce this transudation of fluid. Whole blood may be used until the hemoglobin level is 12.5 gm/100 ml or higher. Albumin, or preferably plasma, should then be given in sufficient quantity so that at least a quarter of the fluids given are colloids. If severe shock or tissue damage has occurred, relatively more colloids may be required (Chaps. 5, 7, and 10).

Although there may be some value to preventing severe hypoproteinemia, excessive administration of albumin may also cause problems. In patients with increased capillary permeability due to severe sepsis or shock, the albumin may rapidly enter the interstitial space of the lungs and draw fluid with it, thereby increasing the interstitial edema. Consequently, if albumin is given, it must be given with careful attention to the fluid intake and output, using small doses of diuretics as necessary to prevent fluid retention.

MAINTAIN A HEMOGLOBIN BETWEEN 12.5 AND 14.0 GM/100 ML. Hemodilution to a hemoglobin less than 10.0 gm/100 ml causes a rapid deterioration in pulmonary function in isolated lung preparations.[21] Our clinical studies have also shown significant improvements in physiologic shunting in the lung when the hemoglobin is raised from below 10.0 to above 12.5 gm/100 ml. Another advantage of higher hemoglobin levels is the increased oxygen-carrying capacity of the blood; this is particularly important in patients who have cardiac or respiratory failure and those who have had multiple transfusions of old blood. If the patient may already be overloaded with fluid, increasing the hematocrit is best done with slow transfusions of packed red blood cells.

Drugs

BRONCHODILATORS. Although bronchospasm or wheezing is not usually a prominent feature in respiratory failure following trauma, it should be treated aggressively if it is found.

Aminophylline should not be used if the patient is hypotensive and should be given cautiously if the patient has arrhythmias, urinary obstruction or renal failure. It may be given: (1) by direct I.V. injection in doses of 250 to 500 mg over a 10- to 20-minute period for acute severe bronchospasm, (2) by slow I.V. infusion of 250 to 500 mg in 50 to 200 ml of fluid over a 1- to 2-hour period, repeated once or twice a day, or (3) as a 250- or 500-mg rectal suppository every 6 to 8 hours.

Isoproterenol should not be used if the patient has arrhythmias or a pulse rate more than 120/minute. The I.V. dose is usually about 5 to 15 gtt/minute of a 0.2 mg/100 ml solution. For inhalation, 0.25 to 0.50 ml of a 1:200 solution can be given in 3 to 5 ml of saline through a nebulizer. Isoetharine (Orcipenaline B.P.), albuterol (Salbutamol, B.P. Schering), beta$_2$ inhalant solutions supposedly can produce bronchodilation similar to that of isoproterenol with less effect on the heart. Salbutamol, which is also effective orally, may well prove to be the ideal agent.

Ephedrine may be very useful if the patient's blood pressure is low. The usual dose is 25 to 50 mg I.M. every 4 to 6 hours as needed. If the bronchospasm is on an allergic basis, Adrenalin (0.2 to 0.5 cc of 1:1000 solution subcutaneously), Benadryl (50 mg I.M. every six hours as needed), and/or hydrocortisone (100 mg I.V. every 4 to 8 hours) may be used.

DIGITALIS (Chap. 32). One of the digitalis preparations should be given if the CVP is excessively elevated, if the lungs are severely congested or if there is any other evidence of cardiac failure. Any condition which increases pulmonary venous pressure, whether it is heart failure or excessive blood volume, will increase pulmonary vascular congestion and aggravate any tendency to respiratory failure. By improving myocardial contractility and reducing left atrial pressure, digitalis may decrease the amount of blood and edema fluid in the lung parenchyma and bronchial mucosa, thereby improving ventilation and gas exchange.

DIURETICS. Relatively large doses of I.V. diuretics may occasionally be required on an emergency basis to prevent or correct pulmonary insufficiency in injured patients with heart failure or evidence of fluid overloading. Great care must be taken, however, to prevent hypovolemic shock as a result of an excessive diuresis, hyponatremia, or hypokalemia.

Not infrequently, efforts to dehydrate an injured patient by fluid restriction alone are unsuccessful because the patient develops severe oliguria. Under such circumstances, furosemide given in doses of 5 to 10 mg by intermittent injection or by continuous infusion in the patient's I.V. fluids may be used to maintain an adequate tissue perfusion and urine output while at the same time providing a progressive dehydration of the patient.

SODIUM BICARBONATE, TRIS BUFFER. If at all possible, the arterial pH should be kept at a relatively normal range of 7.35 to 7.50. Most injured patients initially have a respiratory alkalosis. If shock or hypovolemia persists, however, a metabolic acidosis may develop. If this metabolic acidosis continues in spite of efforts to improve tissue perfusion and the pH is less than 7.35, sodium bicarbonate should be given. In the very late stages of respiratory failure, the patient may eventually also develop a combined respiratory and metabolic acidosis.

The use of sodium bicarbonate at this point may be dangerous because, although it may partially correct the metabolic acidosis, it may result in increased CO_2 retention and a more severe respiratory acidosis. Under such circumstances, tris-hydroxymethylaminomethane (tris buffer) may temporarily restore the pH and P_{CO_2} to a more normal range.

STEROIDS. Two widely differing doses of steroids are currently used in the treatment or prevention of a number of respiratory problems. The smaller doses, equivalent to 50 to 100 mg of hydrocortisone every 4 to 6 hours, may greatly reduce the inflammatory response in the lungs to smoke, aspirated gastric content or allergic bronchospasm, particularly if given prophylactically and maintained for several days. Ashbough also found that steroids given early, in doses of 100 mg cortisone t.i.d. for five days,[34] might prevent the full-blown fat embolism syndrome by decreasing the permeability of the cell membrane to toxic products and by inhibiting access of fatty acids to the endothelial cell. In an occasional patient with a tracheostomy, or with an endotracheal tube and a very irritable trachea causing constant bucking or coughing, a mixture of 25 to 50 mg of hydrocortisone and 25 to 50 mg of lidocaine with 5 to 10 ml of saline may relieve the problem

Massive steroids, in doses equivalent to 150 mg of hydrocortisone per kg body weight, given every 4 to 24 hours by intermittent injection, may occasionally reverse, at least temporarily, progressive severe respiratory failure which might otherwise be lethal. Although convincing data from prospective double-blind studies are not available at this time, many clinicians agree that steroids may be of great help in preventing or treating respiratory failure in some severely injured patients. Much of the benefit of steroids in these very large doses apparently comes from their ability to stabilize lysosomal and cellular membranes,[35] thereby not only decreasing the local release of hydrolytic enzymes and vasoactive substances but also correcting the increased permeability of the endothelium and alveoli. Other effects attributable to massive steroids, such as improved cell metabolism,[36] are harder to confirm in clinical studies. This membrane stabilization effect, which is particularly important in preventing or treating respiratory failure due to sepsis, is apparently dose dependent and is much less apt to occur with even slightly smaller doses.

The earlier the massive steroids are given, the more effective they are likely to be. Tidal volume, respiratory rate, inflation pressures, and blood gases (physiologic shunting in the lung or alveolar-arterial oxygen differences) should be measured carefully before and serially for 1 to 4 hours after the steroids are given. If objective improvement is noted, the dose may be repeated every 4 to 12 hours for a total of 24 to 48 hours, depending on the patient's response. Administration of large doses of steroids for longer periods of time may increase the incidence of stress gastric bleeding and complications from impaired reticuloendothelial function.

OTHER DRUGS. Other drugs that might be of some value in preventing or treating respiratory problems after trauma, particularly in patients with suspected fat emboli, include dextran, heparin, and alcohol. Low-molecular-weight dextran has been recommended to increase blood flow, and heparin has been recommended to reduce the release of serotonin and vasoactive substances by platelets. Results with dextran and heparin, however, are questionable and both these agents may be detrimental in patients with multiple injuries, particularly if there is any suspicion of intra-abdominal or intracranial bleeding. Alcohol may increase the solubility of neutral fat; however, it is rarely used now.

Inhalation Therapy

OXYGEN. The arterial P_{O_2} should be kept above 60 mm Hg and preferably at 80 to

100 mm Hg. The initial efforts to raise the arterial Po₂ should be directed toward improving the patient's ventilation; however, if hypoxia persists in spite of normal or increasing ventilation, oxygen should be administered using the lowest concentration possible to achieve the desired Po₂. Inhaled oxygen concentrations of 40% or less are relatively safe, but prolonged use of higher concentrations, particularly if they exceed 70%, may be associated with an increased tendency to atelectasis and an increased physiologic shunting in the lungs.

AXIOM

IF MORE THAN 40% OXYGEN IS REQUIRED TO MAINTAIN THE ARTERIAL PO₂ OF A SERIOUSLY INJURED PATIENT ABOVE 60 MM HG THE PATIENT SHOULD NORMALLY BE PUT ON A RESPIRATOR.

If the patient is on a respirator and requires more than 40% O₂ to maintain an arterial Po₂ above 80 mm Hg, we will usually be content with a Po₂ of 70 to 79 mm Hg. If more than 70% oxygen is required, we will be content with any Po₂ above 60 mm Hg. Although the inhaled oxygen concentration is an important factor in the development of oxygen toxicity, the arterial Po₂ is probably also important.

Several methods are available for administering oxygen including nasal prongs, nasopharyngeal catheters, masks, nebulizers and ventilators. Nasal prongs are relatively inefficient and seldom supply oxygen concentrations to the patient greater than 40%, but they are generally well tolerated by the patient. Nasopharyngeal catheters can readily provide inhaled oxygen concentrations up to 60%, but if the nasal passage is narrowed or crooked they may be uncomfortable. The tip of the catheter should be visible just above the soft palate; if it protrudes further into the pharynx, it may make the patient gag. Masks can provide oxygen concentrations up to 80 to 100% depending on the minute ventilation of the

patient; however, anxious or restless patients may not tolerate the mask for more than a few minutes at a time.

Oxygen tents usually leak a great deal and seldom provide inhaled oxygen concentrations greater than 30 to 40%. Moreover, they tend to isolate the patient from the nurse and physicians and some patients experience claustrophobia. However, some patients find them very comfortable and the atmosphere inside the tent can be humidified rather well if desired.

AEROSOLIZATION AND NEBULIZATION. Aerosolization or nebulization refers to the introduction of droplets of fluid, mechanically mixed with air or oxygen, into the respiratory tract with or without other medications. The purposes of nebulization include humidification and transport of various medications into the lungs. Humidification may be of benefit by (1) reducing insensible water loss from the lungs, (2) decreasing, by dilution and absorption, the viscosity of mucoid material in the respiratory tract, thus permitting the cilia to function more efficiently, and (3) counteracting the drying effects of the various gases introduced by ventilator.

The most important medications that may be introduced by aerosolization or nebulization include bronchodilators (such as isoproterenol or epinephrine), mucolytics (such as acetylcysteine, potassium iodide, sodium ethasulfate [Tergemist]), surfactants (such as alcohol, propylene glycol), and antibiotics.

Although aerosolization and nebulization may be beneficial, some problems may develop with their use. Ultrasonic nebulizers may provide the large quantities of fluid particles of very small size (0.5 to 3.0 μ) that may cause fluid overload, especially in infants and emphysematous patients. Tergemist carries an inherent danger from occasional severe allergic reactions to the potassium iodide which it contains. The use of proteolytic agents may cause severe bronchospasm and, rarely, may cause sloughing of large areas of infected trache-

TABLE 1. PARTICLE SIZE PRODUCTION OF NEBULIZERS

Equipment	O₂ Concen. Obtainable	Particle Size	Disposition in Airway
Adult tent	45–55% at 12–15 lpm	17–30 μ	Upper airway
Croupette	30–50% at 10 lpm	15–25 μ	Upper airway and bronchi
Cascade	Used in conjunction	Adds water vapor to gas stream	Delivered air is 100% humidified at body temp.
Jet	Rel. hum. 40% 10 lpm 67% at 3 lpm	20–40 μ	Used only in the humidification of gas to the upper airway
Nebulizers			
Bubble	Rel. hum. 28% at 10 lpm 43 at 3 lpm	20–40 μ	
Ultrasonic	Ultrasonic will put out a volume of 3–6 cc per minute	0.5–3 μ	Will deposit in periphery and alveoli
Puritan all purpose	100%–70% 40% by adjustment of air entrainment opening	Aerosol 0.5–5 μ range—100% humidity	Upper airway and bronchi

obronchial tree; indeed, complete casts of segmental bronchi may occasionally be coughed up or may require bronchoscopic removal.

The value of antibiotics in aerosol solutions is controversial. The results reported in the literature range from great enthusiasm to total rejection from the viewpoint of either local therapeutic effect or establishment of adequate blood levels. We have, moreover, evidence of minute granulomas forming in areas of antibiotic deposition, and the risk of sensitizing the respiratory tract as the end-organ in antigen-antibody reaction patterns must always be kept in mind.

An important consideration in aerosolization or nebulization is the particle size. Each nebulizer has its own advertised characteristics of particle size production (Table 1). Unfortunately, no manufacturer will guarantee the particle size produced by his machine under specific conditions. Furthermore, these instruments will vary in their output relative to the physical substance nebulized, gas flow through the instrument, fluid properties, temperature of the gases, age of the instrument, and the mechanics of nebulization or aerosolization. Widely differing estimates of the site of the ultimate deposition of particles of various sizes while breathing through the mouth have been reported; however, our experience suggests a distribution as shown on Table 2. When the patient is breathing through an endotracheal or tracheostomy tube, larger particle sizes penetrate into more peripheral areas of the lung.

When making a choice of nebulizers, the physician must keep in mind not only the area where he desires the droplets to deposit but the problems of fallout if the

TABLE 2. PARTICLE SIZE AND SITE OF DEPOSITION

Particle Size (microns)	Deposition Site
100–25	May not enter respiratory tract
25–10	Trapped in nasopharynx
10–5	Fallout in larynx
5–1.5	Carlina to alveoli
2–0.5	Can enter alveoli with 95% retention of those down to 1 μ
1–0.5	Stable with minimal settling

delivery tubes are too long and shunting back and forth in the valvular system of the instrument. Most nebulizers, however, with adequate aerodynamic propulsion will rain out at the desired levels, assuming no obstructive areas or changes in patterns of air flow.

INTERMITTENT POSITIVE PRESSURE BREATH-ING (IPPB)

PITFALL

THE ROUTINE USE OF IPPB MAY BE EX-CESSIVELY RELIED UPON TO DECREASE THE INCIDENCE OR SEVERITY OF PULMONARY COM-PLICATIONS AFTER TRAUMA OR SURGERY.

IPPB may be beneficial if used thoughtfully in selected patients to achieve specific results; otherwise it is expensive and time consuming and may decrease other efforts at maintaining a clear airway and optimal ventilation. IPPB may be used to stimulate the patient to breathe and cough more deeply or to bring moisture or medication down into the smaller bronchioles where it can be most effective.

AXIOM

THE VALUE OF IPPB DEPENDS TO A LARGE EXTENT ON THE ENTHUSIASM AND EFFORTS OF THE THERAPISTS OR NURSES ADMINISTER-ING IT.

Some of the substances or medications that can be given with IPPB include water, saline, alcohol, mucolytic agents and bronchodilators. Water is more irritating than saline and, therefore, tends to stimulate a better cough and more sputum production. Alcohol may reduce the stability of bubbles and help break them up; this may be particularly important in the treatment of pulmonary edema.

Mucolytic agents are indicated if the tracheobronchial secretions are too thick to be removed adequately by coughing or suction. A frequent drug combination used in IPPB treatments includes 2 to 4 cc saline, 0.5 to 1.0 cc acetylcysteine (Mucomyst) and 0.24 to 0.50 cc of 1:200 isoproterenol (Isuprel). Some of the mucolytic activity of Mucomyst is lost from mechanical denaturation when it is given with the nebulizer, and it is generally more effective if given directly into a tracheostomy or endotracheal tube, starting with 1 to 2 ml of a 1:2 dilution. Since acetylcysteine may cause severe bronchospasm in some individuals, it should be used cautiously in patients with asthma or emphysema.

If the bronchial mucosa is excessively dry and secretions very thick, the trachea may be irrigated with saline, 3 to 5 ml at a time. Greater amounts of saline may wash out surfactant and increase atelectasis. Occasionally, a slow drip of saline at 1 to 3 drops per minute into a tracheostomy or endotracheal tube may supply an appropriate amount of moisture to the tracheobronchial tree.

All drugs instilled directly into the tracheobronchial tree, except for sympathomimetic agents such as epinephrine and isoproterenol, have a bronchoconstrictor effect. It is, therefore, important to add bronchodilators in inhalation therapy. Unfortunately, if the pulse is over 120 to 130/minute or is irregular, isoproterenol even in minute amounts may cause severe tachycardia or arrhythmia.

The effective dose of Isuprel by intermittent positive pressure is extremely variable. In some individuals, two drops of a 1:200 solution in 5 cc of saline will produce a significant bronchodilatation. In other patients, more than 0.5 cc will have to be given. We have generally found no decrease in ventilatory resistance with isoproterenol unless there has also been a significant increase in the pulse rate during its administration.

Maintenance of an Open Airway

The airway must be kept clean and clear at all times. False teeth and any foreign material must be removed from the mouth and pharynx as soon as the patient is seen, and constant vigilance, thereafter, must be maintained by all concerned.

POSITIONING THE PATIENT. In extremely lethargic or unconscious patients, the tongue may fall back into the pharynx occluding the airway. If there are no contraindications to placing the patient on his side (such as possible fracture of the spine, ribs, extremities, etc.), this is the best position. Unnecessary tracheostomies can be avoided in some inebriated or unconscious individuals simply by turning them to the side. Patients with bilateral or severely fractured jaws may present a similar problem.

ORAL AIRWAY. If no other convenient reliable method for supporting the tongue and jaws is available, the jaw can be pulled up and forward until an oral airway is inserted. These plastic or rubber airways may also help to prevent the patient from biting his tongue or an orotracheal tube. The size of the airway can be important, because if it is too long it may irritate the back of the throat and cause vomiting. If the patient is awake or alert, he may not be able to tolerate an oropharyngeal tube, and some other method of maintaining the airway will be needed.

NASOPHARYNGEAL AIRWAY. Occasionally a large tube inserted through one nostril into the pharynx may be used to maintain an adequate airway. This nasopharyngeal airway also allows frequent suctioning of the pharynx, larynx and trachea without repeatedly traumatizing the nasal mucosa.

NASOTRACHEAL SUCTION. Properly performed, nasotracheal suction provides several benefits. It may not only directly remove secretions from the trachea but may also cause the patient to cough much more forcefully and frequently.

The technique of nasotracheal suction is relatively simple, and all nurses and physicians in intensive care units should be trained to do it well. After a well-lubricated, sterile suction catheter with a side-arm is passed through the nose, the head is tilted forward and the tongue is grasped with a gauze 4 × 4 and pulled forward gently. The patient is asked to take deep breaths, and the catheter is advanced rapidly through the glottis while the patient is inhaling. In many instances the presence of the catheter in the trachea causes such forceful coughing that only minimal secretions will be left there for suctioning.

Suction is applied intermittently by covering and uncovering the side-arm of the catheter while the catheter is moved up and down inside the trachea. Suction should not be applied for more than five seconds at a time so as to prevent severe hypoxia during the procedure. Since severe agitation and hypoxia may develop during this procedure, the patient must be monitored closely and the procedure terminated immediately if the EKG or pulse suddenly deteriorates.

BRONCHOSCOPY. If there are excess secretions in the tracheobronchial tree which cannot be removed by coughing or tracheal aspiration, bronchoscopy is indicated. In most instances, bronchoscopy is best done in the operating room with experienced personnel and equipment. In many instances, however, endoscopy can be much more readily and rapidly performed at the bedside with a portable bronchoscope. Although there is usually a need for topical or general anesthesia to perform an adequate examination, in some patients, especially those who are less responsive, effective endoscopy can often be performed with little or no anesthesia. If a tracheostomy is present, the procedure is much easier.

Some physicians feel that the flexible fiberoptic endoscopes have greatly improved our ability to remove secretions from more distal portions of the tracheobronchial tree. These bronchoscopes can be generally passed through the nose or mouth with relative ease and minimal discomfort to the patient. The flexible bronchoscope can also be passed through a side-arm attached to a tracheostomy or endotracheal tube so that the patient may be ventilated during the procedure.

ENDOTRACHEAL TUBES. If an adequate airway cannot be maintained in any other way or if ventilatory assistance is required, an orotracheal or nasotracheal tube may have to be inserted. The orotracheal tube generally has a larger lumen and, since it can generally be inserted more rapidly and accurately, this is the type usually used in emergencies. Because of the relatively small size of the nasal passages, nasotracheal tubes have a narrow lumen, increasing the resistance to ventilation and passage of suction catheters. Trauma to the turbinates or the adenoids during passage of the tube can produce massive hemorrhage which may occasionally require postnasal packing and blood transfusions. In addition, prolonged use of this tube may cause a severe pansinusitis. Many intensivists prefer nasotracheal intubation because it is generally better tolerated by the patient. With practice it can be inserted blindly with minimal manipulation and only mild discomfort to most patients.

The greatest problem with the use of any endotracheal tube is the inadequate removal of secretions. The suction catheter must extend beyond the tip of the tube down to and including the main stem bronchi. The suction catheter can coil or kink during passage, and use of the stethoscope to hear the clicking of the catheter as it passes right or left into the main stem bronchi is the only sure way to determine that the catheter has reached its desired location.

Another problem or hazard with any tracheal tube is the trapdoor clot or crust which may be extremely difficult to diagnose or correct unless the tube is removed. The suction catheter may pass through the endotracheal tube very easily, pushing the attached plug of debris aside; however, on withdrawing the suction catheter, the clot or crust is drawn back onto the distal tip of the endotracheal tube, partially or completely occluding it again. If a one-way valve effect is produced, a progressive entrapment of respiratory gases may occur in the lungs during the expiratory phase, resulting in progressive hypercarbia, hypoxia, distension of the lungs and chest cage.

Additional problems may be caused by the cuff which is usually present on both tracheostomy tubes and the anesthesia type of endotracheal tubes when they are inflated to obtain a relatively airtight system for proper inflation of the lungs by most of our positive pressure respirators. When this cuff is inflated, it may press against the trachea causing mucosal erosions and/or necrosis of the tracheal cartilages, with eventual formation of a tracheal stenosis or stricture. The incidence of tracheal stenosis following long-term intubation with cuffed tubes has been reported to be as high as 20% in patients requiring the tubes for two weeks or longer.[37]

These complications can be reduced by using soft, very compliant cuffs. Another way to reduce the pressure against the tracheal cartilages is to inflate the balloon only partially, allowing a slight leak around it during inflation. Alternately, a large lumen tube can be used without a cuff and the leak can be compensated for with large volumes of introduced gases via the respirator.

Since tracheal stenosis often does not cause any clinical signs or symptoms until it has occluded about 80% of the cross-section of the trachea, it has been advocated that laminagrams of the trachea be obtained on anyone who has been on a respirator for more than 4 to 5 days.[38]

If ventilatory assistance is required for more than 48 to 72 hours, the decision must be made to continue endotracheal intubation or to perform a tracheostomy. This decision depends primarily upon the skill of the individuals taking care of the patient. In centers where physicians have special interest and experience in this area and dedicated and enthusiastic care can be provided, endotracheal tubes have been kept in place with relatively few complications for four weeks or longer, particularly in children. In our own experience, if it appears that the patient will probably require only 48 to 96 hours of airway or ventilatory support, if the patient is tolerating the tube well, and if there are only minimal secretions, we will leave the endotracheal tube in place. On the other hand, if it appears that the patient will need a respirator for more than five days, if he is tolerating the tube poorly, or if there are excessive tracheal secretions, we will perform a tracheostomy after 48 to 72 hours.

TRACHEOSTOMY. Some of the more frequent indications for performing a tracheostomy include:

1. damage to the larynx or trachea,
2. inability to establish an adequate airway in any other manner,
3. excessive secretions which cannot be removed adequately in any other way, and
4. prolonged ventilatory support, particularly if excessive secretions are present or if the patient tolerates the endotracheal tube poorly.

Although a tracheostomy is often life-saving, it can cause a number of serious complications including bleeding, pneumothorax, infection, tracheal stenosis and fistulae. The bleeding may occur at the time that the tracheostomy is performed or during the next few days if vessels in the area are not adequately ligated or if a coagulation problem develops. Rarely, a rigid tracheostomy tube, particularly if the tracheal opening is below the third ring and the tip of the tube is angled forward, may cause catastrophic erosion of the innominate artery where it crosses the trachea. If the tracheostomy is performed through the second and third tracheal cartilages, a rubber or plastic tube is used, and the tip of the tube is angled posteriorly, there is less likelihood of this problem developing. The presence of a "pulsating tracheostomy" suggests that the tip

of the tracheostomy tube is pressing against a large artery and its position should be changed. Withdrawing the tracheostomy 1 to 2 cm and angling the tip posteriorly will usually eliminate or greatly reduce the pulsations.

Any dissection laterally away from the trachea during the performance of the tracheostomy may result in penetration of the adjacent pleura and development of a pneumothorax; this is especially apt to occur in infants and children in whom the pleural reflections closely approach the trachea. X-rays of the chest should be taken immediately after the tracheostomy is completed and then daily for at least two days to be sure that any pneumothorax which may develop is diagnosed early.

Infection may occasionally occur in the mediastinum and surrounding tissues, particularly if the tube must be replaced blindly within 48 to 72 hours. Use of a tracheal flap hinged distally and sutured to the skin provides direct and ready access to the tracheal lumen. The skin should be sutured only loosely around the tracheostomy tube so that air and secretions can drain around the tube readily. Eventually, virtually all tracheostomies will develop positive bacterial cultures. If the patient has been receiving multiple antibiotics, Pseudomonas organisms can often be cultured from the tracheostomy after a few days. The careful use of sterile technique and new catheters each time the tracheostomy is suctioned may prevent or forestall many of these infections.

Occasionally, a small opening into the trachea at the tracheostomy site may persist for several weeks or months after the tracheostomy tube is removed. In general, it will eventually close if there is no supervening disease or obstruction. If the fistula persists in spite of an open trachea and larynx, various plastic procedures may be used to close the opening.

The material used in making the tracheostomy tubes may be important. Aluminum tubes are very light weight, thin walled and somewhat less expensive; however, the distal end tends to be sharp and may lacerate the trachea; in addition, since the adapter edges are easily dented at the site of attachment to the respirator, leaks often develop at this site. Chrome-plated tubes have an additional hazard of "flaking" so that chromium particles dropping into the tracheobronchial passages may cause a foreign-body reaction. Plastic tubes appear to be very useful, and are currently our favorite. One disadvantage is that they tend to collect thick secretions and crusts distally, similar to those found on endotracheal tubes.

Ventilators

To avoid any confusion in terminology, the terms "ventilator" and "respirator" should be clarified. Many physicians use these terms interchangeably; however, "ventilator" is more accurate and is preferable. The process of respiration includes not only the mechanical transport of gases to the level of the alveolar-capillary membrane but also the entire sequence of physiologic mechanisms related to their exchange and utilization in the tissues. Ventilators, on the other hand, only introduce gases into the respiratory tract at varying pressures and volumes. In other words, they are mechanical transport mechanisms in the most basic sense, and will be considered so for the balance of this discussion.

Proper use of ventilators requires constant attention by specially trained nurses and other personnel, preferably in intensive care units. In addition to careful frequent auscultation of the lungs, tidal volume, respiratory rate and blood gases must also be closely monitored. Since the amount of effective alveolar ventilation is difficult to evaluate clinically, it is important to measure tidal volume directly. Rapid and around-the-clock availability of blood gas determinations is also mandatory.

TYPES OF VENTILATORS. Classically, all in-line ventilators have been divided into two main groups: pressure-limited and volume-limited. These instruments act directly through the normal pathway of gas flow (naso-oropharyngeal or tracheal) and, in general, utilize positive pressure mechanisms, though negative phases are available. The advantages of the in-line ventilators include their ability to provide gas flows directly into the lungs, with minimal interference to access to the patient by the physicians and nurses. In patients with multiple fractured ribs, the ability of these ventilators to stabilize the chest wall internally is of major importance. The main disadvantage of the in-line machines is the increased hazard of bacterial contamination of the respiratory tract because of interference with the cough reflex and with the activity of the mucociliary blanket and alveolar macrophages. Other hazards include increased intrapulmonary pressures (which may cause rupture of alveoli, resulting in a pneumothorax with or without mediastinal and cervical emphysema) and increased intrathoracic pressure (leading to a decreased venous return to the right side of the heart).

INDICATIONS FOR USING VENTILATORS. A ventilator should be used whenever the clinical situation or laboratory studies suggest that the patient cannot ventilate adequately by himself or has frank or impending respiratory failure.

PITFALL

IF VENTILATORY ASSISTANCE IS DELAYED IN INJURED PATIENTS UNTIL THERE IS CLINICAL EVIDENCE OF RESPIRATORY FAILURE, THE LUNG CHANGES ARE OFTEN IRREVERSIBLE.

It is important, therefore, to anticipate the need for ventilator assistance in those clinical situations which are often followed or accompanied by respiratory failure. Some of the more frequent clinical indications for early ventilatory assistance in injured patients may include:

1. flail chest, particularly involving seven or more ribs,
2. severe CNS depression due to trauma, drugs or infection,
3. traumatic injury to three or more organs,
4. generalized peritonitis involving the sub-diaphragmatic areas,
5. previous severe pulmonary disease,
6. severe prolonged shock, or
7. massive smoke inhalation or aspiration of vomitus.

Some of the laboratory values which may indicate a need for ventilatory assistance in injured patients include:

1. arterial Po_2 less than 50 mm Hg on room air,
2. arterial Pco_2 greater than 50 mm Hg (in the absence of a metabolic alkalosis),
3. alveolar-arterial oxygen difference on room air greater than 55 mm Hg,
4. physiologic shunting in the lung of 40% or more,
5. need for more than 40% O_2 to maintain an arterial Po_2 of at least 60 mm Hg.

These guides should not be followed blindly; therapy for critically injured patients must be individualized and correlated with all available clinical and laboratory data. In many instances, even a tendency for the patient's laboratory values to approach those mentioned above may also be an indication for ventilatory assistance.

HOW TO ORDER VENTILATOR CARE. The ordering of ventilatory assistance is extremely important, but unfortunately this is often left to the respiratory therapist. Ventilator therapy requires just as careful consideration by the physician as the ordering of digitalis, insulin and other important therapy. The ordering of ventilatory assistance should include:

1. the ventilator to be used,
2. the pressure ranges to be used,
3. the volume range to be used,
4. the concentration of gases to be delivered,
5. the respiration rates to be used,
6. the frequency of sighing,
7. nebulization and humidification,
8. added dead space, if any, and
9. positive end-expiratory pressure, if any.

Since the status of the patient requiring respirator care may change frequently and rapidly, these orders should be reviewed several times a day.

The Ventilator to be Used. As a general rule, when critically ill or injured patients require ventilatory assistance we prefer the volume-limited machines. Pressure-limited ventilation can be used if the patient's pulmonary difficulty is minimal, if he is alert and cooperative, if the chest wall is stable and if the lung compliance is relatively normal. If the pressure-limited ventilator does not significantly and rapidly improve ventilation, a volume-limited machine should be employed. The volume-limited ventilators are especially valuable if there is significant respiratory difficulty or increased resistance to airflow; however, peak flow rates must be adjusted to levels that will not cause excessive turbulence.

It is generally much easier for the patient to synchronize with the pressure-limited ventilators, but this often limits the amount of ventilation that can be obtained and, if bronchospasm or a partial bronchial obstruction develops, the tidal volume may fall to dangerous levels before it is detected. The actual brand of ventilator to be used will be determined largely by the experience of the personnel involved. In general, the ventilator with which they have had the most experience is the best one to use.

Pressure Ranges to be Used. The pressure required to inflate the lungs properly varies greatly from patient to patient and is largely dependent on the tidal volume to be used, the cooperation of the patient and the resistance of the airway, lungs and chest wall. In general, inflation pressures below 30 cm H_2O are relatively safe, whereas if inflation pressures greater than 40 to 45 cm H_2O are used there is an increased risk of alveolar rupture and a resultant pneumothorax. However, in patients with severe bronchospasm, interstitial fibrosis or congestive atelectasis, higher pressures may be required, hopefully only temporarily, to provide an adequate tidal volume.

The Volume Ranges to be Used. In general, we would like our patients with severe trauma, sepsis or shock to have a tidal volume of at least 12 to 15 ml/kg body weight. However, if a pressure of 40 cm H_2O or higher is required to achieve this amount of inflation, we will generally settle for a lower tidal volume. Although much lower tidal volumes would frequently provide adequate blood gases, we feel that the higher tidal volumes may help prevent or reverse the progressive atelectasis that often develops in critically injured or septic patients.

The Gases to be Delivered. The gases most frequently used in ventilation are oxygen and compressed air. Wherever possible, the oxygen concentration is limited to the minimum required to provide reasonable oxygenation of the blood. Although there is some controversy in the literature about the toxicity of high concentrations of inhaled oxygen, we feel that high concentrations can be damaging to the lungs if given for long periods of time.

AXIOM

IN MOST SITUATIONS THE INJURED PATIENT NEEDS VENTILATORY ASSISTANCE, AND ADDITIONAL OXYGEN IS USUALLY ONLY A SECONDARY CONSIDERATION.

We generally attempt to keep the arterial Po_2 in the range of 80 to 100 mm Hg, using as little oxygen in the inhaled gas mixtures as possible. As mentioned earlier in this chapter, we are quite content with an arterial Po_2 of 80 to 100 mm Hg if it can be achieved with 40% or less oxygen. If 41 to 70% oxygen concentrations are required, we are satisfied with a Po_2 of 70 to 79 mm Hg, and if 70 to 100% oxygen is required, with a Po_2 of 60 to 69 mm Hg.

Helium, with an atomic number of 1, lowers the specific gravity and the effective density of gaseous mixtures. This is of value where air flow is very turbulent, as in obstruction in the larger air passages, where the pressure required is proportional to the square of the rate of flow and the density of the mixture. An 80% helium: 20% oxygen mixture has a density of 0.33 compared to 1.00 for air. However, such a mixture is useful only in obstructive disease of the larger upper airways, not in obstruction of smaller airways as seen in asthma. The use of helium has ebbed and flowed with theorists for many years, but the physical properties of this agent (low molecular weight and diameter, and lack of chemical interaction) make it ideally suited for prevention of atelectasis.

The Respiratory Rates to be Used. We have found that a respiratory rate of 12 to 16 per minute is ideal in most patients, particularly if high tidal volumes are used. Unfortunately, many patients, particularly those with sepsis, delirium tremens or brain damage, will be severely tachypneic regardless of the minute ventilation and blood gases. In some instances, I.V. diazepam (Valium) or morphine will successfully correct the tachypnea and will allow the patient to synchronize properly with the respirator. Occasionally, however, severe tachypnea cannot be controlled until or unless the patient is paralyzed with succinylcholine or curare—which may cause additional problems.

The Frequency of Sighing. Under normal circumstances, individuals unconsciously and involuntarily take several deep breaths each hour. This hyperinflation of the lungs, referred to as sighing, inflates many of the alveoli that are not expanded with the usual tidal volumes. When a patient is put on a respirator, especially of the volume-limited type, the resultant fixed tidal volume, if provided for prolonged periods, will allow atelectasis to develop in those areas which are poorly ventilated. To prevent this from occurring, it is important to hyperinflate the lungs for two to three breaths with a tidal volume which is 1½ to 2 times greater, providing of course, that the inflation pressures do not exceed 50 to 60 cm H_2O. The optimal frequency of sighing varies from patient to patient, but 6 to 12 times per hour appears to be satisfactory for most patients.

Nebulization and Humidification. In general, we give the maximum humidity possible because of the drying effect that most ventilators have on the tracheobronchial tree. In small patients, however, particularly those with heart disease, some of the newer machines can provide so much moisture that the quantity of fluid absorbed through the alveoli and bronchial mucosa may overload the circulation and cause congestive heart failure. If the gases are warmed by the machine to temperatures approaching those of the patient, they will have a higher relative humidity and less moisture will be needed. Careful observation of the thickness or dryness of the bronchial secretions, correlated with the patient's weight and vital signs, should allow the physician to determine the ideal amount of humidification.

With some ventilators, various medications can be conveniently nebulized and introduced intermittently into the patient's tracheobronchial tree with the inhaled gases. Pressure-limited ventilators have traditionally been employed for this purpose (see the section on IPPB).

Added Dead Space. When large tidal volumes are used, particularly if the patient's respiratory rate is high, the resultant high minute ventilation may cause a severe respiratory alkalosis. In addition to the acid-base problems that may result, an arterial Pco_2 below 20 to 25 mm Hg may cause severe vasoconstriction in cerebral vessels. On the other hand, if the Pco_2 is allowed to rise above 40 to 45 mm Hg, the hypercarbia may stimulate the patient's respiratory center causing him to take extra breaths out of phase with the ventilator. As a consequence, we attempt to maintain an arterial Pco_2 of 30 to 35 mm Hg.

In many patients, particularly those with sepsis, it may be extremely difficult to keep the arterial Pco_2 above 30 mm Hg. The three possible methods currently available for correcting such hypocarbia include reducing the tidal volume, reducing the respiratory rate, or adding dead space between the ventilator and the patient. Since we prefer to maintain a high tidal volume, and since many patients will remain tachypneic in spite of large doses of diazepam, morphine and $MgSO_4$, we are frequently forced to add dead space. The dead space is added in increments of 50 ml and is adjusted according to the arterial Pco_2, allowing at least 15 minutes for the blood gases to stabilize after each increment is added. Although we frequently use 100 to 200 ml of dead space, more than 300 ml is seldom tolerated by the patient, perhaps because of the additional pressure required to expel the gas from the lung through the increased length of tubing.

Positive End-expiratory Pressure (PEEP). In an effort to prevent or treat the atelectasis which almost inexorably develops in many critically ill and injured patients, a number of investigators have proposed various methods for keeping the alveoli inflated during the expiratory phase. In many patients, positive end-expiratory pressure (PEEP) performs this function very well. Although some ventilators have adjustable PEEP built into the machine, it can also be provided with virtually any ventilator by attaching tubing to the expiratory port and then placing the other end of the tubing under 5 to 10 cm H_2O. Although some investigators have used 15 or more cm H_2O of PEEP, pressures exceeding 10 cm H_2O are not tolerated by our patients and our best results have been obtained with 5 to 8 cm H_2O. The patient generally tolerates increasing PEEP if only 1 to 2 cm H_2O pressure are added at a time.

GETTING THE PATIENT ON THE VENTILATOR. When the patient is first placed on the ventilator, there may be difficulty in synchronizing the machine with his efforts to breathe, particularly if a volume respirator is used. The initial step to be taken under such circumstances is to attempt to remove the patient's drive or stimulus to breathe. This may include lowering the Pco$_2$ to less than 20 to 25 mm Hg and raising the Po$_2$ to over 100 mm Hg. In some cases, large doses of sedatives such as diazepam, morphine, chlorpromazine, and MgSO$_4$ may be required. If these maneuvers and drugs are not successful, muscle paralyzers such as succinylcholine or curare may occasionally be required. In general, it is easier for patients to synchronize with the pressure-limited ventilators, but these respirators may not provide adequate ventilation if partial obstruction develops.

STERILIZATION OF EQUIPMENT. Sterilization of nebulizers and ventilators is of great importance. Various chemical soaks have been recommended; however, the basis of all sterilization lies in vigorous mechanical cleansing including scrubbing with a brush and rinsing with copious amounts of water as soon after use as possible. The use of ethylene oxide sterilization has been somewhat limited by the great diversity of plastics now being used and the problem of "washout" time. Many of the plastics retain the ethylene oxide in solution and it becomes necessary to flush out the gas chamber for prolonged periods of time (18 to 24 hours, and even up to 72 hours). The effects this produces in regard to engineering design, costs, and equipment stores are obvious. The best solution in this regard is the use of disposable tubing and other parts that may be exposed to bacterial and viral contamination. Unfortunately, the cost factor for these disposable items remains significant.

Special Problems

THE OBESE PATIENT. Some of the most difficult respiratory problems are found in the treatment of extremely obese patients. Because of the high inflation pressures required to overcome the weight of the thoracic cage and abdominal viscera, none of the ventilatory equipment currently available will adequately ventilate these pa-

tients without the hazards of rupture of the lungs and decreased venous return.

The extremely obese patient should be placed either on his side or in the semi-Fowler position to decrease the pressure of the abdominal contents on the diaphragm. The erect position also helps to distribute the blood inside the lungs to the areas which are ventilated best. The use of ventilators which can serve as assistor or controller with automatic phase controls (e.g. Engstrom ventilators) may be helpful. The early and long-term use of endotracheal tubes and tracheostomy to decrease the dead space and the aerodynamic resistance through the upper respiratory tract may also reduce the pressures required.

HYPERINFLATION OF THE LUNG. An infrequent but important hazard of mechanical ventilation is expansion rupture of the lungs. Although early diagnosis may be difficult, any delay in treatment may have fatal consequences. Cyanosis and inflation difficulties may precede the appearance of subcutaneous emphysema and circulatory arrest by only a few minutes. These changes are most apt to occur while the patient is receiving inhalation anesthesia; however, careful consideration of this syndrome is urged whenever patients are being ventilated with volume-limited instruments, particularly if high tidal volumes or inflation pressures are used. Studies by Lenaghan et al.[39] revealed that expansion rupture of the dog lung may occur with sustained mean airway pressures as low as 40 mm Hg. However, if any lung damage has occurred (e.g. shock lung syndrome) the lung may rupture with much lower pressures. Lesions are usually found bilaterally, with evidence of tension pneumothorax, interstitial emphysema and mediastinal and pericardial emphysema. Although the arterial pressure may fall abruptly, the central venous pressure may increase only gradually. Treatment includes placing the patient in a head-down position, opening the pericardium and pleural spaces (to relieve the pneumothorax and pericardial emphysema), and performing open cardiac massage. In rare situations, it may be possible to patch the larger leaks in the lung.[40]

Prevention is best accomplished by an awareness that this grave complication can occur during the use of controlled or assisted ventilation. Equipment manufacturers can also help by providing reliable relief valves to prevent sustained pressures exceeding 40 mm Hg in the airway system.

SUDDEN REVERSAL OF RESPIRATORY ACIDOSIS. One of the special hazards of respiratory therapy is the sudden reversal of the chronic respiratory acidosis in patients with severe chronic lung disease and/or chronic obstruction of the larynx or trachea. Such patients gradually adapt to the altered intrathoracic pressures and compensate for the respiratory acidosis by developing a metabolic alkalosis with high blood bicarbonate levels. If endotracheal intubation or tracheostomy is performed and the patient is ventilated vigorously, the arterial Pco_2 may fall abruptly from high to subnormal levels. Since the blood bicarbonate concentrations change rather slowly, the patient's acid-base status will change rapidly from a compensated respiratory acidosis to a severe combined respiratory and metabolic alkalosis. This sudden rise in pH will cause an abrupt fall in the ionized calcium levels, which in turn may cause severe arrhythmias or cardiac arrest. In addition, the hypocarbia may cause enough cerebral vasoconstriction to produce unconsciousness.

The sudden changes in intrathoracic pressure may abruptly alter venous return and cause hypotension or pulmonary edema. With the sudden decrease in Pco_2 and change in pH, the secretion of catecholamines may decrease with a concomitant failure of the stress-reaction peripheral vascular and cardiac responses, which may also cause hypotension, arrhythmias or cardiac arrest.

After a chronic airway obstruction is relieved the sudden return of intrapulmonic pressures to normal may result in a definitive lag in the return of the Hering-Breuer reflexes to normal activity. This, coupled with a decreased CO_2 stimulus to the central nervous system, removes the two most potent elements in the control of respiration and may cause prolonged apnea; provisions must be made to provide adequate ventilation in such patients after the airway problem is corrected. Thus, it is clear that sudden changes in pulmonary function or dynamics, even if they are in the direction of normal, may cause a cardiorespiratory collapse. Unless the patient with chronic pulmonary or airway problems is deteriorating rapidly, correction of the abnormality should be gradual and facilities should

TABLE 3. TEN FREQUENT ERRORS IN THE MANAGEMENT OF POST-TRAUMATIC RESPIRATORY FAILURE

1. Forgetting that even relatively mild non-thoracic trauma may be associated with significant pulmonary changes.
2. Failing to use adequate in-line filters, particularly when giving massive transfusions to patients in shock.
3. Delaying ventilator assistance until there is obvious clinical evidence of severe pulmonary insufficiency.
4. Assuming that a patient's lungs are functioning well if the patient is in no distress, has "good color," and has a relatively normal chest x-ray.
5. Failing to realize that, if an acutely injured patient is not hyperventilating, he is likely to have damage to brain, airway, lungs or chest wall or cerebral depression from drugs or alcohol.
6. Failing to realize that an injured patient with only a mild to moderate reduction in his arterial Po_2 but a large reduction in his Pco_2 may actually have a severe alveolar-arterial O_2 difference associated with significant pulmonary changes.
7. Relying on absolute values rather than trends in the patient's ventilation and blood gases.
8. Relying on oxygen rather than ventilation to improve a reduced arterial Po_2.
9. Delaying or performing inadequate or excessively rapid dehydration of patients with respiratory failure.
10. Routinely ordering and relying on unsupervised IPPB treatments to prevent or correct respiratory failure.

be immediately available for treatment of arrhythmias, cardiac arrest or apnea.

SUMMARY (TABLE 3)

Respiratory failure after trauma must be anticipated and treated prophylactically. The primary condition, especially if it is shock or sepsis, must be rapidly and aggressively controlled.

If the clinical situation suggests that there is a reasonable possibility that respiratory failure may develop or if the A-aDO$_2$ or physiologic shunting is above 55 mm Hg or 40% respectively, ventilatory assistance is usually mandatory. Once respiratory failure in critically ill or injured patients becomes obvious clinically, the process is seldom reversible.

REFERENCES

1. Wilson, R. F., et al.: Clinical respiratory failure after shock or trauma: prognosis and methods of diagnosis. Arch. Surg., 98:539, 1969.
2. Wilson, R. F., et al.: Clinical respiratory failure in clinical shock and trauma. J. Surg. Res., 1:361, 1969.
3. Wilson, R. F., et al.: Physiologic shunting in the lung in critically ill or injured patients. J. Surg. Res., 12:571, 1970.
4. Simmons, R. L., et al.: Acute pulmonary edema in battle casualties. J. Trauma, 9:760, 1969.
5. McNamara, J. J., and Stremple, J. F.: Causes of death following combat injury in an evacuation hospital in Vietnam. J. Trauma, 12:1010, 1972.
6. Burford, T. H., et al.: Traumatic wet lung; observations on certain physiologic fundamentals of thoracic trauma. J. Thorac. Surg., 14:415, 1945.
7. Burke, J. F., et al.: High output respiratory failure. Ann. Surg., 158:4, 1963.
8. Henry, J. N., et al.: The effect of experimental hemorrhagic shock on pulmonary alveolar surfactant. J. Trauma, 5:691, 1967.
9. Pattle, R. E., et al.: Properties, function, and origin of the alveolar lining layer. Proc. Roy. Soc. London, 148:217, 1958.
10. Levin, S. E., et al.: Surface active alveolar lining material and pulmonary disease. Surg. Gynec. Obstet., 123:53, 1966.
11. Greendyke, R. M.: Fat embolism in car deaths. New York J. Forums Sci., 9:201, 1964.
12. Gauss, H.: The pathology of fat embolism. Arch. Surg., 9:593, 1924.
13. Lehman, E. P., and Moore, R. M.: Fat embolism. Arch. Surg., 14:621, 1927.
14. Peltier, L. F.: Fat embolism: the toxic properties of neutral fat and free fatty acids. Surgery, 40:665, 1956.
15. LeQuire, V. S., et al.: A study of the pathogenesis of fat embolism based on human necropsy material and animal experiments. Amer. J. Path., 35:999, 1959.
16. Bergentz, S. E.: Studies on the genesis of post-traumatic fat embolism. Acta Chir. Scand., 282 (Suppl.):1, 1961.
17. Attar, Safuh, et al.: Alterations in coagulation and fibrinolytic mechanisms in acute trauma. J. Trauma, 9:939, 1969.
18. McCarthy, B., et al.: Subclinical fat embolism: A prospective study of 50 patients with extremity fractures. J. Trauma, 13:9, 1973.
19. Wilson, R. F., et al.: Respiratory and coagulation changes after uncomplicated fractures. Arch. Surg., 106:395, 1973.
20. Robb, H. J.: The role of microembolism in the production of irreversible shock. Ann. Surg., 158:685, 1963.
21. Stallone, R. J., Lim, R. C., Jr., and Blaisdell, F. W.: Pathogenesis of the pulmonary changes following ischemia of the lower extremities. Ann. Thorac. Surg., 7:539, 1969.
22. Swank, R. L.: Platelet aggregation. Its role and course in surgical shock. J. Trauma, 8:872, 1968.
23. Sukhnandan, R., and Thal, A. P.: Effect of endotoxin and vasoactive agents on dibenzyline pretreated lungs. Surgery, 58:185, 1965.
24. Wilson, R. F.: Unpublished data.
25. Wilson, J. W., Ratliff, N. R., and Harkel, D. B.: The lung in hemorrhagic shock. In vivo observations of pulmonary microcirculation in cats. Amer. J. Path., 58:337, 1970.
26. Swan, H. J. C., et al.: Catheterization of the heart in man with a flow-directed balloon-tipped catheter. New Eng. J. Med., 283:447, 1970.
27. Civetta, J. M., Gabel, J. C., and Laver, M. B.: Disparate ventricular function in surgical patients. Surg. Forum, 22:136, 1973.
28. Berger, R. L.: Circulatory assistance with intra-aortic balloon counter pulsation. In The Manual of Critical Care Medicine (Vinocour, B., Artz, J. S., and Sampliner, J., Eds.). Boston, Little, Brown & Co., in press.
29. Sankaran, S., and Wilson, R. F.: Factors affecting prognosis in patient with flail chest. J. Thorac. Cardiov. Surg., 60:402, 1970.
30. Wilson, R. F., et al.: Severe alkalosis in critically ill patients. Arch. Surg., 105:197, 1972.
31. Berggsen, S. M.: The oxygen deficit of arterial blood caused by non-ventilating parts of the lung. Acta Physiol. Scand., 4 (Suppl. II):1, 1941.
32. Wilson, R. F., et al.: Oxygen consumption in critically ill surgical patients. Ann. Surg., 176:801, 1972.

33. Hill, D. J., et al.: Prolonged extracorporeal oxygenation for acute post-traumatic respiratory failure (shock lung syndrome). New Eng. J. Med., 286:629, 1972.

34. Ashbaugh, D. G., and Petty, T.: Use of corticosteroids in the treatment of respiratory failure associated with massive fat embolism. Surg. Gynec. Obstet., 123:493, 1966.

35. Janoff, A., et al.: Pathogenesis of experimental shock: IV. Studies of lysosomes in normal and tolerant animals subjected to lethal trauma and endotoxemia. J. Exp. Med., 116:541, 1962.

36. Schumer, W.: Dexamethasone in oligemic shock. Physiochemical effects in monkeys. Arch. Surg., 98:259, 1969.

37. Pearson, F. G., and Andrews, M. J.: Detection and management of tracheal stenosis following cuffed tube tracheostomy. Ann. Thorac. Surg., 12:371, 1971.

38. Westgate, H. D., and Roux, K. L.: Tracheal stenosis following tracheostomy, incidence and prediction. Anesth. Analg., 49:393, 1970.

39. Lenaghan, R., Silva, Y. J., and Walt, A. J.: Hemodynamic alterations associated with expansion rupture of the lung. Arch. Surg., 99:339, 1969.

40. Arbulu, A., Belmaric, J., and Norton, M. L.: Hyperinflation interstitial rupture of the lung. Ann. Otol., 81:825, 1972.

32 CARDIOVASCULAR FAILURE FOLLOWING TRAUMA

I. J. SCHATZ
R. F. WILSON

Of the many causes of death or complications in injured patients, cardiac failure is increasingly significant. In some patients, the cardiac failure develops suddenly after trauma because of pericardial tamponade or rapid severe fluid overloading. In some it develops over several hours during the course of treatment or recovery from shock. In others, it develops insidiously over several days as tissue breakdown, sepsis, and renal or hepatic failure place increasing demands on the cardiovascular system. If the physician is not well grounded in cardiovascular physiology and is not aware of the early signs and symptoms of cardiovascular failure, he may not appreciate the problem until it is irreversible or extremely difficult to correct.

PITFALL

IF THE PHYSICIAN FOCUSES ALL OF HIS ATTENTION ON OBVIOUS INJURIES, HE MAY FAIL TO APPRECIATE CONCOMITANT CARDIOVASCULAR DETERIORATION, THEREBY DELAYING IMPORTANT SUPPORTIVE MEASURES.

Since the effects of preexisting cardiac disease may be profound during resuscitation and later during recovery, evidence of the problem must be sought carefully during the initial examination, especially in the elderly.

The purpose of this chapter is to draw attention to the general principles underlying normal functioning of the cardiovascular system and to emphasize important points in the diagnosis and treatment of the many varied and sometimes subtle changes associated with cardiovascular failure after trauma.

ETIOLOGY

Most patients with cardiovascular failure following trauma have preexisting cardiovascular disease; however, many previously healthy patients develop cardiac failure because of direct trauma to the heart or because of reduced coronary blood flow following severe hemorrhage. In addition, any damage to the respiratory system may produce severe hypoxia which can compound the myocardial dysfunction. In children, evidence of congestive heart failure should stimulate a search for a congenital heart defect or rheumatic carditis. In young adults, valvular defects should be sought. In older adults, previous cardiac damage due to hypertension and coronary artery disease are the most frequent preexisting problems, but valvular defects must also be considered.

AXIOM

ALTHOUGH HYPOTENSION AND SEVERE IN-
JURIES MAY BE TOLERATED WELL BY YOUNG
PATIENTS WITH NO UNDERLYING HEART DIS-
EASE, OLDER PATIENTS AND THOSE WITH PRE-
EXISTING CARDIAC PROBLEMS MAY DEVELOP
SEVERE HEART FAILURE WITH MINIMAL
TRAUMA.

The causes of cardiovascular failure can be divided into cardiac failure, peripheral vascular failure, and circulatory overload.[1]

Cardiac Failure

Cardiovascular failure due to the heart itself may be caused by muscular failure, mechanical interference with diastolic filling, arrhythmias, and electrolyte abnormalities.

MYOCARDIAL (MUSCULAR) FAILURE. Myocardial failure is either a primary muscular problem or secondary to an excessive work load placed on the heart by systemic hypertension, valvular disease, or severe vasoconstriction. Examples of primary myocardial failure include: cardiomyopathies, metabolic abnormalities such as those associated with thyroid disease or beriberi, inadequate quantity of myocardium due to myocardial infarction, and decreased efficiency of contraction due to ventricular aneurysms or dyskinesia.

INTERFERENCE WITH DIASTOLIC FILLING. Preexisting disorders which may limit the normal diastolic stretch of the ventricle and thereby reduce cardiac output include cardiac tamponade, pericardial effusions, constrictive pericarditis and endocardial or myocardial fibrosis. Acute pericardial tamponade following penetrating wounds of the heart is interesting because, although it interferes with filling of the heart, it may also help the patient by reducing the hemorrhage from a penetrating cardiac wound (Chap. 21). Removal of as little as 5 to 10 ml of blood from a cardiac tamponade may improve the stroke volume by an equivalent amount and not infrequently restores the patient's vital signs to normal, at least temporarily.

CARDIAC ARRHYTHMIAS

AXIOM

ANY CARDIAC TACHYARRHYTHMIA THAT
DOES NOT ALLOW ADEQUATE VENTRICULAR
FILLING OR EMPTYING MAY PRECIPITATE
HEART FAILURE.

In most instances, atrial arrhythmias do not by themselves produce clinical heart failure unless a significant reduction of ventricular function is already present.[2] Even when the ventricular response rate is controlled by digitalis, atrial fibrillation will decrease cardiac output and increase any tendency to congestive failure, presumably by causing loss of the normal "booster-pump" function of the atrium. Restoration of normal sinus rhythm in these patients usually results in a marked improvement in cardiac output and function.

ELECTROLYTE AND ACID-BASE ABNORMALITIES. Certain electrolyte and acid-base abnormalities may seriously interfere with the conductive system and with the function of the myocardial muscle fibers, thereby increasing the tendency to arrhythmias and impaired myocardial function. Severe hypokalemia or hypercalcemia tends to make the heart stop in systole while hyperkalemia and hypocalcemia tend to make the heart stop in diastole. Mild acidosis may slightly improve cardiac action, but severe acidosis with a pH of less than 7.2 tends to depress myocardial function.

Peripheral (Noncardiac) Failure (Chap. 5)

Peripheral or noncardiac cardiovascular failure exists when there is a significant reduction in the effective circulating blood volume. This may be caused by decreased intravascular volume due to hemorrhage, fractures, contusions or decreased venous tone, causing increased vascular capacity and a relative hypovolemia, particularly during general anesthesia or after taking narcotics.

Failure Caused by Circulatory Overload

AXIOM
THE MOST COMMON PRECIPITATING CAUSE OF CARDIAC FAILURE IN PATIENTS WITH TRAUMA IS EXCESSIVE ADMINISTRATION OF SODIUM-CONTAINING FLUIDS.

The causes of circulatory overload may be divided into those conditions that increase blood volume and those that are associated with an increased venous return.

INCREASED BLOOD VOLUME. The most frequent cause of an increased blood volume in the injured patient is excessive administration of blood and other fluids during the initial resuscitation. The margin of safety between hypovolemia and fluid overloading may be greatly reduced in the critically injured patient in shock, particularly while under anesthesia. Hypervolemia during the recovery phase may also be due to salt-retaining steroids and renal or hepatic failure.

AXIOM
IT SHOULD BE STRESSED THAT CARDIAC FAILURE FROM FLUID OVERLOAD IS RARE IN PATIENTS WHO DO NOT HAVE CARDIAC TRAUMA OR PREVIOUS CARDIAC DISEASE.

INCREASED VENOUS RETURN. An increased or more rapid venous return may be associated with severe anemia or cirrhosis and rarer conditions such as arteriovenous fistulae and beriberi. Because the cardiac output is generally elevated in these conditions, they are often referred to as types of high-output cardiac failure.

PHYSIOLOGIC CHANGES ASSOCIATED WITH CARDIOVASCULAR FAILURE

Reserve Mechanisms

The reserve mechanisms or adjustments of the body to cardiovascular failure may be divided into acute, subacute, and chronic, depending on the length of time required for the adjustment to become effective.

ACUTE. Increased sympathetic nervous system activity and increased oxygen extraction develop rapidly following most types of circulatory failure due to acute blood loss, cardiac trauma, or acute myocardial infarction.

PITFALL
IF HYPOTENSION IS REGARDED AS A CRITERION FOR DIAGNOSIS OF MYOCARDIAL INFARCTION, VITAL HOURS OF TREATMENT MAY BE LOST.

Patients with acute myocardial infarction or cardiac trauma often have decreased cardiac output and stroke volume, but their arterial blood pressures are generally maintained at normal or only slightly decreased levels because of an increased arteriolar vasoconstriction.

If hypotension does develop following an acute myocardial infarction, not infrequently the cardiac output is normal or only slightly reduced; the arterial hypotension in such individuals is related primarily to inadequate peripheral arteriolar vasoconstriction.[3]

The increased autonomic sympathetic stimulation helps to maintain blood flow to essential organs such as the brain and heart, but does so at the expense of the skin, kidneys, splanchnic organs, and skeletal muscles where the arteriolar vasoconstriction is greatest. The sympathetic stimulation of the veins and augmented venous tone may improve cardiac output by reducing vascular capacity and thereby increasing venous return to the heart. Because of increased sympathetic and decreased parasympathetic stimulation, the heart usually increases its rate and contracts more forcefully and rapidly than it otherwise would for the same diastolic load.

PITFALL

FAILURE TO ADMINISTER OXYGEN TO A PA-
TIENT WITH ACUTE CARDIOVASCULAR FAILURE
OR AN ACUTE MYOCARDIAL INFARCTION WILL
RESULT IN PROGRESSIVE HYPOXIA AND IN-
CREASING CARDIAC DEMANDS.

The tissues of the body that receive less blood because of the redistribution of the available blood flow may be forced to extract more oxygen from the blood. This "venous oxygen reserve" is important in most of the vital organs but is less useful to the myocardium, which normally extracts up to 70 to 75% of the oxygen coming to it.[4] If the available oxygen is still inadequate, the tissues may be forced to resort to anaerobic metabolism. Under such circumstances, progressive peripheral and myocardial cell death may occur.

SUBACUTE. The subacute mechanisms in heart failure are principally those which cause the retention of salt and water by the kidneys. The resultant increased blood volume, together with an increased vasomotor tone, tends to increase venous return. The increased ventricular diastolic filling and stretching of the myocardial fibers may then improve the contractility of the heart. Unfortunately, this salt water retention often overloads the heart further, thereby increasing the severity of the cardiac failure.

CHRONIC. The principal chronic hemodynamic adjustment of heart failure is hypertrophy of the ventricular myocardium. This change, however, has little relevance to the patient who first develops heart failure following acute trauma, since it usually requires weeks or months to develop. In the patient with preexisting hypertrophy, however, hypotension due to trauma may be especially damaging because of the greatly reduced blood flow to the endocardium and inner layers of the myocardium.

Organ Changes in Cardiovascular Failure

HEART. In ventricular failure, the myocardium fails to contract with sufficient force to eject a stroke volume which is appropriate for the filling load upon the ventricle. The abnormal elevation of both end-diastolic volume and pressure which results is reflected in significant elevation of the pulmonary capillary "wedge" pressure.

It might seem advantageous to have a greater end-diastolic ventricular volume and fiber length because each ventricular fiber then has to shorten less to eject a given volume of blood. However, according to the law of LaPlace, as the radius increases more tension must be developed by each fiber to produce a given intraventricular pressure with a proportional increase in myocardial oxygen requirements. A further disadvantage of dilatation is that the increased tension required to develop a given pressure results in a decrease in the rate of myocardial fiber shortening and a decreased ability of the ventricle to eject blood.[5]

LUNGS. The space in the thorax available for ventilation may be decreased during cardiac failure by pleural effusions, increased blood in the pulmonary vasculature and increased fluid in the alveoli and pulmonary interstitial tissues. The increased fluid and congestion in the lungs make the lungs stiffer and thereby increase the work of breathing. The presence of fluid in the alveolar spaces further increases the tendency to atelectasis by inactivating surfactant (Chap. 31).

Pulmonary edema from transudation of fluid out of the pulmonary capillaries into the alveoli occurs when the pressure in the capillaries (normally 7 to 12 mm Hg) exceeds the plasma oncotic pressure (normally 25 to 30 mm Hg). If the lungs have been damaged by the direct or indirect effects of trauma or if the serum oncotic pressure is reduced because of a low concentration of serum proteins, transudation of fluid across the pulmonary capillaries occurs at even lower capillary pressures.[6]

ENDOCRINE ORGANS. Renin, angiotensin, aldosterone, vasopressin, and norepinephrine are often present in normal amounts in patients with congestive failure except during periods of acute severe decompensation when they are elevated.[7] Following trauma, all these substances are usually present in much greater amounts, thereby increasing the likelihood of heart failure in acutely injured patients.

KIDNEYS. The most quantitatively important site for salt and water retention in congestive heart failure is the proximal tubule, and the distal and collecting tubules may be regarded as "fine tuning" devices for further adjustments of fluid excretion (Chap. 30). Trauma, anesthesia, and blood loss may activate the juxtaglomerular cells to produce renin, which stimulates the production of angiotensin, which in turn stimulates the adrenal cortex to elaborate aldosterone. The resultant sodium retention tends to expand the functional extracellular fluid volume and improve renal perfusion; however, this additional salt and water retention may cause or aggravate congestive heart failure.

DIAGNOSIS OF CARDIOVASCULAR FAILURE

Symptoms

Most types of heart disease first affect the left side of the heart. Although the left ventricular end-diastolic pressure may remain elevated for many days or weeks after an acute injury, clinical signs of an isolated left ventricular failure are usually only temporary. Some degree of right heart failure eventually develops after left heart failure, but the time of onset is extremely variable and may occur within minutes, hours or days. The patient with left-sided heart failure classically complains of "shortness of breath" or weakness, whereas failure of the right side of the heart is characteristically associated with systemic venous hypertension, edema, hepatomegaly, and ascites.

PITFALL

IF IT IS ASSUMED THAT ABDOMINAL SYMPTOMS IN THE INJURED PATIENT WITH HEART FAILURE ARE DUE TO CONGESTION OR DIGITALIS TOXICITY, IMPORTANT INTRA-ABDOMINAL DAMAGE MAY BE OVERLOOKED.

Some of the symptoms that may develop from the gastrointestinal tract because of severe congestion include anorexia, nausea, vomiting, and abdominal distension and pain. These symptoms of heart failure also can occur with overdigitalization and may be difficult to differentiate from intra-abdominal injury or infection.

Physical Findings

HEART. A sinus tachycardia is almost invariably present with any cardiovascular failure. Pulsus alternans, although uncommon, is a reliable sign of severe left ventricular failure. Palpation may reveal a hyperactive precordium with or without any cardiac enlargement. Enlargement of the heart, however, usually develops only after prolonged cardiac failure and seldom is found following trauma, unless preexisting cardiac disease was present. Although frequently overlooked by the noncardiologist, a gallop (third heart sound) should be sought for diligently because this is a hallmark of left ventricular failure (Fig. 1).

LUNGS. In early left ventricular failure rales may be present only at the lung bases, but as the decompensation increases the rales usually become more generalized. The rales of congestion, however, may be difficult to differentiate from those of atelectasis, particularly in patients with chest trauma.

PITFALL

IF ALL WHEEZING IS THOUGHT TO BE DUE TO ASTHMA, SERIOUS CARDIAC FAILURE MAY BE OVERLOOKED.

Wheezing, often considered to be due to bronchial asthma, may occur with cardiac failure, in the absence of pulmonary disease, because of swelling and congestion in the smaller bronchioles. Pleural effusions

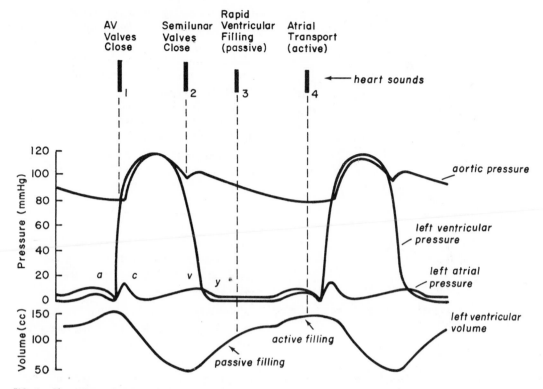

| AV Valves Close | Semilunar Valves Close | Rapid Ventricular Filling (passive) | Atrial Transport (active) |

← heart sounds

FIG. 1. The active and passive filling phases of the cardiac cycle are correlated with the occurrence of heart sounds and changes in aortic, left ventricular, and left atrial pressures.

due to heart failure usually occur predominately or solely on the right, whereas a left hydrothorax suggests pulmonary infarction. In patients with chest trauma, these effusions are often considered to be due to injury to the lungs or chest wall, and, unless the fluid is aspirated and examined, the true cause may be difficult to determine.

NECK VEINS. One of the most readily available signs of cardiac failure is distension of the deep jugular veins to at least 3 cm above the sternal angle when the patient is sitting at a 45° angle. Hepatomegaly and a positive hepatojugular reflux are important corroborative signs of congestive failure.

Hematomas in the upper mediastinum may press on the innominate veins or superior vena cava, hindering venous return from the head and upper extremities. If the pressure on these large mediastinal veins is high, the neck veins may be greatly distended and the head and neck may appear swollen and cyanotic.

Radiographic Signs of Heart Failure (Fig. 2)

Pulmonary clouding due to congestion of the lung and increased density of the central lung markings can often be detected on x-ray examination long before cardiac failure becomes apparent clinically. Accumulation of fluid in the interlobar fissures and blunting of the costophrenic angles by free pleural fluid should also be looked for carefully, especially on the right. Such radiologic changes can also occur after chest trauma; however, thoracic injuries are generally confined to one side.

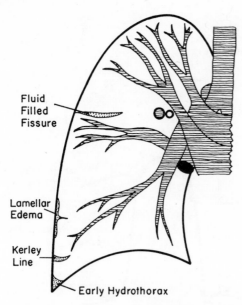

Fluid
Filled
Fissure

Lamellar
Edema

Kerley
Line

Early Hydrothorax

FIG. 2. The radiographic features of congestive heart failure include edema, Kerley lines, and pleural effusion.

Electrocardiogram (EKG)

PITFALL

PHYSICIANS MAY FAIL TO APPRECIATE THAT SEVERE CARDIAC FAILURE CAN OCCUR IN THE PATIENT WITH A NORMAL EKG.

No EKG finding indicates the presence or absence of congestive heart failure per se, but signs of a conduction disturbance, tachy- or bradyarrhythmias, or chamber abnormalities may provide clues to the etiology of the heart failure.

Venous Pressure

In most patients with only mild to moderate trauma and no intrathoracic disease or injuries, there is a relatively good correlation between the central venous pressure (CVP) and the blood volume or the quantity of fluid needed to maintain optimal tissue perfusion. In critically injured patients, however, particularly those with cardiac or mediastinal involvement, the level of the CVP may be deceptively high.

When blood volumes, fluid administration, and the CVP were measured in 124

critically ill and injured patients at Detroit General Hospital, no correlation between these values was found.[8] The CVP response to the administration of fluid appeared to be much more reliable than isolated central venous pressure readings in evaluating the amount of fluid needed; however, none of the single parameters studied (blood volume, central venous pressure, or clinical impression) correlated consistently with the load required to restore normal tissue perfusion.

PITFALL

PHYSICIANS MAY FAIL TO APPRECIATE THAT SEVERE LEFT VENTRICULAR FAILURE CAN OCCUR WITH A NORMAL OR LOW CVP.

Although the central venous pressure is usually elevated in patients with heart failure, it may be normal (4 to 8 cm H_2O), especially if the decompensation is primarily left sided. Five of our patients with acute left ventricular failure following cardiac arrest or acute myocardial infarction developed acute severe pulmonary edema in spite of a CVP less than 5.0 cm H_2O.

PITFALL

PHYSICIANS MAY FAIL TO APPRECIATE THAT A PATIENT WHO IS HYPOVOLEMIC CAN HAVE A HIGH CVP.

Not infrequently, particularly in patients with mediastinal or pulmonary trauma or disease, the CVP may be greater than 12 to 16 cm H_2O in spite of rather severe hypovolemia. This is particularly apt to occur during general anesthesia and with the use of volume-cycled respirators. Under such circumstances, blood and fluid must be given very cautiously; however, if these fluids improve the patient's vital signs and tissue perfusion with little or no rise in CVP or evidence of increasing pulmonary congestion, additional fluids may be given (Chap. 5).

Because of the poor correlation between the CVP and filling pressures in the left heart, especially following ischemic damage to the myocardium, clinicians have become increasingly interested in monitoring pulmonary artery mean, diastolic, and wedge pressures. The Swan-Ganz catheter is a soft balloon-tipped catheter which can be passed through a peripheral venous cutdown into the pulmonary artery until the catheter tip lodges in a distal portion of the pulmonary arterial tree.[9] Inflation of the balloon then allows the monitoring of the pulmonary artery wedge pressure, which reflects the left atrial and left ventricular end-diastolic pressures (LVEDP) quite well. If the pulmonary artery wedge pressure is above 20 to 25 mm Hg or rises abruptly, fluid administration should be stopped and aggressive treatment for congestive heart failure initiated.

Circulation Time

Patients with congestive heart failure usually have a prolonged circulation time; however, since the circulation time reflects not only the cardiac output but also the volume of the pulmonary vascular bed and the heart, patients with acute heart failure induced by a recent myocardial infarction may occasionally have a normal circulation time. Furthermore, patients with high-output cardiac failure often have a shortened circulation time.

Cardiac Catheterization

AXIOM

CARDIAC CATHETERIZATION SHOULD BE OB-TAINED WITH SEVERE PROGRESSIVE CARDIAC FAILURE OF UNKNOWN ETIOLOGY.

Although cardiac catheterization is only rarely indicated in the immediate post-trauma period, severe progressive congestive heart failure may occasionally be caused by injuries which cannot be diagnosed with certainty without cardiac cathe-

terization. Following blunt trauma, such injuries might include rupture of a papillary muscle, sinus of Valsalva, valve cusp, or septum. Damage due to penetrating trauma might include similar injuries as well as lacerations of major coronary arteries and tamponade due to localized collections of blood in the pericardium.

TREATMENT (Table 1)

The treatment of congestive heart failure is primarily concerned with reduction of the work load of the heart, increase of myocardial contractility, and correction of arrhythmias (Fig. 3).

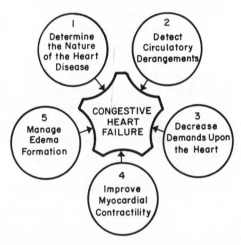

FIG. 3. Principles in the management of congestive heart failure.

Reduction of Work Load

The work load on the heart can be diminished by reducing the venous return to the heart, supplying oxygen, decreasing the metabolic needs of the body, and reducing the amount of peripheral vascular resistance against which the heart must pump.

DECREASING VENOUS RETURN. Venous return can be reduced by elevation of the head and chest, salt and water restriction, the use of tourniquets, diuretics and vasodilators, and occasionally phlebotomy. The patient while in bed should be placed in the "head up–legs down" position. The decreased venous return achieved by this

TABLE 1. TREATMENT OF MODERATE TO SE-
VERE CONGESTIVE HEART FAILURE

1. "Head up—legs down" position.
2. Salt and water restriction.
3. Diuretics.
4. Analgesics, especially morphine, for severe pain.
5. Sedatives for excess anxiety.
6. Oxygen to maintain an arterial Po_2 of 80-100 mm Hg.
7. Hypothermia if febrile.
8. Digitalis preparations.
9. Calcium if massive transfusions and hypotension.
10. Isoproterenol if slow weak pulse.
11. Glucagon (?) if continued severe failure.
12. Thiamine for severe alcoholics.
13. Correction of arrhythmias.
14. Anticoagulants if suspect venous thromboses or pulmonary emboli.
15. Vasodilators if excessive vasoconstriction.

position may improve cardiac efficiency, and edema fluid may accumulate in the dependent parts of the body rather than in the lungs. Reduction of the intake of fluid and salt, especially intravenously, also helps to reduce blood volume; this relieves the load on the heart relatively slowly, but is very important.

Properly applied rotating tourniquets, such as blood pressure cuffs, promptly reduce the venous return from the compressed extremities. This technique is of great value in treating acute heart failure, especially pulmonary edema. The tourniquets, however, must be released intermittently to prevent ischemia to the distal portions of the limbs.

Diuretics, especially I. V. furosemide or ethacrynic acid, can often decrease intravascular volume by 100 to 500 ml within 30 to 60 minutes, thereby improving cardiac efficiency and cardiac output. Osmotic diuretics such as mannitol and urea are rarely used in the treatment of heart failure because they often expand the intravascular volume temporarily and later may increase fluid retention.

Furosemide and ethacrynic acid are extremely potent diuretics and are especially useful in refractory edema. The initial I.V. dose is generally 10 to 40 mg for furosemide and 50 to 100 mg for ethacrynic acid. Furosemide is usually preferred because ethacrynic acid may cause deafness in some critically ill patients. The dose of furosemide is generally doubled every 15 to 30 minutes until a urinary output of 50 to 100 ml/hr or more is obtained or until the total dose exceeds 1000 to 2000 mg. Once a diuresis is obtained, slow infusion of furosemide at 2 to 10 mg/hr may help maintain a high urine output. In an occasional patient, however, the addition of mannitol (12.5 to 25.0 gm I.V. slowly) or ethacrynic acid appears to greatly increase the response to furosemide.

PITFALL

IF EXCESSIVE DOSES OF DIURETICS ARE USED, THE PATIENT WHO IS OVERHYDRATED MAY QUICKLY BECOME HYPOVOLEMIC, PARTICULARLY IF HE HAS HAD MAJOR TRAUMA.

The margin of safety between fluid overloading and hypovolemia, particularly in patients with multiple severe injuries, may be very small. If the diuresis is excessive, severe fluid deficits may rapidly ensue, and the patient may suddenly become hypotensive. Severe electrolyte problems such as hypokalemia, hypochloremia, and metabolic alkalosis may also develop quickly and alter the cardiac response to digitalis or precipitate dangerous arrhythmias.

Removal of 50 to 100 ml of blood every 5 to 10 minutes may be helpful in the urgent management of acute pulmonary edema while waiting for the various drugs to become effective. This may be especially important when excessive quantities of fluid have been given while the surgeon is struggling to get control of a major arterial or venous bleeding point. Close attention must be paid, however, to the patient's vital signs and central venous pressure, so that sudden severe hypovolemia can be avoided.

OXYGEN. Most patients with congestive

heart failure benefit greatly from the administration of sufficient oxygen to maintain an arterial Po$_2$ of 80 to 100 mm Hg, particularly if they have had recent severe injuries. Trauma and pulmonary congestion can greatly reduce the oxygenation of blood in the lungs. This, together with a reduced cardiac output, may cause severe myocardial hypoxia resulting in a vicious cycle of decreasing oxygen supply and increasing oxygen needs.

DECREASING METABOLIC NEEDS. The metabolic needs of the patient can be lowered by reducing pain, apprehension, physical effort, and body temperature. Analgesics, sedatives, and hypothermia, particularly if the patient is febrile, may all be useful in this regard. Shivering from hypothermia can be reduced with chlorpromazine. Intravenous morphine in doses of 3 to 5 mg every 30 to 60 minutes is usually very effective for relieving pain and, by reducing venous return to the heart, may decrease the heart failure and pulmonary congestion. Great care must be taken when using any narcotic, however, particularly after trauma, to maintain adequate ventilation and blood volume.

REDUCING PERIPHERAL VASCULAR RESISTANCE. Vasodilators such as chlorpromazine, by reducing the peripheral vascular resistance against which the heart must pump, allow an increased cardiac output and more complete emptying of the heart with each contraction. Simultaneous dilatation of the capacitance veins may increase vascular capacity by 2 to 3 liters and thereby reduce venous return. Vasodilators may be of particular value in treating cardiac failure in patients who have a normal or high blood pressure with a cold clammy skin and oliguria as evidence of a severe generalized vasoconstriction.

PITFALL

IF A VASODILATOR IS ADMINISTERED TO A HYPOVOLEMIC PATIENT, SEVERE HYPOTENSION MAY DEVELOP.

The vital signs must be watched extremely carefully whenever a vasodilator is given. If the blood pressure in a normotensive patient suddenly falls by more than 15 to 20 mm Hg after administration of a vasodilator, the patient probably is or has become hypovolemic and needs additional fluids.

Chlorpromazine in doses of 1 to 2 mg every 2 to 5 minutes until a satisfactory response is obtained may be of special value in these circumstances. Narcotics, particularly morphine, and massive doses of corticosteroids may have a similar but less intense effect.

Increasing Myocardial Contractility and Cardiac Output

DIGITALIS PREPARATIONS. The signs and symptoms of congestive heart failure can be improved dramatically by digitalis. The major actions of this drug are to increase myocardial contractility and slow the ventricular rate when atrial fibrillation is present. An excellent response to digitalis therapy may be expected in patients with heart failure due to mitral stenosis with atrial fibrillation, aortic valvular disease, mitral regurgitation, and coronary artery disease. A less satisfactory response can be expected in patients with mitral stenosis with sinus rhythm, diffuse myocardial disease, chronic cor pulmonale, constrictive pericarditis, or congestive heart failure associated with thyrotoxicosis, anemia, or peripheral arteriovenous fistulae.[10] Digitalis is useful in the conversion of ectopic rhythms, especially atrial and nodal tachycardia, and in the control of the ventricular rate in other arrhythmias, such as atrial fibrillation and flutter, in which an uncontrolled ventricular rate may produce or aggravate heart failure.

In the administration of digitalis, several points should be emphasized:

1. It is important to know how much and what type of digitalis the patient has had within the past 7 to 14 days.

2. Digitalis should generally be avoided in patients with atrioventricular block.
3. The maintenance dosage may be greatly reduced if renal function is impaired. The specific gravity of fresh urine may provide some initial information, but the BUN, serum creatinine, and serum potassium should also be determined as soon as possible.
4. The optimal digitalizing dose varies greatly in critically injured patients and may be only half the usual dose.
5. Beneficial hemodynamic responses to digitalis may be obtained without administering a dose large enough to cause EKG changes or minor toxic symptoms. The EKG does not indicate when an optimum dosage is reached and it may not change until toxic effects are produced.
6. When digitalis is used to slow a sinus tachycardia due to sepsis or hypovolemia, toxicity may develop before any hemodynamic benefit occurs.
7. Potassium loss and calcium administration increase the chances of digitalis toxicity; conversely, hyperkalemia and hypocalcemia increase the amount of digitalis needed to produce a therapeutic effect.

Digoxin may be given orally for routine digitalization when the failure is not severe; its maximum effect is reached in about six hours and the duration of action is 3 to 6 days. The total oral dose is usually about 2.0 mg given over a period of 48 hours. Most patients tolerate a maintenance dose of 0.25 mg digoxin once daily.

When rapid digitalization is required, the digoxin may be given in divided doses intravenously. The effects of intravenous digoxin begin within 5 to 10 minutes and reach a peak in 1 to 2 hours. In the patient who has received no prior digitalis preparation, an initial dose of 0.5 mg may be given slowly intravenously. Additional increments of 0.125 to 0.25 mg may be given I.M. or I.V. every 1 to 4 hours until there is evidence of adequate digitalization; this usually requires 1.25 to 1.50 mg within 12 to 24 hours.

PITFALL

PHYSICIANS MAY FAIL TO APPRECIATE THE TREMENDOUS VARIABILITY IN THE RESPONSES TO DIGITALIS OF CRITICALLY INJURED PATIENTS.

Digitalis, like all drugs, has toxic effects, including anorexia, nausea, vomiting, and diarrhea. Although paroxysmal atrial tachycardia with varying A-V block may occur in the absence of digitalis administration, most patients with this arrhythmia have digitalis toxicity. Abdominal pain and mesenteric venous occlusion may also rarely be related to digitalis toxicity.

CALCIUM. The injured patient receiving massive blood transfusions may not be able to mobilize calcium rapidly enough to maintain the ionized calcium levels which are optimal for myocardial function. This is particularly true if the patient has been severely hypotensive. If the patient is alkalotic, the ionized calcium levels will fall even further. Administration of 2.5 ml of 10% calcium chloride slowly I.V. after each unit of transfused blood may prevent this problem. If the patient has been digitalized, the calcium must be given very carefully because it increases the tendency to digitalis toxicity.

ISOPROTERENOL. In the rare patient with cardiac failure in whom the pulse rate is less than 80 to 90 per minute with no premature ventricular beats or other evidence of ventricular irritability, isoproterenol may be given. Doses of 1 to 2 μg per minute, given by slow I.V. infusion of a solution containing 0.2 mg per 100 ml, may dramatically increase the force of myocardial contraction and the cardiac output under such circumstances. This drug is especially useful for stimulating the slow, weakly beating heart after cardiac arrest or cardiac surgery.

In some patients, the isoproterenol may cause severe sinus tachycardia and increase the likelihood of developing other tachyarrhythmias, especially if the patient is acidotic or hypoxic. Many physicians feel that isoproterenol is contraindicated if the pulse rate exceeds 120/min.

GLUCAGON. Glucagon has been reported to be a particularly attractive inotropic agent because of antiarrhythmic properties, additive effect with digitalis glycosides, and secondary coronary vasodilation.[11] The usual dosage is 4 to 5 mg directly I.V. or by I.V. infusion at 4 to 12 mg per hour. Glucagon acts by activating adenyl cyclase which converts ATP to cyclic AMP which in turn activates the contractile mechanism. Disturbing side effects are nausea and vomiting, especially with large doses. Authors have reported varying success with the use of glucagon; in our own experience, about a third of the patients show at least a transient improvement.

DOPAMINE. This drug, recently approved for clinical use, is now the positive inotropic agent of choice in cardiogenic shock. Started in doses of about 2 to 5 μg/kg/min, it has a distinct advantage over other positive inotropic agents in that it can increase cardiac output and blood pressure while at the same time increasing renal blood flow. Except for occasional tachyarrhythmias, it has few side effects.

Correction of Arrhythmias

Atrial fibrillation is a common arrhythmia in patients with cardiac failure, and the resultant loss of a synchronized atrial contraction may reduce the cardiac output up to 20%.[12] Reversion of this rhythm to normal, using either small amounts of quinidine sulfate or DC synchronized electrical cardioversion, may be of considerable benefit to patients with heart failure. Atrial tachycardias may respond to quinidine, beta blockers or electroversion, and ventricular tachycardias may respond to I.V. lidocaine, procainamide, Dilantin, or electroversion. Digitalis is of greatest value in slowing the ventricular response to atrial fibrillation.

Beta-blocking agents such as propranolol may occasionally be helpful, especially if the pulse rate is above 150/minute. These drugs can, however, cause significant bradycardia and cardiac depression and should generally be avoided in patients with congestive heart failure.

AXIOM

BETA-BLOCKING AGENTS ARE CONTRAINDICATED IN CARDIAC FAILURE AND LOW-OUTPUT STATES UNLESS THE PROBLEMS ARE DUE SPECIFICALLY TO A TACHYARRHYTHMIA THAT IS UNRESPONSIVE TO OTHER THERAPY.

If the pulse rate is less than 50/minute and unresponsive to atropine or isoproterenol, a temporary intravenous pacemaker may be of value.

Anticoagulants

Deep venous thromboses and pulmonary emboli are common in patients with congestive heart failure and may in themselves precipitate or aggravate congestive heart failure. Anticoagulant therapy may decrease these thromboembolic complications in such circumstances and has been recommended particularly for elderly patients with fractured hips.

Acute Pulmonary Edema

The treatment of acute pulmonary edema consists of:

1. Upright sitting position.
2. Oxygen by mask, nasal catheter, or respirator.
3. Morphine sulfate, 10 to 15 mg slowly I.V. or I.M., with careful observation for respiratory depression or hypotension. Morphine may be contraindicated in patients with pulmonary edema if there is increased intracranial pressure or severe pulmonary disease.
4. Furosemide, 20 to 40 mg I.V.
5. Aminophylline, 250 to 500 mg I.V. over 10 to 30 minutes, as needed for bronchospasm.
6. Cardioversion if supraventricular ectopic tachycardia or ventricular tachycardia does not respond to the usual antiarrhythmic drugs, preferably before digitalis is given.

7. Tourniquets to three extremities rotated every 15 minutes to reduce venous return.
8. In the undigitalized patient, 0.5 to 1.0 mg digoxin may be given I.V. followed by additional increments as indicated if renal function and serum potassium are normal.
9. Positive-pressure breathing with a tight-fitting mask, or preferably through an endotracheal tube, may improve ventilation and reduce the accumulation of fluid in the alveoli.

SUMMARY

Cardiac failure seldom develops in the acutely injured patient unless the patient has preexisting heart disease or has suffered cardiac trauma or prolonged severe shock. The enthusiasm to give adequate quantities of fluid during the initial resuscitation can easily be overdone; once the initial hypotension has been corrected, further fluids should be given cautiously with careful attention to the patient's vital signs, central venous pressure, intake and output. If cardiac failure develops, it should be treated vigorously to prevent further myocardial depression or respiratory failure.

REFERENCES

1. Schlant, R. C.: Altered physiology of the cardiovascular system in heart failure. In: *The Heart* (Hurst, J. W., and Logue, R. B., Eds.). New York, McGraw-Hill, 1966.
2. Brill, I. C., et al.: Congestive failure due to auricular fibrillation in an otherwise normal heart. JAMA, 173:784, 1960.
3. Hughes, J. L., et al.: Abnormal peripheral vascular dynamics in patients with acute myocardial infarction: Diminished reflex arteriolar vasoconstriction. Clin. Res., 19:321, 1971.
4. Messer, J. V., and Neill, W. A.: The oxygen supply of the human heart. Amer. J. Cardiol., 9:384, 1962.

5. Fry, D. L., et al.: Myocardial mechanics: tension-velocity. Length relationships of heart muscle. Circ. Res., 14:73, 1964.
6. Finlayson, J. K., et al.: Hemodynamic studies in acute pulmonary edema. Ann. Intern. Med., 54:244, 1961.
7. Tuttle, E. P.: Humoral factors in the edema of heart failure. In: *The Heart* (Hurst, J. W., and Logue, R. B., Eds.). New York, McGraw-Hill, 1966.
8. Wilson, R. F., et al.: Central venous pressure and blood volume determinations in clinical shock. Surg. Gynec. Obstet., 132:631, 1971.
9. Swan, H. J. C., et al.: Catheterization of the heart in man with use of a flow-directed balloon-tipped catheter. New Eng. J. Med., 283:447, 1970.
10. Logue, R. B., and Hurst, J. W.: The treatment of heart failure. In: *The Heart* (Hurst, J. W., and Logue, R. B., Eds.). New York, McGraw-Hill, 1966.
11. Lvoff, R., and Wilcken, D. E. L.: Glucagon in heart failure and in cardiogenic shock: Experience in 50 patients. Circulation, 45:534, 1972.
12. Morris, J. J., Jr., et al.: Cardiac output in atrial fibrillation and sinus rhythm. Circulation, 28:772, 1963.

Suggested Reading

1. Hurst, J. W., and Logue, R. B. (Eds.): *The Heart*. New York, McGraw-Hill, 1966.
2. Mueller, H. S., et al.: The evaluation and treatment of cardiogenic shock. Med. Times, 96:137, 1970.
3. Gunnar, R. M., and Loeb, H. S.: Use of drugs in cardiogenic shock due to acute myocardial infarction. Circulation, 45:1111, 1972.
4. Hewitt, R. L., et al.: Protective effect of myocardial glycogen on cardiac function during anoxia. Surgery, 73:444, 1973.
5. Hinshaw, L. B., et al.: Prevention and reversal of myocardial failure in endotoxin shock. Surg. Gynec. Obstet. 136:1, 1973.
6. Macnicol, M. F., Goldberg, A. H., and Clowes, G. A.: Depression of isolated heart muscle by bacterial endotoxin. J. Trauma, 13:554, 1973.
7. Wilson, J. M., Gay, W. M., and Ebert, P. A.: The effects of oligemic hypotension on myocardial function. Surgery, 73:657, 1973.
8. Hewitt, R. L., et al.: Protective effect of glycogen and glucose on the anoxic arrested heart. Surgery, 75:1, 1974.

33 GASTROINTESTINAL COMPLICATIONS FOLLOWING TRAUMA

C. E. LUCAS
R. F. WILSON

The most frequent gastrointestinal complications following trauma include severe ileus, bowel obstruction, enterocutaneous fistulae, stress gastric bleeding and hepatic failure. Although a large percentage of these problems are caused by or are related to injury to the gastrointestinal tract, some are the indirect result of severe extra-abdominal injuries or sepsis. These complications are usually relatively mild and transient; however, if diagnosis and treatment are delayed, they may become severe and lead to significant morbidity and even death.

ILEUS

Etiology

Although the exact etiology of adynamic ileus has long been debated by surgeons and physiologists, there are several well-recognized clinical situations that either cause or greatly aggravate this problem. These include shock, trauma or ischemia to the bowel, sepsis (particularly peritonitis and pneumonitis), electrolyte imbalances (rarely), acid-base abnormalities, retroperitoneal hematomas and respiratory failure. From a physiologic point of view, adynamic ileus appears to be caused by sympathetic storm; however, parasympathetic blockade may be a contributing factor.[1] Following injury, the condition most frequently associated with subsequent development of adynamic ileus is severe, prolonged hypovolemic shock. Moreover, the extent of the adynamic ileus is often directly proportional to the severity and duration of the shock. The mechanism by which adynamic ileus occurs under these circumstances is not clear, but it may be related to prolonged mucosal ischemia during the hypovolemia as blood flow is diverted to the outer layers of the bowel.

A second factor frequently associated with adynamic ileus is contamination of the peritoneum by bowel content at the time of the initial trauma. Patients with multiple perforations in the small bowel with moderate to massive spillage can generally be expected to have an adynamic ileus for at least 7 to 14 days. If the contamination is due to colon injury, the ileus is usually worse. If an intra-abdominal abscess develops, the ileus is even more prolonged, and bowel function often does not return to normal for at least 3 to 4 weeks.

A theoretically preventable factor which may cause adynamic ileus is trauma to the viscera by the surgeon at the time of the initial operation. Excessive or rough handling of the bowel during harried attempts to obtain the exposure needed to stop massive bleeding from multiple sources may cause multiple bowel contusions or hematomas and, occasionally, may result in serosal tears. All such injuries delay the return of normal bowel function.

Pelvic and vertebral fractures causing retroperitoneal bleeding are often followed by adynamic ileus even when there is no associated intra-abdominal injury. The cause of the ileus under these circumstances is unclear, but may be related to local irritation or trauma to the neurovascular supply to the bowel.

PITFALL

EARLY REMOVAL OF THE NASOGASTRIC TUBE OR FEEDING OF A PATIENT FOLLOWING RETROPERITONEAL OR INTRAPERITONEAL HEMORRHAGE OR INJURY WILL FREQUENTLY RESULT IN A MORE SEVERE PROLONGED ILEUS.

One patient with a fractured pelvis developed a rupture of the cecum secondary to an increasing adynamic ileus after multiple attempts were made to feed him during the first five days following trauma.

Severe distension of all the hollow viscera, including the stomach, small bowel and colon, by the adynamic ileus invariably leads to diaphragmatic elevation. The resultant increased ventilatory difficulty may in turn cause a more severe ileus, and a vicious cycle of respiratory failure and ileus is established. Premature attempts to remove the nasogastric tube or begin oral feedings may further aggravate the situation if vomiting and aspiration occur. In some patients without intra-abdominal injury, pulmonary insufficiency alone can be a cause of severe adynamic ileus. This is particularly true in patients with post-traumatic respiratory failure. If sepsis also develops, the duration and severity of adynamic ileus are greatly increased.

Diagnosis

The most important factor in the diagnosis and treatment of adynamic ileus is anticipation of the problem. Any patient with one or more of the injuries or complications mentioned earlier is likely to develop adynamic ileus. During the early postinjury period one of the infrequently mentioned, but very important, clues to recognizing this problem is the patient's face, which under these circumstances will often exhibit some degree of anxiety and discomfort similar to that seen with viral gastroenteritis.

Examination of the abdomen generally reveals an obvious severe distension, so that the abdomen often protrudes beyond the rib cage when the patient is supine. After moderate to severe distension has developed, bowel sounds can seldom be heard. However, careful auscultation should be continued for at least three minutes because mechanical bowel obstruction—which is important to differentiate from ileus—is characterized by varying periods in which bowel sounds are absent alternating with episodes in which they are hyperactive.

On radiographic examination, adynamic ileus is characterized by a diffuse distension of the small and large bowel by fluid

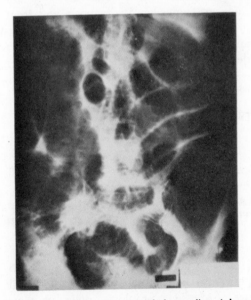

FIG. 1. The diffuse distension of the small and large bowel as demonstrated on this x-ray of the abdomen with the patient recumbent is characteristic of an adynamic ileus.

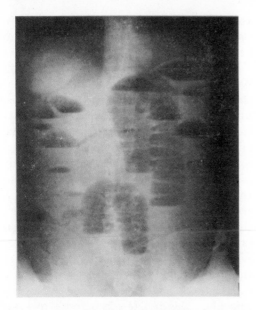

FIG. 2. Differential air-fluid levels with the patient in an upright position are roentgen signs frequently seen with mechanical small bowel obstruction.

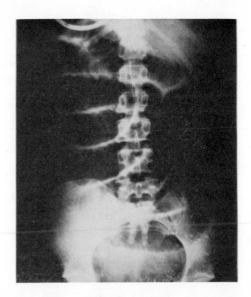

FIG. 3. The distension of several loops of small intestine in a horizontal position, producing a "stepladder" pattern while the patient is recumbent, is characteristic of mechanical obstruction.

and gas (Fig. 1). On the upright films, the air-fluid levels in the same loop will generally be at approximately the same height. This is in contrast to the differential air-fluid levels where two separate levels can be identified within the same loop of bowel, indicating active peristalsis against resistance or an obstruction (Fig. 2). Frequently, distended obstructed small bowel will lie transversely across the abdomen, producing a "stepladder" pattern on the films (Fig. 3).

PITFALL

IT IS OFTEN ASSUMED THAT AIR-FLUID LEVELS IN DISTENDED BOWEL ARE DUE TO A MECHANICAL OBSTRUCTION.

Since fluid must take a dependent position to air, regardless of the etiology of the bowel distension, any patient with distended bowel will have air-fluid levels on an upright film.

Symptomatically, adynamic ileus rarely produces the colicky or spasmotic abdominal pain which typically occurs in patients with a mechanical obstruction. At the time when the adynamic ileus is beginning to resolve, however, the patient may have some pain and increased bowel sounds, passage of gas per rectum and occasional diarrhea, making the differentiation between adynamic ileus and mechanical obstruction somewhat difficult. Frequent re-evaluation over a 6-hour period, however, should resolve this confusion. In general, the patient with ileus will improve after such a period of observation.

Functional Significance

The most frequent physiologic change occurring with adynamic ileus is the fluid and electrolyte loss which occurs into the lumen of the distended bowel. This sequestration of fluid may exceed 4 to 8 liters and may produce a major depletion of the effective extracellular fluid space and circulating blood volume. Although such a deficit is not reflected in the daily weights, this fluid is relatively inaccessible to the functional extracellular fluid space.

PITFALL

IF IT IS ASSUMED THAT AN ACUTELY IN-
JURED PATIENT WITH INCREASING ILEUS WHO
IS GAINING WEIGHT IS BECOMING OVERLOADED
WITH FLUID, DANGEROUS HYPOVOLEMIA MAY
BE ALLOWED TO DEVELOP.

The acid-base problems associated with adynamic ileus usually consist of a metabolic acidosis secondary to the hypovolemia and resultant poor tissue perfusion. On the other hand, these patients not infrequently develop a severe metabolic alkalosis due to prolonged, excessive drainage of gastric fluid high in hydrochloric acid.

Probably the most serious functional derangement caused by adynamic ileus is impaired ventilation. The distended bowel may markedly elevate the diaphragm, increase intrathoracic pressure, and decrease the thoracic cavity volume to less than half of normal. The increased pressure against the diaphragm also increases the work of respiration. The resultant decrease in tidal volume may initiate a vicious cycle of inadequate ventilation, atelectasis and pneumonitis which, in turn, may make the adynamic ileus more prolonged and severe.

The decreased ventilation and increased intrathoracic pressure may cause the central venous pressure to rise to rather high levels. Not only will the high CVP tend to create a false impression of fluid overloading but the resultant decrease in venous return to the right heart may significantly reduce cardiac output, blood pressure and urine flow. Use of loop diuretics to improve urine output under such circumstances may cause disastrous hypovolemia.

Severe adynamic ileus also greatly increases the incidence of wound complications. As the bowel becomes more distended, greater pressure is exerted against the wound. Even if the pressure against the wound were constant, the increased diameter of the abdomen, according to the law of LaPlace, would increase the wound tension. This has led to a significantly in-

creased number of wound dehiscences in patients who have had premature removal of nasogastric tubes.

The incidence and severity of wound complications are further increased in patients who develop necrotizing fasciitis, often associated with or due to a combination of hypovolemic shock plus massive spillage of bowel content into the peritoneal cavity. As the necrotizing fasciitis progresses the wound margins separate, so that the retention sutures span the open wound like banjo strings. When this occurs, the underlying distended intestines push and rub against the exposed sutures. This will eventually cause erosion of the sutures through the bowel wall even if the retention sutures have been placed extraperitoneally. This problem can result in leakage of bowel content onto the surrounding tissues in less than 24 hours. The resultant increased intra-abdominal and wound sepsis and necrosis promote a more severe and prolonged bout of adynamic ileus.

Another complication which may be caused by or related to adynamic ileus, particularly in the presence of sepsis and respiratory insufficiency, is the development of stress gastric bleeding. This is discussed in more detail later in this chapter.

Treatment

The most important aspect of the treatment of adynamic ileus is its prevention. Any patient with severe injury to the small bowel or colon with severe hypotension and massive intraperitoneal spill of intestinal content will require prolonged nasogastric decompression. Return of the normal intestinal function under such circumstances will often be delayed for at least 2 to 3 weeks.

The proper duration of nasogastric decompression is best determined by studying the subtle, progressive changes in facial expression throughout the early postinjury period, noting the degrees of anxiety, fear, discomfort and fatigue which are signs that the patient is not ready for oral feedings.

Another important indication of the appropriate time to remove the nasogastric tube is change in abdominal girth. This may be evaluated with a tape measure; however, inspection alone will reveal that the abdomen, even in an obese patient, protrudes less than the thorax when the patient is in a supine position unless he has ascites, adynamic ileus or bowel obstruction.

AXIOM

ANY PATIENT WHOSE ABDOMEN WHILE SUPINE PROTRUDES BEYOND HIS CHEST WITHOUT ASCITES MUST BE CONTINUED ON NASOGASTRIC DECOMPRESSION FOR ADYNAMIC ILEUS.

Additional factors to help determine when the nasogastric tube may be removed are the more classic signs of return of gastrointestinal function, including active bowel sounds, and the passage of flatus and bowel movements. However, even if the patient has active bowel sounds and is passing flatus and having bowel movements, he should not be fed if he still has moderate abdominal distension and appears anxious or uncomfortable. When this policy is not adhered to rigidly, premature removal of the nasogastric tube is followed by abdominal distension, deteriorating pulmonary function and an increasingly severe adynamic ileus. In addition, premature removal of the nasogastric tube often leads to the development of acute erosive gastritis. Under these circumstances, operative intervention to control the stress bleeding is more likely to be required than if the tube were left in place.

Other factors which are important in the treatment of adynamic ileus include correction of any underlying sepsis and provision of intensive ventilatory and respiratory support. This includes frequent coughing, turning of the patient if he is confined to bed and ambulation, if possible. Reduction in the amount of narcotics given may also help the return of bowel function. Finally, rectal examination is important to rule out the occasional fecal impaction that may develop in these patients. Such an examination may also reveal a pelvic abscess which may be causing the ileus.

BOWEL OBSTRUCTION

Etiology

The most common cause of bowel obstruction following trauma is adhesions between loops of bowel or other intra-abdominal organs. These adhesions are usually filmy and easily broken in the first few days, but, with time, gradually become stronger and tighter. Adhesions developing at or near any infection are often especially dense and may surround a loop of bowel and gradually constrict it over a period of weeks, months or years. Another not infrequent cause is the inadvertent suturing of a loop of small bowel into the wound. Intra-abdominal hernias, especially in mesenteric defects, are uncommon but may occasionally cause sudden severe obstruction or strangulation if the bowel which has passed through the opening becomes distended.

Diagnosis

PITFALL

IF IT IS ASSUMED THAT ALL POST-TRAUMATIC BOWEL DISTENSION IS DUE TO AN ADYNAMIC ILEUS, A MECHANICAL BOWEL OBSTRUCTION MAY BE OVERLOOKED UNTIL STRANGULATION OR PERFORATION OCCURS.

Mechanical bowel obstruction may be extremely difficult to differentiate from adynamic ileus in the immediate postinjury or postoperative period. Since adynamic ileus is a much more frequent cause of bowel distension and absence of bowel movements during this time, mechanical obstruction might easily be missed until complications have developed. As mentioned in the previous section, small bowel obstruction, as contrasted with adynamic or paralytic ileus, produces hyperactive bowel sounds and colicky pain. On x-ray the distension due to obstruction by adhesions usually involves only the small bowel, and differential air fluid levels in the same loop may often be seen on upright films (Fig. 3). Unfortunately, if the bowel obstruction is allowed to persist, the bowel sounds will eventually disappear and, if the bowel perforates or strangulates, x-ray signs of adynamic ileus will also develop. Such patients, however, appear more toxic, suggesting a worsening general condition.

If the usual causes of paralytic ileus are absent or resolving, continued or progressive increase of bowel distension should suggest the possibility of a partial or complete mechanical obstruction. Passage of a long tube into the small bowel for both decompression and injection of a radiopaque material to outline the area in question may be helpful in borderline cases.

Treatment

Prevention is the most important aspect in the treatment of mechanical bowel obstruction. Great care must be taken to handle the intestines gently, decrease bowel spillage as much as possible, and reperitonealize large serosal tears (taking care not to kink the bowel while closing these tears). All mesenteric or omental defects must be closed; however, when the serosal tear cannot be closed without causing kinking, it should be left open. At the end of the operation, the bowel should be placed in the abdomen in smooth orderly loops. Any local collections of blood and debris should be evacuated and the involved or contaminated areas irrigated generously. Copious saline lavage of the peritoneal cavity at the end of the operative procedure helps decrease the incidence and severity of later inflammatory adhesions.

Once bowel obstruction develops, patients with mild incomplete obstruction can generally be handled adequately with nasogastric decompression alone. If the bowel is already distended, long tubes may sometimes decompress it until the edema and inflammation in the adjacent tissue and bowel subside. When all else fails, especially if there is clinical or laboratory evidence of increasing toxicity, an exploratory laparotomy is mandatory.

If at all possible, the distended bowel should be decompressed preoperatively or intraoperatively before it is handled or manipulated during the surgery. A single adhesion can usually be quickly lysed with good reestablishment of intestinal blood flow and return of normal bowel activity. Multiple adhesions require more extensive surgery, which should be supplemented by passing a long intestinal tube (such as a Leonard or Baker tube) down to the cecum. Such tubes are best passed orally or transnasally; rarely is a gastrotomy or jejunostomy needed to achieve this purpose.

GASTROINTESTINAL FISTULAE

Etiology

The most common cause of gastrointestinal fistula formation is traumatic perforation of the bowel, particularly if its mesentery or blood supply is also damaged. The most frequent fistulae arise from colon injuries and occur even after the site of injury is exteriorized or a proximal colostomy is performed. Small bowel fistulae are less common and not infrequently are caused by or related to the use of retention sutures and sump tubes. Gastric fistulae seldom occur after trauma, except following massive wounds from rifle bullets or shotgun blasts which destroy large areas of the stomach and/or its blood supply.

The development of a fistula in the small bowel where it has not been damaged by the injury per se is particularly distressing. As indicated earlier, severe adynamic ileus predisposes to small bowel fistulae as a result of erosion of the distended bowel against the sutures used to close the abdomen. This is particularly true in patients with intraperitoneal sepsis and necrotizing fasciitis following a massive spill of small bowel or colon content into the peritoneal cavity. Under such circumstances, the wound edges tend to separate, exposing the underlying sutures even when they have been placed extraperitoneally. As the distended bowel rubs against the sutures, a fistula can develop in less than 24 hours.

Another cause of small intestinal fistulae, and occasionally gastric fistulae, is erosion of the bowel by sump tubes which have been inserted to function as drains. This is particularly apt to occur if the sump tube is stiff and left in place for a long period of time. Consequently, it is our current policy to remove the tube after 5 to 7 days, and in its place insert a small red Robinson catheter through which daily irrigations can be performed.

AXIOM

GREAT CARE MUST BE TAKEN DURING PARA-CENTESIS OR PERITONEAL LAVAGE TO AVOID AREAS OF PREVIOUS INCISIONS AND ADHESIONS.

A less frequent cause of leakage from the small bowel or colon is diagnostic paracentesis or peritoneal lavage. We have had at least two patients who had a negative paracentesis and peritoneal lavage at the time of their initial injury and, thus, did not require abdominal exploration. Both patients, however, had multiple other injuries which led to the development of adynamic ileus which progressively became worse when the nasogastric tube was prematurely removed. Later both patients developed signs of diffuse peritonitis, and at the time of exploration had large amounts of pus in the peritoneal cavity with thick layers of fibropurulent peel over the intestines, but no evidence of perforation. It is presumed that in both patients the paracentesis or peritoneal lavage caused perforation of the intestine. When the adynamic ileus developed, the small puncture wounds increased

in diameter with leakage of bowel content and subsequent development of peritonitis. Both patients died.

AXIOM

ANY INJURY TO THE PANCREAS GREATLY IN-CREASES THE RISK OF FISTULA, NOT ONLY FROM THE PANCREAS BUT ALSO FROM ANY ADJACENT INJURED BOWEL.

Splenic injuries not infrequently result in iatrogenic damage to the tail of the pancreas during the attempts to rapidly remove the spleen when it is bleeding massively. At the same time, it is possible also to injure both the greater curvature of the stomach, while the short gastrics are being taken down, and the splenic flexure of the colon. If any of the above technical problems occur, the patient may develop a gastric, pancreatic or colonic fistula following splenectomy. Patients with combined pancreatic and duodenal injuries are very likely candidates for the development of duodenal fistula, particularly if the vascularity of the duodenum is impaired by the injury to the head of the pancreas which is closely associated with the blood supply to the duodenum.

Diagnosis

The diagnosis of gastrointestinal fistulae is usually made when there is evidence of leakage of gastrointestinal contents out of abdominal drain sites or through the operative incision. Such leakage is usually also associated with the signs and symptoms of peritonitis, wound infection (with or without necrotizing fasciitis), and intra-abdominal abscesses, particularly in the subphrenic or pelvic spaces. Under such circumstances, it may be impossible to determine whether the drainage is from an intra-abdominal abscess or from a communication with the gastrointestinal tract. The origin of the fistula is easily determined if it is from the biliary tract or pancreas by the observation or measurement of bile or

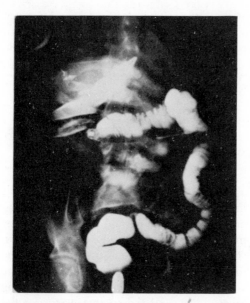

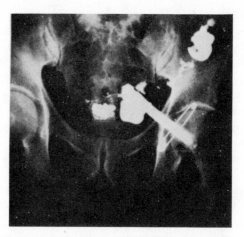

FIG. 5. A fistula of the large bowel following a gunshot wound to the groin is demonstrated by a sinus tract injection of contrast material which fills the distal colon.

FIG. 4. A fistula involving the transverse colon following a gunshot wound is seen on barium enema and demonstrates complete obstruction to retrograde flow with extravasation of barium.

amylase in the fistula drainage. It is particularly noteworthy that patients who develop wound infections and drainage before the fourth day have a high incidence of later enterocutaneous fistulae.

X-ray studies are often of great value for diagnosing the presence and location of gastrointestinal fistulae. Colon fistulae are usually identified by a barium enema (Fig. 4). Upper gastrointestinal fistulae will often be revealed by a Gastrografin swallow, but false negatives are not infrequent. Dilute barium swallows may be more accurate, but if the barium gets into the peritoneal cavity and stays there it can cause local granulomas or severe inflammatory changes.

PITFALL

IT IS EASY TO ASSUME THAT A GASTROIN-TESTINAL FISTULA IS NOT PRESENT IF IT CANNOT BE SEEN WITH A BARIUM ENEMA OR UPPER GASTROINTESTINAL SERIES.

A very accurate method for demonstrating the location of a fistula is injection of Gastrografin or barium through a red Robinson catheter which has been inserted into the opening from which suspected gastrointestinal fluid is draining (Fig. 5).

When there continues to be some question as to whether or not a fistula is present, 5 to 15 ml of Evans blue dye or charcoal can be administered by mouth or through the nasogastric tube. Both will appear quickly at the site of external drainage if the fistula is still open.

Treatment

ESOPHAGEAL FISTULAE (Chap. 20). The treatment of esophageal fistulae varies with their location. A fistula in the cervical esophagus or in the area of the thoracic outlet is usually managed quite simply with drainage of the area to control the local sepsis and with tube feedings through a nasogastric or gastrostomy tube while the fistula heals.

Fistulas involving the intrathoracic and lower esophagus are much more difficult to manage. These fistulas generally drain into the mediastinum and occasionally into the peritoneal cavity beneath the left diaphragm.

Much of the severe inflammation and necrosis caused by middle and lower esophageal injuries is due to regurgitation or reflux of gastric secretions into the esophagus and then into the adjacent tissues. Sepsis in the mediastinum is especially severe and not infrequently is lethal.

Surgical drainage of the mediastinum is best accomplished with closed tube thoracostomy; formal thoracotomy is usually not required. Collections of pus or fluid in the subphrenic spaces are usually best approached for drainage by an incision through the bed of the excised left twelfth rib; occasionally, however, anterior drainage through a left subcostal incision is required.

If the patient with a middle or lower esophageal fistula continues to be severely septic in spite of adequate gastrointestinal decompression and drainage of the mediastinum or subphrenic spaces, it may be necessary to explore the area of the leak to be sure that adequate drainage has been accomplished. If severe sepsis persists, a proximal cervical esophagostomy is helpful to divert swallowed fluid and air from the site of the fistula.

With all types of gastrointestinal fistulae, the appropriate antibiotics should be administered on the basis of the culture and sensitivity reports. In most instances, multiple bacteria are involved so that broad-spectrum antibiotics are usually indicated. Since relatively resistant gram-negative organisms are often involved, gentamicin is generally an appropriate agent to use in critically ill patients while waiting for the culture and sensitivity reports (Chap. 29).

Unfortunately, the prolonged sepsis which typically occurs in patients with distal esophageal fistulae may greatly interfere with attempts to maintain adequate nutrition. Furthermore, if tube feedings are provided through a nasogastric tube or a gastrostomy tube, there is often reflux of gastric juice and food up across the cardioesophageal junction and out the fistula site, increasing the drainage and the sepsis.

Another problem associated with reflux is the aspiration pneumonitis which frequently occurs in patients who are fed through either a nasogastric or a gastrostomy tube. This may also occur in patients who appear to be doing quite well and are thus encouraged to take some of their nutrition orally. In some instances, the aspiration pneumonitis has been so severe that tracheostomy and temporary ventilatory support were required.

Because of these multiple problems, lower esophageal fistulae tend to heal very slowly, and it may take many weeks or months before the fistula closes and the patient is able to tolerate a regular diet. Intravenous hyperalimentation has been used with increasing frequency and success in these patients. Unfortunately, intravenous hyperalimentation under such circumstances is also associated with significant morbidity, particularly from yeast infections (Chap. 4).

GASTRIC FISTULAE. Unfortunately, patients with proximal gastric fistulae are usually extremely ill and cannot tolerate the major gastric resections that might be needed for definitive treatment. In addition, patients with proximal gastric fistulae usually have severe infections, frequently with necrotizing fasciitis, and their anastomoses often heal poorly and break down within a few days of surgery.

In patients with distal gastric fistulae, distal gastrectomy and gastrojejunostomy are the usual procedures of choice. When operative intervention is not appropriate, treatment consists of continuous nasogastric decompression, antibiotics and I.V. hyperalimentation.

DUODENAL FISTULAE. The treatment of duodenal fistulae varies with their type and site (Fig. 6). Fistulae which occur in the duodenum following a distal gastrectomy and gastrojejunostomy are referred to as "end fistulae" and will usually heal if the patient is treated with nasogastric decompression, local drainage of the area, antibiotics and, on occasion, I.V. hyperalimentation. In contrast, duodenal fistulae which

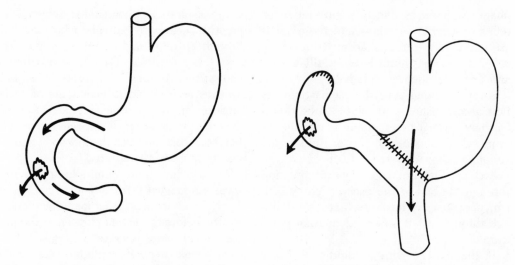

FIG. 6. *Left:* A fistula of the duodenum when it is in normal continuity with the stomach is referred to as a "side fistula." Since a side fistula is exposed to all of the gastrointestinal contents formed proximal to it, it is associated with severe complications and seldom closes spontaneously. *Right:* In contrast, a fistula of the duodenum in patients who have had a gastrojejunostomy is referred to as an end fistula. End fistulas are exposed to much smaller amounts of gastrointestinal fluid, are much less dangerous, and much more apt to heal.

occur when the duodenum is in continuity with the stomach are referred to as "side fistulae" and are less likely to heal spontaneously because of the continued flow of gastrointestinal contents past the fistula site.

Poor healing and infections are particularly apt to occur in patients who have side duodenal fistulae secondary to combined pancreatic and duodenal injuries. In such instances, the duodenal fistula is best treated by resecting the distal stomach and performing a gastrojejunostomy, thereby converting the side duodenal fistula to an end duodenal fistula. At the same time, the site of the duodenal closure proximally should be decompressed by means of a tube duodenostomy, and a vagotomy should be performed to diminish the likelihood of developing acute erosive gastritis in the postoperative period, particularly since most of these patients have severe sepsis.

FISTULAE OF THE SMALL INTESTINE. Most fistulae of the distal small bowel can be treated conservatively by local drainage of the peritoneal cavity, nasogastric decompression, appropriate antibiotics and intravenous hyperalimentation. Occasionally, large fistulae of the proximal or middle jejunum will require more aggressive treatment with operative intervention to resect or bypass the fistula site. In many instances, however, early operation upon patients with diffuse peritonitis and a fistula of the small bowel will only result in another fistula, because of inadvertent injury to edematous friable bowel. Furthermore, there is a high risk of breakdown of anastomoses performed on edematous, inflamed bowel.

On occasion, when the fistula is large and it appears to be scarred into an abscess cavity which cannot be dissected free for fear of causing multiple other small bowel perforations, the area can be excluded by anastomosing proximal uninvolved bowel in an end-to-side fashion into distal uninvolved bowel. The fistula site will then become defunctionalized and gradually heal.

When intestinal surgery is performed in the presence of diffuse peritoneal inflammation, the intestines should be internally decompressed by a long intestinal tube for an extended period of time. We have had good success with the Leonard tube, which has been left in place for up to 2 to 3 weeks following resection and reanastomosis of small bowel in the presence of diffuse peritonitis.

PITFALL

IF ADEQUATE NUTRITION WITH I.V. HYPERALIMENTATION IS NOT MAINTAINED IN PATIENTS WITH UPPER GASTROINTESTINAL FISTULAE, THE CHANCES OF HEALING ARE GREATLY REDUCED.

The use of I.V. hyperalimentation has enhanced our ability to sustain patients with small bowel fistulae through the worst period of illness. Recently, we carried a patient on I.V. hyperalimentation for approximately nine months while multiple enterocutaneous fistulae either healed spontaneously or were removed by operative intervention.

COLONIC FISTULAE. Small colonic fistulae with minimal infection or inflammation and no associated injuries will frequently heal spontaneously with little or no treatment other than adequate drainage of the area. In the patient with peritonitis or other severe injuries, the involved colon should be exteriorized. Later, after all local inflammation has resolved and the other injuries have healed, the involved colon can be resected and a primary anastomosis performed.

If the involved colon is severely inflamed and can be exteriorized only after difficult or hazardous dissection, a proximal colostomy should be performed with complete drainage of the area of the fistula. After the inflammation has resolved and the patient has recovered from his other injuries, the involved area can be resected. Several weeks later, after the anastomosis is well healed, the proximal colostomy can be closed.

If the fistula involves the rectum, a proximal colostomy should be performed and the involved area of the rectum debrided if necessary and drained. Later, after the rectum has healed, the colostomy can be closed.

Nasogastric drainage should be continued until the local inflammation has been controlled. I.V. hyperalimentation may be used to maintain the patient's nutrition until oral alimentation is safe.

STRESS GASTRIC BLEEDING

Stress gastric bleeding following trauma is one of the most frequent causes of acute upper gastrointestinal hemorrhage in emergency hospitals.[2] The incidence of this complication is particularly high in patients who develop a combination of sepsis and respiratory insufficiency following initial trauma. The hemorrhage in these patients is usually from multiple erosions in the body and fundus of the stomach; rarely, a single ulcer of the antrum or duodenum may be the source of bleeding. An unusually high incidence of erosive gastritis occurs in patients with severe head injuries and those suffering shotgun blasts with multiple bowel perforations and extensive soft-tissue destruction. The combination of intra-abdominal injury with peritoneal spill, thoracic injury with respiratory insufficiency and head injury almost invariably leads to severe bleeding from acute erosive gastritis in the postoperative period.

Etiology

The exact etiology of stress gastric bleeding or acute erosive gastritis is controversial, but it is probably related to a severe decrease in gastric mucosal blood flow during the period of hypovolemia and hypotension. This is followed by an increase in acid production 2 to 4 days later, leading to acid peptic digestion and erosions in the areas of previously ischemic gastric mucosa. Although experimental studies in animals suggest that impaired mucin production or release is an important cause of acute erosive gastritis,[3] most well-controlled clinical studies indicate that mucin production and release are normal or increased in traumatized and septic patients who later develop acute erosive gastritis. The patients treated and studied at Detroit General Hospital uniformly had an increase in the total amount of mucous production compared to patients who did not bleed, and they had no evidence of mucous or mucin deficiency on the basis of histologic studies.[4]

AXIOM

GASTRIC ACID PRODUCTION FOLLOWING TRAUMA, PARTICULARLY IN THE PRESENCE OF SEPSIS, MAY BE GREATLY INCREASED.

Although it has generally been assumed that acid production by the stomach soon after trauma is reduced, many severely injured patients have a marked increase in the volume and degree of acid production by the third day following injury, especially if postoperative complications such as respiratory insufficiency or sepsis occur. During this period, the pH of the gastric juice often falls below 2 and as low as 1. This is important because the patients with the lowest pH in the gastric juice have the greatest chance of developing clinically significant bleeding which will require multiple transfusions.

This increased gastric acid production in severely injured patients only began to be appreciated when a prospective study of gastric secretion following trauma was instituted. Since acid is neutralized by blood, it may be difficult to demonstrate hyperacidity during or immediately following gastric hemorrhage. The acid production will also decline during and soon after a hypotensive episode, but, if the underlying insult persists, it will reach prebleed status again after another 2 to 3 days. Another misleading factor is the frequent appearance of a green color in the nasogastric juice shortly before the bleeding episode begins, giving the false impression that the gastric juice contains large amounts of bile, and is, therefore, alkaline. Even small amounts of bile, however, will cause a pronounced color change, so that a dark green nasogastric aspirate in the postinjury period will commonly have a pH as low as 1.0.

Serial gastric endoscopy on patients on the emergency surgical division of Detroit General Hospital has revealed mottled areas of pallor with tiny petechiae as early as 2 to 4 hours following the initial injury.[2] This reticular pattern of pallor, mixed with hyperemia, persists for the first 36 hours, by which time small 5-mm red-based erosions frequently appear. These changes are usually confined to the proximal two-thirds of the stomach, particularly along the greater curvature near the fundus, with little or no change in the antrum. By the third postinjury day, multiple red- and black-based erosions are present throughout the proximal two-thirds of the stomach. Occasionally, white erosions also occur. The size of these erosions gradually increases so that by 4 to 5 days, when actual bleeding occurs, some are 10 to 15 mm in diameter. The larger erosions will frequently lose their concentric appearance and develop various geometrical shapes—linear, oval and round, with pseudoprojections. If the etiologic problems have been treated adequately, the erosions will gradually resolve over the next 7 to 14 days by progressively becoming more superficial and less red until the color approximates that of the surrounding mucosa.

The histologic appearance of the early erosions, obtained either by direct gastric biopsies during surgery for acute erosive gastritis or else by endoscopic biopsy in patients not undergoing surgery, shows mucosal edema beneath the gastric pits (Fig. 7). Later there is diapedesis of red cells into this space which, as it increases in amount, gives the appearance of gross mucosal hemorrhage. At this time, the superficial portion of the mucosa appears normal and the mucin content of superficial mucosal cells and the mucin layer overlying

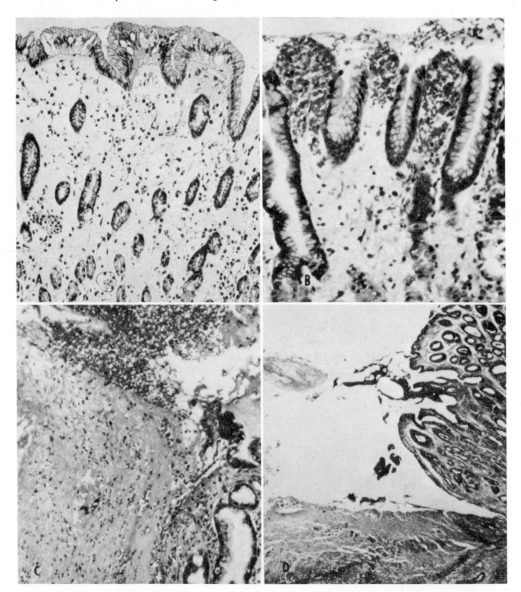

FIG. 7. A: Biopsy of gastric mucosa showing marked interstitial edema. (H & E × 40.) B: Hemorrhage in the superficial zone of the mucosa, with loss of surface epithelium between foveola. (H & E × 64.) C: Coagulative necrosis involving most of mucosal thickness in this endoscopic biopsy. Intact gastric glands are seen to the right. (H & E × 64.) D: Slough of the area of coagulative necrosis leaving the ulcer, which extends down to the muscularis mucosa. (PAS × 10.) (These light photomicrographs were supplied by Dr. Barbara Rosenberg, Department of Pathology, Wayne State University School of Medicine, Detroit, Michigan.)

the mucosa is intact as judged by PAS stains and electron microscopy. This appearance is in contrast to the acute erosive gastritis produced in experimental studies in animals by the administration of drugs such as aspirin or histamine. In these studies, the superficial mucin layer and the intracellular mucin content along the apex of the cells in the animals are greatly diminished or disappear.

As the stress gastritis in the injured patient progresses, the mucosa develops areas of focal necrosis which gradually deepen and widen. This is followed by slough of

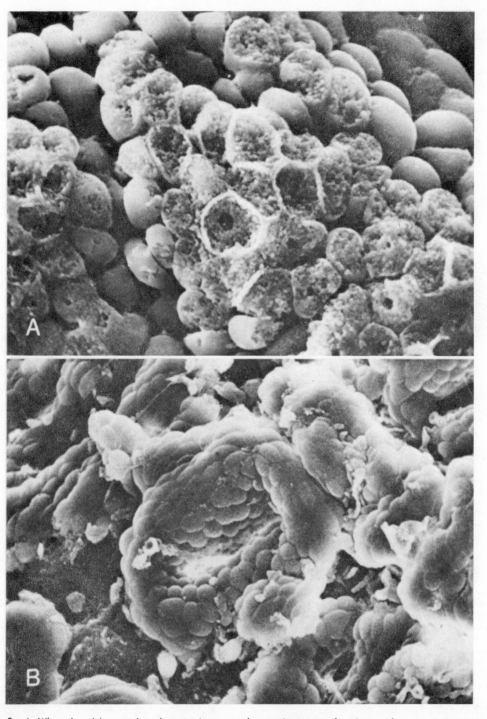

FIG. 8. A: When viewed by scanning electron microscopy, the gastric mucosa of patients with acute erosive gastritis displayed focal areas in which a group of epithelial cells showed loss of their apical portion with dissipation of the internal cellular contents. (× 2700.) B: Further cell disruption was evidenced by a partial denudation of the gastric mucosa so that intact epithelial cells were seen only in association with the gastric glands when the architecture was viewed in 3-D. (× 840.)

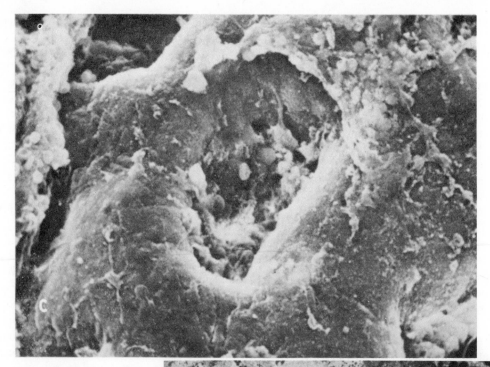

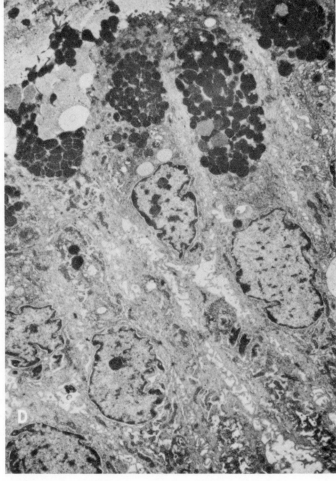

FIG. 8. C: The process of denudation progressed with destruction of even the surface epithelial cells which lined the gastric glands. ($\times$ 940.) D: Using the transmission electron microscope, individual gastric epithelial cells showed intracellular vacuolization in the absence of apical disruption in some cells and with apical disruption in other cells. The morphology of the mucin granules varied. ($\times$ 12,500.) (The electron micrographs for Figure 8 were supplied by Dr. Jeanne M. Riddle, Department of Pathology, Wayne State University School of Medicine, Detroit, Michigan.)

the involved tissue down to the muscularis mucosa. Occasionally this process will extend below the muscularis mucosa into the submucosa and rarely the necrosis will extend into a submucosal vessel. In most instances, the bleeding is diffuse and appears to be coming from a large number of erosions; only rarely does the major bleeding seem to come from a single erosion which has extended below the muscularis mucosa into a submucosal vessel.

On transmission electron microscopy, the earliest changes consist of intracellular and intercellular vacuolation with minimal other cellular injuries (Fig. 8). The superficial apical mucin layer appears to be normal and intact, supporting the concept that stress gastritis in man occurs without change in mucin production or release. Later, the cell loses its apex and discharges its mucin granules into the gastric lumen. When this focal process involves multiple cells in the same area, the area develops a honeycomb appearance. Later, the involved area collapses and necrosis down to the muscularis mucosa is apparent. Direct electron microscopy confirms that the areas immediately adjacent to the well-defined erosions are essentially normal, emphasizing the focal nature of this disease.

Diagnosis

Any patient with severe shock, massive peritoneal contamination and respiratory insufficiency or head injury should be recognized as a likely candidate for the development of acute erosive gastritis. This is a particularly frequent complication in patients with close-range shotgun blasts to the abdomen with destruction of large quantities of soft tissue.

On physical examination, the patients likely to develop this problem appear to be anxious, diaphoretic and tachypneic. If the nasogastric tube has been removed prematurely or has not been functioning adequately, severe adynamic ileus is usually also present. The volume of gastric secre-

tions will generally be increased to more than 1,000 ml in 12 hours and the acidity will be increased to a pH in the range of 1 to 2. By the third to fourth day, the gastric secretions contain black flecks due to superficial bleeding with oxidation of the red cells by gastric acid. As the stress gastritis becomes worse, bright red blood is noted in the nasogastric aspirate, indicating clinically significant hemorrhage. It may take several hours before a significant drop in the hemoglobin or hematocrit occurs.

Upper gastrointestinal x-rays are essentially useless because of the superficial location of these lesions. If there is some question about the diagnosis, endoscopy should be employed to confirm the presence of the typical lesions in the proximal two-thirds of the stomach with absence of changes in the antrum and to rule out coincident gastric or duodenal ulcer disease.

AXIOM

ENDOSCOPY SHOULD BE EMPLOYED TO OBTAIN AN ACCURATE DIAGNOSIS OF THE CAUSE OF POST-TRAUMATIC UPPER GASTROINTESTINAL HEMORRHAGE.

Treatment

The most important aspect of treatment of acute erosive gastritis is prevention. This includes an aggressive initial resuscitation with rapid correction of any hypovolemia and hypotension.

Another aspect of prevention includes the aggressive treatment of any tendency to sepsis, adynamic ileus or respiratory insufficiency. If these problems become well established and cannot be reversed, operative intervention is often required to control the stress gastric bleeding. Occasionally, severe hemorrhage due to acute erosive gastritis has been stopped simply by the drainage of an intra-abdominal abscess.

Another important factor in the prevention of bleeding from acute erosive gastritis is use of a nasogastric tube to provide complete gastric decompression, thereby removing the acid produced by the parietal cells before further injury to the already ischemic gastric mucosa is produced. By the third or fourth postinjury day, it may also be wise to use antacids to neutralize the excess acid.

PITFALL

IF TOO MUCH RELIANCE IS PLACED ON LARGE DOSES OF ANTACIDS TO PREVENT STRESS GASTRIC BLEEDING, THE ANTACIDS MAY BE USED IN EXCESSIVE QUANTITIES CAUSING INCREASED COMPLICATIONS WITHOUT NECESSARILY PREVENTING BLEEDING.

The aggressive use of large volumes of Maalox to prevent stress gastric bleeding may be effective in some injured patients,[5] but it has also caused other problems such as severe metabolic alkalosis, abdominal distension from ileus, and diarrhea. In some instances, the metabolic alkalosis achieved by this regimen has resulted in the development of an arterial pH exceeding 7.55. Consequently, usage of excessive quantities of Maalox is now essentially contraindicated.

A compromise approach which seems reasonable is nasogastric suction with the intermittent administration of 30 to 60 ml of Maalox on an hourly basis whenever the gastric pH is less than 3.5. After the Maalox is administered through the nasogastric tube, the suction is discontinued for approximately 5 minutes so that any acid that had not been removed by the previous suctioning will be neutralized. The nasogastric tube is then immediately attached back to suction to remove the Maalox. When this procedure is followed, it is important to check the patency of the nasogastric tube frequently. If the tube becomes occluded, large amounts of acid are left to bathe the ischemic gastric mucosa.

PITFALL

IF IT IS ASSUMED THAT A NASOGASTRIC TUBE CAN CAUSE STRESS GASTRIC BLEEDING, THE TUBE IS APT TO BE REMOVED AT A TIME WHEN IT IS MOST NEEDED.

A frequently expressed myth in the area of acute erosive gastritis in injured and septic patients is that trauma to the mucosa caused by the nasogastric tube itself is an important cause of acute erosive gastritis and subsequent bleeding. Our own experience, however, indicates that early removal of the nasogastric tube is more likely to cause clinically significant bleeding from acute erosive gastritis than is the continuation of the nasogastric decompression.

AXIOM

SEPSIS MUST BE CONTROLLED BEFORE PERFORMING A GASTRECTOMY TO CONTROL POSTTRAUMATIC STRESS GASTRIC BLEEDING.

In many patients who have active hemorrhage from acute erosive gastritis, control of sepsis by drainage of any collections of pus and vigorous lavage of the stomach with iced saline will often control the bleeding and the nasogastric aspirate will begin to clear. At this point, if the sepsis, adynamic ileus and respiratory failure are controlled, the nasogastric drainage may be continued for long periods of time with gradual healing of the acute erosive gastritis. In contrast, in a few patients in whom no nasogastric tube was ever inserted but who developed abdominal sepsis and acute erosive gastritis, the acute erosive gastritis was still confined to its usual position in the proximal two thirds of the stomach.

Once acute erosive gastritis has developed and clinical bleeding is significant, ice-saline lavage has been our most successful method for controlling active bleeding. Although large volumes of ice-saline are often required to achieve this result, the procedure will stop the bleeding in over 80% of the patients so treated. According to some reports, bleeding which persists in spite of vigorous ice-saline lavage may occasionally respond to gastric hypothermia. In our experience, however, this procedure has not been beneficial.

PITFALL

IF CLOTTING ABNORMALITIES IN PATIENTS WITH STRESS GASTRIC BLEEDING ARE NOT PREVENTED OR ARE NOT CORRECTED PROMPTLY, IT MAY BE VIRTUALLY IMPOSSIBLE TO CONTROL THE BLEEDING, EVEN WITH SURGERY.

While transfusing the patient to replace the volume loss, it is crucial also to provide fresh blood. Not infrequently, an infusion of fresh platelets has caused cessation of stress gastric bleeding which was continuing in spite of all other therapy. When more than 6 units of blood are required in a 24-hour period to replace the blood loss, despite vigorous ice-saline lavage and other measures, some type of operative intervention is generally indicated.

AXIOM

GASTRODUODENOSCOPY PRIOR TO AND/OR DURING EMERGENCY SURGERY FOR MASSIVE UPPER GASTROINTESTINAL HEMORRHAGE MAY PROVIDE INFORMATION ON THE SOURCE OF THE BLEEDING THAT MIGHT NOT OTHERWISE BE AVAILABLE.

At the time of surgery, intraoperative fiberoptic endoscopy helps confirm that the source of bleeding is erosions in the proximal two thirds of the stomach. Following the laparotomy, a noncrushing clamp is placed on the proximal jejunum to prevent inflated air from causing small bowel distension. The fiberoptic endoscope is then passed transorally while the balloon of the endotracheal tube is temporarily released. Once the endoscope has been inserted into

the stomach, the balloon on the endotracheal tube can be reinflated. Most patients with acute erosive gastritis on whom this technique has been employed have had previous nasogastric decompression and ice-saline lavage, so that large amounts of clot within the stomach have not been a problem. Occasionally, a large Ewald tube may be required to empty the stomach of large clots.

Once the diagnosis of acute erosive gastritis is confirmed, the operative procedure for uncontrolled bleeding consists of a vagotomy, followed by some type of gastric drainage or a distal gastric resection. The vagotomy is done as the initial procedure because it often provides a temporary decrease in gastric mucosal blood flow at surgery and reduces acid secretion postoperatively. Indeed, in two patients, the vagotomy alone was observed by endoscopy to cause a dramatic cessation of bleeding from the erosions.

The decision to perform a simple drainage procedure as opposed to a distal gastrectomy is related to how well the underlying causes of bleeding have been controlled. Patients who have minor pulmonary problems or a single isolated intraabdominal abscess will require only a pyloroplasty if the bleeding stops immediately following the vagotomy. However, patients who have severe uncontrolled respiratory insufficiency or diffuse multiple intraloop intraperitoneal abscesses will require removal of at least 50 to 75% of the distal stomach. Unfortunately, the patients with severe respiratory problems and multiple intraperitoneal abscesses are often so sick that the surgeon is reluctant to perform a gastric resection. As a consequence, many patients who were extremely ill had only a vagotomy and pyloroplasty for the acute bleeding episode; these patients have had a very high incidence of severe rebleeding in the postoperative period.

Total gastrectomy is best reserved for those patients who have unusually large volumes of acid secretion in the prebleed-ing phase, for example more than 100 mEq of free hydrochloric acid in 12 hours. Total gastrectomy in patients with acute erosive gastritis from trauma and sepsis is technically more difficult than it is in patients with alcoholic or aspirin-induced gastritis. The gastric mucosa in the severely injured patient with sepsis is thicker, more edematous and much more likely to crack when the gastric clamp is applied. Furthermore, larger sutures are generally required to approximate this edematous gastric wall and obtain a tension-free anastomosis.

AXIOM

OPERATIVE INTERVENTION TO CONTROL SEVERE STRESS GASTRIC BLEEDING IS FREQUENTLY UNSUCCESSFUL IF THE INCITING OR PRIMARY PROCESS HAS NOT BEEN CORRECTED.

The prognosis following operative intervention for acute erosive gastritis in patients with trauma or sepsis is related primarily to how well the underlying disease process and the associated illnesses can be controlled. Patients with severe respiratory failure and diffuse peritonitis requiring vagotomy and 70% gastric resection will have a high mortality rate, primarily because of continued respiratory failure, renal failure or overwhelming sepsis. However, if these other factors can be controlled, the prognosis is usually good and the incidence of rebleeding is very low.

LIVER FAILURE

Etiology

The causes of liver failure following trauma may be divided into three main groups: prehepatic, hepatic and posthepatic. Prehepatic liver failure is the result of hypoperfusion to the liver during the period of hypovolemia and hypotension during and following trauma or surgery. This causes a variable degree of degenerative changes and areas of focal necrosis

within the liver. An important predisposing factor to the development of liver failure in such patients is prior Laennec's cirrhosis.

AXIOM

SEVERE PROLONGED SHOCK IN PATIENTS WITH ADVANCED CIRRHOSIS IS GENERALLY FATAL.

Hepatic or intrahepatic causes of liver failure following trauma are results of direct damage to the liver from the injury, drugs or sepsis. In most instances, the injury to the liver itself is not likely to cause liver failure unless severe associated problems such as shock and sepsis are also present. Normally only about 20 to 30% of the liver tissue is required to sustain life, but if the remaining liver has been insulted or damaged by shock or sepsis it may be totally inadequate.

Hepatic failure due to drugs may be caused by a wide variety of agents, particularly anesthetics and street drugs such as heroin and other intravenously administered narcotics. One of the most frequently implicated anesthetic drugs in the development of hepatic failure is Fluothane, particularly if it is given on two separate occasions several days or weeks apart. It is difficult to determine, however, whether this drug has been important in the development of liver failure in any of our injured patients.

"Septic jaundice" or hepatic failure due to or associated with sepsis is being seen with increasing frequency in patients who survive extremely severe trauma and shock and later become septic. We have shown, both by light and electron microscopy, that sepsis produces a nonspecific change in both Kupffer cells and hepatocytes which results in impairment of enzymatic function and bile transport. This is recognized experimentally by impairment in glucose metabolism similar to that seen following experimental hepatic transplantation.

19

Posthepatic causes for liver failure following trauma are very rare. They would most often be related to damage to the common bile duct or ampulla of Vater by the trauma itself, or by the surgeon while repairing an injury to the biliary tract, pancreas or duodenum. Injury to the liver itself rarely, if ever, causes extrahepatic biliary obstruction and such a complication has not been identified in the past 500 patients with liver injuries who were treated at Detroit General Hospital.[6]

Diagnosis

The diagnosis of liver failure after trauma is made primarily by observing the alterations in liver function studies. This is true whether the patient has had preexisting liver disease or a previously normal liver; however, the severe alterations in liver function studies occur much earlier and are much more severe in patients with cirrhosis.

Typical laboratory abnormalities include elevation of the bilirubin, LDH, alkaline phosphatase, SGOT and prothrombin time with a fall in the serum albumin. The serum bilirubin in "septic jaundice" has risen as high as 37 mg/100 ml and is usually about 50% direct or conjugated. Jaundice due to massive transfusions, hemolysis or transfusion reactions usually causes an elevation primarily in the indirect fraction of the bilirubin, with minimal changes in the other liver function tests.

The alkaline phosphatase frequently rises proportionally more than the bilirubin in patients with post-traumatic or septic jaundice. The SGOT tends to be in a range of 100 to 500 units, whereas the LDH generally rises to 500 to 1,500 units. The albumin typically falls below 3 gm/100 ml and may be associated with an increase in the prothrombin time to greater than 5 seconds above control in spite of vitamin K therapy. Little data has been obtained on BSP retention in these patients.

The differential diagnosis between intrahepatic and posthepatic jaundice is rarely a problem in our critically injured patients because the latter is so uncommon. If, however, there is some question, the diagnosis of extrahepatic biliary obstruction can be confirmed or ruled out by peroral endoscopic cannulation of the ampulla of Vater and retrograde cholangiography. Percutaneous transhepatic cholangiography should be avoided since it is likely to cause bile leakage or hemorrhage which may require operative intervention, and these patients are very poor risks for emergency surgery.

Treatment

The treatment of impaired liver function depends upon its cause. If the tissue perfusion is inadequate, it must be improved by administration of additional blood or other fluids and inotropic agents such as digitalis as needed. Hepatic failure due to or associated with sepsis requires debridement and drainage of any necrotic tissue or pus and administration of appropriate antibiotics based on smears and culture and sensitivity studies. Extrahepatic biliary obstruction, although rare in trauma patients, requires some type of decompression of the biliary tract or correction of the obstruction. I.V. hyperalimentation may be important to maintain nutrition while the liver function is poor; however, the intravenous catheters must be watched and managed carefully to prevent further sepsis.

SUMMARY

The incidence and severity of most gastrointestinal complications can be reduced by rapid resuscitation with blood and fluids

TABLE 1. FREQUENT ERRORS IN THE MANAGEMENT OF GASTROINTESTINAL COMPLICATIONS FOLLOWING TRAUMA

1. Late insertion and/or early removal of a nasogastric tube in severely injured patients, particularly those with peritoneal contamination by small bowel or colon contents.

2. Inadequate attention to ensuring that a nasogastric tube is functioning and emptying the stomach properly.

3. Inadequate appreciation of the increased fluids that a patient with severe ileus requires.

4. Assuming that a fistula is not present just because it cannot be seen on appropriate x-ray contrast studies.

5. Failure to maintain adequate nutrition, using I.V. hyperalimentation as needed, in patient with gastrointestinal fistulae.

6. Inadequate removal and/or neutralization of gastric acid in patients with peritoneal sepsis, massive tissue destruction, respiratory failure, and/or severe head injury.

7. Excessive reliance on antacids to neutralize post-traumatic gastric hyperacidity leading to combined respiratory and metabolic alkalosis and control of concomitant sepsis.

8. Failure to use flexible gastroduodenoscopy to determine the cause of upper gastrointestinal hemorrhage.

9. Inadequate attention to control of sepsis in patients with post-traumatic or septic jaundice.

and early operation to keep the peritoneal contamination from bowel leakage to a minimum. Copious irrigation of the peritoneal cavity and careful complete drainage of the involved areas probably reduce the likelihood and severity of peritonitis. Continuous complete decompression of the stomach with a nasogastric tube until bowel activity is normal is particularly important for preventing adynamic ileus, small bowel fistulae and stress gastric bleeding.

Anticipation of gastrointestinal complications in patients with severe prolonged shock, massive tissue destruction or extensive peritoneal contamination may allow appropriate procedures to be begun early when they are most effective. Once the complications have developed, prolonged supportive care, including gastrointestinal decompression, ventilatory support, I.V. hyperalimentation and antibiotics, is generally required. Surgical intervention is rarely required except to drain collections of pus, to control massive unrelenting upper gastrointestinal bleeding or to lyse adhesions.

Frequent errors in the management of post-traumatic gastrointestinal complications are listed in Table 1.

REFERENCES

1. Landman, M. D., and Langmire, W. P., Jr.: Neural and hormonal influences of peritonitis on paralytic ileus. Amer. Surg., 33:756, 1967.
2. Lucas, C. E., et al.: Natural history and surgical dilemma of "stress" gastric bleeding. Arch. Surg., 102:266, 1971.
3. Zimmerman, B., and Gerwig, W. H., Jr.: The large and small intestine. In: Physiologic Principles of Surgery (Zimmerman, L. M., and Levine, R., Eds.). Philadelphia, W. B. Saunders, 1964.
4. Lucas, C. E., et al.: Therapeutic implications of disturbed gastric physiology in patients with stress ulcerations. Amer. Surg., 123:25, 1972.
5. Skillman, J. V., et al.: Respiratory failure, hypotension, sepsis, and jaundice: A clinical syndrome associated with lethal hemorrhage from acute stress ulceration of the stomach. Amer. Surg., 117:523, 1969.
6. Lucas, C. E., and Walt, A. J.: Critical decisions in liver trauma. Experience based on 604 cases. Amer. Surg., 101:277, 1970.

34 COAGULATION ABNORMALITIES IN TRAUMA

E. F. MAMMEN

Abnormally functioning hemostatic mechanisms in the injured patient, unless recognized promptly and treated appropriately, may lead not only to excessive bleeding and possible death but also to poor wound healing or thromboembolic complications. Whenever a patient develops excessive bleeding following trauma or in the intra- or postoperative period, it must be immediately determined whether the bleeding is caused by a technical problem (open vessels which must be sutured, tied or coagulated) or whether it is a result of a defect in the hemostatic mechanisms.

AXIOM

INTRAOPERATIVE AND POSTOPERATIVE BLEEDING, ESPECIALLY WHEN LIMITED TO THE SITE OF TRAUMA, IS USUALLY DUE TO INADEQUATE SURGICAL EFFORTS AND ONLY RARELY WILL AN ABNORMALITY BE FOUND IN ANY OF THE CLOTTING MECHANISMS.

The objective of this chapter is briefly to outline the factors involved in normal hemostasis, the diagnostic procedures used for detecting hemostatic abnormalities, and the methods used to diagnose and treat the most frequent congenital and acquired bleeding disorders.

NORMAL HEMOSTASIS

Normal hemostasis is accomplished by the harmonious interplay of blood vessel wall, platelets and the coagulation mechanism.

Primary Hemostasis

Following any trauma, injured blood vessels promptly respond with local vasoconstriction which appears to be chiefly mediated by the autonomic nervous system, greatly reducing blood flow in that area. The exposure of collagen fibers or basement membrane initiates "platelet adhesion," resulting in the deposition of a single layer of platelets at the site of injury. This adhesion of platelets is followed by a "release reaction" in which adenosine diphosphate (ADP) and serotonin are released from the adhered platelets. These substances mediate "platelet aggregation" or "cohesion," which lead to the clumping of platelets at the site of injury. The serotonin helps to maintain local vasoconstriction. If the vessel is 50 μ or smaller in diameter, platelet aggregation leads to the formation of a "first hemostatic plug" or "platelet plug" which facilitates "primary hemostasis." At this time, no fibrin can yet be demonstrated.[1-4]

The Coagulation Mechanism (Secondary Hemostasis)

The coagulation mechanism is initiated by the release of phospholipids in micellar form from platelets (platelet factor 3) which sets in motion a series of protein interactions resulting in the formation of fibrin. Fibrin then replaces the first hemostatic plug to form the "second hemostatic plug." This process of fibrin formation, also referred to as "secondary hemostasis," can be divided arbitrarily into (1) the formation of activated Factor X (Factor Xa), (2) the formation of thrombin, and (3) the formation of fibrin.

FORMATION OF ACTIVATED FACTOR X (FACTOR xa). The formation of activated Factor X from Factor X, its precursor, can be accomplished either by an intrinsic pathway or an extrinsic pathway.

The Intrinsic Pathway (Fig. 1). In the intrinsic pathway, a complex is formed between platelet phospholipids in micellar form serving as surfaces, calcium ions serving as binders, activated Factor IX (Factor IXa) as the enzyme and Factor VIII (antihemophilic Factor A) which seems to determine the reaction specificity between enzyme and substrate. This reaction may be depicted as follows:

$$\left.\begin{array}{l}\text{Phospholipids}\\\text{Calcium ions}\\\text{Factor IXa}\\\text{Factor VIII}\end{array}\right\}\text{Complex}\longrightarrow \begin{array}{c}\text{Factor X}\\\downarrow\\\text{Factor Xa}\end{array}$$

Factor IX is produced in the liver and, like that of prothrombin and Factor X, its synthesis requires the presence of vitamin K. Factor VIII is the only clotting factor *not* synthesized in the liver. The mechanisms by which Factor IXa is formed from Factor IX are presently subject to speculation, but two factors seem to be involved: Factor XII (Hageman factor) and Factor XI or plasma thromboplastin antecedent (PTA), both produced in the liver.

It is assumed that Factor XII is activated to Factor XIIa on phospholipid surfaces or collagen fibers, and Factor XIIa in turn activates Factor XI to Factor XIa. Factor XIa then is supposed to convert Factor IX to Factor IXa. The details of this sequence are not known.

The Extrinsic Pathway (Fig. 1). The extrinsic pathway is marked by the involvement of tissue thromboplastin. All forms of tissue contain a clot-promoting activity called tissue thromboplastin. Tissue thromboplastin can be separated into a protein portion and a lipid portion. The active principle of the lipid portion consists of phospholipids in micellar form. Like the platelet phospholipids, the tissue phospholipids also seem to serve as surfaces for formation of a complex between "enzymes" (apparently located in the protein portion), Factor VII (a plasma protein which is produced in the liver in the presence of vitamin K, and which seems to determine the reaction specificity between enzyme and substrate) and calcium ions (acting as binders). The extrinsic pathway can thus be depicted as follows:

$$\left.\begin{array}{l}\text{Phospholipids}\\\text{Calcium ions}\\\text{Enzyme(s)}\\\text{Factor VII}\end{array}\right\}\text{Complex}\longrightarrow \begin{array}{c}\text{Factor X}\\\downarrow\\\text{Factor Xa}\end{array}$$

FORMATION OF THROMBIN. Thrombin is formed from prothrombin, which is synthesized in the liver parenchymal cell with the aid of vitamin K. The conversion of prothrombin to thrombin is facilitated by a complex formed between platelet phospholipid micelles (acting as surfaces), calcium ions (acting as binders), activated Factor X (acting as an enzyme) and Factor V (also known as Ac-globulin, a protein produced in the liver without vitamin K, which seems to determine the reaction specificity between enzyme and substrate). Thus, the formation of thrombin from prothrombin can be depicted as follows:[5,6]

$$\left.\begin{array}{l}\text{Phospholipids}\\\text{Calcium ions}\\\text{Factor Xa}\\\text{Factor V}\end{array}\right\}\text{Complex}\longrightarrow \begin{array}{c}\text{Prothrombin}\\\downarrow\\\text{Thrombin}\end{array}$$

FORMATION OF FIBRIN. Fibrin is formed from fibrinogen, a plasma protein produced by the liver parenchymal cells. Normally there are between 200 and 300 mg of clottable fibrinogen in every 100 ml of plasma.

The formation of fibrin can be divided into (1) the proteolytic phase, (2) the polymerization phase, and (3) the stabilization phase.

The Proteolytic Phase. The fibrinogen molecule circulates in a dimer form and is composed of three chains called α, β, and γ. The proteolytic phase of fibrin formation is marked by the cleavage of an A and B peptide from the N-terminal end of the α and β chains respectively. This cleavage is facilitated by the proteolytic enzyme thrombin. Since fibrinogen circulates in a dimer form, a pair of A peptides and a pair of B peptides are released. The fibrinogen dimer now minus its fibrinopeptides A and B is called a "fibrin monomer."

The Polymerization Phase. The polymerization phase is characterized by the spontaneous polymerization of the fibrin monomers, whereby α chains polymerize with α chains and β chains with β chains forming an end-to-end and side-to-side polymerized fibrin network composed of individual fibrin monomers. This polymerization occurs spontaneously without the participation of an enzyme.

The Stabilization Phase. During the stabilization phase, the polymerized fibrin monomers are covalently bonded by a "fibrin stabilizing factor" also called Factor XIII. Factor XIII is produced in the liver in a proenzymic form and becomes activated to its enzymatic form by thrombin.[7-10]

Clot Retraction

After the fibrin fibers have formed, they begin to shorten, causing the clot to retract. This fibrin shortening is due to thrombosthenin, a protein found in platelets. The

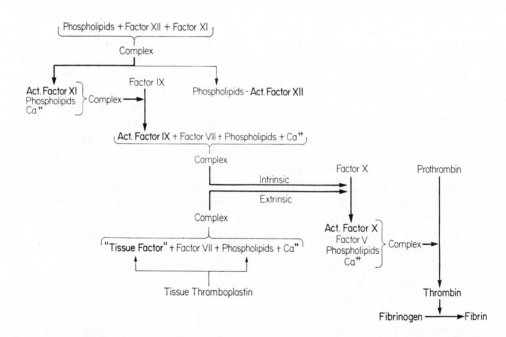

FIG. 1.   Simple coagulation scheme describing the formation of fibrin or the formation of the "second hemostatic plug."

actual mechanisms of shortening of fibrin fibers is analogous to that involved in the shortening of actinomyosin in muscle. Calcium ions and ATP must be present in both reactions. The ATP required as the energy source for clot retraction comes from platelets.[11]

Fibrinolysis

Clot retraction is followed by fibrinolysis, which serves to remove fibrin in order for the fibroblasts to repair the injured tissue. Fibrinolysis is accomplished by a proteolytic enzyme called plasmin or fibrinolysin, which is derived from a precursor called plasminogen or profibrinolysin. Plasminogen is produced in the liver and also carried (or produced) in the eosinophilic granulocytes. It is converted by activators into its enzymic form.[12,13]

Several plasmin activators of uncertain biochemical nature are recognized in tissues, particularly in the intima of blood vessels, and in the blood itself. All of these substances convert plasminogen directly to the plasmin by what appears to be an enzymatic process. One of the plasmin activators, urokinase, found normally in urine, is well defined, and has been used clinically to treat thromboembolic diseases. Another well-known and clinically important plasmin activator is streptokinase, which is obtained from streptococci.[14-16]

Plasmin is a protease which, like trypsin, digests a variety of proteins including fibrin

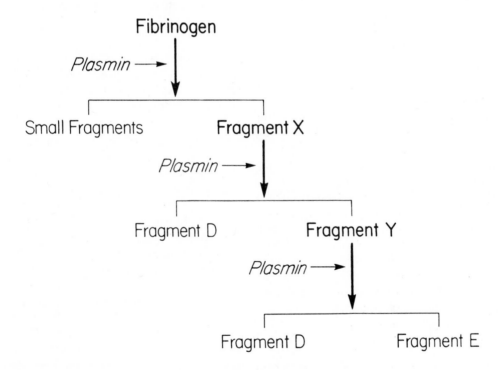

FIG. 2. Proteolytic digestion of fibrinogen and its fragments by plasmin into so-called early and late fibrinogen split products.

and fibrinogen, thus causing fibrinolysis and fibrinogenolysis. Fibrin and fibrinogen are digested or broken down into so-called fibrin or fibrinogen split products (FSP) or fibrin or fibrinogen degradation products (FDP), initially, large-molecular-weight split products (called fragments X and Y or "early split products") (Fig. 2). The "early fibrin(ogen) split products" act as anticoagulants in that they inhibit the polymerization phase of fibrin formation, competitively inhibit thrombin, and coat the surface of platelets, thereby rendering them unaggregable. FSP thus block both primary and secondary hemostasis.[17-19]

DIAGNOSTIC PROCEDURES FOR THE DETECTION OF BLEEDING DISORDERS

Prior to any type of surgery, the possible existence of a bleeding tendency should be ruled out. This precaution will eliminate many problems that otherwise may catch the surgeon by surprise.

History

A good history obtained from the patient or from the relatives will give a clue to the existence of most cases of congenital or acquired bleeding disorders. Many patients with known bleeding problems wear an identification tag or have some other notification in their wallets. On the other hand, it must be recognized that many injured patients, for a variety of reasons, may not spontaneously mention an increased bleeding tendency. Therefore, direct questions related to bruising tendency, epistaxis, hemorrhage following minor trauma or operations, melena, hematuria, joint swellings, and prolonged menstrual periods or postpartum bleeding are important.

PITFALL

IF A DILIGENT EFFORT IS NOT MADE TO OB-
TAIN A HISTORY OF ANTICOAGULANT DRUGS IN
BLEEDING PATIENTS, APPROPRIATE THERAPY
MAY BE DANGEROUSLY DELAYED.

An effort should always be made to determine if the injured patient has been taking anticoagulants, particularly if surgery is contemplated. It should also be determined whether he has been taking drugs which contain acetylsalicylic acid or other compounds which interfere with platelet function.

Physical Examination. The physical examination should include a thorough search for bleeding manifestations in the skin and joints (hemorrhagic arthropathies).

Laboratory Studies. If there is any suggestion of a bleeding tendency on the basis of the history or physical examination, a proper laboratory diagnosis of the underlying problem should be obtained prior to any surgery, if time allows. This is best done in consultation with a hematologist who has access to a laboratory that can perform sophisticated coagulation tests.

PITFALL

IF LABORATORY TESTS ARE RELIED UPON
TO RULE OUT COAGULATION ABNORMALITIES,
MILD TO MODERATE DISORDERS MAY BE COM-
PLETELY OVERLOOKED.

The usefulness of screening all patients with certain coagulation tests prior to surgery is a matter of debate. In most instances, the number and type of tests are inadequate to diagnose all possible coagulation problems. Relatively mild congenital or acquired bleeding disorders are easily overlooked because most of the procedures currently available are not as sensitive as one might wish them to be. Nevertheless, any hospital in which surgery is performed should be capable of performing the following six tests on a routine basis. If these tests are performed by adequately trained individuals, most aspects of the hemostatic mechanisms can be screened and any serious abnormality will become apparent.

1. A *platelet count*, performed by means of phase contrast microscopy[20,21] or Coulter counter techniques, gives a quantitative

assessment of the number of circulating platelets, a decrease of which is one of the most common causes for excessive surgical hemorrhage.

2. A *bleeding time,* preferably performed according to the procedure described by Ivy,[22] will be abnormal not only in patients with thrombocytopenia, but also with many forms of thrombocytopathy, especially those which affect the formation of the first hemostatic plug or platelet plug. Mild thrombocytopathies, however, may not be discovered.

3. *Partial thromboplastin times (PTT),*[23] activated or nonactivated, will screen the activity of all coagulation factors involved in the formation of thrombin via the intrinsic pathway (Factors II, V, VIII, IX, X, XI, XII) (Fig. 1). Only Factor VII activity is not measured by the PTT.

   This test is not very sensitive, however, and the factors involved have to be reduced to less than 40% of normal before an abnormality in the PTT is apparent. Unfortunately, excessive bleeding during major surgical procedures can occur from relatively mild reductions in these clotting factors.

4. The *prothrombin times*[24] screen the activity of all coagulation factors involved in the extrinsic formation of thrombin (Factors II, V, VII, X), but the same sensitivity criteria apply as with the PTTs. Using both the PTT and prothrombin time, however, one can screen for *all* the coagulation factors involved in thrombin formation, and any major abnormalities should become apparent with one or both tests.

5. *Fibrinogen determinations*[25] give information concerning the quantity of fibrin that can be expected to be formed. If the fibrinogen levels are above 100 mg/100 ml and are not associated with other defects, they will maintain adequate hemostasis. Unfortunately, low levels of fibrinogen are usually associated with other defects, expecially fibrinolysis or disseminated intravascular coagulation (D.I.C.).

6. *Thrombin times*[26] are most helpful in determining defects associated with the actual formation of fibrin from fibrinogen by thrombin. They are abnormal if the fibrinogen level is below 50 mg/100 ml, if heparin is present, if abnormal plasma proteins (paraproteinemias) are present, and, most importantly, if fibrinogen split

products (especially the early ones) are present. Thrombin times, in the absence of heparin and in the presence of more than 50 mg/100 ml fibrinogen, are highly sensitive to the presence of split products and thus can be highly sensitive indicators of the presence of fibrinolysis.

In summary, platelet counts and bleeding times screen for most of the serious quantitative and qualitative platelet abnormalities; partial thromboplastin times and prothrombin times screen for all serious clotting factor deficiencies involved in the formation of thrombin; and fibrinogen determinations plus thrombin times screen for the presence of increased fibrinolytic activity.

A reptilase time, if available, can be used to differentiate hyperheparinemia from increased split products. A normal reptilase time combined with a prolonged thrombin time is an indication of hyperheparinemia. In the presence of fibrin(ogen) split products both tests will be prolonged.[27]

CONGENITAL BLEEDING DISORDERS

PITFALL

ATTEMPTS TO MANAGE INJURED PATIENTS WITH KNOWN CONGENITAL BLEEDING DISORDERS IN SMALL COMMUNITY HOSPITALS ARE OFTEN UNSUCCESSFUL.

Elective surgery on patients with known congenital bleeding disorders should be performed only in those centers where excellent hematologic services are available. This entails not only a "hemostasiologist" but also the services of a well-functioning coagulation laboratory which is capable not only of diagnosing the defects but also of following the effects of specific therapeutic regimens. It must be remembered that in spite of our advances in component therapy, which have unquestionably prolonged the life expectancy of many patients with congenital bleeding disorders, surgery or trauma is still the most frequent cause of

TABLE 1.   CONGENITAL COAGULATION DISORDERS AND THEIR EFFECT ON
SCREENING TESTS

Coagulopathy	Factor Involved	Platelet Count	Bleeding Times	PTT	Pro L-Times	Fibrinogen	Thrombin Times
Afibrinogenemia	Fibrinogen	−	−	+	+	+	+
Hypoprothrombinemia	Prothrombin	−	−	+	+	−	−
Parahemophilia	Factor V	−	−	+	+	−	−
Factor X deficiency	Factor X	−	−	+	+	−	−
Factor VII deficiency	Factor VII	−	−	−	+	−	−
Hemophilia A	Factor VIII	−	−	+	−	−	−
Hemophilia B	Factor IX	−	−	+	−	−	−
PTA deficiency	Factor XI	−	−	+	−	−	−
Hageman trait	Factor XII	−	−	+	−	−	−
Factor XIII deficiency	Factor XIII	−	−·	−-	−	−-	−

− = Normal
+ = Abnormal

death for these patients. Even in cases of emergency, these patients should be referred to centers specializing in the treatment of these problems if at all possible.

Most congenital bleeding disorders are diagnosed relatively early in life, and a good history and physical examination will usually provide clues to the problem in those cases where no diagnosis has been established. In all cases, an accurate diagnosis should be made prior to surgery, if at all possible. Successful treatment of intra- and postsurgical bleedings in these patients, especially with blood components, requires accurate diagnosis and accurate follow-up of the therapeutic attempts.

The congenital bleeding disorders can be divided into three major categories, coagulopathies (disturbances in the classic clotting factors), thrombocytopathies (qualitative and quantitative platelet abnormalities) and telangiopathies (congenital vascular abnormalities).[28-30] Careful performance of the six standard screening coagulation tests will generally indicate which type of disorder is present (Table 1).

Congenital Coagulopathies

DIAGNOSIS: As a general rule, only one factor is abnormal in the congenital coagulopathies; combined congenital· deficiencies are very rare. The platelet count and bleeding times are always normal (Table 1), indicating an uncomplicated formation of the first hemostatic plug. As a consequence, although these patients usually do not ooze excessively from small vessels during the surgery, rather severe bleeding can occur postoperatively. Only Factor XIII deficiencies have normal partial thromboplastin times and prothrombin times; in all other cases, either one or both of these tests are usually abnormal. It should be pointed out that all patients with moderate to severe coagulopathies have a bleeding problem, except those with Hagemen trait, which, as a general rule, is not associated with a hemostatic abnormality.

AXIOM

NORMAL RESULTS ON THE SCREENING TESTS IN A PATIENT WITH A HISTORY OF BLEEDING DO NOT EXCLUDE THE PRESENCE OF A CONGENITAL BLEEDING PROBLEM.

To have abnormal partial thromboplastin times and prothrombin times, a rather significant degree of factor abnormality must be present.

TREATMENT. The following five general rules must be followed if a patient with a congenital coagulopathy is to undergo surgery:[27]

TABLE 2.   PRESENCE OF CLOTTING FACTORS IN BLOOD AND BLOOD COMPONENTS

	Factors									
	I	II	V	VII	VIII	IX	X	XI	XII	XIII
Fresh whole blood	+	+	+	+	+	+	+	+	+	+
Bank blood (< 5 days old)	+	+	−	+	−	+	+	+	+	+
Fresh frozen plasma (FFP)	+	+	+	+	+	+	+	+	+	+
Cohn Fraction I	+	−	+?	−	+?	−	−	−	−	+
Cryoprecipitate	+	−	+	−	+	−	−	+	+	+
Factor VIII concentrates	−	−	−	−	+	−	−	−	−	−
Factor IX concentrates	−	+	−	+	−	+	+	−	−	−
Fibrinogen concentrates	+	−	+?	−	+?	−	−	−	−	+

1. Determine the plasma level of the factor prior to surgery.
2. Exclude the presence of a possible inhibitor.
3. Infuse the factor in question and be certain that its plasma level rises.
4. Raise the concentration of the factor in the plasma to its desired level immediately prior to surgery.
5. Maintain sufficient levels until wound healing is complete.

Although whole blood contains a number of coagulation factors (Table 2), the method of choice for treating congenital coagulopathies is component therapy rather than whole blood. Whole blood is needed only when the hematocrit so indicates. Component therapy requires an accurate diagnosis of the factor missing in the patient in order to be effective. Components used for the treatment of hemophilia A and B, the two most frequently occurring congenital coagulopathies, are expressed in units. A unit factor is the amount of activity found in 1 ml of fresh plasma. In major surgical procedures, the plasma levels of Factors VIII or IX should be raised to 30 to 60% of normal immediately prior to and during surgery and should be maintained at a level of 20 to 30% of normal in the postoperative period.[27] Similar rules also apply to the other coagulation factors. The fibrinogen level should be maintained at about 100 mg/100 ml at all times.[31]

In order to reach appropriate levels of Factors VIII and IX, several formulas have been published. Blombäck and Blombäck[32] have suggested the following formula to reach the suggested initial levels of both factors prior to surgery:

$$\frac{A \times V}{100}$$

where A is the desired rise of factor in percent of normal and V the plasma volume in milliliters. Rizza and Biggs[33] have suggested:

$$\frac{A \times G}{2}$$

where A is the desired rise of factor level in percent of normal and G the body weight in kilograms. Both groups suggest that one-half of the calculated dose should be given every 6 to 8 hours to maintain adequate plasma levels.

Pool[34] has recommended one unit of cryoprecipitate per 6 kg of body weight for the initial dose, and one unit per 12 kg every 12 hours for maintenance.

Johnson and co-workers[35] recommended 3,000 units as the initial dose, followed by 1,500 units every 8 hours during the first postoperative day, 1,500 units every 12 hours for the next 6 days, and then 750 units every 12 hours until completion of wound healing.

AXIOM

NO FORMULA CAN SUBSTITUTE FOR CAREFUL REPEATED SERIAL AND CLINICAL OBSERVATION.

It must be kept in mind that most blood components can carry the hepatitis virus; consequently the patient or his family must be advised of the possibility of this complication and serial laboratory tests performed.[27] The presence of an immune antibody to any of the coagulation factors, a phenomenon diagnosed today in many patients with hemophilia A and B, absolutely requires an expert hematologist to prevent disastrous complications.

Congenital Thrombocytopathies

DIAGNOSIS. The most important congenital thrombocytopathies can be fairly well diagnosed by the standard screening tests listed in Table 3. Von Willebrand's syndrome, the most frequent congenital thrombocytopathy, almost as frequent as both hemophilias, is characterized by prolonged bleeding times and prolonged partial thromboplastin times, due to an associated clotting factor deficiency, usually Factor VIII.[36]

In all of the congenital thrombocytopa-thies, except pure forms of platelet factor 3 release disturbance, the bleeding times are abnormal, indicating that one of the defects lies in the formation of the first hemostatic plug. For this reason, these patients often display severe intraoperative oozing in addition to excessive postoperative hemorrhage. The platelet factor 3 release disturbances, however, act more like a coagulopathy because of the role that platelet factor 3 plays in the formation of thrombin (Fig. 1).

TREATMENT. The exact mechanism of the defect must be determined accurately in order to initiate and follow the proper therapeutic regimen. Von Willebrand's syndrome, although characterized by lack of platelet adhesion, should be treated with fresh frozen plasma or cryoprecipitate and not platelet concentrates.[36,37] Highly purified Factor VIII concentrates will *not* correct the abnormal bleeding times.

All other thrombocytopathies can be treated with platelet concentrates, provided the concentrates are prepared from whole blood less than 24 hours old, and provided they are used within 4 hours after their preparation.[29] Without these precautions, the concentrates may contain platelets that neither adhere to the vessel wall nor aggregate, thus not contributing to the formation of the first hemostatic plug. Normali-

TABLE 3. CONGENITAL THROMBOCYTOPATHIES AND THEIR EFFECT ON SCREENING TESTS

Thrombocyto-pathies	Function Disturbed	Platelet Count	Bleeding Times	PTT Pro	L-Times	Fibrinogen	Thrombin Times
Von Willebrand's syndrome	Adhesion plus occasional aggregation	−	+	+	−	−	−
Aggregation abnormalities	Aggregation	−	+	−	−	−	−
Platelet factor 3 availability	Phospholipid release	−	−	−	−	−	−
Thrombasthenia	Aggregation and clot retraction	−	+	−	−	−	−
Thrombocytopenia	All above	+	+	−	−	−	−

− = Normal
+ = Abnormal

zation of the prolonged bleeding times and the platelet count can serve as indicators for successful substitution therapy. Again it is advisable to have an expert hematologist available for advice.

Congenital Telangiopathies

Congenital telangiopathies are not only difficult to diagnose, unless associated with prolonged bleeding times, but are also extremely difficult to treat specifically.

ACQUIRED BLEEDING DISORDERS

Acquired bleeding disorders are much more frequently encountered than those of congenital origin, particularly in adults. These disorders can but need not always manifest themselves in an overt clinical bleeding tendency prior to surgery. In most instances, the defects can be detected preoperatively by conducting a careful history and physical examination and by performing some screening tests. Some bleeding disorders, however, develop intra- and postoperatively in patients who have no hemostatic defects prior to surgery.

Preoperatively Acquired Bleeding Disorders

LIVER DISEASE. Disturbances in liver parenchymal cell function, especially cirrhosis, invariably lead to major disturbances in the hemostatic mechanisms. Since all blood coagulation factors, except Factor VIII (antihemophiliac Factor A), are synthesized in the liver, they will, depending upon the degree of parenchymal cell damage, be decreased in patients with cirrhosis. The vitamin-K dependent clotting factors (Factors II, VII, IX and X) are particularly sensitive to any impaired liver cell function and are, therefore, often found in decreased concentrations in plasma, even in patients with mild liver diseases.[29,38]

Other problems may also be encountered in cirrhosis. The splenomegaly which often develops because of the increased portal pressure, for example, may cause a thromboctyopenia.[39] These patients may also develop a fibrinolysis, either of the primary type (i.e. not associated with disseminated intravascular coagulation) or of the secondary type (associated with D.I.C.).[40]

If significant liver disease is present, the patient's hemostatic potential should be assessed carefully preoperatively if at all possible. Prolonged partial thromboplastin times and prothrombin times are usually found in such patients, and decreased platelet counts, decreased fibrinogen levels and prolonged thrombin times may also occur. Therapeutically, fresh frozen plasma will correct all the clotting defects seen in these patients, except for platelet deficiencies. If thrombocytopenia is also present, fresh whole blood may be used or platelet concentrates may be given with the fresh frozen plasma. If D.I.C. has developed, heparin may also be required.

THROMBOCYTOPENIA. Thrombocytopenia is one of the most frequently encountered acquired bleeding disorders. An inadequate number of circulating platelets can be a reflection of either inadequate platelet production in the bone marrow or increased peripheral platelet utilization or destruction. Impaired platelet production may be caused by drugs, chemicals, or myeloproliferative diseases. Increased utilization or destruction of platelets may be caused by immune antibodies, isoantibodies, drugs, infections, splenomegaly, anaphylactoid reactions, and disseminated intravascular coagulation.[27,29,41]

Thrombocytopenia may cause disturbed primary hemostasis, defective secondary hemostasis (due to the unavailability of platelet factor 3) and impaired clot retraction. In general, thrombocytopenia will not cause a bleeding disorder if 30,000 to 50,000/cu mm or more normally functioning platelets are present.

PITFALL

IT IS SOMETIMES ASSUMED THAT PATIENTS WITH A PLATELET COUNT ABOVE 50,000/CU MM CANNOT HAVE BLEEDING DUE TO A PLATELET DEFICIENCY.

Patients with multiple transfusions of blood that has been stored for more than 24 to 48 hours may contain a significant number of platelets which are incapable of adhesion or aggregation.[29,42] Thus, such patients may have platelet counts exceeding 80,000/cu mm and still have a significant bleeding problem due to the inadequate number of adequately functioning platelets. Properly prepared platelet concentrates or fresh whole blood will usually correct any platelet deficiency.

VITAMIN K MALABSORPTION. Vitamin K malabsorption, as occasionally observed in long-standing biliary-tract obstruction and some forms of sprue, can cause a decrease in the vitamin-K dependent clotting factors (Factors II, VII, IX, X). Consequently, the partial thromboplastin times and prothrombin times will be abnormal. The parenteral administration of vitamin K will often correct this defect rather promptly unless there is coincident liver-cell damage. This malabsorption syndrome is functionally identical to the defect intentionally caused by treatment with coumadin or similar drugs.[28]

PARAPROTEINEMIAS. Patients with diseases such as Waldenström's macroglobulinemia, cryoglobulinemia, multiple myeloma and hypergammaglobulinemia, which cause the formation of abnormal proteins, occasionally display a defect in primary and secondary hemostasis. Coating of the platelets by the abnormal proteins may interfere with their aggregation and, therefore, cause prolonged bleeding times. Secondary hemostasis may also be impaired on the basis of a disturbed polymerization of the fibrin monomers resulting in abnormal fibrin formation.[28] Abnormal thrombin times and, if the defect is rather severe, abnormal partial thromboplastin and prothrombin times may be observed. Therapy is difficult, but platelet concentrates, fresh frozen plasma or purified fibrinogen may be helpful.

CIRCULATING ANTICOAGULANTS. Immune antibodies against coagulation factors can be found not only in patients who have been treated for congenital coagulopathies but also in previously healthy individuals after blood or plasma transfusions. Most of these antibodies are directed against Factor VIII, but other clotting factors have also been found to be inhibited by immune antibodies. Because of the severity and complexity of the problem, these patients should, if possible, be referred to centers experienced in their management.

Intra- or Postoperatively Acquired Bleeding Disorders

PITFALL

IF IT IS ASSUMED THAT EXCESSIVE BLEEDING AFTER TRAUMA OR SURGERY IS USUALLY DUE TO A COAGULATION ABNORMALITY, THE ATTEMPTS TO OBTAIN GOOD LOCAL HEMOSTASIS ARE APT TO BE LESS VIGOROUS.

Occasionally, hemostatic defects develop during or immediately following surgery in patients with no known prior bleeding problem or hemostatic defect. However, most such intra- and postoperative hemorrhages, especially when limited to the operative site, are due to technical problems and should be corrected surgically by suturing, ligation, or coagulation of the open vessels. Nevertheless, if the bleeding is diffuse and involves previously dry areas, and if bleeding occurs from other sites such as needle punctures, Foley catheter, Levin tube, tracheostomy, etc., a major breakdown in the hemostatic mechanisms must be considered. Disseminated intravascular coagulation (with or without secondary fibrinolysis) and primary fibrinolysis are the most likely reasons for this hemostatic breakdown, both leading to a "consumption coagulopathy."

CONSUMPTION COAGULOPATHY. A consumption coagulopathy can present itself in one of the following three forms: (1) a generalized intravascular activation of the coagulation system (D.I.C.) with no appreciable simultaneous activation of the fibrinolytic system, (2) disseminated intravascular coagulation associated with an activation of the fibrinolytic system (secondary fibrinolysis), and (3) activation of the fibrinolytic system without an associated intravascular clotting episode (primary fibrinolysis).

Etiology. In disseminated intravascular coagulation (D.I.C.), a generalized activation of prothrombin to thrombin occurs with subsequent conversion of fibrinogen to fibrin. In this process, not only are fibrinogen and prothrombin consumed but also platelets, Factor V and Factor VIII. Thus, patients with D.I.C. develop hypofibrinogemia, hypoprothrombinemia, thrombocytopenia, and Factor-V and Factor-VIII deficiencies. As these factors are "consumed," their concentration in the blood falls below those needed for maintenance of normal hemostasis, and a breakdown in the hemostatic mechanism results, hence the name "consumption coagulopathy." This subject matter has been reviewed in numerous publications and details should be obtained from these.[19,27,28,36,41,43-46]

When a generalized intravascular activation of the fibrinolytic system occurs, the resulting plasminemia not only produces fibrinolysis, thus opening up previously coagulated vessels, but also causes fibrinogenolysis with resulting formation of split products. The consumption of fibrinogen plus the anticoagulant action of the split products on the primary and secondary hemostasis results in a hemorrhagic diathesis.

Consumption coagulopathy is never a disease per se but a complication of another underlying disease which triggers it. There are two principal mechanisms initiating clotting, the intrinsic and extrinsic pathways (Fig. 1). The intrinsic pathway depends upon the availability of phospholipids from platelets, due to either a generalized intravascular platelet release reaction or to a breakdown of platelets following intravascular platelet aggregation. Since

erythrocyte stroma contains phospholipids identical to those in platelets,[5] a generalized hemolysis can also trigger intravascular clotting. The extrinsic pathway for initiating clotting involves the contact of blood with tissue thromboplastin (Fig. 1); thus, major trauma could also provide the proper stimulus.

There are a number of clinical situations which may precipitate D.I.C. Endotoxin from gram-negative microorganisms or septic shock due to other organisms may cause intravascular platelet aggregation (the human equivalent of the generalized Shwartzman reaction). Antibody-antigen interactions associated with transfusion of mismatched blood, severe anaphylactoid reactions due to drug or antitoxin hypersensitivity, or hyperacute rejection of transplanted organs and severe burns[47] may also cause intravascular platelet aggregation. Acidosis may cause intravascular platelet breakdown, thus explaining D.I.C. in nonseptic shock conditions.[48]

Massive invasion of the circulating system by tissue thromboplastin may occur in abruptio placentae, dead fetus syndrome, amniotic fluid embolism, cancer, massive trauma and fat embolism. Some forms of accelerated intravascular coagulation can occur in all forms of surgery, probably explaining, in part, the increased postoperative tendency for thromboembolic complications. However, the body's defense mechanisms, especially the phagocytosis capacity of the RES, can, as a general rule, defend the organism against D.I.C. Impairment of the RES due to poor liver function during shock can thus contribute greatly to the development of D.I.C. if the appropriate stimuli are present.[48] This probably explains the frequent development of D.I.C. during hepatic coma or liver transplantation.

The trigger mechanisms for the activation of the fibrinolytic system are less well understood. Since the tissue activator of plasminogen is located in the vessel intima, damage to organs such as the placenta, lung or liver which are rich in blood vessels may release not only tissue activators of the clotting system (tissue thromboplastin) but also activators of the fibrinolytic system. Severe hypoxia, as encountered during shock or improper anesthesia, is also recognized as a powerful stimulus for plasminogen activation to plasmin. Some organs, such as the prostate gland, pancreas and lungs, contain proteases which can directly or indirectly activate plasminogen and thus cause fibrinolysis. Last, but not least, stress has also been identified as an activator of the fibrinolytic system.[49] As in coagulation, however, powerful defense mechanisms are present. These are in the form of antiplasmins which have to be overcome before free circulating plasmin in plasma can produce fibrinolysis and fibrinogenolysis. This again explains why insults such as those described above do not always produce hyperfibrinolysis.

Thus, the potential for producing generalized intravascular coagulation or fibrinolysis is found with many disease states and with many surgical procedures; however, a series of additive circumstances must generally be present to allow this syndrome to develop fully.

Diagnosis. Proper therapy of consumption coagulopathy requires an accurate diagnosis. An early diagnosis can occasionally be made in the operating room by a very simple clotting test of placing 1 to 2 ml of blood in two test tubes without addition of an anticoagulant and observing them for clotting. If no clot forms spontaneously within 30 minutes, thrombin should be added. If a clot still does not form, the patient probably has very little or no fibrinogen in the plasma. If a clot forms either spontaneously or after the addition of thrombin, it is advisable to look not only at the quantity of clot formed (in hypofibrinogenemia only a small blood clot may form), but also at how well the clot persists, for rapid dissolution of the clot may be an indicator of excessive fibrinolysis.

PITFALL

FAILURE TO DIFFERENTIATE NORMAL PHYSIO-LOGIC CLOT RETRACTION FROM DISSOLUTION OF THE CLOT DUE TO FIBRINOLYSIS MAY RESULT IN ADMINISTRATION OF ANTIFIBRINO-LYTIC DRUGS WHICH MAY CAUSE SERIOUS COMPLICATIONS.

Coagulation tests are extremely important and necessary if the diagnosis of a consumption coagulopathy is to be made early and accurately. The partial thromboplastin time and prothrombin time should be prolonged in D.I.C. due to the consumption of constituents needed for coagulation. For the same reason, the fibrinogen level and platelet count will be reduced. At times, it may be necessary to repeat these studies after one or two hours to look for a further decrease in the fibrinogen level and platelet count which would be expected with D.I.C. The simple inspection of a peripheral blood smear is also helpful because macerated red cells (schistocytes) are, as a general rule, present in D.I.C. especially when fibrin is formed intravascularly.

PITFALL

IF BLOOD FOR COAGULATION TESTS IS DRAWN FROM AN INDWELLING ARTERIAL OR VENOUS CATHETER, THE HEPARIN IN THE LINE MAY PRODUCE EXTREMELY ERRONEOUS RESULTS.

A prolonged thrombin time may indicate the presence of fibrin and fibrinogen split products which are the result of fibrinolysis or fibrinogenolysis, respectively. Since heparin, even in minute quantities, also prolongs the thrombin time, drawing of blood samples from arterial lines or indwelling catheters which have been flushed with heparin solutions may destroy the accuracy of this test. Therefore, blood for coagulation studies should always be obtained by a fresh venipuncture.

Although differentiating between the three forms of consumption coagulopathy may be extremely difficult at times, an accurate diagnosis is absolutely essential for proper treatment. The platelet count and ethanol gelation test[50] can be extremely helpful in this regard. Primary fibrinolysis is generally associated with a normal platelet count. However, the platelet count may drop as increased quantities of blood are given so that this criterion is valid only early in the syndrome. The ethanol gelation test, as modified by Glueck,[50] may be positive in the presence of fibrin monomers which are the product of the action of thrombin on fibrinogen. Unfortunately, since this test may occasionally be falsely negative or even falsely positive, its usefulness is somewhat limited. Nevertheless, when considered in conjunction with the usual clinical manifestations, and other typical coagulation changes, one will rarely be misled by an erroneous result on the gelation test.

Treatment. The treatment of consumption coagulopathy depends on the type of hemostatic breakdown and must, generally speaking, not only be directed toward correction of the coagulation defect but also toward elimination of the underlying disease mechanism which triggered the process.

If the source of the trigger mechanism in a patient with D.I.C. (with or without secondary fibrinolysis) can be eliminated within an hour or two, as for example by evacuating the uterus in patients with abruptio placentae, massive replacement of lost blood volume and clotting factors with fresh blood, or fresh frozen plasma and platelet concentrates, will usually restore normal hemostasis. As a general rule, secondary fibrinolysis will end when the intravascular clotting is arrested. If the source of the trigger mechanism cannot be eliminated quickly, then anticoagulant therapy with heparin must be considered.

PITFALL

ATTEMPTS TO PREVENT INTRAVASCULAR CLOTTING WITH INTERMITTENT OR INADEQUATE DOSES OF HEPARIN ARE SELDOM EFFECTIVE AND TEND ONLY TO CONFUSE THE CLINICAL AND LABORATORY PICTURE.

D.I.C. can generally be interrupted in an adult by rapidly administering 30 to 50 mg of heparin I.V. as a primary dose, followed by 150 to 300 mg given by continuous I.V. infusion over the next 24 hours, preferably by an infusion pump. Any bleeding which is already present will obviously not be arrested by the heparin, but within hours one will be able to measure a rise in the fibrinogen levels and platelet counts. This restoration of the hemostatic mechanisms can and should be aided by infusion of fresh whole blood or fresh frozen plasma with platelet concentrates. As the hemostatic potential returns to normal values, the bleeding will generally decrease in spite of the continued heparin infusion. As a general rule, fibrinolysis will subside when the intravascular clotting has been successfully blocked, and drugs to specifically block the fibrinolytic system are only rarely required.

PITFALL

IF ANTIFIBRINOLYTIC DRUGS ARE USED TO TREAT FIBRINOLYSIS SECONDARY TO D.I.C., THE INTRAVASCULAR CLOTTING MAY PROCEED AT A MUCH MORE DANGEROUS RATE.

Patients with D.I.C. without secondary fibrinolysis usually have the poorest prognosis. This is because the fibrin which is formed in D.I.C. is deposited in the microcirculation, causing multiple thromboses or microemboli, leading to organ necrosis. Bilateral renal cortical necrosis is probably the best known, but by no means the only pathologic finding in D.I.C.[43] Renal failure with anuria which cannot be explained on the basis of hypotension is often an early sign of D.I.C., even before a generalized bleeding tendency becomes apparent. Furthermore, administration of additional blood or plasma will result in even more fibrin deposition, unless the intravascular clotting is blocked by anticoagulant therapy. Thus, heparin treatment is imperative in these patients, and the earlier it is initiated the better the prognosis.

AXIOM

IF PATIENTS WITH DISSEMINATED INTRAVASCULAR COAGULATION ARE NOT HEPARINIZED BEFORE AN ATTEMPT IS MADE TO RESTORE CIRCULATING FACTORS WITH FRESH BLOOD OR FRESH FROZEN PLASMA, THE AMOUNT OF INTRAVASCULAR FIBRIN FORMATION MAY BE GREATLY INCREASED.

Antifibrinolytic therapy with epsilon-aminocaproic acid (EACA) should be considered only for patients in whom the diagnosis of primary fibrinolysis is properly established beyond any doubt. In most instances, however, this is very difficult to achieve. The indiscriminatory use of epsilon-aminocaproic acid in consumption coagulopathy must be strongly discouraged. If there is any doubt as to the type of fibrinolysis present in a patient, heparinization is recommended prior to antifibrinolytic therapy.

AXIOM

ANTIFIBRINOLYTIC THERAPY SHOULD NEVER BE GIVEN TO PATIENTS WITH D.I.C. UNLESS IT IS GIVEN IN CONJUNCTION WITH HEPARIN.

MASSIVE BLOOD TRANSFUSIONS. The development of a hemorrhagic diathesis during or following massive blood transfusions is a well-known phenomenon.[29,51] During massive transfusions, the patient's blood quickly comes to resemble the donor blood. Blood stored in a blood bank undergoes a number of important changes in its hemostatic constituents, primarily as a result of decreased quantities of Factor V, Factor VIII, fibrinogen, and platelets and as a result of increased fibrinolysis.[52] Certain coagulation factors, such as Factor V (accelerator globulin) and Factor VIII (antihemophilia Factor A) are often referred to as "labile factors" because they lose their biological activity rapidly during storage, and after 21 days generally less then 10% of their original activity can be found in the plasma. About 50% of the activity of Factor V is lost within the first six days of storage. The gradual decrease in the concentration of fibrinogen in the stored blood is associated with an increased fibrinolytic activity and increased levels of fibrinogen split products which can also cause increased bleeding.[52]

From the bleeding point of view, probably even more serious are the functional changes in the platelets. Although the number of platelets may not change significantly within the first 48 hours of storage, their aggregability or their ability to form a first hemostatic plug has virtually disappeared.[29,42,51] Thus, patients receiving massive volumes of blood which is 48 hours or older will eventually have a circulating platelet population which is unable to form the first hemostatic plug which is necessary for hemostasis in the small-diameter vessels. This, in turn, explains the clinical observation that the excess bleeding in patients with massive transfusion is often of the diffuse oozing type.

Thus, only fresh blood, less than 48 hours old, should be used in patients receiving massive blood transfusions. However, since this is not generally possible, some type of a compromise must be made. In our experience we have found that bleeding in patients with massive transfusions can be minimized if every third unit of blood given is less than 48 hours old.[52] The use of calcium to promote hemostasis must be discouraged because the bleeding has no relationship to the level of calcium in plasma. The citrate received by the patients during massive blood replacement is usually metabolized quite rapidly. In the newborn and in patients with severe liver

TABLE 4. FREQUENT ERRORS IN THE MANAGEMENT OF COAGULATION ABNORMALITIES IN INJURED PATIENTS

1. Assuming that excessive intraoperative or postoperative bleeding is due to a coagulation abnormality rather than realizing that such bleeding is usually due to inadequate surgical efforts to obtain local hemostasis.
2. Failing to obtain appropriate coagulation tests in patients with possible coagulation abnormality.
3. Assuming that a clinical coagulation disorder cannot be present if the coagulation tests are normal.
4. Failing to obtain an adequate history concerning drugs with possible anticoagulant effects in preoperative or bleeding patients.
5. Attempting to manage patients with known congenital or unusual bleeding disorders in a hospital with an inadequate coagulation laboratory.
6. Assuming that a platelet count greater than 50,000/cu mm rules out a bleeding disorder due to platelet deficiencies.
7. Drawing blood for coagulation tests from indwelling venous or arterial catheters, particularly if the catheter may have been flushed with heparin.
8. Failing to provide adequate quantities of fresh blood and fresh frozen plasma to patients receiving massive transfusions.
9. Using antifibrinolytic drugs in patients who may have fibrinolysis secondary to D.I.C.
10. Attempting to restore clotting factors in patients with D.I.C. without first heparinizing adequately.

damage or shock, however, the level of ionized calcium might fall to levels less than those needed for optimal cardiovascular function.

In summary, the bleeding diathesis associated with massive blood transfusions is usually a combination of a qualitative and quantitative platelet defect, decreased clotting factors and an increased fibrinolytic activity. Occasionally, because of the shock and massive tissue trauma which may also be present, D.I.C. may further complicate the situation.

REFERENCES

1. Horowitz, H. I., and Spielvogel, A. R.: Hemostasis. In: *Thrombosis and Bleeding Disorders* (Bang, N. U., Beller, F. K., Deutsch, E., and Mammen, E. F., Eds.). New York, Academic Press, 1971.
2. Marcus, A. J., and Zucker, M. B.: *The Physiology of Blood Platelets*. New York, Grune and Stratton, 1965.
3. Walsh, P. N.: Platelets, blood coagulation and hemostasis. In: *Platelets and Thrombosis* (Sherry, S., and Scriabine, A., Eds.). Baltimore, University Park Press, 1972.
4. Johnson, S. A.: Platelets in hemostasis and thrombosis. In: *The Circulating Blood Platelet* (Johnson, S. A., Ed.). New York, Academic Press, 1971.
5. Mammen, E. F.: Physiology and biochemistry of blood coagulation. In: *Thrombosis and Bleeding Disorders* (Bang, N. U., Beller, F. K., Deutsch, E., and Mammen, E. F., Eds.). New York, Academic Press, 1971.
6. Seegers, W. H.: Role of platelets in blood clotting. In: *The Circulating Blood Platelet* (Johnson, S. A., Ed.). New York, Academic Press, 1971.
7. Laki, K.: Introduction and summary. In: *Fibrinogen* (Laki, K., Ed.). New York, Marcel Dekker, 1968.
8. Blombäck, B.: Fibrinogen to fibrin transformation. In: *Blood Clotting Enzymology* (Seegers, W. H., Ed.). New York, Academic Press, 1967.
9. Murano, G.: The molecular structure of fibrinogen. Seminars Thromb. Hemost. 1:1, 1974.
10. Finlayson, J. S.: Crosslinking of fibrin. Seminars Thromb. Hemost., 1:33, 1974.
11. Lüscher, E. F., and Bettex-Galland, M.: Thrombosthenin. In: *The Circulating Blood Platelet* (Johnson, S. A., Ed.). New York, Academic Press, 1971.
12. Kline, D. L.: Physiology of fibrinolysis. Thromb. Diath. Haemorrh., 45(Suppl.):5, 1971.
13. Robbins, K. C., and Summaria, L.: Biochemistry of fibrinolysis. Thromb. Diath. Haemorrh., 47 (Suppl.):9, 1971.
14. Mammen, E. F., Anderson, G. F., and Barnhart, M. I., Eds.: Thrombolytic therapy. Thromb. Diath. Haemorrh., 47 (Suppl.):165–324, 1971.
15. Kakkar, V. V., and Flute, P. T.: Treatment of deep vein thrombosis with streptokinase. In: *Thromboembolism: Diagnosis and Treatment* (Kakkar, V. V., and Jouhar, A. J., Eds.). Edinburgh, Churchill Livingstone, 1972.
16. Sasahara, A. A., et al.: NHLI urokinase pulmonary embolism trial: Phase I results of a controlled study. In: *Thromboembolism: Diagnosis and Treatment.* (Kakkar, V. V., and Jouhar, A. J., Eds.). Edinburgh, Churchill Livingstone, 1972.
17. Marder, V. J., Matchett, M. O., and Sherry, S.: Detection of serum fibrinogen and fibrin degradation products. Amer. J. Med., 51:71, 1971.
18. Deykin, D.: The clinical challenge of disseminated intravascular coagulation. New Eng. J. Med., 283:636, 1970.

19. Nalbandian, et al.: Consumption coagulopathy. Mich. Med., Sept. 1971, 793.

20. Brecher, G., and Cronkite, E. P.: Morphology and enumeration of human platelets. J. Appl. Physiol., 3:365, 1950.

21. O'Brien, J. R.: Platelet count techniques, platelet adhesiveness and aggregation tests. In: *Thrombosis and Bleeding Disorders* (Bang, N. U., Beller, F. K., Deutsch, E., and Mammen, E. F., Eds.) New York, Academic Press, 1971.

22. Borchgrevink, C. F.: Bleeding time techniques. In: *Thrombosis and Bleeding Disorders* (Bang, N. U., Beller, F. K., Deutsch, E., and Mammen, E. F., Eds.). New York, Academic Press, 1971.

23. Langdell, R. D.: Partial thromboplastin time techniques. In: *Thrombosis and Bleeding Disorders* (Bang, N. U., Beller, F. K., Deutsch, E., and Mammen, E. F., Eds.). New York, Academic Press, 1971.

24. Rizza, C. R., and Walker, W.: One-stage prothrombin time techniques. In: *Thrombosis and Bleeding Disorders* (Bang, N. U., Beller, F. K., Deutsch, E., and Mammen, E. F., Eds.). New York, Academic Press, 1971.

25. Huseby, R. M., and Bang, N. U.: Fibrinogen. In: *Thrombosis and Bleeding Disorders* (Bang, N. U., Beller, F. K., Deutsch, E., and Mammen, E. F., Eds.). New York, Academic Press, 1971.

26. Ingram, G. I. C., and Matchett, M. O.: The serial thrombin time method for measuring fibrinogenolytic activity of plasma. Nature, 188:674, 1960.

27. Deutsch, E.: Gerinnungsstörungen. In: *Chirurgische Operationslehre* (Breitner, B., Kern, E., Kraus, H., Zuckschwerdt, L., Eds.). Munich, Urban and Schwarzenberg, 1973.

28. Mammen, E. F.: Irregular blood coagulation. In: *Blood Clotting Enzymology* (Seegers, W. H., Ed.). New York, Academic Press, 1967.

29. Salzman, E. W., and Britten, A.: *Hemorrhage and Thrombosis, A Practical Clinical Guide.* Boston, Little, Brown and Co., 1965.

30. Shulman, N. R.: Surgical care of patients with hereditary disorders of blood coagulation. In: *Treatment of Hemorrhagic Disorders* (Ratnoff, O. D., Ed.). New York, Hoeber, 1968.

31. Britten, A. T. H., and Salzman, E. W.: Surgery in congenital disorders of blood coagulation. Surg. Gynec. Obstet. 123:1333, 1965.

32. Blombäck, M., and Blombäck, B.: On the preparation and use of fraction I–O. Thromb. Diath. Haemorrh., 35(Suppl.):21, 1969.

33. Rizza, C. R., and Biggs, R.: Treatment of congenital deficiencies of Factor VIII and Factor IX. Thromb. Diath. Haemorrh., 35 (Suppl.):73, 1969.

34. Pool, J. G.: Cryoprecipitated Factor VIII concentrate. Thromb. Diath. Haemorrh., 35 (Suppl.):35, 1969.

35. Johnson, A. J., Karpatkin, M. H., and Newman, J.: Clinical investigation of intermediate and high-purity antihaemophilic Factor VIII concentrates. Brit. J. Haemat., 21:21, 1971.

36. Owen, C. A., Bowie, E. J. W., Didisheim, P., and Thompson, J. H.: *The Diagnosis of Bleeding Disorders.* Boston, Little, Brown and Co., 1969.

37. Breckenridge, R. T., and Ratnoff, O. D.: Therapy of hereditary disorders of blood coagulation. In: *Treatment of Hemorrhagic Disorders* (Ratnoff, O. D., Ed.). New York, Hoeber, 1968.

38. Lasch, H. G.: Pathophysiologie. Thromb. Diath. Haemorrh., 55(Suppl.):37, 1973.

39. Havemann, K., and Egbring, R.: Leber und Blutplättchen. Thromb. Diath. Haemorrh., 55(Suppl.):115, 1973.

40. Loo, van de, J.: Leber und fibrinolytisches System. Thromb. Diath. Haemorrh., 55 (Suppl.):77, 1973.

41. Lasch, H. G., Heene, D. L., and Mueller-Eckhardt, C.: Pathophysiologie und Klinik der haemorrhagischen Diathesen. In: *Klinische Haematologie* (Begemann, H., Ed.). Stuttgart, Thieme, 1970.

42. Joerin, H. W.: Platelet aggregation in normal stored blood. Master's thesis, Wayne State University Library, 1969.

43. McKay, D. G.: *Disseminated Intravascular Coagulation. An Intermediary Mechanism of Disease.* New York, Hoeber, 1965.

44. Hardaway, R. M.: *Syndromes of Disseminated Intravascular Coagulation.* Springfield, Charles C Thomas, 1966.

45. Horowitz, H. I.: Treatment of defibrination syndromes (other than those of pregnancy) and fibrinolytic disorders. In: *Treatment of Hemorrhagic Disorders* (Ratnoff, O. D., Ed.). New York, Hoeber, 1968.

46. Mammen, E. F., Anderson, G. F., and Barnhart, M. I., Eds.: Disseminated intravascular coagulation. Thromb. Diath. Haemorrh., (Suppl.) 36: 1, 1969.

47. McManus, W. F., Eurenius, K., and Pruitt, B. A.: Disseminated intravascular coagulation in burned patients. J. Trauma, 13:416, 1973.

48. Broersma, R. J., Bullemer, G. D., and Mammen, E. F.: Acidosis induced disseminated intravascular microthrombosis and its dissolution by streptokinase. Thromb. Diath. Haemorrh., 24:55, 1970.

49. Ulin, A. W.: Bleeding in the surgical patient: Stress and the vasculature. Exp. Med. Surg., 28:281, 1970.

50. Breen, F. A., and Tullis, J. L.: Ethanol gelation test improved. Ann. Intern. Med., 71:422, 1969.

51. Johnson, S. A., and Greenwalt, T. J.: *Coagulation and Transfusion in Clinical Medicine.* Boston, Little, Brown and Co., 1965.

52. Wilson, R. F., Mammen, E. F., and Walt, A. J.: Eight years of experience with massive blood transfusions. J. Trauma, 11:275, 1971.

Part 6
MEDICOLEGAL IMPLICATIONS OF TRAUMA

35 LEGAL ASPECTS OF TRAUMA PATIENT CARE

M. L. NORTON

PITFALL

MANY PHYSICIANS FAIL TO LEARN THEIR LEGAL RESPONSIBILITIES IN THE PRACTICE OF MEDICINE.

The antipathy of physicians toward the legal aspects of health care is, in part, a reflection of a lack of knowledge and understanding,[1,2] partly an emotional response to the novelty of being required to justify their professional actions to laymen[3] and, in large measure, a reflection of the requirements of insurance companies as indicated to the practitioner in his malpractice insurance policy. There is no absolute prescription for avoiding malpractice suits. However, the risk of legal action is reduced when we communicate fully and candidly with our patients and to the best of our ability care for them utilizing all the knowledge and skills that the profession possesses. Nevertheless, we must also learn about our medicolegal obligations.

THE GOOD SAMARITAN SITUATION

Scene of the Accident

The individual injured in an automobile accident generally depends upon the good will of passers-by for his initial first-aid care. In many of our states, statutes[4] have been enacted as a matter of public policy to encourage professionals to stop and render assistance without undue concern for litigation. These laws are popularly known as "Good Samaritan acts," and for the most part protect the assisting individual (physician, nurse, ambulance driver and other personnel) from civil suits for damages except in cases of gross negligence, willful misconduct or abandonment. It is interesting to note that the Law Division of the American Medical Association reportedly has been unable to locate either a single adjudicated case involving a Good Samaritan situation or a test of such laws.

The provisions of the statutes vary from state to state, and in some apply only to licensed physicians[5] "under . . . circumstances that suggest that the giving of aid is the only alternative to death or serious bodily injury." In other states[6] ". . . any person or persons, or group of persons" is included within the statutory protection. In most jurisdictions, the provision applies only outside the confines of a hospital or the doctor's office. The physician responding to the emergency is obligated to provide care in accord with the facilities and situations at hand. However, some feel that the limitation of legal recourse to circumstances of gross, willful or wanton negligence implies a lesser standard of care than is otherwise acceptable.[7]

PITFALL

THE PHYSICIAN MAY ASSUME THAT HIS ONLY RESPONSIBILITY AT THE SCENE OF AN ACCIDENT IS TO PROVIDE FIRST AID.

"Good Samaritan" provisions do *not* relieve the physician from responsibility to see that the accident victim receives continuous and necessary professional attention subsequent to the roadside first aid. It should also be pointed out that standards as to the quality of first-aid care expected will be different for the physician than for other persons. In other words, what may be perfectly acceptable on the part of the ambulance attendant might be considered gross negligence on the part of the physician.

Transfer to the Hospital

A "Good Samaritan" physician must take measures to ensure that the patient is transported to the hospital under circumstances of due care.[8] His responsibility ends only when the patient's care has been transferred to and accepted by another physician. Thus, the doctor would presumably be subject to legal action for abandonment if he does not make sure the accident victim receives adequate continuing care. This may involve proceeding to the hospital with or after the patient for that purpose.

At the Hospital

Hospitals would be well advised not to turn away emergency care patients.[9] At the hospital, the Board of Trustees, administrators and medical staff may all be responsible for various aspects of patient care, including the personnel and equipment that are involved. All individuals involved are responsible for certain standards of care determined by the local conditions.

PRINCIPLES OF THE LAW

Standard of Care

"Standard of care" refers to that level of professional service that would be required of other institutions with equivalent facilities and personnel, or physicians of equivalent training and experience, under the circumstances of the situation.[10] It also includes the need for consultations and referrals to individuals with special or superior training and experience which the reasonable physician would be expected to consider.[11]

The physician providing the first aid is required only to assure the patient the best care that is available in that situation. It is impossible to state what each individual must or must not do, since each individual situation must be met in its own distinctive manner. However, this does not relieve the referring physician of responsibility for his acts.[12] The importance of consultation or referral cannot be overstressed. Indeed, when the patient is first brought to the hospital from the scene of the accident, even by the physician, proper recommendations for referral must be noted.

PITFALL

THE PHYSICIAN MAY ASSUME THAT HE WILL BE FREE OF MEDICOLEGAL LIABILITY IF HE REQUESTS MANY CONSULTATIONS, X-RAYS OR TESTS.

It is prudent to obtain x-rays of any region where there is a possibility of a fracture or foreign body (Chap. 12). Many physicians who are "suit conscious" complain that they order many more x-rays and tests than are absolutely necessary because of the fear that otherwise they might be sued. However, mere ordering of more x-rays or tests does not ensure less liability. The physician would spend his time and effort more productively by examining and talking with the patient.

AXIOM

CAREFUL EXAMINATION OF THE PATIENT, PRECISE NOTATION OF THE FINDINGS AND DE-TAILED WRITTEN INSTRUCTIONS FOR PROPER FOLLOW-UP ARE THE BEST GUARANTEES AGAINST LEGAL ACTION.

Locality Rule

The concept of the locality rule was originally developed[13] in recognition of the limitations of practice in specific areas (e.g. rural) where facilities, informational exchange and the availability of professional personnel were not comparable to those found in large cities and medical centers. It must be noted, however, that with improved communications and increased attention to provision of health services to the general population, the standard has changed to that of a "similar locality,"[14] and now seems to be progressing toward the point where local factors will not modify the required level of professional excellence,[15] despite an occasional unenlightened retrogressive decision.[16]

PITFALL

MEDIOCRITY IN THE MEDICAL PRACTICES IN A PARTICULAR AREA CANNOT BE RELIED UPON TO PROTECT THE PHYSICIAN WHO HAS FALLEN BEHIND IN HIS KNOWLEDGE OF MEDICAL PROGRESS.

Respondeat Superior

AXIOM

THE PHYSICIAN IS RESPONSIBLE FOR THE ACTS OF ALL HIS EMPLOYEES IN RELATION TO HIS PATIENTS.

The term "respondeat superior" indicates responsibility of the supervisor. It represents the view that the acts of the employee are, or should be, under the control of the employer in a master-servant relationship.

On a more prosaic level, this is the "deep pocket" concept[17] of making the employer financially responsible because he is the one most likely to have the funds. The salutary effect of this concept is that it has forced institutions to ensure the qualifications, training and activities of each category of employee in order to meet the standards of care required for their professional activities. Thus, it becomes vital for the physician to become involved in the inner workings of the hospital to ensure optimum professional competence at all levels.[18]

It is important to warn the employee, however, that under the concept of "joint and several liability"[19] he may still be sued by the patient for his actions. In addition, the employee may also be subject to an action for "contribution" or "indemnification," i.e. a secondary suit by the employer for the tortious acts of the employee.[20] An example of this application is found where the hospital and a resident have lost in a suit charging negligence on the part of the resident. The dollar judgment against the resident by the patient would be covered by the professional liability policy provided by the hospital. However, this would not protect the resident from a suit by the hospital for "contribution" or "indemnification" for the hospital's monetary loss.

Consent

When an injured patient is admitted to the hospital and it is determined that surgery is required, the problem of obtaining consent for the treatment is presented.[21] For elective situations, the physician is faced with concepts of legal age for consent, the "emancipated minor," informed consent, express vs. implied consent and special problems (e.g. the Jehovah's Witness).

Justice Cardozo eloquently stated[22] that "Every human being of adult years and sound mind has a right to determine what shall be done with his own body." Thus, even if we believe that the patient is mak-

ing a decision contrary to our best judgment, he has the right to do so.

INFORMED CONSENT. Informed consent
implies, regardless whether it is oral or
written,[23] that the patient understands
what is to be done and the risks involved[24]
and the alternative methods of treatment
and the consequences thereof.[24a]

PITFALL

CONSENT FORMS OBTAINED BY INDIVIDUALS
OTHER THAN THE RESPONSIBLE PHYSICIAN
SHOULD NOT BE RELIED UPON.

The physician has a duty to inform his
patient of the dangers inherent in any proposed surgery or treatment before he seeks
permission to treat or operate upon him.
This is the concept of "informed consent."
Unless the patient has been properly informed, his consent to treatment will not
prevent him from suing the physician for
any damages or losses caused by that
treatment. Thus, the specifics of the procedure planned should be explained, including the significant risks and alternatives.
The explanation may be limited, however,
if such details would adversely affect the
pathophysiologic or psychologic status of
the patient.[25] Procedures specifically forbidden by the patient are absolutely prohibited, as are any extensions of the operation beyond the scope of the proposed surgery.[26] However, if in the course of surgery
the surgeon finds another condition which
materially or substantially endangers the
life, limb or health of the patient, he would
seemingly be justified in extending the procedure.[27]

PITFALL

THE CONSENT FORM CANNOT BE REGARDED
AS A GENERAL AUTHORIZATION FOR ANY TYPE
OF TREATMENT OR OPERATION THE PHYSICIAN
MAY FEEL IS NECESSARY.

The medicolegal climate in which we
live indicates increasingly that consent is
given for specific treatments or surgery
and cannot be extended unless an emergency or serious documentable situation develops.[28]

AGE OF CONSENT. The matter of "age of
consent" is essentially one of statutory control. This, in most states, means the age of
18 years for purposes of contract.[29] Any
adult of "sound mind" may agree to the
procedure as regards himself. The phrase
"sound mind" involves the ability to understand alternatives and implications as well
as the specifics of the therapeutic means to
be used. This has been even more broadly
interpreted to include "sufficient capacity
to understand the significance" of one's
acts.[30]

A parent or guardian must sign for the
legal minor. However, a child who is below legal age of consent but is either mar-
ried or living apart from parental support
and control would be considered as an
"emancipated minor," and in most states
would be entitled to grant permission as if
he were of adult age. It appears wisest,
however, to obtain consent from both the
emancipated minor and the parent or
guardian wherever possible.

There are also problems involved in obtaining consent from patients who are mentally incompetent.[31] Under these circumstances the problem may be particularly
confusing, since such a patient might be
considered capable of making a value
judgment in one situation and not so en-
dowed in other situations.[32]

TYPES OF CONSENT. There are various
forms of consent in addition to oral or
written, both of which are contractually
acceptable. "Express" consent signifies a
formal acceptance of the proposed procedure. "Implied" consent signifies acceptance by action, e.g. the person who know-
ingly holds up his arm for vaccination.[33]
This obviously presupposes that the patient: (1) knows that he can either agree
to or refuse the surgery, (2) has been fully
and fairly informed as to what is to be
done, and then (3) cooperates with the

physician without duress.[34] Note that oral consent is ordinarily supplemented and reinforced by implied consent.

It is also acceptable to obtain permission for surgery or other treatment by telephone or telegram where the parent or guardian would be unavailable in a reasonable period of time to personally sign the usual forms. Telephone consent, however, should be obtained by two individuals (e.g. one on an extension) who request the parent or guardian to identify himself and his relationship to the patient. After the planned procedure is explained, the consent can be requested. The guardian consenting should also be requested to send a follow-up confirmatory letter or telegram, although it is not an absolute requirement. Telegraphed consent alone is also acceptable. Both forms of documentation, however, should indicate that every effort has been made, within the limitations imposed by the nature of the emergency, to obtain consent in the standard manner.

EMERGENCY PROCEDURE. The medicolegal situation as regards emergency surgical or medical therapy is much simpler than that for elective procedures. Here we deal with a matter of public policy, because there are no sharply defined legal principles applicable to all emergency situations. First, we have the issue relative to consent to emergency treatment when the patient is a legal minor. Under such circumstances, it may be permissible to treat the patient without consent if there is evidence that diligent efforts were made to locate the parents for the purpose of obtaining consent.[35] For example, if treatment includes amputation of a mangled arm under extreme emergency circumstances, the courts have shown a recognition of the need to do the procedure without delaying for express consent.[36] Review of a series of cases dealing with consent for minors[37,38] indicates many varied interpretations, but all are based on the concept that the reasonable man would consent to save his life or limb, and that, furthermore, it is in the public

interest to encourage the medical profession to do what is needed under such emergency situations. This is not carte blanche, however, since this liberal approach holds only in situations where it is *impossible* to obtain the usually required consent because of the patient's status (unconsciousness, legal minority coupled with the unavailability of the legal guardian, etc.) and insufficient time to remedy the situation. It is definitely clear[39] that operations without consent will be allowed only in cases involving a true emergency. In such instances, written consultations or notes by one or more other qualified physicians agreeing that the situation is a bona fide emergency will generally remove any doubt on this question.

AXIOM

THE PRESENCE OF AN EMERGENCY NEEDS ADEQUATE DOCUMENTATION.

EFFECT OF MEDICATION. In this matter of consent, we occasionally find a patient who has received premedication but has not yet signed the consent form. In an emergency situation, this is not a problem. However, in less urgent situations it is definitively established that one who is under the influence of drugs is incompetent to give consent.[40] The temptation to proceed under the doctrine of implied consent is very great but should be resisted because action under such circumstances is not legally supportable.[40a]

PITFALL

PERFORMANCE OF NONEMERGENCY SURGERY ON MINORS WITH PERMISSION OF NEXT-OF-KIN OTHER THAN FATHER OR MOTHER IS RISKY BUSINESS.

Obtaining the consent of the available next-of-kin is valid only under very limited circumstances.[41] The determination of "next-of-kin" qualifications is extremely complex and would take an entire chapter to discuss. As a practical guide, in the absence of a legally appointed guardian, only a mother or father would definitely qualify as next-of-kin.

Next, we have the problematic situations of the adult alcoholic, drug taker and mentally unsound. Unless a legal guardian is appointed, there is no basis for obtaining consent from anyone except the patient himself. On the other hand, these people cannot be reasonably considered to have the full understanding necessary to consent to surgery. The law has not given us any guide as to how to overcome this obstacle. Consent from next-of-kin, including sisters, brothers or whoever so presents himself, is acceptable if there is evidence that the physician did everything reasonable to inform the patient and his family.

In some situations, it is very tempting for the physician personally to attempt to act for the patient. This is unacceptable, and was one of the most important issues in the landmark Mohr case,[24] despite the reliance on the implied consent concept.

Captain of the Ship

During the conduct of the surgical procedure, it is well recognized that there will be unnecessary confusion if there are too many individuals attempting to direct the procedure. This was the basis for the doctrine known as "captain of the ship."[43] It developed during the era when the surgeon was the only physician in the operating room, and was also based on the fact that there is a special relationship between patient and surgeon. The presence of assistants, no matter how well qualified, does not alter this relationship.

With the entry of physician anesthesiologists into clinical practice, a new element was introduced. The concept of the "captain of the ship" was modified to the concept of the "team" with the surgeon and the anesthesiologist jointly and severally responsible for their interrelated functions.[44] It is now well recognized that the anesthesiologist has an independent contractor relationship with the patient based on his special knowledge and his licensure as an independent practitioner. The surgeon can no more relieve the anesthesiologist of his responsibility to exercise his independent judgment than the anesthesiologist can replace the surgeon.

AXIOM

DISAGREEMENTS CONCERNING THERAPY SHOULD BE RESOLVED PRIOR TO SURGERY.

Communication among all members of the patient-care team before, during and after the procedure is absolutely essential. In the event that there are any differences of opinion concerning any aspect of the operation, they should be resolved preoperatively. No one practitioner, although equal in professional status, can serve his patient to the best of his ability without fully understanding his colleagues' plan of action.

The Nurse Anesthetist

The nurse anesthetist's position varies according to the situation of her employment. If she is employed by the hospital, is supervised by the anesthesiologist, but functions alone at times (e.g. nights and weekends), then all three parties share in the responsibility for her actions. The hospital is responsible because of the qualifications and guidelines it established for the function of nurse anesthetist when they hired her. The anesthesiologist is responsible for her management of the patient's care while he is in direct control, as well as for allowing her to function professionally during his absence.

PITFALL

THE SURGEON MAY FAIL TO COMMUNICATE ADEQUATELY WITH THE NURSE ANESTHETIST IF A SUPERVISING ANESTHESIOLOGIST IS NOT PRESENT IN THE O.R. SUITE.

If the anesthesiologist is absent, the surgeon bears a measure of liability since during this time he, as a physician, is in direct and immediate control of her duties. The byword for all three supervising parties is "control." In a situation where there is an officially appointed director of a department of anesthesiology, it is clear that he has a definite responsibility for the nurse anesthetist's activities under the "borrowed servant" doctrine. The same is true for the surgeon.

Blood Transfusions

Blood transfusions, particularly if given in a nonemergency situation, always present great legal risks if a reaction occurs. The entire problem is compounded by the large number of individuals who handle the blood from the time it is collected from the donor until it is administered to the patient. In addition, there are issues of "express warranty."[48] Although now generally limited to warranty as to goods and not services,[49] this cannot be entirely relied upon.

The problems encountered with blood transfusions are particularly complex if the patient is a member of the religious denomination called Jehovah's Witnesses. This group bases its objection to the infusion of blood and its by-products or fractions on Biblical admonition.[45] Since every person has the right, as a matter of law, to say what may or may not be done to his body, such agents cannot be administered if the patient specifically refuses. The best procedure, under ordinary circumstances, is to obtain a release from the patient absolving the hospital, surgeon and anesthesiologist from liability for any complications that might arise because of the patient's refusal to accept a blood transfusion.[46] With legal minors, some courts have assumed jurisdiction in the form of temporary guardianship in order to permit transfusion, stating "the welfare of the child is paramount." If, according to medical science, blood transfusions are necessary to preserve the child's life, the courts have stated that the child should not be deprived of such treatment because the parent's religious persuasion opposes such transfusions. "The child has a right to survival and a chance to live, and the court has a duty to extend its protecting arm to the child."[47]

Privacy

The right of privacy is very precious to our society.[52] The physician may not take a picture of a patient without specific consent,[53] even if the patient is not identifiable or the picture is not published. Indeed, allowing a layman or other individual not ordinarily permitted in the surgical suite to invade the privacy of the operating room is likewise actionable,[55] as is unconsented disclosure of confidential communications[56] or information from medical records. The patient has at all times the right to receive "decent and respectful treatment."[57]

Postoperative Care

The physician, once he has entered into the management of the patient's problem, has the responsibility of following it until no further care is needed. Case law[42] indicates that the surgeon and the anesthesiologist both have the duty to make adequate postoperative visits. Relegating this responsibility to others, as to interns or residents, does not relieve the surgeon of his duty, and he is liable for their actions under the doctrine of respondeat superior.

Statutes of Limitation

Each state has its own provisions concerning the statutes of limitations for "malpractice or negligence actions."[58] One of the greatest problems is determining when the statute of limitations begins. Most states hold that, barring special circumstances, the statute commences at the time of the wrongdoing. However, there appears to be a trend toward modifying this stand to have the statute begin at the time of discovery.[59] Other concepts now suggested are that the statute should begin at the end of the last treatment,[60] or at the end of the physician-patient relationship.

The justice of these situations is often explained as protecting the common law recourse of the patient from the time he discovers or should have discovered the wrongful act. One of the other arguments favoring a later beginning time for the statute of limitations is that this also gives the physician time to discover his error, advise his patient and provide necessary corrective measures. This is often referred to as the "discovery rule" and relates particularly to foreign objects,[62] although it is not necessarily so limited.[63] The analogous concept of the doctrine of "continuous treatment"[64] includes that period of time wherein the patient is under the professional care of the practitioner for the specific condition in question. These extensions of time for beginning the statute of limitations benefit the plaintiff patient, but work to the procedural disadvantage of the defendant physician.

PITFALL

A FALSE SENSE OF SECURITY MAY LULL THE PHYSICIAN INTO THINKING THAT THE RISK OF MALPRACTICE WILL DISAPPEAR WITH THE PASSAGE OF TIME.

THE FUTURE

Forensic Duties

The physician must, in addition to keeping up with the knowledge in his own field, be aware of his forensic responsibilities. If the trauma inflicted on his patient is due to another individual or may involve a legal action, the physician may be called upon to present his findings in court. Law enforcement, as it has become more scientific, has demanded more scientific investigation of violent trauma. The purpose of such enquiry is to determine exactly the mechanism and extent of the injury, the type of treatment and the manner of death.

The importance of preserving all medicolegal evidence, maintaining proper records, and filing proper reports for law enforcement agencies must be stressed. Unfortunately, medical schools and residency programs offer very little in medicolegal instruction.[51]

New Areas of Liability

With the development of schools of allied health sciences and the introduction of physician's assistants into the practice of medicine, increasing legal hazards will be found. Computerization and other biomedical instrumentation, coupled with revised concepts of "ordinary care," will almost certainly modify the liability of hospitals in the near future. Malpractice rulings have increasingly required hospitals to prove that the most modern electronic equipment is available to their patients. Juries, no doubt, will also stretch the principle of "ordinary care" to include strict liability for the safety of the electronic monitors and other electrical equipment. Greater emphasis will be placed on utilization of safety devices and preventive maintenance.[65]

AXIOM

EQUIPMENT THAT IS USED ON PATIENTS MUST BE TESTED FREQUENTLY FOR SAFETY AND ACCURACY.

The hospital, as well as the physician (in whose hands the utilization of such equipment rests), will bear increasing responsibility in regard to the equipment used on patients. The growing field of products liability and warranty will become closely interrelated with physicians' efforts and interests, forcing them to work more closely with the biomedical engineers and other research and development professionals.

SUMMARY

Society, through statute and medicolegal precedent, has provided physicians with several parameters to help them police their own profession. Although it often seems to the physician that a multitude of legal technicalities have been developed to trap him and force him into requesting excessive x-rays, tests or consultations, all that he is being asked to do is provide good medical care with due respect for the rights of the patient and the public good.

It is important to realize that, when discussing such topics as the standard of care, it is the physician as a generic entity who must determine the standards. Thus, all physicians, in large measure, determine the standards to which they are held by society as represented by "the law." There will, however, always be risks and gray areas relative to these principles. In the final analysis, we must accept these responsibilities, doing what is best for our patients according to the evergrowing body of knowledge called medical science.

REFERENCES

1. Louisell, D., and Williams, H.: *Medical Malpractice*, Vol. I., Cumulative Series. New York, Matthew Bender, 1969.
2. Curran, W. J., and Shapiro, E. D.: *Law and Medicine*, 2nd ed. Boston, Little, Brown and Co., 1970.
3. Evarard v. Hopkins, 2 Bulst 332, Court of King's Bench, 1615.
4. Louisell, D., and Williams, H.: *Medical Malpractice*, Vol. II. XXI. New York, Matthew Bender, 1969.
5. Alaska Stat. § 08.64.365, 1962.
6. Idaho Code § 5-330, Supp. 1965.
7. Bryan, W. W.: Good Samaritan laws—good or bad? Mercer L. Rev., 15:477, 1964.
8. Vogreg v. Shepard Ambulance Co., 47 Wash. 2d 659, 289 P.2d 350, 1955. Minimal Equipment for Ambulances, Committee on Trauma, Bull. Amer. Coll. Surg., 52:92, 1967. Brown, R.: Emergency care and transport of the injured. J. Med. Assoc. Georgia, 56:467, 1967.
9. Wilmington General Hospital v. Manlove, 54 Del. 15, 174 A.2d, 135, 1961. Williams v. Hospital Authority of Hall County, State Report 168 S.E.2d 336, 1969.
10. Prosser, W. L.: *Law of Torts*, 4th ed. St. Paul, West Publishing Co., 1971.
11. Principles of medical ethics. Amer. Med. Assoc. Rev. 1957, § 8.
12. Ferrara v. Galluchio, 152 N.E.2d, 249 (Ct. of App. N.Y.), 1958.
13. McCoid, A. H.: Vanderbilt L. Rev. 12:549, 1959.
14. Small v. Howard, 128 Mass. 131, 35 Am.Rep. 363, 1880.
15. Viita v. Fleming, 132 Minn. 128, 136; 155 N.W. 1077, 1081, 1916. Geraty v. Kaufman, 115 Conn. 563, 162A 33, 1932. Cavallaro v. Sharp, 84 R.I. 67, 121 A.2d 669, 1956. Stewart, W.: The locality rule in medical malpractice cases. Cal. Western L. Rev. 4:124, 1968.
16. Murphy v. Dyer, 409 F.2d 747, 1969.
17. Prosser, W. L. and Smith, Y.: *Torts, Cases and Materials*, 4th ed., Brooklyn, Foundation Press, 1967.
18. Toth v. Community Hosp., @ Glen Cove 239 N.E. 2d 368, 1968.
19. Prosser, W. L.: *Torts*, 4th ed. St. Paul, West Publishing Co., 1971.
20. Knell v. Feltman, 174 F.2d 662 (D.C.Cir.) 1949.
21. Norton, M. L.: Consent—A problem in medicine. Mich. Med. 69:111, 1970.
22. Schloendorf v. New York Hospital, 211 N.Y. 125, 105 N.E. 92, 1914.
23. Maerchlein v. Smith, 129 Colo. 72, 266 P.2d, 1095, 1954.
24. Natanson v. Kline, 186 Kan. 393, 350, P.2d 1093, 1960. Kinney v. Lockwood Clinic Ltd., 4 D.L.R. 906 (Ont.), 1931.
24a. Cobbs v. Grant, 8 Cal 3d 229; Sup., 104 Cal. Rptr. 505, 1972.
25. Williams v. Menehan, 191 Kan. 6,379 P.2d 292, 1963.
26. Mohr v. Williams, 95 Minn. 261, 271 104 N.W. 12, 1905.
27. Delahunt v. Fenton, 244 Mich. 226, 221 N.W. 168, 1928.
28. Kennedy v. Parrott, 243 N.C. 355, 90 S.E.2d 754, 1956.
29. Norton, M. L.: In Ref. 19.
30. Bakker v. Welsh, 144 Mich. 632, 108 N.W.94, 1906.
31. Pratt v. Davis, 224 Ill. 300, 79 N.E.562, 1906.
32. Aiken v. Clary, 396 S.W.2d 668 Mo., 1965.
33. O'Brien v. Cunnard S. S. Co., 154 Mass. 272, 28 N.E. 266, 1891.
34. Knowles v. Blue, 209 Ala. 27, 95 So. 481, 1923.
35. Jackovach v. Yocom, 212 Iowa 914, 237 N.W. 444, 1931.
36. Meyer v. St. Paul-Mercury Indem. Co., 61 So. 2d 901, 1952, 225 La. 618, 73 So. 2d 781, 1953. Robinson v. Wirts, 387 Pa. 291 127 A.2d 706, 1956.
37. Bishop v. Shurly, 237 Mich. 76, 211 N.W. 75. Luka v. Lowrie, 171 Mich. 122, 136 N.W. 1106, 1912. Sullivan v. Montgomery, 155 Misc. 448, 279 N.Y.S. 575, Annotation. 26 A.L.R. 1036, 53 A.L.R. 1056.
38. Chayet, N.: *Legal Implications of Emergency Care*. New York, Appleton-Century-Crofts, 1969.
39. Bonner v. Moran 126 F.2d 121, 1941. *See also* 139 A.L.R. 1366.

40. Wheeler v. Barker, 92 Cal. App. 2d 776, 208 P.2d 68, 1949. Stone v. Goodman, 241 App. Div. 290, 271 N.Y.S. 500, 1934.

40a. Demers v. Gerety, 515 P.2d 645 (N.M. Ct. of App.), 1973.

41. Barnett v. Bachrach, 34 A.2d 626 (D.C. Mun. App.) 1943. Roth v. Hull, 352 Mo. 926, 180 S.W.2d 7, 1944.

42. Jackson v. Burton, 226 Ala. 483, 147 So. 414, 1933. Moeller v. Hauser, 237 Minn. 368, 54 N.W.2d 639; Gross v. Pratt 190 Wash. 489, 68 P.2d 1034, 1957. Young v. Nordau, 106 W. Va. 139 145 S.E. 41, 1958.

43. Wasmuth, C.: *Anesthesia and the Law.* Springfield, Charles C Thomas, 1961.

44. Kennedy v. Gaskel, 78 Cal. Rptr. 753, 1969. Bergen, R. P.: Nurse anesthetist. JAMA 211: 1591, 1970. Jackson v. Joyner, 236 N.C. 259, 72 S.E. 2d 589, 1952.

45. Genesis 9:3,4; Leviticus 3:17, 17:10; 17:13, 14; Deut. 12:23-25, I Samuel 14:32, 33 (King James version).

46. Hayt, E., and Hayt, J.: *Manual of Therapy Consents and Legal Forms,* Form No. HA-19. Hospital Association of New York, 1961.

47. Battaglia v. Battaglia, 172 N.Y.S.2d 361, 1958.

48. Napoli v. St. Peters Hosp., Sup. Ct., Kings City, N.Y.L.J. May 7, 1969.

49. Carter v. Interfaith Hosp. of Queens, 304 N.Y.S. 2d 97 (N.Y.), 1969. Cunningham v. MacNeal Memorial Hosp., 25 N.E. 2d 733 Ill., 1969.

50. Hendrix, R.: Seminars on medico-legal investigations. Ann Arbor, Univ. of Michigan, Department of Pathology, 1969-1970.

51. Fisher, R.: Teaching medical law. Comm. on Medicolegal Problems. JAMA, 205:245, 1968; Norton, M. L.: Development of an integrated program of instruction in law and medicine. J. Med. Educ., 46:405, 1971; Norton, M. L.:

Biomedical instrumentation and liability. J. Amer. Assoc. Adv. Med. Instr., 5:3, 1971.

52. Warren, S. D., and Brandeis, L. D.: The right to privacy. Harvard L. Rev. 4:193, 1890.

53. Barber v. Time, Inc., 348 Mo. 1199, 159 S.W.2d 291, 1942. Clayman v. Bernstein, 38 Pa. D. & C. 543, 1940. Griffin v. Medical Soc'y, 11 N.Y.S.2d 109 (Sup. Ct.), 1939. Feeney v. Young, 191 App. Div. 501 181 N.Y.S. 481, 1920.

54. Banks v. King Features Syndicates, 30 F Supp. 352 (S.S.N.Y.) 1939. *See also* Medical practice and the right to privacy. Minn. L. Rev. 43:943, 1959.

55. Carr v. Shifflett, 82 F.2d 874 (D.C. Cir.) 1936. DeMay v. Roberts, 46 Mich. 160, 9 N.W. 146, 1881.

56. Boyd v. Wynn, 286 Ky. 173, 150 S.W.2d 648, 1941.

57. Stone v. Eisen, 114 N.E. 44 (N.Y.) 1916.

58. Louisell, D., and Williams, H.: Vol. I, Cumulative Series. New York, Matthew Bender, 1969.

59. Arizona, Florida, Hawaii, Idaho, Louisiana, Maryland, Michigan, Montana, Nebraska, New Jersey, North Dakota, Oklahoma, Oregon, Texas, West Virginia, and Federal Torts Claims Act.

60. DeHaan v. Winter, 262 Mich. 192, 247 N.W. 151, 1933.

61. Schmit v. Esser, 183 Minn. 354, 236 N.W. 622, 1931.

62. Flanagan v. Mt. Eden Hosp., 248 N.E.2d 871 N.Y., 1969.

63. Frohs v. Greene, 452, p.2d 564 Ore., 1969.

64. Wear v. State of N.Y., 299 N.Y.S. 2d 469, 1968.

65. Weeks v. Latter-Day Saints Hosp., 418 F2d, 1035, 1969.

INDEX

Page numbers followed by f indicate figures; those followed by t indicate tables.

20